CASUALTY CARE
for Fire and Rescue

Simon Todd,
Kris Lethbridge
and
Richard Pilbery

Disclaimer

Class Professional Publishing have made every effort to ensure that the information, tables, drawings and diagrams contained in this book are accurate at the time of publication. The book cannot always contain all the information necessary for determining appropriate care and cannot address all individual situations; therefore, individuals using the book must ensure they have the appropriate knowledge and skills to enable suitable interpretation. Class Professional Publishing does not guarantee, and accepts no legal liability of whatever nature arising from or connected to, the accuracy, reliability, currency or completeness of the content of Ambulance Care Practice. Users must always be aware that such innovations or alterations after the date of publication may not be incorporated in the content. Please note, however, that Class Professional Publishing assumes no responsibility whatsoever for the content of external resources in the text or accompanying online materials.

The information presented in this book is accurate and current to the best of the authors' knowledge.

The authors and publisher, however, make no guarantee as to, and assume no responsibility for, the correctness, sufficiency or completeness of such information or recommendation.

Printing history

This edition first published 2018

The authors and publisher welcome feedback from the users of this book. Please contact the publisher:

Class Professional Publishing,
The Exchange, Express Park, Bristol Road, Bridgwater TA6 4RR
Telephone: 01278 427 826
Email: post@class.co.uk
www.classprofessional.co.uk

Class Professional Publishing is an imprint of Class Publishing Ltd

A CIP catalogue record for this book is available from the British Library

Paperback ISBN: 9781859596579
eBook ISBN: 9781859596586

Line illustrations by David Woodroffe
Cover design by Hybert Design Limited, UK
Designed and typeset by S4Carlisle
Printed in the Czech Republic by FINIDR

About the Editors

Editors:

Simon Todd has worked for the Fire and Rescue Service for 22 years. He is currently a Crew Manager for Dorset & Wiltshire Fire and Rescue Service and a paramedic for South Western Ambulance Service NHS Foundation Trust (SWAST). He has a passion for pre-hospital education, technical rescue and an interest in advanced life support.

Kris Lethbridge lives in the West Country and also works for South Western Ambulance Service NHS Foundation Trust (SWAST). He is a paramedic and clinical educator. Kris has a passion for all aspects of pre-hospital care, with a particular focus on acute medical and resuscitation care.

Richard Pilbery, FCPara, is a Research Paramedic employed by Yorkshire Ambulance Service NHS Trust and Associate Lecturer at Sheffield Hallam University. He is the editor of the College of Paramedics *British Paramedic Journal* and co-author of *Ambulance Care Practice*, *Ambulance Care Essentials* and *First Responder Care Essentials*.

Editorial Advisor:

Mark Bryers, MCPara, GIFireE, has worked within the Fire and Rescue Service and pre-hospital arena for over 30 years. He is currently the Trauma Care Coordinator for Leicestershire Fire and Rescue Service (LFRS) and a Paramedic Medical Responder and Associate Clinical Tutor for East Midlands Ambulance Service NHS Trust (EMAS). Mark is the National Casualty Care lead for CFOA and as such is part of the NFCC Health Coordinating Committee. He also represents CFOA/NFCC on the boards for the FPHC, RCsEd and the ALSAR Medical Advisory board.

Contents

List of Abbreviations

ABC	airway, breathing, circulation
ABCDE	airway, breathing, circulation, disability, exposure/environment
ACP	advance care plan
ACS	acute coronary syndrome
ADRT	advance decision to refuse treatment ('living will')
AED	automated external defibrillator
AHF	acute heart failure
AIC	ambulance incident commander
AMHP	approved mental health professional
ANS	autonomic nervous system
ATMIST	age, time of incident, mechanism of injury, injuries, signs and symptoms, treatment given/immediate needs
ATP	adenosine triphosphate
AV	atrioventricular
AVPU	alert, voice, pain, unresponsive
BLS	basic life support
BP	blood pressure
BVM	bag-valve-mask
CABCDE	catastrophic haemorrhage, airway, breathing, circulation, disability, exposure/environment
CAD	coronary artery disease
CAP	Community-acquired pneumonia
CBRNE	chemical, biological, radiological, nuclear, explosive
CCO	casualty clearing officer
CCP	critical care paramedics
CCS	casualty clearing station
CNS	central nervous system
CO	carbon monoxide
COPD	chronic obstructive pulmonary disease
COSHH	control of substances hazardous to health
CPR	cardiopulmonary resuscitation
CQC	Care Quality Commission
CRT	capillary refill time
CSF	cerebrospinal fluid
DKA	diabetic ketoacidosis
DoH	Department of Health
DNA	deoxyribonucleic acid
DNACPR	do not attempt cardiopulmonary resuscitation
DRA	dynamic risk assessment
DSH	deliberate self harm
DVT	deep vein thrombosis
ECG	electrocardiogram
ED	emergency department
EMR	emergency medical responder/response
EOC	emergency operations centre
EPRR	emergency preparedness, resilience and response
ETA	estimated time of arrival
$EtCO_2$	end-tidal carbon dioxide
FAST	face, arm, speech test
FGM	female genital mutilation
FRS	fire and rescue service
GDPR	General Data Protection Regulations
GI	gastrointestinal
GSL	general sales list
GTN	glyceryl trinitrate

HART hazardous area response team
HCAI healthcare-associated infection
HCPC Health and Care Professions Council
HHS hyperosmolar hyperglycaemic state
HIV human immunodeficiency virus
HSE Health and Safety Executive
HSWA Health and Safety at Work Act 1974
IM intramuscular
IPAP intent, plans, action, protection
IV intravenous
JESIP Joint Emergency Services Interoperability Principles
kPa kilopascal
LAD left anterior descending artery
LCA left coronary artery
LOC level of consciousness
LOLER Lifting Operations and Lifting Equipment Regulations 1998
LPA lasting power of attorney
MCA Mental Capacity Act 2005
METHANE major incident, exact location, type of incident, hazards, access, number of casualties, emergency services
MHA Mental Health Act
MHFA mental health first aid
MHOR Management of Health and Safety at Work Regulations 1999
MHSWR Manual Handling Operations Regulations 1992
MI myocardial infarction
MILS manual in-line stabilisation
MIU minor injuries unit
mmHg millimetres of mercury
MOI mechanism of injury
MSC motor, sensory, circulation [function]
MTA marauding terrorist attack
NAI non-accidental injury
NEWS National Early Warning Score
NHS National Health Service
NIBP non-invasive blood pressure measurement
NICE National Institute for Health and Care Excellence
NILO National Inter-Agency Liaison Officer
NNBC National Network for Burn Care
NOI nature of illness
NPA nasopharyngeal airway
NSTEMI non-ST-segment elevation myocardial infarction
OCD obsessive compulsive disorder
OPA oropharyngeal airway
PAT paediatric assessment triangle
PD personality disorder
PDA posterior descending artery
PE pulmonary embolism
PEA pulseless electrical activity
PEF/PEFR peak expiratory flow/peak expiratory flow rate
PNS peripheral nervous system
POM prescription only medicines
pPCI primary percutaneous coronary intervention
PPE personal protective equipment
PPV positive pressure ventilation
PUWER Provision and Use of Work Equipment Regulations 1998
RCA right coronary artery
REAP Resource Escalation Action Plan
RNA ribonucleic acid
ROSC return of spontaneous circulation
RSV respiratory syncytial virus
RTC road traffic collision
SA sino-atrial
SAD supraglottic airway device
SAMPLE signs and symptoms of presenting complaint, allergies, medications, past medical history, last oral intake,

	events leading to current illness/injury
SaO_2	arterial oxygen saturation
SARS	severe acute respiratory syndrome
SBAR	situation, background, assessment, recommendations
SCENE	safety, cause including NOI/MOI, environment, number of patients, extra resources needed
SCI	spinal cord injury
SOBOE	shortness of breath on exertion
SOCRATES	site, onset, character, radiation, association, timing, exacerbating/relieving factors, severity
SpO_2	blood oxygen saturation
SPUC	specialist paramedic (urgent care)
STEMI	ST-segment elevation myocardial infarction
SW	support worker
T2DM	type 2 diabetes mellitus
TBI	traumatic brain injury
TBSA	total body surface area
TEP	tracheo-oesophageal puncture
TETRA	terrestrial trunk radio
TILEE	task, individual, load, environment, equipment
UA	unstable angina
USAR	urban search and rescue
UTI	urinary tract infection
VF	ventricular fibrillation
VT	ventricular tachycardia
VTE	venous thromboembolism
VZV	varicella-zoster virus
WHO	World Health Organization

Acknowledgements

The following images are © Richard Pilbery:

- Figure 6.2 Non-latex disposable gloves
- Figure 6.3 Face masks
- Figure 12.7 An ambulance station medical gas cylinder store
- Figure 13.7 An example of a 12-lead ECG
- Figure 13.8 Basic components of an ECG complex
- Chapter 16 Procedure - Accu-Chek® Aviva blood glucose meter images
- Figure 19.1 Infant positive pressure ventilation
- Figure 19.2 An infant with the airway in neutral alignment
- Figure 18.6 Ventricular fibrillation
- Figure 18.7 Ventricular tachycardia following a 200 J shock
- Figure 18.8 Asystole

We would like to thank the following for their kind permission to publish material:

- Figure 1.2 A dispatcher in the emergency operations centre. Courtesy of Yorkshire Ambulance Service NHS Trust
- Chapter 6 Alcohol Handrub Procedure. Based on the 'How to Handrub' poster © World Health Organization 2009. All rights reserved
- Chapter 6 Handwashing Procedure. Based on the 'How to Handwash' poster © World Health Organization 2009. All rights reserved
- Figure 6.5 Clinell wipes. Republished with permission of GAMA Healthcare Ltd. Best practice guidance for infection control wet wipes developed by Clinell and GAMA Healthcare Ltd © 2016
- Figure 9.1 Dynamic Risk Assessment Model (National Ambulance Resilience Unit: National Ambulance Service Command and Control Guidance). Reproduced by the kind permission of the National Ambulance Resilience Unit (NARU)
- Figure 9.2 JESIP joint decision-making model taken from 'Joint Doctrine – The Interoperability Framework Edition Two'. Reproduced by the kind permission of JESIP
- Figure 9.3 An incident command structure showing examples of the additional support roles that may be required. Reproduced by the kind permission of the National Ambulance Resilience Unit (NARU)
- Figure 9.4 The triage sieve. Copyright National Ambulance Resilience Unit, 2014. Reproduced by the kind permission of the National Ambulance Resilience Unit (NARU)
- Figure 10.6 Reproduced from: Royal College of Physicians. *National Early Warning Score (NEWS) 2: Standardising the assessment of acute-illness severity in the NHS*. Updated report of a working party. London: RCP, 2017
- Chapter 11 salbutamol, Chapter 12 salbutamol and Chapter 13 aspirin and GTN drugs guidelines are republished with permission of AACE
- Figure 11.9 Mechanical suction device. Image reproduced by the kind permission of Laerdal Medical
- Figures 11.17, 11.18 Tracheostomy tubes. Images reproduced by the kind permission of Kapitex Healthcare Ltd
- Figure 12.16 A Firesafe. Image reproduced by the kind permission of BPR Medical
- Figure 12.18 Bag-valve-mask with oxygen reservoir bag attached and inflated. Image reproduced by the kind permission of Ambu A/S

- Chapter 12 Instructions for use of oxygen images. © BOC Ltd 2014. Image reproduced by the kind permission of BOC healthcare
- Figure 12.25 Normal adult peak flow values. Image reproduced by the kind permission of Clement Clarke International
- Figure 13.14 An aneroid sphygmomanometer. Image reproduced by the kind permission of Welch Allyn
- Figure 14.8 Petechial non-blanching rash. Courtesy Meningitis Research Foundation www.meningitis.org
- Figure 14.9 Maculopapular rash with scanty petechiae. Courtesy Meningitis Research Foundation www.meningitis.org
- Figure 15.5 Swift water rescue. Image reproduced with the kind permission of the photographer, Arfon Huband
- Chapter 16 Procedure for Jext® Auto-Injector. Images reproduced with the kind permission of ALK
- Figure 17.1 A close-range gunshot wound to the right knee, with a shotgun. By DiverDave (Own work) [CC-BY-SA-3.0 or GFDL], via Wikimedia Commons
- Figure 17.2 An explosion, with visible blast wave. By D.R. Richmond/United States Army [Public domain], via Wikimedia Commons
- Figure 18.1 The chain of survival. Image reproduced by the kind permission of Laerdal Medical
- Figure 19.3 A newborn with intercostal recession. By Bobjgalindo (Own work) [CC-BY-SA-3.0-2.5-2.0-1.0], via Wikimedia Commons
- Figure 21.3 The Abbey pain scale. Reproduced by permission of MA Healthcare Ltd

Every effort has been made to secure permission to reproduce copyright images. If any have been inadvertently overlooked, the copyright holders are invited to contact Class Professional Publishing and the omission will be rectified in the next printing as well as all further editions.

Foreword

The Fire and Rescue Service (FRS) has seen many changes over recent times, particularly with the introduction of the Fire and Rescue Services Act (2004) which replaced the original Fire Services Act (1947). This, along with the developing role of the firefighter has meant a shift in the types of incidents and duties that the FRS responds to or undertakes.

These shifts have seen the progression from a firefighter being trained in basic first aid, to the need for a more in-depth knowledge of pre-hospital casualty care. The Chief Fire Officers Association (CFOA) and the National Fire Chiefs Council (NFCC) are currently developing guidelines for a national standard of casualty care for the FRS. This, along with the appropriate governance, will assist in providing guidance to the FRS as to the level of training a firefighter should receive.

The FRS can be the first emergency response to arrive at an incident. In those developing moments, the firefighters' medical knowledge and training can make the difference to a casualty's outcome. The need for more Interprofessional Collaboration (IPC) and education between the FRS and the Ambulance Service is increasing, along with a synergy between the emergency services and the way we deliver our casualty care.

Class Professional Publishing have produced a range of books based around Ambulance Practice, such as *Ambulance Care Essentials* (Pilbery and Lethbridge, 2015) and *Ambulance Care Practice* (Pilbery and Lethbridge, 2016). This book uses the information for casualty care as used by the Ambulance Service and translates this to the pre-hospital setting for the FRS. It provides relevant information that is consistent to that available to the Ambulance Service, and therefore delivers some form of constructive alignment for Interprofessional Education (IPE) for all concerned.

Mark Bryers
GIFireE, MCPara
May 2018

Chapter 1

Introduction

Introduction

This textbook is designed to help prepare you to work as a Fire and Rescue Service Emergency Medical Responder (EMR). It is designed to be read from start to finish on the first reading, as concepts introduced later on in the book assume that you already have knowledge of the content that has been covered in earlier chapters. However, this workbook will be a useful reference to which you can return again and again, reflecting on the learning points that are highlighted.

Each chapter comprises a number of topics centred by a theme, such as health and safety, or the airway. The learning objectives for each chapter have been mapped to objectives from a range of courses that are used by fire services to prepare their staff for the role of emergency medical responder.

Background

This text has been specifically written for firefighters already employed or undertaking training within a fire and rescue service (FRS). A certain amount of pre-existing knowledge is expected, particularly fire service operations, which will not be covered in this book. If you are not employed by, or familiar with, the workings of a UK fire and rescue service, then other texts in the Ambulance Care series may be more appropriate reading material. These are *Ambulance Care Essentials*, for support workers, *First Responder Care Essentials*, for volunteers and *Ambulance Care Practice*, the highest level in the series.

The Fire Service Role in Pre-Hospital Care

Fire and rescue services have always worked closely with pre-hospital medical providers in the aim of saving life. Since around the turn of the century, fire services have become increasingly involved in the delivery of medical care through various co-responding schemes where firefighters respond to emergency medical calls, normally on behalf of the ambulance service, to provide immediate care and support until other health professionals can get to the scene (Fire Brigade Union, 2015).

In recent years, the demand on the ambulance service has risen by around 6% per year, while fire service activity has fallen by a similar amount per year (AACE and CFOA, 2016). Ambulance services receive over 10 million calls per year, while fire services receive a little under 500,000.

It is not surprising that ambulance services (and the health service in general) are looking for new and innovative ways to help meet this rising demand,

and various initiatives are being explored to help overcome the challenges this presents. Firefighters have become more involved in the delivery of pre-hospital care in recent years and these roles are continuing to develop. Below are examples of situations in which firefighters are currently contributing to pre-hospital care:

- co-responding
- marauding terrorist attack
- cardiac response
- falls response
- safe and well visits.

Co-Responding

FRS have been operating co-responder schemes in partnership with NHS ambulance services for many years now. The scheme is designed to mobilise personnel alongside the ambulance service providing an effective, rapid response to immediately life-threatening medical emergencies.

The training and skills enable the co-responders to attend a variety of medical emergencies within the community. These firefighters then provide initial assessment and care to patients, while awaiting the arrival of the ambulance.

In addition to their skills for patient assessment and care, co-responders are trained to undertake more advanced skills of pain relief and lifesaving interventions when managing a cardiac arrest.

Each FRS will work with an NHS ambulance trust to lay down a specific scope of working practices that will be governed by the NHS trust, ensuring the guidelines are clear when treatment is provided by firefighters.

Marauding Terrorist Attack

A marauding terrorist attack (MTA) is a terrorist attack that may or may not include firearms. A specialist team of firefighters forms part of the national resilience response to a terrorist attack or other mass casualty event. Incidents of this nature are designed to inflict large numbers of casualties and would represent a major incident for the emergency services.

The rapidly changing and unique features of all types of attacks require a more dynamic and collaborative approach to that adopted in standard major incident response planning. FRS involved in this response are working closely with their partner agencies incorporating the Joint Emergency Services Interoperability Principles (JESIP) approach.

Cardiac Care Response

Cardiac care response is lifesaving intervention within the community, providing early cardiopulmonary resuscitation (CPR) and defibrillation to increase the chances of survival from an out-of-hospital cardiac arrest.

Firefighters are mobilised to provide high-quality life support as part of a team approach. The focus of this work allows paramedics to prioritise critical advanced life support interventions and patient care. This collaborative work by FRS and NHS ambulance trusts is aimed at delivering high-quality care to the most critical of incidents.

Falls Response

FRS and NHS ambulance services are working together to provide a rapid response for falls patients. Where it has been identified through clinical triage that a response is required, a multi-skilled falls response will be mobilised to support patients.

Appropriately trained and equipped firefighters will provide a collaborative approach to patients within their community. This approach to support high-risk groups who have fallen does not only help reduce hospital admissions but can also reduce the likelihood and severity of future falls. FRS working in this area have been able to identify and implement specific fall prevention work, helping to support and provide a better life for the more vulnerable within the community.

Safe and Well Visits

Safe and well visits are a variation on the work fire services have been doing for some time in providing home safety assessments. They are an extension of these visits and may include giving health advice on diet, weight management, smoking, alcohol use and trip hazards in the home to help prevent falls

(CFOA, 2017). Where necessary, patients may be referred to their GP or other health services.

The Future of Casualty Care

As pressure on the health system continues to rise, and trials of firefighters responding to medical patients have proved successful, it is likely that fire and rescue services will increasingly be asked to take on more medical responding. There will be many factors yet to be agreed that will determine the scale of this additional resource, but it will be welcomed by all sides if it leads to improved patient care.

Getting Started

Each chapter of the book is divided into sections, which are typically laid out in the following way:

- **Learning Objectives**: To clearly highlight what you are expected to learn in the chapter.
- **Introduction**: Setting the scene for the theme of the chapter.
- **Content**: The content!

To help get you orientated to the book and the relevance of the various chapters to clinical practice, the next section of this Introduction will take you step by step through an emergency, highlighting the variety of knowledge and skills that you will require to be an effective emergency medical responder (EMR).

Extended Skills

Look out for the ! extended skill icons throughout the book. These highlight where a skill may be out of your current scope of practice. These are included for your further learning and development. If you are unsure about your role, talk with your local co-ordinator.

Anatomy of an Emergency Call

Introduction

The topics covered in the chapters of this textbook are an essential part of your role as an emergency medical responder. It can be helpful to find out **WHY** you need to learn something. In order to see this in context, let's review a typical clinical scenario to which you may be mobilised (Figure 1.1).

The Emergency Operations Centre

When Emma makes a 999 call, she speaks to a telephone operator who asks her which service she requires. She asks for the ambulance service

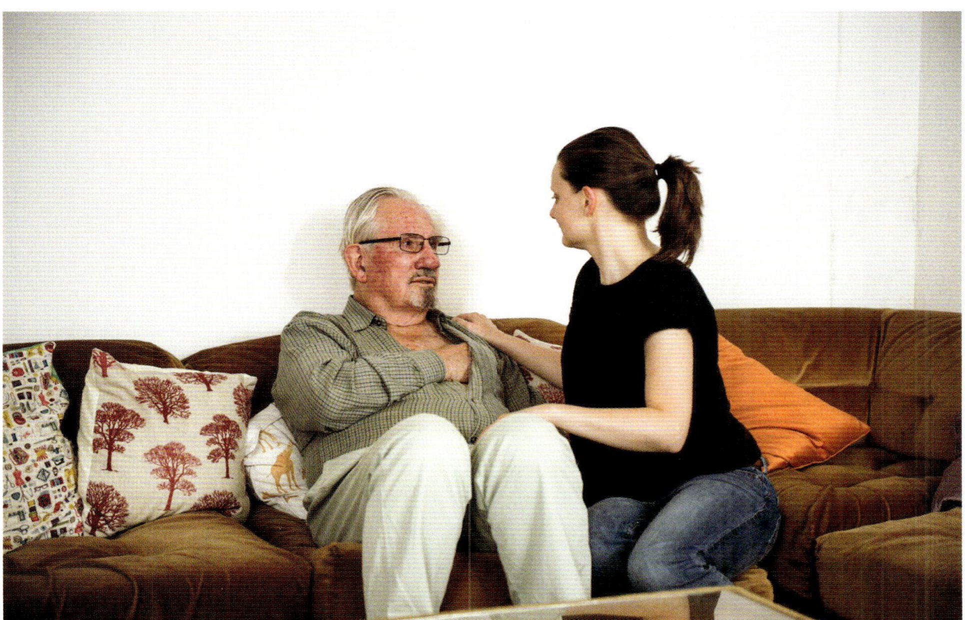

Figure 1.1 *Mr James Brown, a 59-year-old man who has chest pain, with his daughter, Emma.*

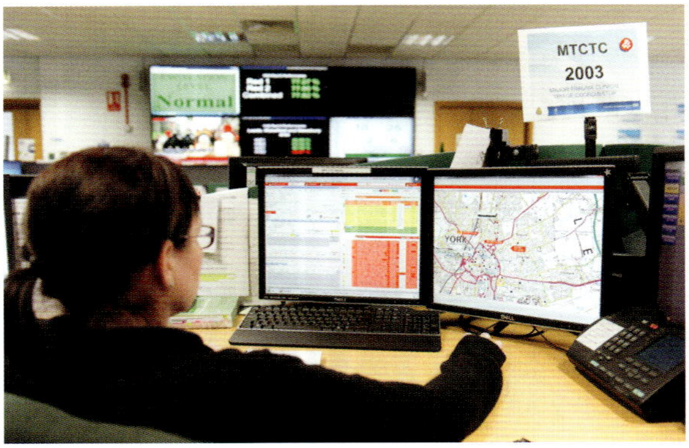

Figure 1.2 *A dispatcher in the emergency operations centre.*

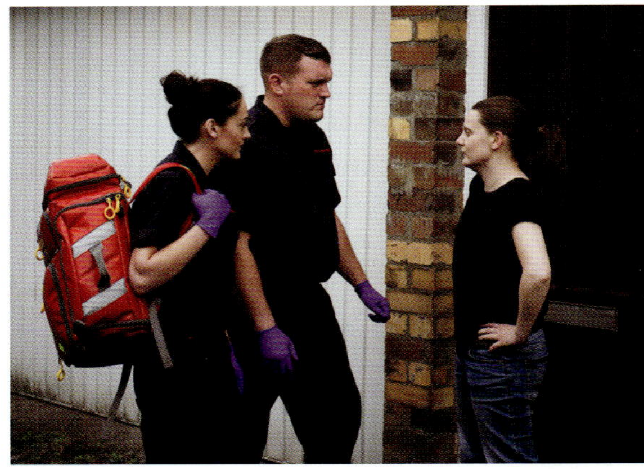

Figure 1.3 *The fire and rescue service EMR arrive at the address.*

and is put through to her local ambulance service's emergency operations centre (EOC) (Figure 1.2).

While she talks to the call handler, the dispatcher allocates an ambulance resource and also activates the nearest fire and rescue service emergency medical response, thereby ensuring that the patient receives a timely response.

Arriving on Scene

You will have been conducting a scene assessment, even before arriving at the address. This will include the location, time of day and type of incident, and is a dynamic process, i.e. it should be constantly reviewed as the scene can change rapidly.

In addition to scene safety, you will consider the need for personal protective equipment. At a residential address, this may be initially limited to a pair of disposable gloves, but could expand to include additional personal protective equipment (PPE) of face masks and aprons for extra protection.

With the help of your colleague, you carry your response bag, oxygen and defibrillator to the front door, where Emma is anxiously waiting (Figure 1.3).

Principles of Communication

You are shown into the living room where Mr Brown is sitting on the sofa, clutching his chest and looking rather grey and sweaty. You introduce yourself and your colleague to Mr Brown and clarify what Mr Brown prefers to be called. He tells you to call him Jim (Figure 1.4).

Communication is a fundamental aspect of all EMR work. However, it is not always easy, as you will have to adapt your communication approach and style appropriately with healthcare professionals, patients, friends and family members. In addition, you cannot communicate the same way with an elderly person as you would a two-year-old child. Some patients cannot, or will not, communicate with you, because they are depressed or don't speak English, for example. This will be covered in more detail in Chapter 3: Communication.

Patient Assessment

Your colleague completes a primary survey of catastrophic haemorrhage, airway, breathing, circulation, disability, exposure/environment (CABCDE) assessment of Jim and asks you to obtain a set of baseline observations to support this. Jim's airway is patent; he is breathing at a rate of 16 breaths per minute, which is in the normal range. After obtaining permission (correctly termed 'consent', an important legal concept, covered in Chapter 4: Clinical Governance, Legal and Ethical Issues) from Jim, you apply a pulse oximeter to one of his fingers. His oxygen saturations are 93% on air and, having excluded the presence of chronic obstructive pulmonary disease (COPD, which you will learn about in Chapter 12: Breathing), you administer oxygen via the appropriate mask.

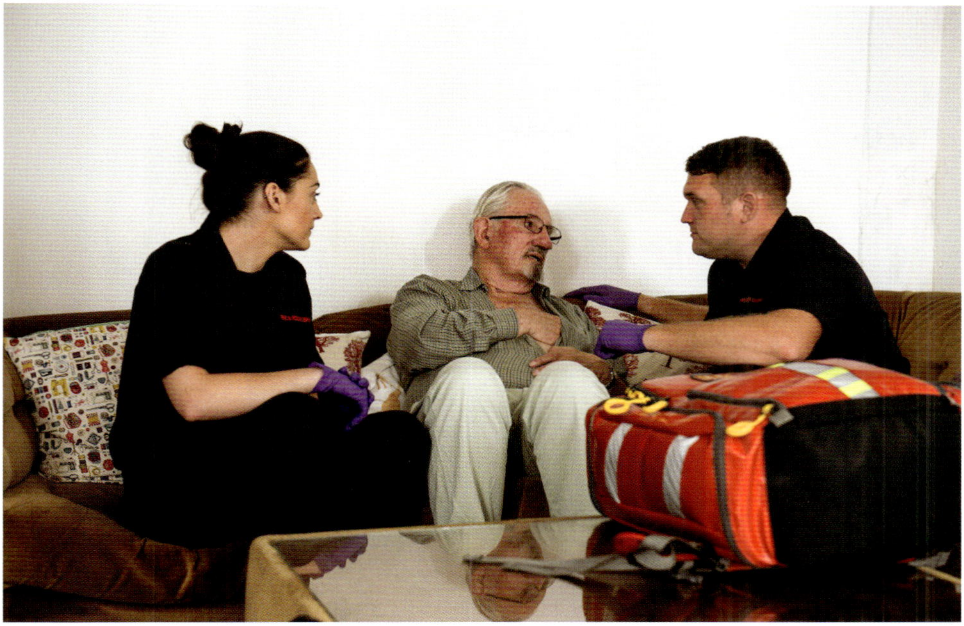

Figure 1.4 *Talking to Jim.*

Continuing with the assessment of Jim's circulation, you measure his blood pressure, put on your disposable gloves to check his blood sugar, record his pain score (covered in the assessment of disability section in Chapter 14: Disability) and, finally, check his temperature.

Patient History

A solo-responding paramedic arrives and asks you for a handover. You pass your observations over and describe Jim's explanation of a sudden onset of central chest pain radiating to his jaw, back and both arms an hour prior to his daughter's 999 call. He states that it feels like a heavy pressure, which he scores a 7 out of 10, and is associated with shortness of breath, nausea and sweating. His daughter states that he has been very pale since the onset of pain. You are asked by the paramedic to prepare the Entonox administration set for Jim to use (covered in Chapter 12: Breathing).

The paramedic asks Jim about his past medical history and is told that he has high cholesterol and hypertension (high blood pressure), both of which he is medicated for. He has never suffered from a heart attack (myocardial infarction, MI), but does admit to suffering from occasional chest pain on exertion over the past month or so.

Manual Handling

An ambulance arrives and its crew bring a carry chair to transfer Jim to the ambulance. After completing a Task, Individual, Load, Environment, Equipment (TILEE) assessment, and explaining to Jim how they would like him to transfer onto the carry chair, the ambulance crew safely assist Jim onto the chair and wheel him out to the ambulance. Jim is wheeled onto the ambulance tail-lift, which is then raised (Figure 1.5). Once at ambulance level, they carefully wheel Jim alongside the ambulance stretcher so that he can transfer onto it.

The TILEE manual handling assessment tool and the equipment used for manual handling are covered in Chapter 7: Manual Handling under the sections Principles of Manual Handling and Moving and Handling Equipment and Techniques.

The solo-responding paramedic thanks you for your assistance and you leave the patient with the ambulance crew.

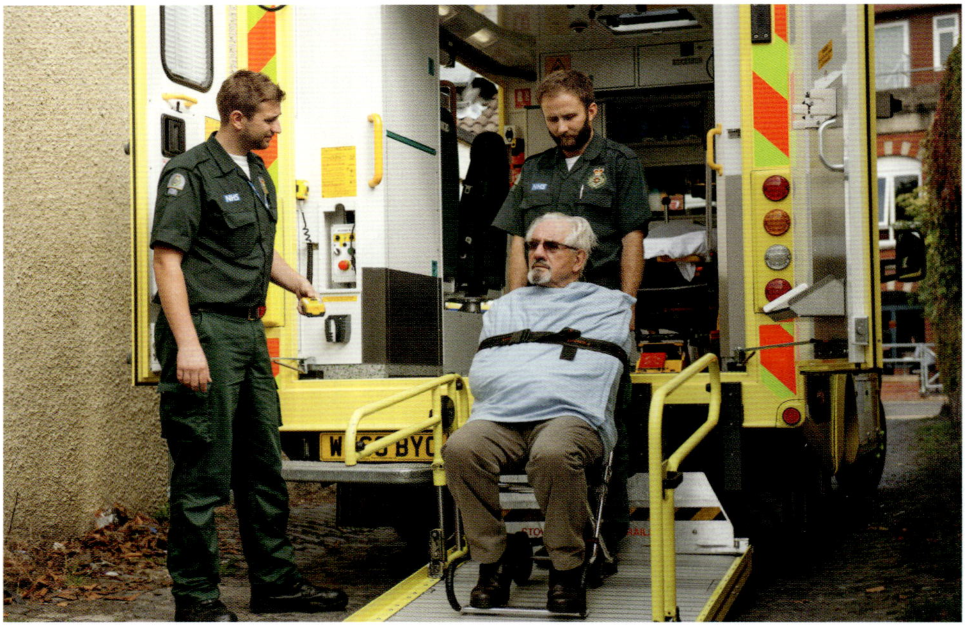

Figure 1.5 *The crew loading Jim onto the ambulance.*

On Board the Ambulance

With the patient safely aboard the ambulance, the paramedic reconnects the monitor/defibrillator so changes in Jim's condition can be observed en-route to hospital.

Due to the fact that Jim is having a heart attack, the paramedic states that blue lights and sirens are required for transfer to the local heart attack centre and not the local emergency department (ED). This is a pathway to a regional centre capable of performing primary percutaneous coronary intervention (pPCI). The paramedic phones through a pre-alert to the hospital to inform and update them.

Hospital Arrival

Traffic was light and good progress was made, arriving at the heart attack centre within 30 minutes. Just as the ambulance pulls up outside the doors to the hospital, the paramedic shouts through that Jim has suffered a cardiac arrest.

The paramedic starts performing chest compressions and connects the defibrillator pads (Figure 1.6). He pauses chest compressions to check the rhythm and recognises it is ventricular fibrillation (VF), one of the shockable rhythms. The paramedic charges the defibrillator and resumes chest compressions.

The tone of the defibrillator informs that it is ready to deliver a shock and, after checking that no one is touching the patient, the shock button is pressed. Jim jolts upwards slightly as his chest muscles contract. As soon as the shock is

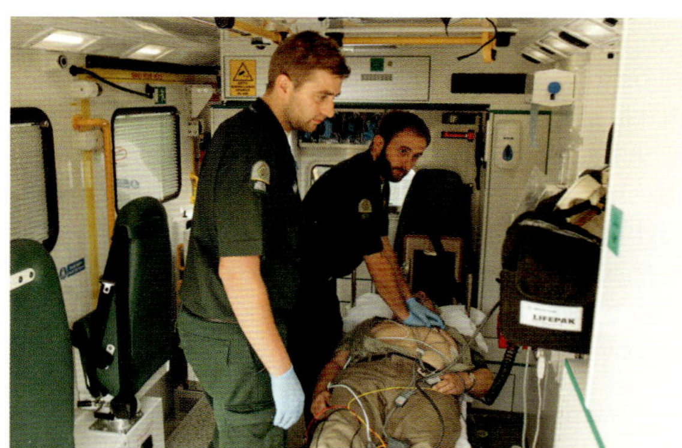

Figure 1.6 *Resuscitating Jim requires good quality basic life support and early defibrillation.*

delivered, the paramedic's colleague takes over chest compressions, while the paramedic inserts an oropharyngeal airway (OPA) and connects the bag-valve-mask (BVM) to high-flow oxygen.

After 2 minutes of cardiopulmonary resuscitation (CPR), a brief pause in chest compressions is made to assess the rhythm. The ECG shows an organised rhythm and a pulse check reveals that Jim's heart is beating again. His breathing is not adequate, however, and en-route to the cardiac catheter lab, the paramedic ventilates Jim with the BVM. And by the time they arrive at the catheter lab, Jim is making some respiratory effort.

The paramedic provides a handover to the waiting staff, explaining Jim's history, findings on examination, treatment administered and the cardiac arrest, for which Jim has just successfully been resuscitated.

Clean Up and Prepare for the Next Call

With Jim safely in the hands of the cardiac catheter lab staff, the paramedic returns to the ambulance to clean up, restock and get ready for the next emergency call. You find out later that Jim had an occluded left anterior descending coronary artery, which was cleared and reopened by the cardiac catheter lab staff. He is recovering well and due to be discharged from hospital soon.

Working as an emergency medical responder will frequently involve meeting patients like Jim, but often it is the non-life-threatening calls that are the most challenging. This book, together with clinical practice and hands-on training, will provide you with the knowledge and skills you require to become a competent EMR and valued member of the pre-hospital team.

Chapter 2

Working with Other Health Professionals

Response to a 999 Call

Learning Objective

By the end of this section you will be able to:

- Explain how the ambulance service manages an emergency call.

Introduction

As an emergency medical responder, it is likely that most of the clinical incidents you attend will be because of a 999 call to the ambulance service. The response to a 999 call can be complex and varies between each incident depending on the degree of need: it is also a very different response from when an emergency call is received by the fire and rescue service. You should understand your role in the process and the other stages that the patient will already have been through and will go on to after your care. The three main stages of a response are:

- call for help and triage
- pre-hospital response
- onward care of the patient.

Call for Help and Triage

When someone calls 999 (or 112) in the UK, they are connected to an operator from the national telephone network. Once the nature of the emergency has been established, the call will be forwarded to the police, fire and rescue service, ambulance service and/or coastguard, depending on the most appropriate response(s) required.

Once the call is connected to the ambulance service emergency operations centre (EOC), a qualified call handler will ask a series of pre-defined questions as part of a triage system. The response to the questions will help to determine those that need an ambulance most urgently. Triage systems can also identify those callers who do not need an ambulance and for whom an alternative care pathway, such as visiting the GP or self-presenting at a minor injuries unit (MIU), would be more appropriate (UKCGC, 2017).

Also during triage, the call handler will identify if there is a need for other emergency services, or whether there may be any dangers to the responding ambulance clinicians present (such as an assailant still at a scene). Where required, other services will be contacted and those responding on behalf of the ambulance service will be made aware of the risk.

Ambulance Service Response

Based on the information gathered during the triage process, the most appropriate response can be determined. There are two main types of response, which are:

- hear and treat
- physical response.

Hear and Treat

'Hear and treat' is where the patient is advised how to look after themselves, or recommended to self-present to a more appropriate care provider, such as a GP or MIU. The average number of patients being managed in England through this route is around 8% of all 999 calls (NHS England, 2015).

Physical Response

For the majority of 999 calls, the ambulance service will send a physical response. Depending on the need of the patient and the scale of the incident, this may include:

- community or emergency medical responder
- rapid response car
- response motorcycle
- emergency ambulance
- air ambulance (including critical care teams)
- specialist practitioner in urgent care
- hazardous area response team (HART)
- ambulance service officer/commander
- specialist operations response team
- medical support such as British Association for Immediate Care (BASICS).

Onward Care

Where necessary, patients will be transported to hospital for emergency care and treatment. This is frequently to emergency departments (EDs) but now also includes an increasing number of specialist emergency care departments, such as stroke units, cardiac wards or major trauma centres.

In addition to this, health professionals now have a range of alternative care pathways available to them, in order to avoid hospital admission where appropriate. In England, in up to 40% of incidents where patients receive a response from the ambulance service, they are not transported to an ED, but instead are either managed at the scene ('see and treat') or taken to an alternative care provider (NHS England, 2015).

Alternative care providers may include:

- specialist paramedics in urgent care – paramedics with additional training who can manage a range of minor injuries and illnesses within the community
- GPs
- GP drop-in centres
- out-of-hours services
- mental health teams
- minor injury units
- pharmacies
- 111
- social services
- 'hospital at home' teams
- emergency residential care
- community hospitals.

Given the current pressure being faced by urgent care services within the UK, it is likely that more routes for referral and additional training in managing more patients in the community will feature prominently in ambulance service development over the coming years (NHS England, 2016).

Roles Within the Ambulance Service

Learning Objectives

By the end of this section you will be able to:

- Identify a number of clinical and commander roles within the ambulance service and briefly explain what each role entails.
- Describe the importance of good working relationships.

Introduction

In your role, you will be working closely with colleagues from ambulance services on a daily basis. Understanding the different roles within ambulance services is important as you will need to integrate into large teams of health providers to help ensure patients receive appropriate care. Below is a brief description of the structure and roles of different clinicians within ambulance services.

There are 11 NHS ambulance trusts in England, as well as NHS ambulance services in Scotland, Wales and Northern Ireland, who are statutory providers of ambulance services for the Government within the UK (NHS Choices, 2011). There are also a range of voluntary services, including St John Ambulance and the British Red Cross, and a variety of independent sector services, ranging from the very small to national scale organisations.

Each service is structured differently, so it is not possible to give a definitive list of the different roles. However, over the following pages are descriptions of some of the roles you may find, which could be broadly divided into:

- clinical
- clinical leadership
- command and control.

Clinical Roles

Community or Emergency Medical Responder

Community responders come from a variety of backgrounds and volunteer their time for the ambulance service. They respond to incidents close to where they live or work, often in remote settings, which can take longer for an ambulance to get to. Responders carry basic life-saving equipment including an automated external defibrillator (AED) and devices for managing a patient's airway. In some places the fire service and other similar agencies may also act as first responders for the ambulance service (SWAST, 2014b).

Support Worker (SW)

SWs work alongside paramedics on front line ambulances. They are trained in providing emergency care, basic emergency interventions and life support, and are qualified emergency drivers. SWs normally work under the supervision of a qualified clinical colleague. SWs may also work on support vehicles that are used to transport patients to hospital when they have been assessed by another healthcare professional and are viewed as needing a less urgent admission to hospital. SWs have different names in different places, though a common name is emergency care assistants or emergency care support workers.

Associate Practitioner

Associate practitioners are non-registered clinicians who normally work alongside a paramedic, but may also work on their own. They have a range of skills relevant to emergency and urgent care and can undertake a number of pre-hospital procedures and administer a range of medications. There is national variation in their skill sets and the way in which they are deployed by different services.

Associate practitioners are similar to, but not the same as, the previous role of technicians, who are also unregistered clinicians that may work independently or under supervision.

Paramedic

Paramedics are qualified and registered clinicians who specialise in working in the urgent and emergency care setting. They are trained in the examination and treatment of emergency conditions, have a wide range of skills and treatment options and are considered specialists in emergency care. Registered with the Health and Care Professions Council (HCPC), paramedics have a degree of autonomy in their practice, and can be held accountable to the HCPC for their actions and omissions that arise from providing clinical care to patients.

Specialist Paramedic – Urgent Care (SPUC)

Specialist paramedics have been known by a range of titles including emergency care practitioner and paramedic practitioner. They have undertaken an enhanced course of learning, usually at post-graduate level, along with a range of placements that equip them with the skills and knowledge to treat urgent care patients. These patients include those with acute illnesses, such as respiratory tract and urinary tract infections or minor injuries and wounds. Specialist paramedics have a broad range of skills in the management of urgent patients and can administer a greater variety of medications (CoP, 2014).

Specialist Paramedic – Critical Care

Also known as critical care paramedics (CCP), these clinicians have also undertaken enhanced study, but with a focus on dealing with the most critically ill or injured. Specialist paramedics in critical care will often work as part of a multidisciplinary team alongside a doctor who specialises in emergency pre-hospital care (CoP, 2014). In teams, they can provide a range of enhanced surgical and medical procedures that may include being able to provide emergency anaesthetics. CCPs often work on air ambulance services, though in some places may also be ground based.

Hazardous Area Response Team (HART)

HARTs are typically comprised of paramedics who have been specially trained to work in difficult situations and alongside the police and fire services at large and dangerous incidents. They have a special set of skills and equipment, which can include swift water rescues, working at heights and use of breathing apparatus. This allows them to safely access patients in remote and difficult settings. There is a network of HART bases around the country and their help can normally be requested through the ambulance EOC.

Clinical Leadership Roles

Running any ambulance service requires a large range of clinical leaders. Some of the common roles include:

- consultant paramedic
- pharmaceutical adviser
- medical director.

Consultant Paramedic

The consultant paramedic is a relatively new role in some ambulance trusts throughout the UK. The role of the consultant is to act as a senior clinical leader involved in service development, clinical leadership, research and evaluation, and education and professional development. Consultants will normally work in a mixed role providing advanced clinical support to operational staff while also undertaking their other responsibilities. After the medical director, a consultant paramedic is normally the most senior clinical leader in an ambulance trust.

Pharmaceutical Adviser

Most organisations will have a pharmacist working for them at least part time. This is to ensure that the use of medications by the service is safe and appropriate and that the relevant laws are being followed.

Medical Director

The medical director, normally a doctor with a background in emergency and/or critical care, is the person ultimately responsible for the clinical care inside an organisation. They are senior clinical leaders and are answerable for clinical errors and omissions within an organisation.

Command and Control Roles

Inside every large organisation is a command and control structure. This structure is required to co-ordinate and effectively deliver the functions of the organisation, but it becomes particularly relevant in emergency services at times of complex or major incidents. All commanders receive specific training relevant to their role. Different command roles do not necessarily indicate rank or seniority within an organisation, but are instead allocated so that those involved understand their role in managing an incident. Following criticism of emergency services not communicating effectively at previous major incidents, the national Joint Emergency Services Interoperability Principles (JESIP) has been launched in the UK so commanders from all the emergency services know better how to work together and communicate at complex and major incident scenes (JESIP, 2013).

Operational Commanders

Operational commanders, broadly equivalent to what were formerly known as 'bronze' commanders, are present at the scene of an incident and are responsible for organising the delivery of care and the safety of those working at a scene. They have to assess what resources are available to them, or have been made available to them by tactical and strategic commanders, and utilise those resources in the most effective way possible.

Depending on the size of the incident, operational commanders work alongside a number of other officers from both the ambulance and other emergency services to ensure services are being provided in an effective and co-ordinated manner. Operational commanders receive direction from tactical commanders, with whom they have to constantly liaise closely to ensure they have the resources they require to manage an incident.

At the scene of an incident the operational commander should be easily recognised, as they will be wearing a tabard detailing their role. If you were to arrive at a large-scale incident in progress, you should make yourself known to the operational commander on arrival.

Tactical Commanders

Formerly known as 'silver' commanders, the tactical commander is responsible for ensuring that all the tactical resources an operational commander requires for the management of the incident are in place. They will communicate closely with other emergency services and agencies, and may or may not be present at the actual incident, depending on the scale and nature of the incident as well as the amount of time it goes on for. At some incidents there may be multiple operational commanders, each dealing with different sections of the incident, in which case the tactical commander will be responsible for co-ordinating their actions.

The tactical commander achieves a level of oversight for an incident that cannot normally be achieved by an operational commander on the ground. From this position, the tactical commander can ensure there is effective joint working of agencies and that the deployment of resources and the tactics being used to manage an incident are appropriate.

Strategic Commanders

Formerly known as 'gold' commanders, strategic commanders are responsible for devising and making available the resources to implement a strategy for managing an incident. The strategic commander usually has control over all of the organisation's resources and is responsible for making these resources available to the tactical and operational commanders.

Strategic commanders, like tactical commanders, get an oversight of the management of an incident and are responsible for ensuring the tactics being used are appropriate, that all services are working effectively together and that clear lines of communication are in place. Where necessary, strategic commanders are responsible for national level communication to make available further resources if they are required.

National Inter-Agency Liaison Officer (NILO)

The NILO is a nominated person who has had specific training and experience to ensure that agencies such as fire, police and ambulance services can communicate effectively during a major or serious incident. They will normally work remotely from the scene of an incident to ensure that all agencies are communicating effectively (NARU, 2012).

Working Relationships

As you can see, there are a large range of roles in the ambulance service and it is likely that you will need to work collaboratively with all of them at some time or another. Key to successful collaborative working will be building successful working relationships.

The key principles of good working relationships are:

- knowledge of the responsibilities and limits of one's own role
- regularly working together
- performance feedback sessions
- opportunities to ask questions so you can develop your skills.

Chapter 3

Communication

Principles of Communication

Learning Objectives

By the end of this section you will be able to:

- Identify the different reasons people communicate.
- Explain how communication affects relationships in the work setting.
- Describe the factors to consider when promoting effective communication.
- Explain how people from different backgrounds may use and/or interpret communication methods in different ways.
- Identify barriers to effective communication.
- Explain how to access extra support or services to enable individuals to communicate effectively.

Introduction

Communication will be at the core of your role in your day-to-day management of patients and when attending incidents. As inter-personal communication forms such a fundamental aspect of our daily lives, we rarely stop to think about how we do it. But, as will be discussed throughout this chapter, effective communication, especially in a high-stress environment, is a skill that requires development and practice.

Poor communication is one of the most frequently received complaints for organisations providing healthcare (HSCIC, 2013). The World Health Organization (WHO) recognises that communication is a key aspect of improving medical safety; poor communication has previously been responsible for disastrous medical and surgical errors, including the removal of incorrect organs and limbs (WHO, 2009).

For an emergency medical responder, effective communication is a key skill for providing effective care and keeping yourself and your colleagues safe.

Who Will You Be Communicating With?

Over the course of one day at work you will probably communicate, through different forms, with many different people, who may include:

- service users
- other health and care professionals
- colleagues
- members of the public
- staff in the ambulance operations centre and fire control room
- other professional services.

This communication is likely to take place through a variety of methods including:

- verbal
- body language
- handwritten

- electronic written (email or electronic patient record)
- radio
- telephone.

This will often be under pressure or personal stress, where poor communication or misinformation can have a detrimental effect on patient outcomes. Therefore, mastering communication in the emergency environment is a core skill for any emergency medical responder.

Basics of Communication

Traditionally, communication has been regarded as the sending of a message from one person to another (Figure 3.1) (Corcoran, 2013). The sender (person A) has a message they wish to pass to the receiver (person B). The message exists within the consciousness of the sender initially; they then decide how to pass on that message. Before it can be passed it must be 'encoded'. This encoding may be the selecting of certain words, certain emphasis during part of the sentence or other verbal or non-verbal features. The receiver must then 'decode' the message as they receive it and try to interpret the original message from all the verbal and non-verbal information they have received. Clearly, this model is not sufficient in healthcare, as it implies a one-way communication, not the two-way communication that is essential for providing best care to patients.

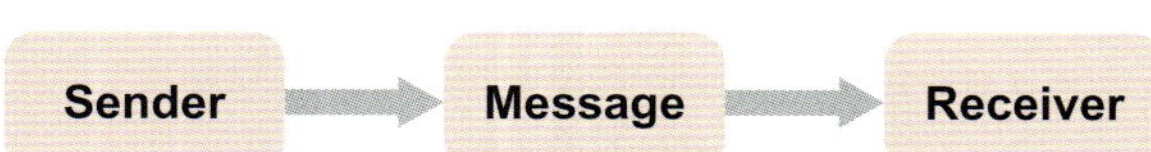

Figure 3.1 *Basic model of communication.*

A modified model has been suggested, which includes the variables of understanding and feedback, and is a cyclic process (Figure 3.2). This inclusion of checking the understanding of the message given, and receiving feedback, is fundamental to ensure that messages have been understood in the way in which they were intended (Corcoran, 2013).

This is particularly important in high-stress situations or when communicating information a person may not understand well (such as a medical complaint), to ensure that the correct message has been received and understood. In these situations, it is very easy for a message to be misinterpreted, with potentially disastrous consequences.

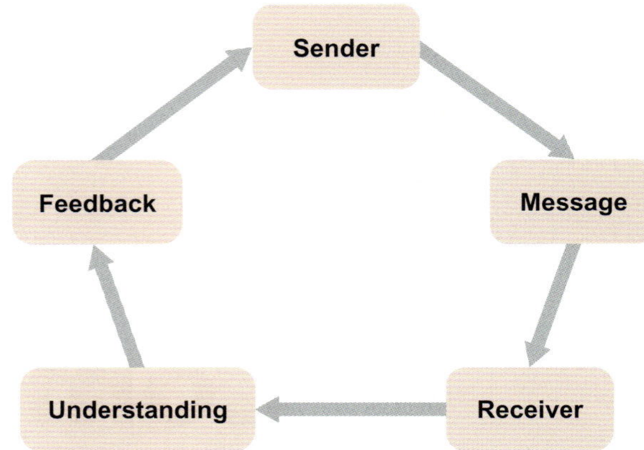

Figure 3.2 *Modified model of communication.*

Verbal Skills

Verbal communication can be divided into two broad areas (Blaber, 2008):

- language and vocabulary
- paralinguistic features of communication.

Language and Vocabulary

Working in healthcare you must be able to adjust your language and vocabulary so that it is suited to the person you are communicating with. When communicating with colleagues and health professionals you will need to use more complex and professional language. However, there will be times when you need to adjust to communicate with those who have a narrower range of language skills, which may include children or those with cognitive impairment, such as dementia patients or those with learning difficulties.

Guidance for ensuring clear verbal communication includes the following key points:

- Do not try to say too much at once; people can only process a certain amount of new information at one time.
- Avoid using jargon.
- Speak in a clear manner and as be concise as possible.

- Frequently check that what you are trying to communicate is being understood.
- Think about what you want to say and then the easiest way to communicate that to someone else.
- Do not use overly complex language to try and appear knowledgeable; lots of medical language can be complicated and similar sounding words have different meanings, which if used incorrectly can cause confusion, i.e. dysphasia (difficulty with language) and dysphagia (problems with swallowing).

Paralinguistic Features

Paralinguistics refers to the modification of the way in which we speak and place emphasis in communication. This includes:

- volume
- timings
- pitch
- accent
- intonation
- tone.

Non-Verbal Communication

Non-verbal communication can have a dramatic impact on the message you are sending and the way that it is then interpreted. It can be possible to communicate entirely by non-verbal means, especially if you know the person well (Blaber, 2008).

Examples of non-verbal communication include:

- eye contact
- facial expression
- gesture and posture
- arm position
- personal space and touch.

All of these should be used in a manner that is appropriate to the situation. For example, when gathering a history from a patient, if you are head down and writing as they speak, the patient may get the impression you are not paying attention to them and might leave out key details. In contrast, if you are making eye contact, nodding your head and acknowledging their communication with small verbal cues, such as 'OK' and 'yes' as they are speaking, known as active listening, then they are more likely to continue communicating and reveal all the information you need to assess them properly.

Equally, you should observe the body language of those with whom you are communicating. If the person you are talking to looks as though they are becoming increasingly agitated and frustrated, you should respond to this visual reaction and change the conversation or method of communication.

Handwritten Communication

It is likely that every patient contact you have will involve some form of communication, most commonly as part of the patient record.

It is important that all handwritten communication is neat, legible, concise, and follows a logical structure. Completing patient clinical records will become a routine part of your role and something you will need to master based on your local record keeping procedures, but some general guidelines include:

- Avoid unnecessary abbreviations.
- Ensure that your writing is legible and, if a carbon copy is being used, has transferred through to the copy sheet.
- Diagrams can be beneficial, but these need to be clear and labelled appropriately.
- Ensure you follow a structure. Most organisations use some form of standardised 'medical model' to aid this.

Social Context

Communication relies heavily on the social context in which it takes place. Consider the two following scenarios and how the changing social context may influence how you communicate (Hartley, 1999):

Scenario A: You attend a small child who has fallen and injured their wrist. As part of your assessment you need to look at the wrist, but the child is wary of letting you get close, due to fear that you will cause more pain.

Scenario B: You are called to give evidence in court at the case of a serious assault you attended. You are placed in the witness box and asked a series of questions by the prosecution, prior to cross-examination by the defence.

In both these scenarios, effective communication is critical to ensure that others receive the message you intend to send; however, the way in which you communicate these messages will be vastly different. Your role is to ensure you encode the message, using both verbal and non-verbal features of communication, in such a way that it is likely it will be decoded in the manner you intended.

This concept extends well beyond the extreme examples cited above and into your daily role. You will, every day, meet people from a wide range of social and cultural backgrounds. Every one of these people will have a different social context in which they exist, and you will need to be mindful of modifying your communication, based on the needs of the individual, to ensure that accurate messages are passed and misunderstanding does not occur.

Barriers to Communication

Barriers to communication are anything that influences your ability to effectively pass on and receive back the message you need. You will frequently encounter difficult-to-manage barriers to communication and will need to think of ways of dealing with them. Here are some examples of barriers to communication and how they can be overcome:

- **Physical obstacles:** Such as distance or your patient being stuck the other side of a closed door. The clear answer here is to remove the obstacle, but in some situations this may not be possible, so you will need to think of novel solutions. Examples may include establishing contact via a phone, using an intermediary to relay messages, or signalling with your hands or other props.
- **Language:** You will inevitably meet people with whom you cannot communicate in their native language. The use of a family member as a translator can be helpful; alternatively, your service may have provided you with other tools, such as phrase books or access to Language Line, a telephone service that provides translators for a wide range of languages over the phone.
- **Emotions:** You will frequently encounter patients and situations where those involved are experiencing extreme emotions. At these times people are less able to understand what is being said to them or asked of them. Use of your verbal and non-verbal skills of communication will be key here to ensure clarity of message.
- **Age:** Young patients in particular will need to be communicated with in a way that is suitable to them and that they can understand. Using pictures, drawings and other props can be an effective means of overcoming barriers to communication.

This is just a short list of examples of barriers that you may experience in communicating. It is worth noting that whenever you adapt your communication to overcome such difficulties there is an increased risk of your message being misinterpreted, so you should make doubly sure that what you wanted to communicate is the message the person has received.

As with all elements of your practice, you should constantly reflect on your communication skills to learn from both positive and negative experiences to continue improving your abilities in this fundamental skill of clinical practice.

Clarify Misunderstandings

In the emergency and urgent care setting it is inevitable that, at times, you will be communicating large quantities of information in a short space of time. Due to the emotions that are frequently present in scenarios that accompany emergency situations it is inevitable that misunderstandings can develop. To combat this you should:

- Observe for non-verbal cues that the person you are talking to has not understood what you are trying to communicate.
- Confirm the person understands what you are saying to them.
- If you suspect misunderstanding, repeat what you are trying to communicate in a different manner.

Summary

Communication is a natural skill that we all use on a daily basis; however, in your operational role you will routinely be faced with challenging and demanding communication scenarios. To help overcome these, having an understanding of the theory of communication and a strong working knowledge of what resources are available to you locally will be helpful. You will also need to be adaptive, creative, responsive and innovative in overcoming barriers to communication on a daily basis. Only when you can overcome barriers can you be sure of providing the right care to your patient.

Long after your patients have forgotten what you did for them, they will remember the way in which you went about doing it. Communication may be one of the most frequently received complaints for healthcare services, but being treated with care and compassion, and effectively communicated with, is also one of the most frequently praised attributes of individual health professionals.

Practical Communication

Learning Objectives

By the end of this section you will be able to:

- Explain the importance of clear, concise reporting of findings to the clinician.
- Explain the importance of recording patient observations.
- Describe the procedure for clinical handover to medical professionals.

Introduction

In your role it is likely that you will frequently need to undertake examinations and record observations.

Keeping accurate records and gaining accurate observations is critical to safe patient care, as it forms a part of the continuity of their care. Changes in observations can indicate a deteriorating or improving patient, so if there are errors in the recorded observations it can create a false perception of the patient's changing state of health.

The following tips will help to ensure patient safety when undertaking this part of your role:

- Pass on, or record, all the information you obtain. If you are not sure of its relevance, pass it on to the clinician responsible for their care.
- If you are asked to undertake procedures, observations or interventions that are outside your skill set, politely inform the responsible clinician that you are not able to do this.
- If you are struggling or unsure, make your supervising clinician aware: sometimes in very poorly patients getting accurate observations can be very difficult and you may not be able to. Just explain this was the case to your supervising clinician; they will understand.
- Never fabricate, estimate or make up observations. Doing so not only exposes the patient to risk but would also be considered unprofessional conduct when discovered.

Handover

The process of a handover is passing on the care of your patient to another healthcare provider(s). During handover, all information relevant to the care of the patient should be provided in a concise and effective manner. The most common situation is handing over a patient to an ambulance crew or hospital staff.

It is well recognised that handovers are a high-risk aspect of a patient's care, where important information can be forgotten or missed (BMA, 2014). This can lead to errors or omissions on the part of the receiving clinician and then harm to the patient as a result.

This risk of error is increased in high-stress situations, for example, where patients are critically ill or injured: just the time when that information needs to be passed on accurately.

There are many models to help facilitate clinical handover and thereby reduce the risk of key information being forgotten. It may be necessary to use different models in different circumstances. Two that are particularly common are SBAR and ATMIST.

Medical Handover

When conducting a handover of a patient whose primary concern is a medical problem, SBAR is usually the most appropriate tool (.Institute for Healthcare Improvement, 2018):

S: Situation

- Identify yourself and your role.
- Identify the patient by name and the reason you have come into contact with them.
- Outline your concerns.

B: Background

- Describe the reason the patient has called for help.
- Describe the history of the presenting condition.
- List any other pertinent information about the patient's background, which may include: medical history, previous illnesses, current medications, allergies, social situation etc.

A: Assessment

- Relate details of the patient's vital signs.
- Pass on your clinical impressions and concerns.

R: Recommendations

- Explain what you need – be specific about the request and time frame.
- Make suggestions.
- Clarify expectations.

In most scenarios you will not need to make recommendations; however, it may be appropriate to describe what you believe the priorities of immediate treatment might be. For example, if you are at a cardiac arrest where you are struggling to ventilate a patient with a BVM and an ambulance crew arrives, it would be appropriate to let them know about the difficulties with the airway so they can focus on trying to correct the problem.

Trauma Handover

The UK Ambulance Services Clinical Practice Guidelines recommend the use of the ATMIST model as a quick and easy way of conducting a handover for trauma patients (JRCALC, 2016):

A: age of patient
T: time of incident
M: mechanism of injury
I: injuries sustained
S: signs and symptoms
T: treatment given/immediate needs.

Other principles to consider when conducting a handover include the following:

- Make sure the person to whom you are handing over is the person responsible for the patient's care.
- Have your handover ready; make notes in advance to help if necessary.
- Make it concise; especially for the critically ill and injured patient, you will have a very limited period of time (often less than 60 seconds) in which to provide a handover.
- Make sure you have everyone's attention prior to beginning your handover (unless the patient is critically unwell, in which case some of the team will still need to be providing interventions).
- Provide written copies of all information as well as a verbal account whenever you hand over the care of your patient.

Pre-Alert

If you become involved in transporting a critically unwell patient to hospital, it is routine practice to call the hospital in advance and provide a pre-alert. Different hospitals will use pre-alert in different ways and you should be familiar with the local expectations. Providing a timely pre-alert allows the hospital to prepare for your arrival. For example, if you are bringing in a major trauma patient, it is common for a 'trauma call' to be placed, which will gather all the correct medical experts in the ED waiting for your arrival.

A pre-alert can be provided via phone or radio. It will follow the same models used for handover, though in addition should also include an estimated time of arrival (ETA). This ETA should be given in a time format, i.e. 'We will arrive at 13:30' and should include the transport method, i.e. ground ambulance or air ambulance. Wherever possible, it should be the person directly caring for the patient that provides the pre-alert and not passed via a third party.

Breaking Bad News

At some point, you may become involved in breaking bad news to patients, relatives or friends of patients. This may be when you attend a cardiac arrest, but recognise that the patient has injuries or a condition unequivocally associated with death, so resuscitation is not started (see Chapter 18: Cardiac Arrest for more detail).

Breaking bad news can be a difficult and very emotive issue. To help prepare yourself for when you need to break bad news, consider the SPIKES mnemonic below (Baile et al., 2000):

- **Setting up**: Consider what you can do in preparation so that the situation goes as smoothly as possible. Do not begin the conversation until you have a plan for what you are going to do. Consider what you are going to say. Turn off or silence your radio and consider how the person or people may react to the news; be prepared to manage this.
- **Perception**: When you begin, try to gain an understanding of what the person thinks is going on already. Often patients or relatives will have good insight into a situation and the bad news will not come as a shock. Sometimes it is, however, and these can be particularly challenging scenarios to manage.
- **Invitation**: As the conversation is progressing, find out how much the person wants to know. Most people want to know a lot of detail, but this is not always the case.
- **Knowledge**: Remember you may be speaking to someone that does not fully understand the situation. Avoid using complex medical language. Try to speak in a way that matches their communication. Most importantly, be sensitive, honest and informative.
- **Emotions and empathy**: Use empathetic statements to respond to emotions. Do not rush to provide reassurance that you cannot be sure will happen. Statements such as 'it will all be ok' are not necessarily helpful and can give false hope.
- **Strategy and summary**: Summarise the situation and come up with concrete next steps for what the person needs to do so they are not in doubt or confused. Continue to clarify using statements such as 'Does this make sense to you?' or 'Are you clear about what to do next?' until you are satisfied that they understand.

Breaking bad news can also be difficult on you, so remember to talk to colleagues afterwards or seek help managing your own emotions.

Summary

Communication is a skill and, like all skills, it can be refined with practice, reflection and improving knowledge. Good communication is a fundamental skill for safe, effective healthcare and ensuring the safety of yourself and others.

In your role as an emergency medical responder, you should frequently critique your own communication skills in order to continue developing them. You will become aware of those considered by colleagues to be good communicators and should observe their methods.

Ultimately good communication will lead to better inter-personal relationships, happier patients and safer, more effective care being provided.

Chapter 4

Clinical Governance, Legal and Ethical Issues

Being a Healthcare Provider

Learning Objectives

By the end of this section you will be able to:

- Explain what it means to have a duty of care.
- Explain how duty of care contributes to the safeguarding or protection of individuals.
- Describe how to respond to complaints.
- Explain the main points of agreed procedures for handling complaints.
- Explain expectations about your work role as expressed in relevant standards.
- Describe how your values, belief systems and experiences may affect working practice.
- Describe why it is important to adhere to the agreed scope of the job role.

Introduction

This section will describe what it means to be a healthcare volunteer, with a focus on:

- values-based healthcare
- duty of care
- scope of practice
- standards
- complaints.

Values-Based Healthcare

Working as a provider of emergency care is an extraordinarily privileged role. As in your main fire service role, you will often be caring for people when they are at their most vulnerable. The majority of people have less than a handful of contacts with the emergency services throughout their lifetime, so when they do call, during extreme life events, patients will look to you for help and support in whatever situation they find themselves. Being in this privileged role, it is important to recognise that you should be patient focused and the attitudes and beliefs that you hold can influence the care you provide to your patient.

Stafford Hospital

Stafford Hospital was an acute hospital that became the focus of a national outcry about standards of care. Following concerns raised by the families of patients around poor standards of care and further concerns around unusually high mortality rates, especially for emergency admission patients (Cure the NHS, 2018), the Healthcare Commission conducted an investigation in 2008 looking into care at the hospital. This uncovered deficiencies at virtually every stage of the pathway of emergency care (HC, 2009).

The resulting public inquiry and report, widely known as the Francis Report, painted a damning picture of a hospital where there were fundamental failures of care. These included (Francis, 2013):

- patients left in excrement-soiled bedclothes for lengthy periods
- no assistance provided for feeding patients who could not eat without help
- water left out of reach
- patients and those close to them treated by staff with what appeared to be callous indifference.

Although a definitive number has never been released, it is suspected that hundreds of patients died unnecessarily and thousands more suffered as a result of poor care.

The final report made 290 recommendations in total, many of which have been adopted nationally. There have been a number of other reports into improving care within the NHS published since, but perhaps the most influential is the one conducted by the National Advisory Group on the Safety of Patients in England (DoH, 2013c). This review made a number of key recommendations including the following:

- The NHS should continually and forever reduce patient harm by embracing wholeheartedly an ethic of learning.
- Patients and their carers should be present, powerful and involved at all levels of healthcare organisations from 'wards to the boards'.

Not only does this philosophy make the NHS an organisation that learns from and builds on its errors, but it puts the patient at the core of all activities. Health professionals must always apply a culture of compassionate care when looking after patients, a culture that is best summarised by the '6 Cs':

- care
- compassion
- competence
- communication
- courage
- commitment.

What Influences Your Values and Attitudes?

There are multiple aspects that influence our own attitudes, but understanding this and understanding how our attitudes impact on the management of our patients is an important distinction to make. Everyone harbours prejudgements about certain people or groups of people. These can be positive or negative, and these stereotypes are used as a form of mental shortcut (Paul, 1998). However, this can also be dangerous, as it can lead to judgements being made about people based on limited information. These judgements can even influence the way in which a patient is treated, which in turn can lead to errors.

Consider the following scenario:

You are on call overnight on a Friday. You have had a long week at work, and already have been out to one incident earlier in the night. Around 02:00 you are dispatched to an incident around half a mile away. You recognise the address: it is an elderly female who frequently calls 999, complaining of chest pain on the phone. Despite lengthy tests and examinations, no-one has ever found anything wrong with the patient, and it is thought that her calls are more due to loneliness and panic attacks than any critical medical need.

Is there a risk of stereotyping influencing your practice in this scenario? The answer is almost certainly yes, particularly if you approach the incident thinking 'here we go again', wondering how long it will take this time. Having a certain amount of pre-judgement is probably unavoidable, but you should recognise that this is the case, and not allow these judgements to bias your thinking, which may in turn lead to you providing less than optimal patient care.

Duty of Care

Duty of care is a civil law concept within the UK and exists to ensure that one party does not allow unreasonable harm or loss to occur to another (Dimond, 2011).

As an emergency medical responder, you owe a duty of care to your patient from the point at which they are accepted as a service user (HCPC, 2016). From that point onward, you must act in a way to prevent harm where a reasonable person could see that harm might occur. If you breach this duty of care and someone suffers as a result, this can lead to the civil wrong of negligence.

Negligence

Negligence occurs when duty of care is breached and reasonably foreseeable harm occurs as a result. If a party is guilty of negligence, they can be pursued through the civil courts for damages.

There are four stages for negligence to be proven (Pilbery, 2013):

- It must be established that a duty of care existed.
- A breach of that duty must be identified.
- It must be confirmed that harm occurred.
- Causation between the breach and the harm must be established.

Establishing a duty is usually straightforward, since as an emergency medical responder you owe a duty to any patient you encounter. **Breach of duty** occurs when a reasonably foreseeable consequence of a person's action leads to harm. The difficult part to measure is what counts as 'reasonably foreseeable', and this is a point that the courts may have to decide upon. **Harm** can take many forms including physical injury, but may also include:

- mental or emotional distress
- loss of earnings or loss of potential future earnings.

Causation is the final step in proving negligence. It is not enough for a duty of care to exist and for that duty to be breached. The breach of duty has to go on to cause harm and it should be evident that this breach was the cause of that harm. Also sometimes referred to as the 'but for' principle, it is applied by asking 'But for the (action or omission) would harm have occurred?' If the answer to this is 'yes', then negligence is not proven; if the answer is 'no', then it is likely that negligence exists.

If negligence is proven, it is likely that the person suffering harm will receive damages for the harm they suffered. This money, likely to run to thousands, if not hundreds of thousands of pounds depending on the nature and severity of the harm caused, will be paid by the ambulance or fire service under their responsibility of vicarious liability (as your employer, they are responsible for your actions and omissions). However, you should note that in certain exceptional circumstances, you can also be found guilty of certain criminal charges if you are grossly negligent in caring for your patient. Therefore, it is important to ensure you act within your scope of practice to ensure your own safety.

Scope of Practice and Standards

Your scope of practice will be established by the service you are linked to through a series of standards. Such standards are treated as the benchmark for determining whether or not a person is working within their scope of practice and also whether or not they are fit to be an emergency medical responder.

Standards can cover a wide range of topics, not just clinical skills. It is not possible to list the standards here, as they will vary from organisation to organisation, but you should be aware of the standards expected of you and what your scope of practice is, i.e. what you can do when responding to a patient. Not everything included in this book will be within the standard scope of practice for all emergency medical responders.

A number of skills, such as taking manual blood pressures, may not be standard skills for all emergency medical responders, and it is the decision of your organisation as to exactly what examination and management skills, including medications, are available to you.

You should not attempt to undertake any activity outside your scope of practice, as you are not likely to have the knowledge, skill or experience to do so safely and would therefore be putting the patient and yourself at risk. What constitutes negligence was outlined earlier, and it should be noted that any activity undertaken outside of your scope of practice, and which leads to harm, is likely to be the grounds for a claim of negligence.

When Things Go Wrong

All healthcare providers strive to be a 'no harm' organisation (i.e. cause no harm to their patients), but it is probably an unavoidable fact that systems as large and complex as modern health services will always have adverse incidents. However, these errors should not lead to patient harm, and lessons should be learnt from mistakes when they do occur.

All health organisations should learn from their mistakes. They should also promote a learning culture where staff are not unnecessarily blamed for mistakes, and where people feel safe in reporting incidents so that the larger organisation can learn from those incidents, even small ones. Only when organisations can learn from their mistakes will they be able to prevent events from being repeated, meaning that overall, a well-functioning complaints system plays a major role in service improvement and preventing patient harm.

Failure to Achieve Standards

This concept of reporting extends to yourself and your own practice as well. If you recognise that in the course of your duty you have failed to achieve the expected standards for someone in your role, then you should make this known.

Different organisations will have different methods of reporting, but most now have a central system for reporting incidents and a dedicated team that deals with those reports. In most health services, this is the 'Datix' system.

Complaints

During the course of your duty it may be the case that someone wishes to make a complaint about you, your colleagues, your organisation, or another organisation. This can be challenging, as the natural response is to be defensive, but remember that the principles of a learning organisation, together with opportunities to reflect, should be seen as a way of improving services and should be welcomed as such.

It is likely that your service will have specific guidelines or a policy on handling complaints, which you should be familiar with, but good general guidelines for the actions you should undertake include the following:

- Record facts and pass them on to appropriate people; do not undertake the investigation yourself.
- If someone wishes to make a complaint, take the details and pass them on to relevant parties, or give the person the contact details of the relevant people inside your organisation.
- Do not challenge facts about a complaint; if necessary this can be done later on, once all the facts have been established.
- Provide contact details so that patients know how to get in touch should they wish to.

If you become involved in an investigation or complaint, you should do all you can to support the investigation. Withholding key information may be seen as a misconduct offence, which is likely to be handled very differently from learning from a genuine error. You should seek advice from managers/union officials to support you if you are a part of an investigation. Remember the aim of investigations in a good organisation is to learn and improve patient safety for future similar events, not to blame and inappropriately discipline individuals.

Additional Sources of Support

Dealing with situations where things have gone wrong can be a challenging time and you may well need further advice and support. In those circumstances, you may find that some of the options listed below are able to assist you:

- organisational policy
- your line manager
- 'Making Experiences Count' (or similar) investigation team within your organisation (DoH, 2007b).

Consent and Capacity

Learning Objectives

By the end of this section you will be able to:

- Describe the components of assessing capacity.
- Gain consent.
- Maintain consent.
- Analyse factors that influence the capacity of an individual to express consent.

Introduction

As an emergency medical responder in a front line role, you will regularly have to seek consent to treat people, and should have a basic understanding of mental capacity and how it impacts on patient treatment.

Having a good understanding of the basic principles will make this easier and help to remove doubt when tackling challenging and potentially confusing scenarios.

Consent

In the United Kingdom, case law has determined that adult patients with mental capacity must give consent before they are touched or treated. Failure to do this leaves those treating them open to civil claims for trespass against the person, which includes assault and battery (Dimond, 2008); therefore, you must seek valid consent to treat your patient.

Valid Consent

In order for consent to be valid, there are three criteria that must be met (NHS England, 2016); they stipulate that consent must fulfil the following three criteria:

- **Given voluntarily**: i.e. free from pressure exerted by relatives, partners, healthcare staff or police officers etc.
- **Informed**: The patient must understand what course of action is being proposed, what the benefits and significant risks are, what alternatives are available, and what the consequences are of doing nothing.
- **Capacity**: The person consenting needs to have the mental capacity to do so. This is usually the patient, but includes someone with parental responsibility in patients less than 18 years of age, or a person who has been given a Lasting Power of Attorney (LPA) or authority by a court to make treatment decisions (DoH, 2009a).

Communicating Consent

Communicating consent may take many forms. Often for elective procedures in hospital it will be written. Working out-of-hospital, the majority of the time it will be verbal, but it may take another form, particularly if the patient has a disability that would make written or verbal communication impossible. Other forms that you may encounter include, but are not limited to:

- sign language
- use of props
- blinking
- movement of limbs
- use of technology, such as speech generators.

Best Interest Decisions

Generally, if your patient is over 18 years of age, only they can consent to any intervention. Lying unconscious in the street after being involved in a road traffic collision does not imply consent but instead you would treat them under a principle of 'best interest', whereby you can apply life-saving treatments without the patient's consent, as long as, to the best of your knowledge, they have not previously made a declaration refusing such treatment, also known as an advance decision to refuse treatment (ADRT).

Advance Decision to Refuse Treatment (ADRT)

An ADRT is an order made by a person over the age of 18 when they still have capacity, to refuse specified medical treatment at a future point in time when they may lack the capacity to consent to or refuse treatment.

If faced with an ADRT you should be confident that it is valid before working to it. For it to be valid you should, where possible, confirm whether the patient:

- has done anything that clearly goes against their advance decision
- has withdrawn their decision
- would have changed their decision if they had known more about the current circumstances
- has subsequently conferred the power to make that decision to an LPA.

Generally, an ADRT does not have to be written – it can be verbal – but if it refers to life-saving treatment then it must:

- be in writing
- be witnessed and signed
- state clearly that the decision applies even if life is at risk.

If you believe an ADRT exists, is valid and applicable, you should follow the instructions contained therein.

Mental Capacity

Case law has clearly laid out the right of a mentally competent adult to refuse any treatment, including life-saving interventions, regardless of the reason, or for no reason at all. This has now been incorporated into several statutory frameworks. In England and Wales, this framework is the Mental Capacity Act 2005 (MCA), and in Scotland, the Adults with Incapacity (Scotland) Act 2000. The purpose of this legislation is to protect the rights of individuals from having treatment forced upon them in all but rare circumstances.

Central to capacity and consent is the concept of personal autonomy, that is, the right of an individual to 'govern themselves' according to their own set of personal values, preferences, commitments and character traits (Freyenhagen, 2009). This can come into conflict with the tendency of healthcare staff towards beneficence (i.e. serving the best interests of patients (Moye, 2007)) and wanting to safeguard their job.

Mental capacity is the ability to make a decision, and covers everything from when to get up, to how much alcohol to drink and whether to go to hospital as advised by a health professional. A lack of capacity is defined as an inability of your patient to make a specific decision at the time they are required to make it, due to an impairment of, or disturbance in the functioning of, the mind or brain. It does not matter if this impairment or disturbance is temporary or permanent. Examples of impairment include:

Temporary:
- post-ictal following a convulsion
- a diabetic suffering a hypoglycaemic event
- ingestion of alcohol or drugs.

Permanent:
- dementia
- significant learning disabilities
- long-term effects of brain damage.

What to Do If You Suspect a Lack of Capacity

As a responder, it is unlikely you will receive the specific training required to undertake a capacity assessment. Instead, if you have a patient that is refusing life-saving treatment you should contact control as soon as possible and inform them about the situation. A clinician in the emergency operations centre (EOC) may be able to assist you, and they can make sure you receive appropriate backup as quickly as possible.

All clinicians that back you up should be able to undertake a capacity assessment and may, in certain circumstances, depending on the immediate risk facing the patient, decide to treat them against their will. While you are waiting for backup, you should explain clearly and simply, in a way the patient will understand, why you want to treat them, what it is you want to do and what risks are associated with their refusing treatment.

Summary

As an emergency medical responder you are subject to the same laws as any other clinician in respect of consent. Be sure that, where possible, you seek valid consent from your patient and that you are not accidentally forcing unwanted treatment on them.

You should also have a general understanding of what mental capacity is and what you should look for when you believe your patient may lack capacity. If you believe your patient may lack capacity, a clinician will undertake an assessment and decide on the best course of action.

Confidentiality and Information Governance

Learning Objectives

By the end of this section you will be able to:
- Explain the meaning of the term 'confidentiality'.
- Demonstrate ways to maintain confidentiality in day-to-day communication.
- Define information governance.
- Explain your role in information governance.

Introduction

Any responders, like other healthcare professions, have a duty of confidentiality to their patients, whereby they must protect all patient information and handle it in an approved manner. Failure to follow strict organisation policies and, where relevant, codes of conduct in relation to handling information can be a source of distress for patients and embarrassment for organisations. It can also result in legal or disciplinary action for both organisations and individuals (NHS England, 2016).

Information governance is broadly defined as the framework organisations have in place to bring together all the legal rules, guidance and best practice that apply to the handling of information (HSCIC, 2015). These rules and guidelines include:

- the Data Protection Act 1998
- General Data Protection Regulations (GDPR) – coming into force during 2018
- the Confidentiality NHS Code of Practice
- the Freedom of Information Act 2000
- the Records Management NHS Code of Practice
- the Information Security Management NHS Code of Practice.

Within your role, you will routinely have access to confidential, patient-identifiable information. This information, or data, should be protected: this means that you should record, handle and store this information in such a way that you are not likely to misplace any information or accidentally breach confidentiality by making an unauthorised or unnecessary disclosure, which could lead to civil or criminal legal proceedings being brought against you or the organisation you work for.

What Should Be Considered Patient-Identifiable Information?

Patient-identifiable information is anything that may enable a patient to be identified, either directly or indirectly (JRCALC, 2016). This includes obvious personal information, such as name, address, date of birth etc. However, it also includes less commonly considered things, such as:

- clinical record numbers
- images or voice recordings of a patient
- rare disease information.

Consider the following scenario:

You work in a small town with a population of around 25,000 people. In this town lives a patient who suffers from Addison's disease: a rare endocrine disorder. The patient frequently suffers from Addisonian crises, and when this happens family members call for an ambulance.

You attend this patient suffering from a crisis one day; as this is not a condition you are familiar with, next time you visit a local ambulance station you ask an ambulance crew for some information about the condition. You are mindful not to disclose the name or location of the patient (to prevent a breach of confidentiality), but instead describe the incident and ask for advice.

Considering that Addison's is a rare disease and this one person, in a small community, frequently requires ambulance assistance, is it reasonable that, on the balance of probabilities, the crews would be able to identify whom you are talking about, just by describing the condition?

Any information that has the potential to identify the patient, however remotely, should be considered as identifiable and managed in such a way as to help avoid a breach of confidentiality from occurring (JRCALC, 2016).

Maintaining Confidentiality

Organisations should have policies in place to describe how they handle information and protect confidentiality. As you have a legal obligation to maintain confidentiality, you should have a good working knowledge of these policies (NHS England, 2016).

During the course of your duties, it may be necessary to discuss or share patient-identifiable information on a number of occasions. Such occasions may include:

- discussing the care of your patient with another healthcare professional
- handing over the care of your patient.

These communications can take many forms including:

- face-to-face
- written
- telephone.

Different systems will have different strengths and weaknesses in their security of managing data. Most records in the out-of-hospital setting are recorded either on paper or, increasingly frequently, on electronic patient record devices. Below are some of the security features of each type of storage:

Electronic record keeping:
- All data is transferred and stored securely. No data is left 'hanging around' once it is no longer required.
- No physical copies of records means it is less likely records will be 'misplaced'.

Physical records:
- Once completed these should be submitted into a secure storage system.
- Copies of the record are only passed to patients or patients' relatives with permission once completed.

Regardless of which system you use, you should consider how best to maintain confidentiality. Your employer or volunteer organisation should make a copy of its policy available, but some good practice guidelines include (NHS England, 2016):
- **Seek consent before sharing information**: Before you share patient information you should seek consent from the patient to do so. However, in a limited range of situations it may be appropriate to share information without the patient's consent, for example:
  - It is not possible to gain consent – this would most likely be due to the patient's condition, i.e. unconscious.
- **Share only that information which is necessary**: If you phone the EOC after an incident to book clear, you are probably going to speak to a dispatcher. It is unlikely that person needs to know all the medical details of the patient, so you should limit your discussion to relevant points and not disclose confidential information unnecessarily.
- **Maintain the physical security of information**: Part of your role is likely to include making notes and records on the patients you attend. It is unlikely that you would keep these records once you have treated the patient; instead they should go with the patient to be passed to the ambulance crew that backs you up.

You may decide to keep a record of incidents that you attend for your own development; however, this must not include any patient-identifiable information.

If you find following an incident that you have accidentally retained a copy of patient-identifiable information, you should immediately inform your line manager and follow their instructions on how to deal with it appropriately.

Key Points

Remember these key points relating to confidentiality:
- Patients are the owners of information or data relating to them.
- Patient-identifiable information comes in many forms and is communicated in a range of ways.
- Patient-identifiable information should not be shared without consent except in specific circumstances.
- Only share information that is necessary.
- Consider how to maintain security of data in order to prevent accidental disclosures.
- Organisations should have policies in place for protecting information and you should be familiar with these.

Equality and Diversity

Learning Objectives

By the end of this section you will be able to:
- Explain what is meant by:
  - diversity
  - equality
  - inclusion
  - discrimination.
- Describe the potential effects of discrimination.
- Explain how inclusive practice promotes equality and supports diversity.
- Explain how legislation and codes of practice relating to equality, diversity and discrimination apply to your own work role.

Introduction

Promoting equality should be at the heart of a healthcare organisation's values. It ensures that organisations work in a way that is fair, so that no community, group or individual is left behind (NHS England, 2015).

It is helpful to understand what the terms 'diversity', 'equality' and 'inclusion' mean:

- **Diversity**: This involves recognising and valuing the differences between individuals across groups. Such differences should be seen as 'assets to be valued and affirmed, rather than as problems to be solved' (Thompson, 2006b).
- **Equality**: In its simplest form, equality is about being treated fairly. Equality recognises that people are different (diversity), but that those differences do not mean that a person should be discriminated against, as everyone should be treated fairly and equally. Equality also recognises that inequality exists and needs to be overcome for a truly fair society.
- **Inclusion**: This involves positively striving to meet the needs of different people and taking deliberate action to create environments where everyone feels respected and able to achieve their full potential (NIHR, 2012).

Equality in Healthcare

At first glance, it may not be obvious how equality and diversity can have an influence on healthcare or outcomes; however, various health inequalities do exist (NICE, 2012a). The King's Fund (2015) discusses how men and women from the richest social groups live an average of 7 years longer than those from the poorest social class.

Issues that are thought to influence health inequalities include:

- employment
- education
- availability and accessibility to healthcare
- housing.

Discrimination

Discrimination occurs when someone treats one person less favourably than they would another, because of a personal characteristic. This is often due to stereotyping.

Under the Equality Act 2010, it is unlawful for a person to discriminate against another with respect to certain protected characteristics. The nine characteristics are:

- age
- disability
- gender
- gender reassignment
- marriage and civil partnership
- pregnancy and maternity
- race
- religion and belief
- sexual orientation.

As well as the Equality Act, the Human Rights Act 1998 also provides direction for ensuring certain equalities, including the:

- right to life
- right to a fair trial
- right to education
- right to participate in free elections.

Discrimination in Your Role

In order to make sense of society and those in it, we naturally group individuals together when they share common characteristics. Based on these characteristics we may expect people within the group to act in similar ways or to have similar responses to the same situations; this is the process of stereotyping (Judd, 1993).

Using these stereotypes is a natural process as it allows us to 'shortcut' our thinking, but often the stereotypes are not accurate. Making such shortcuts in emergency care can be dangerous, as we may make incorrect assumptions about our patients and fail to challenge our own thought processes.

Applying such stereotypes is probably unavoidable, but we must be prepared to challenge our own thinking and the assumptions made on the basis of that thinking. For example, older patients have very varied life expectancies. Some patients may suffer from a multitude of medical conditions in their early seventies and, therefore, have a relatively limited life expectancy, whereas many people will live late into their nineties and beyond with very few medical concerns. If all of these patients were treated the same purely on the basis of their age you would not be treating patients as individuals and would be likely to provide poor care as a result – potentially even leading to the avoidable early death of a patient. Remember that age is a protected characteristic and it is both unethical and unlawful to discriminate against someone on the basis of one of these characteristics.

Further Support

If you observe discrimination then you will need support in understanding how best to resolve the situation. In this instance help would normally be available from your:

- line manager
- organisation Equality and Diversity lead.

If a patient wishes to make a complaint in relation to being discriminated against, you should support them in doing this.

Remember, everyone is responsible for promoting equality, recognising diversity and challenging discrimination. Only by doing this will you be able to ensure your patients are receiving the best care possible and you are practising in a non-discriminatory manner. Do not assume that others will tackle the issue.

Clinical Governance

Learning Objectives

By the end of this section you will be able to:

- Define the term clinical governance.
- Describe why clinical governance is relevant to your role.
- Outline how you should engage in clinical governance procedures.

Introduction

Public Health England (2017) describes clinical governance as: 'the system through which NHS organisations are accountable for continuously improving the quality of their services and safeguarding high standards of care by creating an environment in which clinical excellence will flourish'.

Rather than being a single idea or set of actions, clinical governance and the ethos of improving standards of care should be at every level of health service design, commissioning, and implementation. This means the principles of good clinical governance affects everyone, from the top of government through to the clinicians and support staff working to deliver patient care.

How to Contribute to Clinical Governance

In your role, you should strive to deliver the highest possible standards of care to your patients. The following are examples of how you can contribute to high standards of clinical governance in your organisation:

- **Report incidents and near misses**: As discussed above in relation to being a healthcare provider, you have a responsibility to report any adverse incidents or near misses. This is not so individuals can be blamed but so that lessons can be learned to improve future care.
- **Propose and support service improvement**: Working on the front line, you may be able to identify ways in which care can be delivered more effectively and safely. These don't have to be big changes and can be as simple as changing the layout of equipment in bags. Working operationally, you are best placed to identify how small changes could improve patient care, and you should approach your management or use a staff suggestion scheme to propose improvements.
- **Personal reflection**: Every incident you attend offers opportunity for reflection and learning. You may be familiar with written reflections, but not all reflection needs to be in this format. Simply taking time to think about what went well and what you would do differently in a similar situation is a good way to slowly learn and improve your practice.
- **Team reflection**: As well as reflecting personally, you should support and encourage reflections as a team. Bringing together lots of individuals' personal reflections can be a powerful tool, as others will have ideas that have not occurred to you. From your fire service role, you will already be familiar with debriefing incidents and the same format can be used here.
- **Support the development of others**: As you gain experience as an emergency medical responder, it is likely that you will be asked to work alongside new staff and those with less casualty

care experience than you. You should support these people to develop their skills and offer them potential development ideas based on your own experience.

- **Engage in clinical supervision sessions**: All organisations providing healthcare should offer clinical supervision sessions. These are opportunities for clinicians to come together and discuss cases. These cases may be examples where something has not gone quite as well as hoped, or where really good practice was identified. They might also just be the opportunity for you to ask, 'what would you have done?'. Such sessions are very good learning environments, and give opportunities to ask those little questions that might have been playing on your mind but there has been no other forum to discuss them.
- **Training**: One of the best ways to improve your knowledge and skills is to complete training. This can be formal training, such as your casualty care course, or less formal training, for example a daily drill on station. You should also be sure to regularly complete refresher and mandatory training, which helps to ensure that your skills are always kept up-to-date.

Chapter 5

Safeguarding Adults and Children

Learning Objectives

By the end of this chapter you will be able to:

- Define the various types of abuse.
- Identify the signs and/or symptoms associated with different forms of abuse.
- Describe factors that may contribute to an individual being more vulnerable to abuse.
- Explain the actions to take if there are suspicions that an individual is being abused.
- Explain the actions to take if an individual alleges that they are being abused.
- Identify reports into serious failures to protect individuals from abuse.
- Identify sources of information and advice about your own role in safeguarding and protecting individuals from abuse.
- Describe the action to take if suspected abuse or unsafe practices have been reported but nothing has been done in response.

Introduction

As an emergency medical responder you hold a trusted and privileged position, and one from which you can potentially identify and assist victims of abuse or neglect. In order to do this, you will need to have a good understanding of the forms abuse can take, the signs and symptoms of those suffering, what increases a person's risk of being a victim of abuse, and also how to get help and support for victims.

Before going further, consider some of the key terms associated with safeguarding:

- **Safeguarding**: the process of promoting the welfare of individuals and groups and protecting them from harm, often putting controls and measures in place to do so.
- **Abuse**: any action that causes significant harm to an individual. Harm may take many forms in this definition.
- **Harm**: physical or psychological damage or injury.
- **Maltreatment**: includes all forms of physical and emotional ill-treatment or abuse.

We will mainly be discussing safeguarding for children (according to legal definitions, a child is anyone under the age of 18) and vulnerable adults.

Learning from Previous Cases

The vast majority of abuse and neglect happens behind closed doors and rarely reaches the attention of the public. However, over recent years there have been a number of notable cases, including:

- Winterbourne View: In 2011 a BBC *Panorama* programme showed staff at Winterbourne View, a private hospital caring for patients with disabilities, abusing their patients both physically and psychologically. A national outcry followed, and in the subsequent investigation 11 staff were convicted of criminal offences and the hospital was shut. The investigation also identified that there were serious warning signs evident at the hospital for a long time prior to the discovery of abuse, which had not been properly looked into (DoH, 2013b).
- Daniel Pelka: Daniel died aged 4 years and 8 months following a period of sustained abuse and neglect by his mother and her partner. His death was caused by a serious head injury, but he had been physically beaten and starved for a prolonged period prior to his death. In the serious case review following his death, it was identified that although the family and Daniel were well known to police, social services, healthcare services and his school, the warning signs had not been correctly picked up on or appropriate action taken. The report said that Daniel was 'invisible against the backdrop of his mother's controlling behaviour' and that professionals involved in his case had failed to 'think the unthinkable' (CSCB, 2014).

Sadly, this failure to notice warning signs is not unique and other equally tragic cases, such as the murders of Victoria Climbié and baby Peter Connelly (Baby P), reached very similar findings in their investigations.

Abusers can be skilled at explaining away injuries or unusual behaviour and making professionals feel relaxed about the situation they find. In your role, you may be the only individual that comes into contact with a vulnerable person over a prolonged period of time, so you must be prepared to identify and raise concerns where necessary, in order to help prevent further similar cases like those above. You must be prepared to 'think the unthinkable'.

Vulnerability

People are considered to be vulnerable when they are at a greater than normal risk of abuse. For vulnerable adults, this can include (NHS Choices, 2015a):

- those with learning difficulties
- older people who are isolated
- those with memory problems
- those who are dependent on others for support
- those whose carer is addicted to alcohol or drugs
- those who live with a carer.

Abusers of Vulnerable Adults

Vulnerable adults may be abused by a wide range of people, including relatives and family, professional staff, paid care workers, volunteers, other service users, neighbours, friends and those who deliberately target and exploit the vulnerable (DoH, 2000).

Risk Factors for Child Abuse

All children are vulnerable to abuse, but those who may be more so include those in the following situations (NICE, 2009):

- parental or carer drug or alcohol misuse
- parental or carer mental health problems
- intrafamilial violence or history of violent offending
- previous child maltreatment in members of the family
- known maltreatment of an animal by the carer or parent
- vulnerable and unsupported parents or carers
- pre-existing disability in the child.

What is common to most of these scenarios for both adults and children is that the abused tend to have reduced support networks or social contacts around them to whom they can turn for help and support. The victim tends to have a degree of reliance on the abuser, and this gives the abuser a position of power with which to control and manipulate the victim.

Forms of Abuse

There are four types of abuse common to both adults and children (DfE, 2015; DoH, 2011):

- physical abuse
- psychological/emotional abuse
- sexual abuse
- neglect.

For vulnerable adults there is also (Age UK, 2017):

- financial abuse
- discriminatory abuse.

Additionally, you should also be aware of Female Genital Mutilation (FGM), a form of child abuse.

Physical Abuse

Physical abuse, also known as non-accidental injury (NAI), involves contact intended to cause, or resulting in, pain, injury or other physical harm. It may include striking someone (with or without an object), kicking, grabbing, biting or inappropriate restraint. For older patients in particular, it may also include being handled roughly, or moved in a way that causes pain without the appropriate lifting or moving aids (DfE, 2015; Age UK, 2017).

Physical harm can also be caused when a carer or parent fabricates illness, or induces symptoms of an illness, in an adult or child (Munchausen's syndrome by proxy).

Signs of physical abuse may include:

- bruising at multiple stages of repair
- bruises on children who are not yet crawling
- injuries inconsistent with the age of the patient
- frequent attendance at hospital
- inappropriate history for the injury demonstrated
- specific injuries, such as cigarette burns and 'hand-grip' bruises
- fear of those around them
- fear of making mistakes
- being very withdrawn and quiet
- delays in seeking help for illness or injury.

Psychological/Emotional Abuse

Psychological, also known as emotional, abuse is a form of abuse characterised by damaging a person's psychological well-being. This is often seen in situations of power imbalance, such as abusive relationships. It may include conveying a feeling of unworthiness, unimportance or being unvalued. It may also include causing a person to feel ashamed or humiliated through the words or actions of another person.

Over a prolonged period, this form of abuse can allow the abuser to mentally control the abused person and seriously damage their emotional and psychological development. All forms of abuse usually contain an element of psychological abuse, as abusers will try to control the actions and behaviour of their victim (DfE, 2015; Age UK, 2017). Signs may include:

- lack of social skills
- low self-worth
- depression
- self-harm
- poor relationships with others
- helplessness
- excessive fear or anxiety.

Sexual Abuse

Sexual abuse involves forcing or enticing a person to take part in sexual activity against their wishes, or for which they are not able to consent. Activities may involve physical assault, including penetration (for example, rape or oral sex), or they can be non-penetrative, such as kissing, masturbation or touching the outside of clothing. Sexual abuse can also include non-contact activities, such as indecent exposure, or forcing a person to watch, or to be involved in the production of, explicit sexual material. Grooming a person in preparation for abuse is also a form of sexual abuse (DfE, 2015; Age UK, 2017).

Signs may include:

- physical indications, such as anal or vaginal soreness
- sexually transmitted infection
- unusual discharge
- inappropriate use of sexual language for age
- a child being sexually active at a young age
- guilt or shame
- appearing frightened by or avoiding being near to certain people.

Neglect

Neglect is the persistent failure to meet a person's physical and/or psychological needs. A carer or parent should take reasonable steps to prevent harm from occurring to a dependant, and failure to do so may be neglect. Neglect can be deliberate or accidental, due to not fully understanding the needs of a dependent person.

Neglect may include:
- failure to provide adequate food, warmth or shelter for a dependant
- failure to ensure adequate access to appropriate medical care.

Signs of neglect include:
- poor appearance and hygiene
- untreated injuries or dental issues
- poor physical development for age
- poor language or communication skills for age
- pressure sores
- signs of malnourishment or dehydration
- dirt, urine or faecal smell in the person's environment.

Financial Abuse

This is the unlawful use of a person's property, money or other valuables. It may include an individual being pressured into lending or giving money or other belongings to another person. A carer could start to take control of personal finance and then use that control to gain profitably without consent. It may also include charging excessive amounts of money for simple services or goods. Relatives are often perpetrators of this kind of abuse and may move into a patient's house in order to be able to exert the influence required to take financial control (Age UK, 2017).

Signs of financial abuse can include:
- unexplained loss of money
- unusual bank account activity
- rapid deterioration in a person's standard of living as they can no longer afford essential goods and services
- a relative or carer moving into the home and taking control.

Discriminatory Abuse

A person can be discriminated against on the basis of their age, gender, race, ethnicity, religion, culture, beliefs or some other aspect or value of their life. It could include a failure to take into account personal or religious beliefs in the provision of care, and could impact on the spiritual welfare of a person. Age-related discrimination is an offence under the Equality Act 2010 (Age UK, 2014).

Female Genital Mutilation (FGM)

FGM is the partial, or complete, removal of the female genitalia, also known as female circumcision or cutting. It is a practice most commonly observed in certain African countries and also the Middle East (UNICEF, 2013).

FGM is a deeply rooted tradition that acts as a complex form of control over women's reproductive and sexual rights, and although it can be performed at any age from birth through to marriage or first pregnancy, it most commonly takes place between the ages of 5 and 8 (HO and DfE, 2016). Being subject to FGM can have a long-term impact on physical and mental health and well-being.

FGM is a criminal offence in the UK, and it is also an offence for anyone to take a child abroad in order for FGM to be performed (NSPCC, 2018). You are legally required by the Female Genital Mutilation Act 2003 to report to the police any cases of FGM in those under 18. This should be done by reporting through usual safeguarding procedures, which will involve informing the police and social services (JRCALC, 2017).

Managing Abuse or Disclosures of Abuse

The primary goal in the management of a patient who has suffered abuse should be their long-term safety. The situation may be highly emotionally charged, not least for you, but your actions in the immediate moments on scene may influence the entire course of protecting a vulnerable person.

You should remain calm and professional, and not judge those around you. Situations are rarely as simple as they may initially appear, and in the amount of time you will be in contact with a person, it is unlikely that you will discover the full truth.

As an emergency medical responder, it is likely you will pass your concerns on to an ambulance crew or other health professional responding to the same incident as you, and that they will take on responsibility for making appropriate referrals; however, this may vary between organisations and you should be aware of these key principles in managing a safeguarding concern (JRCALC, 2016):

- Consider not just the patient, but also others present. For example, you may be called to manage an adult with chest pain initially, but if you are concerned about the welfare of a child living in the same house, you have the same duty to report and raise concerns as if that child was the original patient.
- Your first priority should be to manage the presenting condition and ensure medical well-being, i.e. provide the usual clinical management for the presenting complaint.
- Limit your questioning to that which is relevant; stop questioning if your suspicions are confirmed, as unnecessary questioning or probing may affect the credibility of subsequent evidence.
- Accept any given explanation. Even if you do not believe the answer, do not make suggestions to the patient on how an incident may have occurred.
- Do not directly accuse parents or carers of abuse, as to do so may result in refusal of further care or transport, thereby increasing the risk faced by the patient.
- Wherever possible, work in partnership with the parents or carers, and inform them of your concerns and the need to share these concerns with other agencies. The only exemption to this rule is when you believe that doing so may put the patient at greater risk of harm. You will have to exercise professional judgement on this point and should record in detail your justification for not informing, if that is the option you choose.
- Take any and all accusations seriously; it is not your role to decide on their validity or to investigate further, but instead you should refer your concerns to the other health professionals who also attend the incident.
- If a person makes a disclosure, make sure you treat them with respect and dignity, and act in a manner that suggests you believe them. Body language and your words can have a massive influence on a patient's behaviour and confidence in you, and if they feel you do not believe them, they may not disclose what they were previously about to.
- Complete full and accurate records of events. Where possible try to record word-for-word what the patient has disclosed.

Reporting an Urgent Concern

An urgent concern exists where you believe a person may be at immediate risk of further harm. In those circumstances all at the scene should ensure the immediate safety of the patient. This can often be best achieved by transporting the patient to hospital where they can be monitored and assessed while awaiting the support of other services.

In the most serious circumstances it may be necessary to contact the police with your concerns via the emergency operations centre to ensure immediate patient safety. Remember that in certain circumstances, including the prevention or detection of a serious crime, such disclosures can be made to the police without the patient's consent. It would normally be the decision of the most senior clinician on scene to do this.

Safeguarding Referrals

Whenever you believe a person is being abused or neglected, or is at risk of either, a safeguarding referral should be completed. Your organisation will probably have a policy on how this should be achieved, and as a responder you should be aware of your responsibilities in this.

You should be aware of your local policies for making such referrals but should also have a general understanding of these guidelines for making a referral:

- **Report all concerns**: Any concern, however small, should be reported through safeguarding referral pathways. Experienced and qualified safeguarding professionals can judge for themselves whether further investigation or action is required. They will also know whether the patient, place of care or family is known for previous safeguarding concerns, information that may not be available to you.

- **Additional sources of help**: All services should have safeguarding teams including named professionals responsible for safeguarding. These teams are experienced in the management of safeguarding issues and have established relationships with the multidisciplinary teams that work around those issues.
- **Role of social services**: In most areas, social services are the main organisation around which safeguarding concerns articulate. Social workers are experienced in dealing with vulnerable people and with cases of abuse and neglect, and can be a great source of support and advice.
- **Escalating concerns**: All care organisations should be well prepared for managing safeguarding concerns, but in the unlikely event that you do not believe that your concerns are being managed in an appropriate manner, you have a duty to escalate your concern (JRCALC, 2016). To do this you should speak to a senior manager, colleague or a named professional. Ensure you make records of all concerns that you pass on.
- **Preserve evidence**: If you suspect abuse you may need to consider how to preserve evidence. This could take many forms depending on the form of abuse, and might include not touching items you believe have been used to assault a victim, or encouraging a person not to wash or change their clothes if they have been subject to physical or sexual abuse in order to retain evidence (JRCALC, 2016).

Summary

Safeguarding can be a highly emotive topic for all involved, and this should be at the front of your mind when managing a situation where safeguarding is a concern. Try to remain calm, impartial and factual, and keep the immediate safety of patients as your primary goal. Remember the cases of Winterbourne View and Daniel Pelka, where key signs were missed and professionals failed to 'think the unthinkable'.

Be aware of the signs of abuse or neglect and immediately raise any concerns you have through local policy for doing so. Also be mindful that dealing with safeguarding incidents can be emotionally traumatic for all responders and health professionals, and following such incidents you may need to make use of your organisation's counselling or support services.

Chapter 6

Health and Safety

Health and Safety Policies and Legislation

Learning Objectives

By the end of this section you will be able to:

- Identify legislation relating to health and safety when providing casualty care.
- Explain the main points of health and safety policies and procedures.
- Analyse the main health and safety responsibilities for:
    - Yourself
    - Your employer or manager
    - Others in the work setting
- Describe types of hazardous substances that may be found in the work setting.

Introduction

A variety of the legislation that relates to the pre-hospital emergency care has been reviewed in Chapter 4: Clinical Governance, Legal and Ethical Issues, but it is also important that you are aware of the legislation relating to health and safety, and in particular, that you know your and your employer's legal responsibilities.

This section will provide an overview of the following legislation that directly applies to health and safety, including manual handling:

- Health and Safety at Work etc. Act 1974 (HSWA)
- Management of Health and Safety at Work Regulations 1999 (MHSWR)
- Manual Handling Operations Regulations 1992 (MHOR) (as amended 2002)
- Provision and Use of Work Equipment Regulations 1998 (PUWER)
- Lifting Operations and Lifting Equipment Regulations 1998 (LOLER)
- Personal Protective Equipment at Work Regulations 1992
- Control of Substances Hazardous to Health Regulations 2002.

Health and Safety at Work etc. Act

All workers have a right to work in places where risks to their health and safety are properly controlled. Health and safety is about stopping you getting hurt at work, or becoming ill through work. Your employer is responsible for health and safety, but you must help (HSE, 2009).

Employers must do the following in order to comply with the Act (HSE, 2009):

- Decide what could harm you in your job and what precautions could prevent it. This is part of risk assessment
- In a way you can understand, explain how risk will be controlled and tell you who is responsible for this
- Consult and work with staff and the health and safety representatives, to protect everyone from harm in the workplace
- Provide (free of charge) health and safety training and provide equipment and protective clothing that you need to do your job
- Provide toilets, washing facilities, drinking water and adequate first-aid facilities
- Notify the Health and Safety Executive in the event of any major injuries and fatalities at work
- Have insurance that covers staff in the event of injury at work
- Display a physical or electronic copy of the current insurance certificate where you can easily read it
- Work with other employers or contractors sharing the workplace to ensure that everyone's health and safety is protected.

You have a number of responsibilities as an employee too (HSE, 2009):

- Follow the training you have received when using any work item your employer has provided
- Take reasonable care of your own and other people's health and safety
- Co-operate with your employer on health and safety
- Tell someone (for example your employer, line manager or safety representative) if you think that a method of working or inadequate precautions are putting anyone's health and safety at serious risk.

Management of Health and Safety at Work Regulations

The Management of Health and Safety at Work Regulations 1999 require employers to put in place arrangements to control health and safety risks. These include (HSE, 2013a):

- A written health and safety policy
- Assessments of the risks to employees, contractors, customers, partners and any other people who could be affected by work-related activities, and record significant findings in writing
- Arrangements for the effective planning, organisation, control, monitoring and review of the preventive and protective measures that come from risk assessment
- Access to competent health and safety advice
- Providing employees with information about the risks in the workplace and how those employees are protected
- Instruction and training for employees in how to deal with the risks
- Ensuring there is adequate and appropriate supervision in place
- Consulting with employees about their risks at work and current preventive and protective measures.

Manual Handling Operations Regulations

Any transporting or supporting of a load (including the lifting, putting down, pushing, pulling, carrying or moving thereof) by hand or by bodily force is considered to be a manual handling operation by the Manual Handling Operations Regulations 1992.

Employers are required to make a suitable and sufficient assessment of the risks to the health and safety of their employees while at work. Where this assessment indicates the possibility of risks to employees from the manual handling of loads, the Regulations require a hierarchy of measures that must be adhered to. These include avoiding hazardous manual handling operations so far as is reasonably practicable and assessing any hazardous manual handling operations that cannot be avoided so as to reduce the risk of injury, as far as is reasonably practicable.

No doubt you have noticed the term 'reasonably practicable' appearing a couple of times. This means that the employer's duty to avoid manual handling or to reduce the risk of injury can be limited, if the employer can show that the cost of any further preventive steps would be grossly disproportionate to their perceived benefit. Employees are also expected to play their part by following appropriate systems of work laid down by their employer to promote safety during the handling of loads (HSE, 2016).

Emergency services

Preventing all potentially hazardous emergency service manual handling operations would result in an inability to provide the general public with an adequate service. As an employee of an emergency service, you may be asked to accept a greater risk of injury than someone employed to move inanimate objects (like boxes). In this case, additional relevant factors may include:

- The seriousness of the need for the lifting operation
- The service's duty to the public overall and the patient who requires assistance.

Taking these factors into account, the level of risk which an employer may ask an employee to accept may, in appropriate circumstances, be higher when considering the health and safety of those in danger, although this does not mean that employees can be exposed to unacceptable risk of injury (HSE, 2016).

Provision and Use of Work Equipment Regulation

Work equipment as defined by the Provision and Use of Work Equipment Regulations 1998 is any machinery, appliance, apparatus, tool or installation for use at work. This includes equipment which employees provide for their own use at work. The scope of work equipment is therefore extremely wide. The use of work equipment is also very widely interpreted: it covers any activity involving work equipment and includes starting, stopping, programming, setting, transporting, repairing, modifying, maintaining, servicing and cleaning.

Employers must manage the risks from that equipment, including (HSE, 2014d):

- Ensuring equipment is constructed or adapted to be suitable for the purpose it is used or provided for
- Taking account of the working conditions and health and safety risks in the workplace when selecting work equipment
- Ensuring work equipment is only used for suitable purposes
- Ensuring work equipment is maintained in an efficient state, in efficient working order and in good repair.

Lifting Operations and Lifting Equipment Regulations

Lifting equipment includes any equipment used at work for lifting or lowering loads, along with attachments used for anchoring, fixing or supporting it, including hoists and ambulance trolleys. Employers are required to ensure that all lifting equipment is (LOLER, 1998):

- Sufficiently strong, stable and suitable for the proposed use. Similarly, the load and anything attached must be suitable
- Positioned or installed to prevent the risk of injury, e.g. from the equipment or the load falling or striking people
- Visibly marked with any appropriate information to be taken into account for its safe use, e.g. safe working loads. Accessories, e.g. slings, clamps etc., should be similarly marked.

Additionally, employers must ensure that (LOLER, 1998):

- Lifting operations are planned, supervised and carried out in a safe manner by people who are competent
- Where equipment is used for lifting people it is marked accordingly, and it should be safe for such a purpose, i.e. all necessary precautions have been taken to eliminate or reduce any risk
- Where appropriate, before lifting equipment (including accessories) is used for the first time, it is thoroughly examined. Lifting equipment may need to be thoroughly examined in use at periods specified in the Regulations (i.e. at least 6-monthly for accessories and equipment used for lifting people and, at a minimum, annually for all other equipment) or at intervals laid down in an examination scheme drawn up by a competent person. All examination work should be performed by a competent person (someone with the necessary skills, knowledge and experience)
- Following a thorough examination or inspection of any lifting equipment, a report is submitted by the competent person to the employer to take any appropriate action.

You should not use any equipment that 'lifts' if you are not trained and competent in doing so. One of the most common lifting pieces of equipment you will come across is likely to be a patient hoist. There is a large range of these available on the market, all of which look similar, but actually operate in slightly different ways.

For this reason it is unlikely that you will ever be able to be competent on all the different hoists you come across and, instead of using them yourself, you should seek help from others present who are competent in their use.

Personal Protective Equipment at Work Regulations

Personal protective equipment (PPE) is equipment that will protect the user against health or safety risks at work. It can include items such as safety helmets and hard hats, gloves, eye protection, high-visibility clothing, safety footwear and safety harnesses (HSE, 2013c).

PPE should be used as a last resort. Wherever there are risks to health and safety that cannot be adequately controlled in other ways, the Personal Protective Equipment at Work Regulations 1992 require PPE to be supplied. The Regulations also require that PPE is:

- Properly assessed before use to make sure it is fit for purpose
- Maintained and stored properly
- Provided with instructions on how to use it safely
- Used correctly by employees.

Control of Substances Hazardous to Health Regulations

The Control of Substances Hazardous to Health Regulations 2002 cover substances that are hazardous to health. Substances can take many forms and include:

- Chemicals
- Products containing chemicals
- Fumes
- Dusts
- Vapours
- Mists
- Gases and asphyxiating gases
- Biological agents (germs).

If the packaging has any of the hazard symbols then it is classed as a hazardous substance.

Employers have a responsibility to manage and minimise the risks from work activities. They must develop suitable and sufficient control measures and ways of maintaining them by (HSE, 2013b):

- Identifying hazards and potentially significant risks
- Taking action to prevent and control risks
- Keeping control measures under regular review.

To be effective in the long term, control measures must be practical, workable and sustainable.

Good practice in the control of substances hazardous to health can be encapsulated in the eight generic principles set out in the Control of Substances Hazardous to Health Regulations 2002:

- Design and operate processes and activities to minimise emission, release and spread of substances hazardous to health
- Take into account all relevant routes of exposure – inhalation, skin and ingestion – when developing control measures
- Control exposure by measures that are proportionate to the health risk
- Choose the most effective and reliable control options that minimise the escape and spread of substances hazardous to health
- Where adequate control of exposure cannot be achieved by other means, provide, in combination with other control measures, suitable PPE
- Check and review regularly all elements of control measures for their continuing effectiveness
- Inform and train all employees on the hazards and risks from substances with which they work, and the use of control measures developed to minimise the risks
- Ensure that the introduction of measures to control exposure does not increase the overall risk to health and safety.

Regulatory Bodies

The main regulatory body for overseeing health and safety is the Health and Safety Executive (HSE), formed as part of the 1974 Health and Safety at Work Act. The HSE is a national independent watchdog responsible for work-related health, safety and illness, working to reduce work-related death and serious injury across Great Britain (HMG, 2015).

The HSE achieves this by working with employers so that all practicably reasonable steps are taken to ensure health and safety at work. They also undertake research and investigate incidents that result in death or significant injury. If an employer fails to meet their health and safety obligations then the HSE can issue a range of improvement orders, or where necessary file a prosecution, which can result in large fines and custodial sentences for those responsible for allowing health and safety breaches to occur.

Why Health and Safety Matters

Health and safety exists to make work a safer and more enjoyable place for us all. Although sometimes rules and regulations can appear restrictive they exist to protect you and to ensure that you are able to continue working and reduce, so far as is reasonably practicable, the risk you face on a daily basis at work.

As discussed above, you have a responsibility to comply with health and safety regulations at work and to contribute to making your workplace a safer place to be. If you fail to abide by the regulations and protocols put in place by your employer, not only are you making work a less safe place for yourself, your colleagues and ultimately your patients, but you may also be committing an offence that you could be prosecuted for.

Communicating Health and Safety

Health and safety should be considered a dynamic process as it is constantly being reviewed to ensure it is suitable for new ways of working, or that new technologies are being used to their maximum potential to reduce the risk. Because of this, it is likely that there will frequently be updates to your organisation's health and safety procedures. Updates may come in many forms, including: e-mails, standard operating procedures, updates to policy, local posters or as part of statutory and mandatory training. Some updates will be made very evident, while others might be subtler, such as a change in policy.

You should be aware of where you can find all relevant health and safety information and updates, and keep yourself informed of any changes.

Remember, you are responsible for keeping yourself up to date and if you become ill or are injured due to a lack of familiarity with updates, then it may be viewed that you have contributed to your own illness or injury and therefore have to take a proportionally greater amount of responsibility for what has happened.

Risk Assessment

Learning Objectives

By the end of this section you will be able to:

- Define the term 'risk'.
- Describe the process of carrying out a risk assessment.
- Explain the importance of carrying out a risk assessment.
- Compare different uses of risk assessment in health and social care.
- Explain why risk assessments need to be regularly reviewed and revised.

Introduction

As a firefighter, you will already be familiar with the concept of risk and performing risk assessments in your operational duties. You may be less familiar with considering risk in relation to patient treatment and healthcare, so the information below is a brief summary of performing risk assessments and is a refresher to remind you of some of the key principles of risk and how to mitigate it in your new role as an emergency medical responder.

All healthcare staff, including volunteers, have a duty to protect patients, their colleagues and themselves as far as is 'reasonably practicable', by minimising the chance that they are harmed by something, whether that be a procedure, drug administration or dangerous environment.

It is helpful to understand what is meant by the terms 'hazard' and 'risk' (HSE, 2014b; NPSA, 2007):

- Hazard: Anything that might cause harm, such as chemicals, electricity, working from ladders, an open drawer etc.
- Risk: The chance, high or low, that somebody could be harmed by these and other hazards, together with an indication of how serious the harm could be

- Clinical risk: Also known as a healthcare risk, clinical risk is the chance of an adverse outcome resulting from clinical investigation, treatment or patient care. For an organisation providing healthcare, there are also other risks to consider:
- Injury and safety (patients, staff and the public)
- Legal and financial
- Service interruption
- Resource Escalation Action Plan (REAP) level increases
- Regulatory requirements
- Reputation.

Risk Assessment

Risk assessment does not have to be difficult. It can be distilled into five steps (NPSA, 2007):

1. Identify the hazards (What can go wrong?)
2. Decide who might be harmed and how (What can go wrong? Who is exposed to the hazard?)
3. Evaluate the risk (How bad? How often?) and decide on the precautions (Is there a need for further action?)
4. Record your findings and your proposed action, and identify who will lead on what action. Record the date of implementation
5. Review your assessment and update, if required.

Identify the Hazards

This step consists of working out what is likely to go wrong and why. Many hazards can be anticipated in advance, allowing time for a formal written risk assessment to be completed, which is then kept on an organisation and/or departmental risk register. Items suitable for this include:

- Equipment
- Cleaning products
- Industrial action
- Adverse media coverage.

However, some risk assessments will have to be conducted quickly, and mentally, as there will be no time to conduct a formal written risk assessment. This dynamic risk assessment is the type you will perform as you arrive on scene at an incident and may well conduct a number of times during a patient episode, depending on the risk of harm and the volatility of the scene and/or patients and bystanders. You will learn more about this in Chapter 9: Scene Assessment.

Decide Who Might be Harmed and How

Consider who might be harmed by the hazard and the circumstances that might lead to harm occurring. This could be you, for example when assisting a senior clinician with a procedure that involves the use of sharp instruments. Patients can be harmed in many ways, for example during manual handling or the administration of a drug. Your colleagues are also at risk during certain procedures, such as when you are reversing a vehicle.

It is not usually necessary to identify the individual, just groups of people who may be at risk of harm from the hazard you are assessing. In addition to the examples listed above, consider other groups such as (HSE, 2014c):

- Pregnant patients
- Children
- Non-English speakers
- People with a disability.

Evaluate the Risk and Decide on Precautions

Evaluating risk is a skill that becomes easier with practice. To assist with the evaluation, it can be helpful to use a risk matrix (Table 6.1) to quantify the two aspects of risk evaluation (NPSA, 2008):

- Consequence: How severe is the risk?
- Likelihood: How often is the risk likely to arise?

To calculate the risk rating, the consequence score is multiplied by the likelihood score. Consider the example of a staff injury at work. The consequence would be scored as follows:

1 = Negligible injury requiring no medical intervention and no time off work
2 = Minor injury requiring some medical intervention and less than 3 days off work
3 = Moderate injury requiring hospital or other professional intervention and 4–14 days off work
4 = Major injury leaving the staff member with long-term incapacity and/or disability and more than 14 days off work
5 = Catastrophic injury resulting in death.

Table 6.1 Risk matrix

CONSEQUENCE	LIKELIHOOD				
	1	2	3	4	5
	Rare	Unlikely	Possible	Likely	Almost certain
5 Catastrophic	5	10	15	20	25
4 Major	4	8	12	16	20
3 Moderate	3	6	9	12	15
2 Minor	2	4	6	8	10
1 Negligible	1	2	3	4	5

The likelihood scores are allocated as follows:

1 = Rare: Not expected to occur for years
2 = Unlikely: Expected to occur at least annually
3 = Possible: Expected to occur at least monthly
4 = Likely: Expected to occur at least weekly
5 = Almost certain: Expected to occur at least daily.

Precautions

Having identified risks and given them a risk rating, it is necessary to determine what precautions (controls) are most appropriate to try to reduce the likelihood of the risk occurring (NPSA, 2008). It is quite likely that there will already be policies and procedures in place, which as an employee you will be expected to be familiar with, although you may also need training to ensure you can comply with them. In addition, as an employee you are likely to have a responsibility to report any risks and not undertake any action which would knowingly cause harm to you or anyone else, including your employer (SWAST, 2014b).

When assessing the risks and deciding which precautions to take, consider the following (MoD, 2008):

- Can the hazards be eliminated altogether?
- Can the risks be controlled to give the lowest risk rating?
- Is there a less risky alternative?
- Can access to the hazard be eliminated or reduced?
- Can work practices be changed to reduce the risk?
- Is personal protective equipment (PPE) required? This is generally considered a last resort and should not be preferred over other forms of risk elimination.

Finally, once you have decided on the most appropriate precautions to take, you should re-evaluate the risk on the basis that your precautions are undertaken.

Record and Implement Findings

Risk assessments and action plans need to be reviewed periodically (step 5), but this will not be straightforward unless the assessment has been well documented and is able to show that (NPSA, 2007):

- A thorough check was made to identify all hazards and address the significant risks
- The precautions (controls) taken are reasonable and any residual risk is acceptable
- The solutions are realistic, sustainable and likely to be effective.

Dynamic risk assessments also need to be documented and this should take place as soon as possible after the incident. This will provide justification for actions taken in the event of any adverse outcomes as well as providing a starting point for future formal risk assessments if the situation is likely to recur (MoD, 2008).

Review and update

Risk assessments need to be reviewed periodically as things change. New best practices emerge from research, equipment is updated or modified and new hazards may be identified. Examples of when risk assessments should be reviewed include (NPSA, 2007; MoD, 2008):

- When you are planning a change
- When there has been a significant change
- Periodically, at least annually
- Following an accident or near miss.

Infection Prevention and Control

Learning Objectives

By the end of this section you will be able to:

- Explain what is meant by infection and how infections can occur and be transmitted.
- Identify a number of microorganisms, the illnesses they cause and how they can enter the body.
- Describe how to manage and dispose of sources of infection safely while avoiding causing harm to self or others.
- Outline the current regulations, legislation and responsibilities relating to infection control.
- Describe the different types of personal protective equipment (PPE) and how to use them appropriately.
- Explain the role of regulators and other bodies in infection prevention and control.
- Describe the key principles of good personal hygiene.
- Describe the correct sequence for handwashing and when it should be carried out.
- Describe the services that occupational health provide to employees.

Introduction

Infection prevention and control is a collective term for those activities intended to protect people from infections (Dougherty, 2011).

An infection is the body's adverse response to the presence of a pathogen, or disease-causing microorganism (Betsy, 2012). Damage to tissues caused by an infection can either be limited to the site of infection (localised) or spread throughout the body, typically via the blood (systemic).

Sometimes, however, a pathogen in or on the body may not lead to an infection. This is known as colonisation (Weston, 2014).

A healthcare-associated infection (HCAI) is any infection acquired as a result of a healthcare-related intervention or an infection acquired during the course of healthcare that the patient may reasonably expect to be protected from. HCAI has replaced the term 'hospital-acquired infection' since many healthcare interactions take place outside of hospital (such as in the patient's home) (Dougherty, 2011). The scale of the problem is staggering, with an estimated 300,000 patient's each year in England acquiring an HCAI, with a significant number of deaths and a cost to the NHS of around £1 billion (NICE, 2012a).

Your Own and Patient's Health

As well as passing diseases and illnesses on to patients, you as an emergency medical responder can also be made unwell by poor infection prevention and control. Some diseases, such as norovirus, a viral infection which causes gastroenteritis (NHS Choices, 2014b), is very infectious and spreads easily from person to person. In winter, when it is most prevalent, it is likely you will come into contact with patients suffering from this on a frequent basis. If you do not apply adequate infection prevention and controls then it is likely that you may also become unwell and contract the illness. This could mean that you are off sick for several days or weeks from work, impacting not only on your health, but potentially the health of family and friends as well.

Equally, you can spread illness to your patient. If you are not well, then you should not come into work as you might spread illness to already unwell people. For many of our patients, including the elderly, those with chronic lung conditions or receiving chemotherapy, only a small infection will place a major strain on their immune system and an illness that may not be a major issue for a healthy person could kill someone already unwell.

If you are unsure if you are fit to return to work then you should see your GP or contact your occupational health team for advice.

Impact On Organisations

For organisations, an outbreak of an illness such as norovirus can be disastrous. In a healthcare setting, if a large number of staff were all to become ill with gastroenteritis at the same time, there would be a very significant strain put on the remaining workforce to cover the gaps left by sickness.

Regulations and Legislation

At the beginning of the chapter, some of the relevant legislation relating to infection prevention and control was reviewed, in particular the Health and Safety at Work etc. Act 1974. This requires employers to provide training and appropriate personal protective equipment (PPE) to prevent harm, and employees to follow the training that they have received, use PPE provided, and report any situations where they believe that patients' and/or staff's health and safety are at serious risk.

However, the Health and Social Care Act (2008) specifically highlights infection prevention and control and also makes the Care Quality Commission responsible for ensuring that care services meet the requirements of the code of practice that accompanies the legislation. This code specified ten key elements that services must demonstrate that they comply with:

- Systems to manage and monitor the prevention and control of infection. These systems use risk assessments and consider the susceptibility of service users and any risks that their environment and other users may pose to them.
- Provide and maintain a clean and appropriate environment in managed premises that facilitates the prevention and control of infections.
- Ensure appropriate antimicrobial use to optimise patient outcomes and to reduce the risk of adverse events and antimicrobial resistance.
- Provide suitable accurate information on infections to service users, their visitors and any person concerned with providing further support or nursing/medical care in a timely fashion.
- Ensure prompt identification of people who have or are at risk of developing an infection so that they receive timely and appropriate treatment to reduce the risk of transmitting infection to other people.
- Systems to ensure that all care workers (including contractors and volunteers) are aware of and discharge their responsibilities in the process of preventing and controlling infection.
- Provide or secure adequate isolation facilities.
- Secure adequate access to laboratory support as appropriate.
- Have and adhere to policies, designed for the individual's care and provider organisations that will help to prevent and control infections.
- Providers have a system in place to manage the occupational health needs and obligations of staff in relation to infection.

There is also additional legislation that does not apply exclusively to the healthcare setting, but is intent on reducing the risk of infection. This includes regulations relating to food hygiene (Food Safety Act 1990), water supply (DWI, 2012) and waste management (Hazardous Waste Regulations 2005; Control of Substances Hazardous to Health Regulations 2002).

Regulators and Other Bodies

The regulators of healthcare services in the UK, the Care Quality Commission for England, the Care and Social Services Inspectorate in Wales, and the Care Inspectorate for Scotland, are responsible for ensuring that organisations meet required standards in the management of infection prevention and control. If organisations fail to meet required standards they can be prosecuted and have their licence to provide care services taken away.

As fire services become more involved in the delivery of pre-hospital care, it is likely they will either have to register with the CQC themselves or will be inspected by their partner agencies (commonly ambulance services) to ensure thay are meeting the standards described above.

Health Protection

Public Health England are responsible for monitoring and helping to control outbreaks of, and provide protection against, infectious diseases, such as:

- Hepatitis
- Genital herpes
- Measles.

When such outbreaks occur, they provide specialist advice, expertise and equipment to combat the illness and prevent it spreading further (PHE, 2015). In Scotland this is provided by Health Protection Scotland and in Wales by Public Health Wales.

World Health Organization (WHO)

The WHO provides advice to member states on infection prevention and control based on the best available evidence from international studies (WHO, 2015). They also respond to large-scale disease outbreaks to support the local response and prevent spreading of the disease.

Microorganisms

Microorganisms are very small organisms that live outside and inside larger organisms such as the human body. The four main types that enter the body and cause infection are:

- Bacteria
- Viruses
- Fungi
- Parasites.

Bacteria

These are probably the most important microorganisms in relation to infection control as they are responsible for many opportunistic infections in healthcare. There are around ten times as many bacteria as there are cells in the human body and many have functions that are essential, such as the microorganism Escherichia coli (E. coli), which aids digestion in the gut. However, it can cause a urinary tract infection (UTI) if it gains access to the urinary tract (Dougherty, 2011).

Bacteria are fairly simple, single-celled microorganisms and are often classified by their shape. For example, they may be termed bacillus (rodlike), coccus (spherical or ovoid) or spiral (corkscrew or curved). Examples of common bacteria include Group A streptococcus, which can cause throat and ear infections, and Staphylococcus, which can cause impetigo and pneumonia. You may have heard of a particularly troublesome strain of Staphylococcus which is resistant to many antibiotics and is called methicillin-resistant Staphylococcus aureus (MRSA) (Betsy, 2012).

Viruses

Viruses are even smaller than bacteria and have no cellular structure. They typically just consist of a core containing genetic material such as deoxyribonucleic acid (DNA) or ribonucleic acid (RNA) and are sometimes surrounded by a membrane called an envelope. Viruses can reproduce only by using the cellular machinery of other organisms and so are rather like parasites (Tortora, 2013).

Common viruses include the rhinovirus, which is responsible for the common cold, respiratory syncytial virus (RSV) which can cause serious respiratory tract infections in infants and children, and the varicella-zoster virus (VZV), which causes chickenpox and shingles (Betsy, 2012).

Fungi

You are probably most familiar with fungi as mushrooms or as yeast used in bread making and brewing. Some fungi are responsible for opportunistic infections, such as dermatophytes, which can cause athlete's foot, and Candida albicans, yeast that can cause vaginal thrush (Dougherty, 2011).

Parasites

Parasites are organisms that live at the expense of another organism or host. Pathogenic parasites include bacteria, viruses, protozoa (animal-like single-celled microorganisms) and animals such as roundworms, flatworms and arthropods. Examples of parasitic infections include malaria and toxoplasmosis (Betsy, 2012).

Infection and Precautions

Chain of Infection

Transmission of infection is a complex process, involving a number of factors, which must all be present and are collectively known as the chain of infection (Figure 6.1) (Ross, 2014; Dougherty, 2011).

Pathogen

An infectious agent is required, such as a bacterium, virus, fungus or parasite. This link can be broken by cleaning, sterilisation of equipment and the treatment of the patient, using antibiotics for bacterial infections, for example.

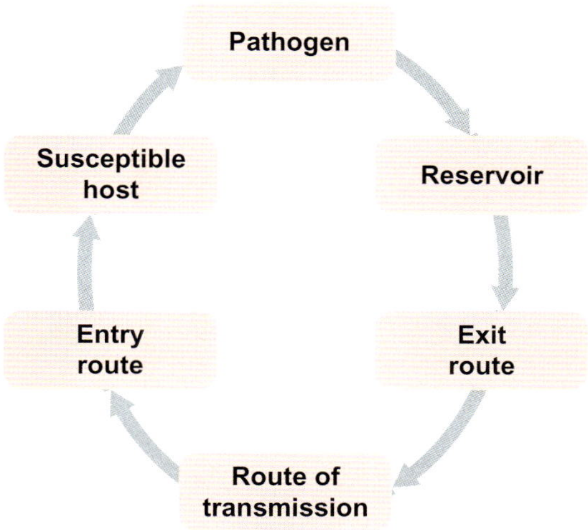

Figure 6.1 *Chain of infection.*

Reservoir

A reservoir is a place where the pathogen can live and replicate; it includes the human body, but also animals, water and the soil, for example. This link can be broken by cleaning equipment and the environment and removing stagnant water.

Exit Route

The exit route is a method for the pathogen to leave its reservoir. In humans, this usually involves urine, faeces, vomit, sputum and in aerosolised form, such as after sneezing or coughing. Asking a patient with active tuberculosis to wear a mask would help break this chain.

Route of Transmission

The transmission route can be direct, such as through touching, sexual intercourse and faecal–oral via ingestion, or indirectly via contaminated bedding, clothing, blood and bodily fluids and then the hands of healthcare workers. One of the most effective ways of breaking this chain is the use of good hand hygiene.

Entry Route

Entry routes include the respiratory, gastrointestinal and genitourinary tracts, but also mucous membranes and via the skin. Direct access to the blood is also possible if the pathogen is inadvertently injected into a person. Covering an open wound with a waterproof plaster would be a good example of breaking the chain by blocking the route of entry.

Susceptible Host

Some people are more vulnerable to infection than others, for example those with a weak immune system due to old age, medication or pre-existing disease. Others may have their natural defences compromised by wounds, surgery, intravenous cannulas and urinary catheters. This chain can be broken by ensuring that healthcare workers are vaccinated and that adequate nutrition and personal hygiene is provided to vulnerable groups.

Universal Precautions

Universal or standard precautions are a group of actions that should be taken in every patient contact to reduce the risk of infection. NHS Professionals (2010) describe the universal precautions as:

Hand Hygiene

Discussed in detail later in this chapter.

Respiratory Hygiene

Respiratory hygiene refers to covering the mouth and nose with single disposable tissues when coughing, sneezing, wiping or blowing noses. These tissues should be disposed of appropriately immediately after use, followed by washing the hands.

Personal Protective Equipment

Use PPE appropriately. More details on the range of available PPE is provided later in this chapter.

Occupational Exposure and Managing Sharps Injury

Sharps injury and splash contamination is discussed later in the chapter.

Management of Care Equipment

Discussed later in this chapter as part of decontamination.

Safe Care of Linen Including Uniform

How to handle linen is described later in this chapter. You should think about how you handle and clean your work uniform. Uniform can harbour a large number of pathogens and should be cleaned after each shift on the hottest wash setting suitable for the fabric. When uniform becomes visibly soiled as part of your duties it should be changed immediately.

Control of Environment

In emergency services, controlling the environment can be very challenging as you will constantly be attending different locations. It is not possible for you to control the environment. Recognise that this presents an additional risk and mitigate it where possible.

Safe Waste Disposal

Management of healthcare waste is discussed in detail later in this chapter.

Personal Hygiene

Personal hygiene is defined as the physical act of cleansing the body to ensure that the hair, nails, ears, eyes, nose and skin are maintained in an optimum condition. It also includes mouth hygiene, which is the effective removal of plaque and debris to ensure that the structures and tissues of the mouth are kept in a healthy condition. In addition, personal hygiene includes ensuring the appropriate length of nails and hair (DoH, 2010b).

Good personal hygiene habits include (DoH, 2010c; Dougherty, 2011):

- Having a shower or bath every day
- Brushing your teeth at least once (but preferably twice) a day
- Washing your hair with soap or shampoo at least once a week
- Washing your hands after going to the toilet
- Washing your hands with soap before preparing and/or eating food
- Wearing clean clothes.

Hand Hygiene

Good hand hygiene is the primary measure to reduce HCAIs. It is a straightforward method and inexpensive, but poor compliance among healthcare workers is a worldwide problem (WHO, 2009a).

You should clean your hands in the following circumstances, known as the 'five moments of hand hygiene' (NICE, 2012b):

- Immediately before every episode of direct patient contact or care, including aseptic procedures
- Immediately after every episode of direct patient contact or care
- Immediately after any exposure to body fluids
- Immediately after any other activity or contact with a patient's surroundings that could potentially result in hands becoming contaminated
- Immediately after removal of gloves.

Use an alcohol-based handrub to decontaminate your hands, except when your hands are visibly soiled or potentially contaminated with body fluids, and when it is suspected that alcohol-resistant organisms (such as Clostridium difficile or other organisms that cause diarrhoeal illness) are involved.

In order to ensure that you can clean your hands while at work, you should (NICE, 2012b):

- Be 'bare below the elbows' when delivering direct patient care
- Not wear any wrist or hand jewellery
- Ensure that fingernails are short, clean and free of nail polish
- Cover cuts and abrasions with waterproof dressings.

Alcohol Handrub

Procedure

This is the World Health Organization's (WHO) recommended procedure for hand hygiene with handrub. This procedure should take 20–30 seconds (WHO, 2009a).

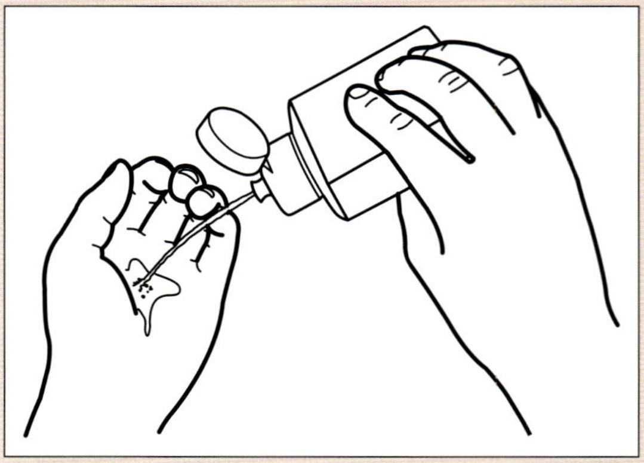

1. Apply a palmful of the alcohol rub in a cupped hand, covering all surfaces

Procedure – *cont*

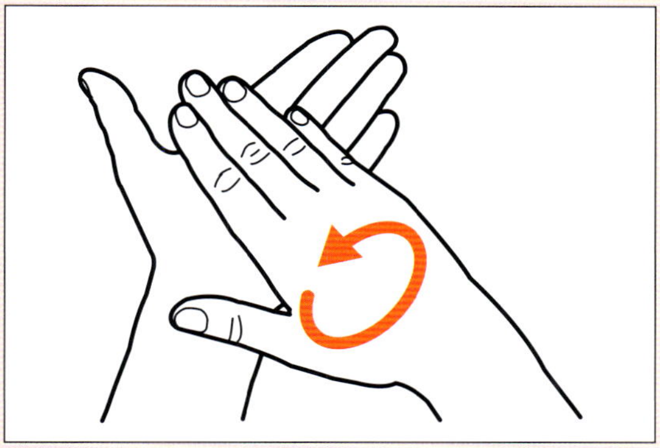

2. Rub hands palm to palm

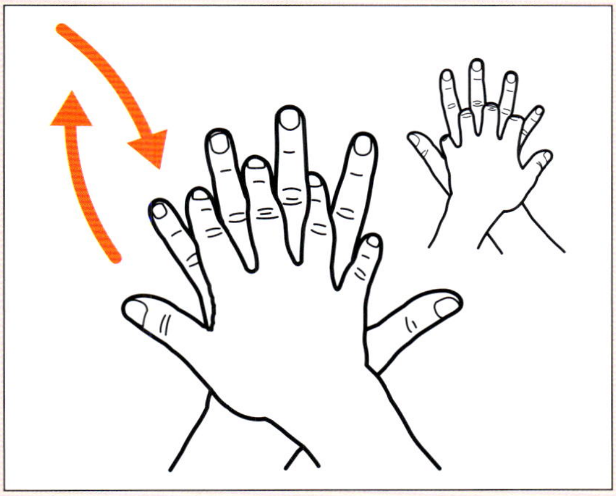

3. Right palm over left dorsum with interlaced fingers and vice versa

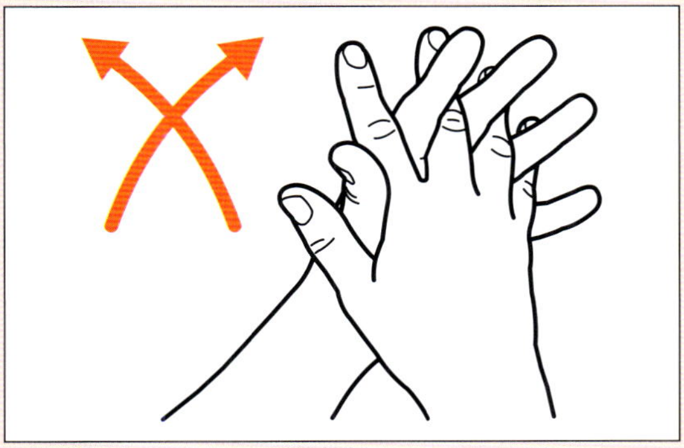

4. Palm to palm with fingers interlaced

Procedure – *cont*

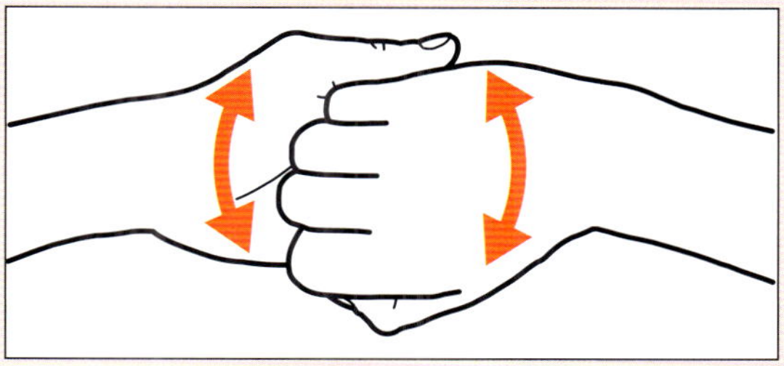

5. Backs of fingers to opposing palms with fingers interlocked

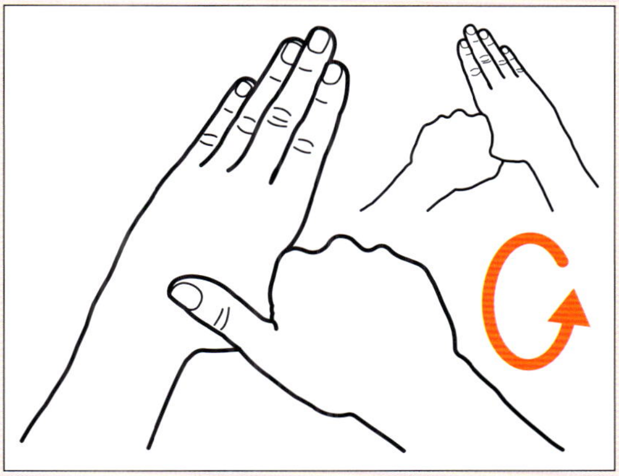

6. Rotational rubbing of left thumb clasped in right palm and vice versa

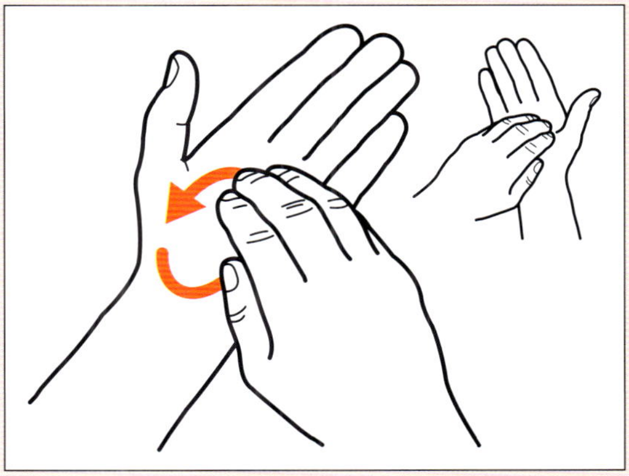

7. Rotational rubbing, backwards and forwards with clasped fingers of right hand in left palm and vice versa

Procedure – *cont*

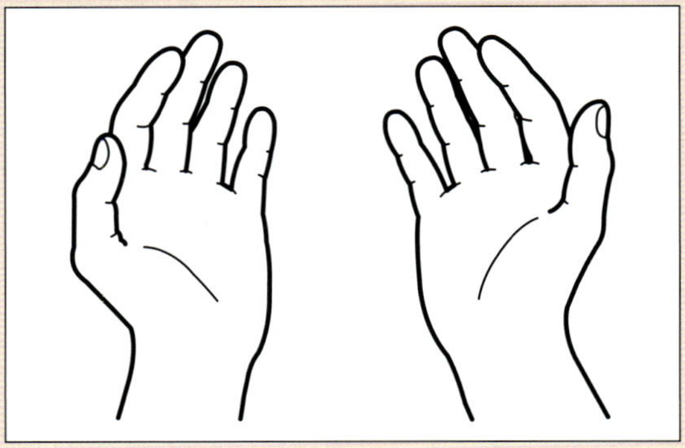

8. Once dry, your hands are safe

Based on the 'How to Handrub' poster. © World Health Organization 2009. All rights reserved.

Handwashing

Procedure

This is the WHO recommended procedure for handwashing. This procedure should take 40–60 seconds (WHO, 2009a).

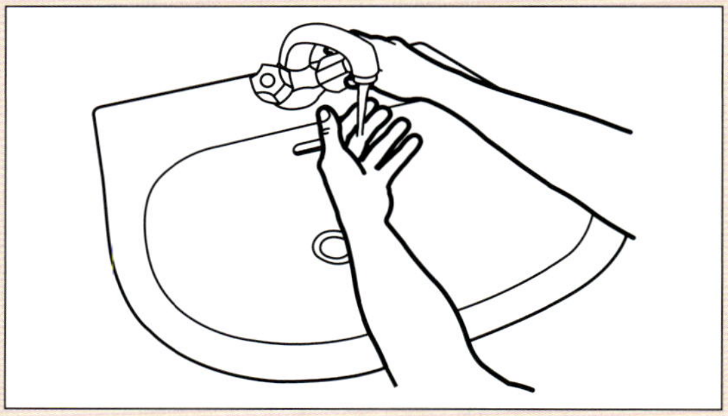

1. Wet hands with water

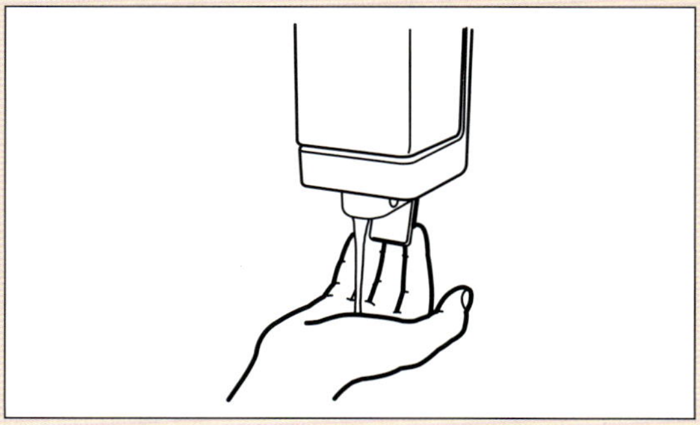

2. Apply enough soap to cover all hand surfaces

Procedure – *cont*

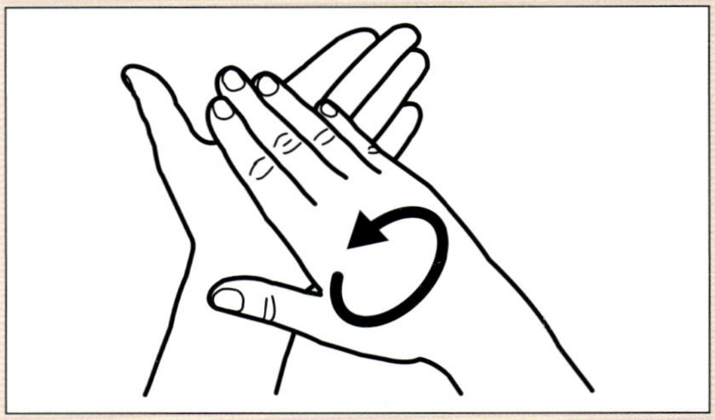

3. Rub hands palm to palm

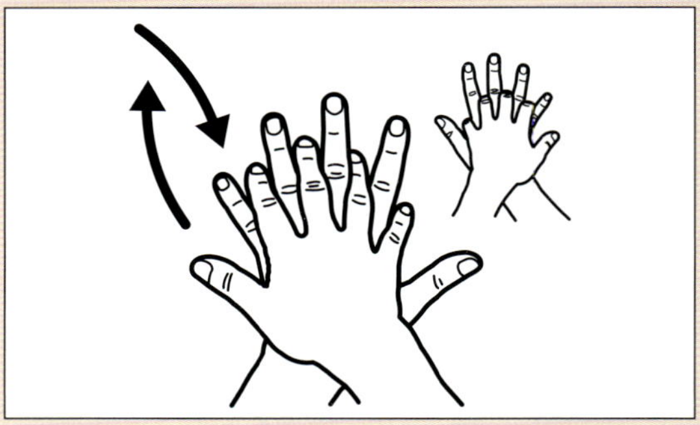

4. Right palm over left dorsum with interlaced fingers and vice versa

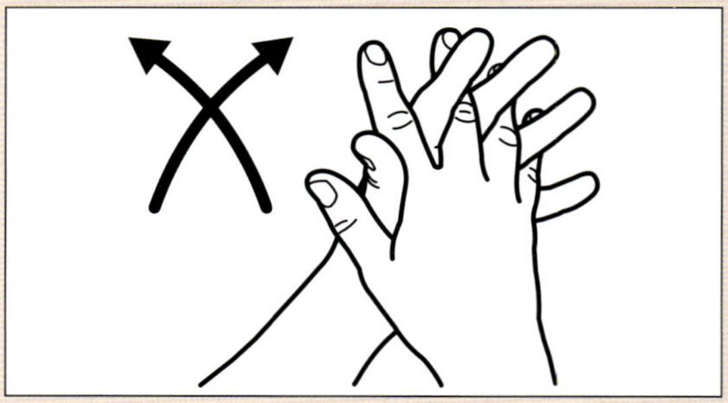

5. Palm to palm with fingers interlaced

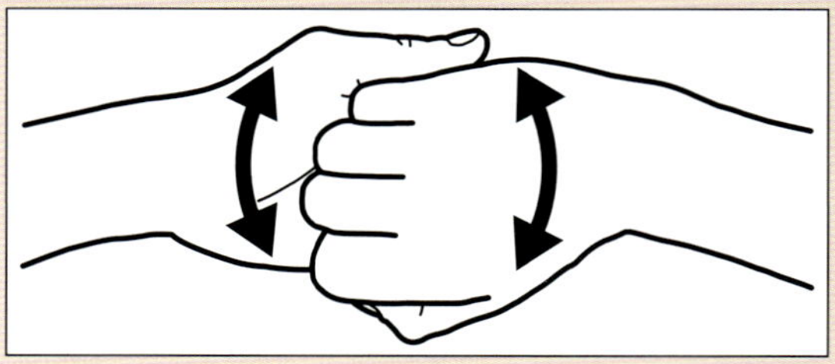

6. Backs of fingers to opposing palms with fingers interlocked

Procedure – *cont*

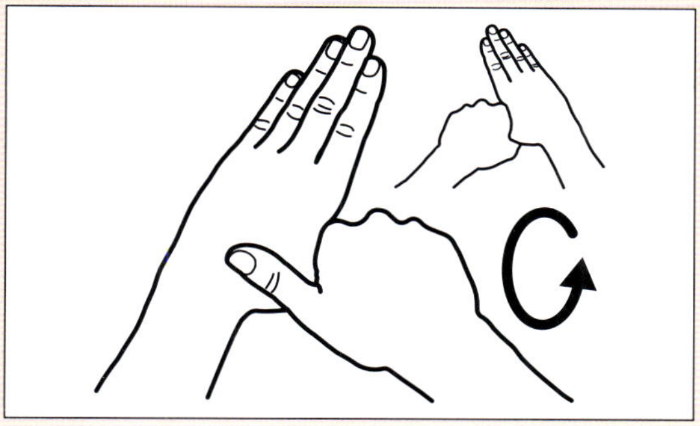

7. Rotational rubbing of left thumb clasped in right palm and vice versa

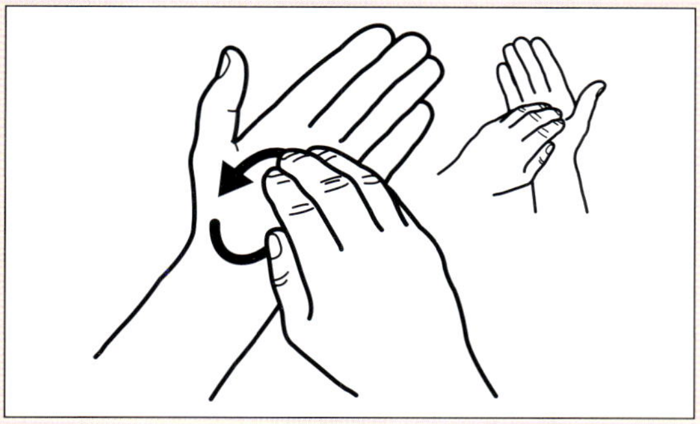

8. Rotational rubbing, backwards and forwards with clasped fingers of right hand in left palm and vice versa

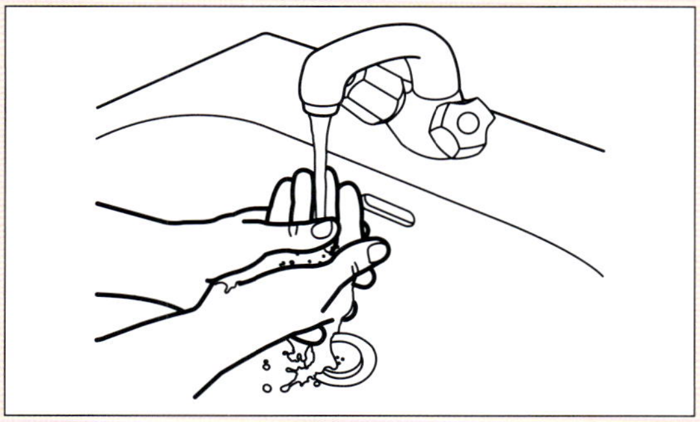

9. Rinse hands with water

Procedure – *cont*

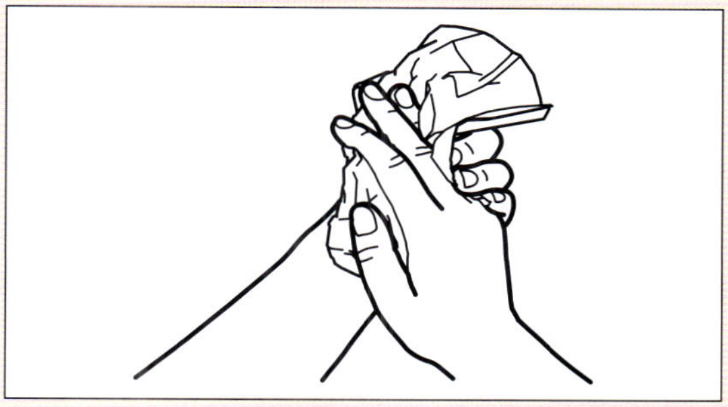

10. Dry hands thoroughly with a single use towel

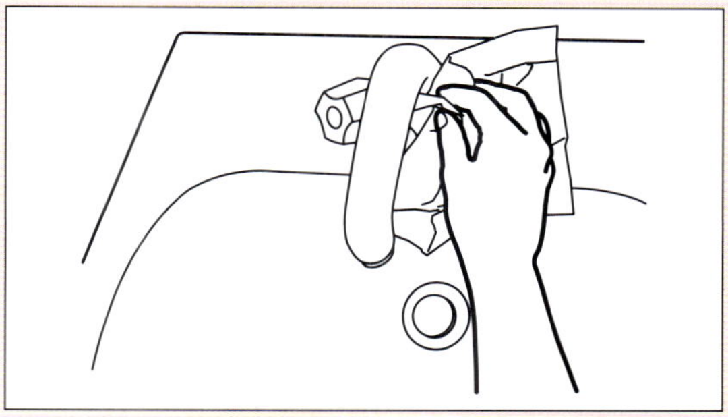

11. Use towel to turn off taps

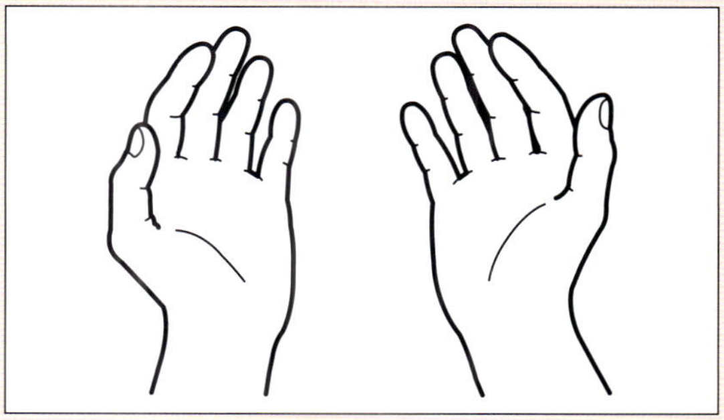

12. Your hands are now safe

Based on the 'How to Handwash' poster.

Skincare

Work-related skin problems are very common, with contact dermatitis being the most common form of work-related skin disease. It is more common in healthcare staff due to their need to wash their hands regularly and skin frequently coming into contact with chemicals or rubber materials as used in personal protective equipment (HSE, 2015d).

When washing your hands frequently it is important to use hand cream to replace the natural oils that are lost in the washing process (HSE, 2015a) and to observe for signs of contact dermatitis developing. These signs include:

- Dry itchy skin
- Reddening
- Flaking, cracks or blisters.

If you suffer from contact dermatitis, or any other form of skin disease, then you should see your GP or occupational health team to try to find a personal solution for improving your skincare.

Personal Protective Equipment

Personal protective equipment (PPE) is used to prevent the spread of infection to you, your colleagues, patients and other members of the public. Your choice of PPE (including not wearing any) should be based on an assessment of the risk of transmission of infection (DoH, 2010d).

Typical items of PPE to prevent infection include:

- Gloves
- Aprons
- Face masks
- Eye protection
- Sleeve protectors
- Protective suits (these are generally only for specially trained personnel, such as hazardous area response team (HART) members, and are not covered in this text).

Gloves

Gloves should only be worn (Figure 6.2):

- If there is a risk of contact with blood and/or bodily fluids
- When sharp and/or contaminated items are handled

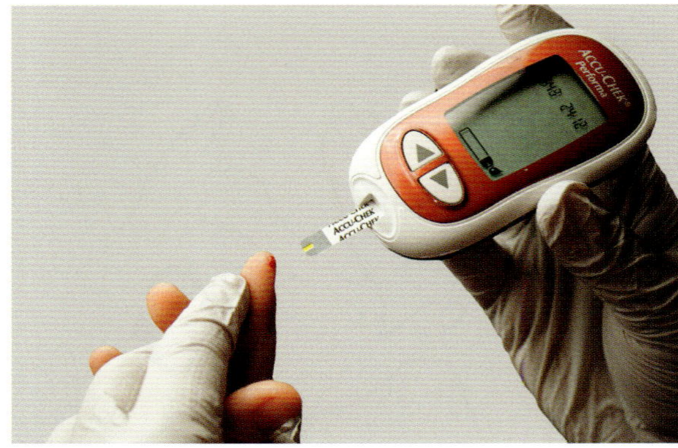

Figure 6.2 *Non-latex disposable gloves should be worn when there is a risk of contact with blood, such as when checking a patient's blood sugar.*

- If there is likely to be contact with non-intact skin or mucous membranes during contact with a patient.

Gloves should not be worn longer than required and never when driving from the scene. Don't forget that hand hygiene is required before and after wearing gloves. Put gloves on immediately prior to patient contact and change them between each patient task, when caring for different patients and as soon as they are contaminated. Once you have removed your gloves, discard appropriately (DoH, 2010d).

Aprons

Aprons should be worn in the following situations:

- Your uniform is likely to be contaminated with blood and/or other bodily fluids
- Carrying out cleaning that may lead to contamination of your uniform
- Transporting infectious patients.

Aprons should be disposed of appropriately following a single use. Unfasten or break the ties and then pull the apron away from your neck and shoulders. Only touch the inside of the apron. Once away from your body, turn it inside out and then fold it into a bundle before discarding appropriately (DoH, 2010d).

Face Masks

There are two types of face mask in common use by healthcare services (Figure 6.3):

- Surgical face mask
- Filtering face piece (FFP3) mask.

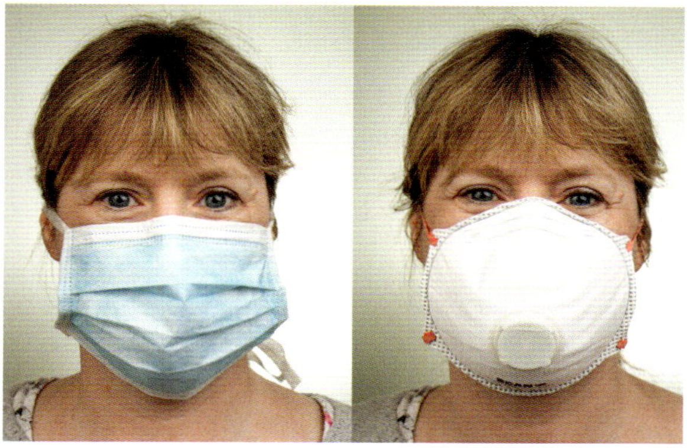

Figure 6.3 *Face masks – (Surgical face mask on left and FFP3 mask on right).*

Surgical face masks are ineffective against airborne infection, but provide protection against splashes of blood and bodily fluids on to the face and into the mouth and nose. In addition, they are also useful for patients who are prone to bouts of coughing and sneezing. Some surgical face masks come with a clear shield to protect the eyes from splash contamination. These should be used if you believe there may be a risk of you being splashed by bodily fluids from the patient.

FFP3 masks, when fitted correctly, provide protection against airborne infections such as severe acute respiratory syndrome (SARS) (NHS England, 2013).

Eye Protection

Eye protection, such as goggles, should be worn if a procedure being undertaken is likely to lead to splashing of bodily fluids, including blood, into the eyes, e.g. when assisting the paramedic with intubation. Ideally, the eye protection used should be single-patient use, but if this is not the case, wash the eye protection in hot soapy water, dry and store for subsequent use (NEAS, 2010).

Sleeve Protectors

Most health services have a 'bare below elbows' policy, making contamination of long-sleeved uniform less likely. However, cross-contamination can occur if you are manual handling multiple patients while wearing long-sleeved clothing such as your high-visibility jacket or fleece. Sleeve protectors can help protect your uniform from wrist to elbow.

They are for single-patient use, can be worn over the top of gloves and should be disposed of as clinical waste (DoH, 2010d).

Wearing and Removing PPE

The amount of PPE required will vary depending on the patient and not all items are always required. In the event that an apron, mask and eye protection are required, adopt the following procedures for putting on and removing PPE (DoH, 2009b):

Procedure – Wearing PPE

Take the following steps when putting on PPE:

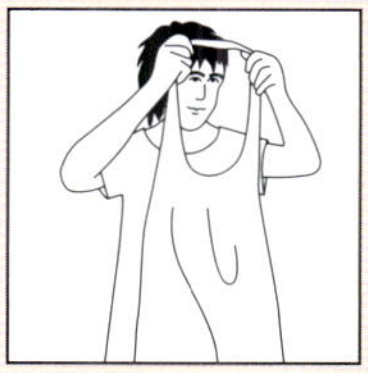

1. Put on apron as shown and fasten at back of waist
2. Apply face mask:
   - Secure ties or elastic bands at middle of head and neck
   - Fit flexible band to nose bridge
   - Fit snug to face and below chin

(NHS England, 2013)

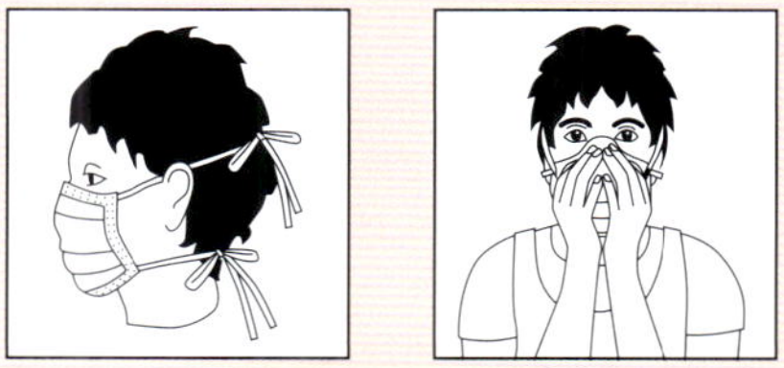

3. Put on eye protection. Place over face and eyes and adjust to fit

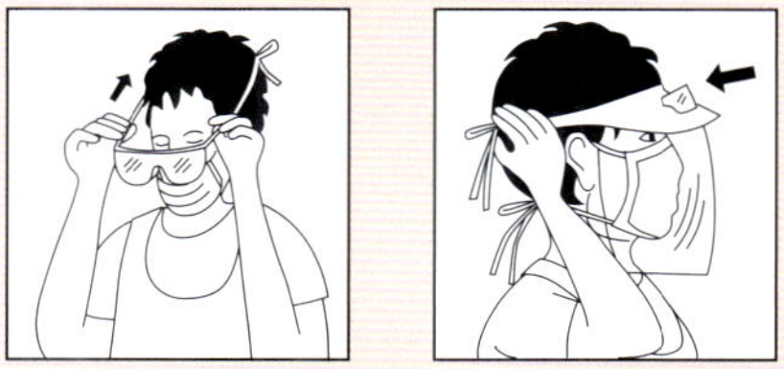

4. Put on disposable gloves. Extend to cover wrists

Procedure – Removing PPE

Take the following steps to remove PPE:

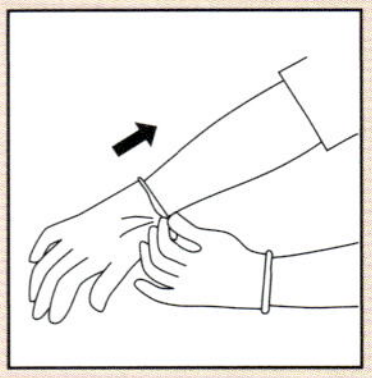

1. Remove gloves:
   - Grasp the outside of the glove with the opposite gloved hand; peel off
   - Hold the removed glove in the gloved hand
   - Slide the fingers of the ungloved hand under the remaining glove at the wrist
   - Peel the second glove off over the first glove and discard appropriately

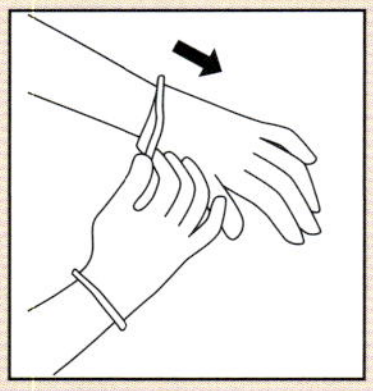

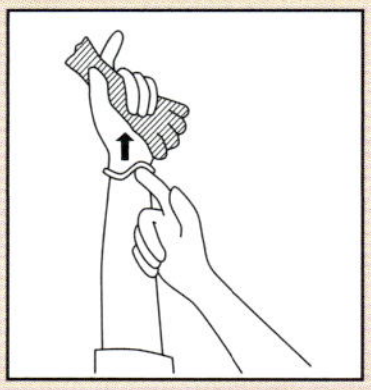

2. Remove apron:
   - Unfasten ties
   - Pull the apron away from the neck and shoulders, touching the inside of the apron only
   - Turn the apron inside out, fold or roll into a bundle and discard

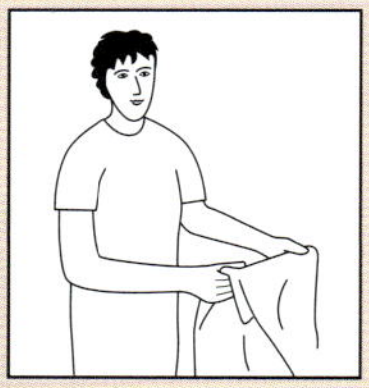

3. Remove eye protection. Handle by headband or earpieces and discard appropriately

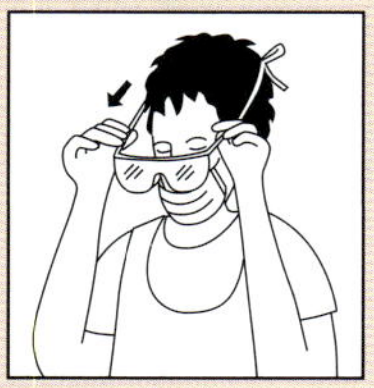

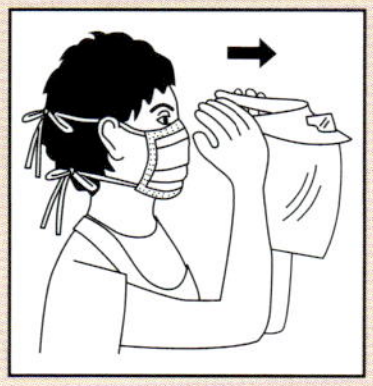

Procedure – Removing PPE – *cont*

4. Remove face mask. Untie or break bottom ties, followed by top ties or elastic. Remove by handling ties only and discard appropriately

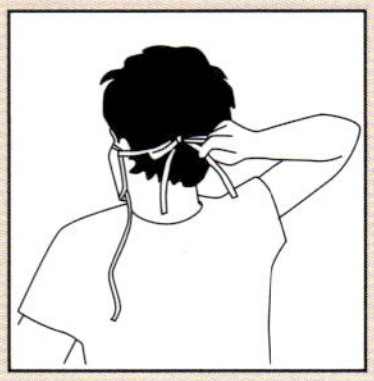

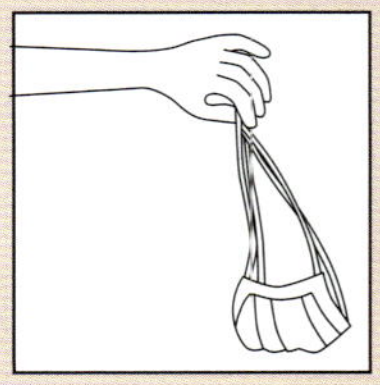

Managing Healthcare Waste

Healthcare waste must be segregated immediately by the person generating the waste into appropriate colour-coded waste disposal bags or containers and labelled, stored, transported and disposed of appropriately (NICE, 2012b).

You should be aware of your organisation's policy on managing healthcare waste, but below are a number of basic principles that apply to most healthcare organisations.

Types of Healthcare Waste

Table 6.2 provides information on the different types of healthcare waste you are likely to encounter. It's very important that all waste is segregated correctly as the way in which different waste is processed varies greatly based on the risk it presents. There are also significant cost variations, with domestic waste being far cheaper to process than infectious waste. Therefore, if infectious waste was filled with unnecessary packaging, it can lead to substantial unnecessary costs.

There are four main types of waste you will encounter:

- Mixed sharps: Sharps are items that could cause cuts or puncture wounds, including: needles, scalpels, knives, broken glass and open drug ampoules.
- Infectious or potentially infectious waste: Items where the concentration of harmful microorganisms is likely to be high enough to

Table 6.2 Types of healthcare waste (DoH, 2013a: SWAST, 2013)

Waste type	Example	Disposal method
Mixed sharps	All needles from injections or cannulation, as well as used medicine ampoules	Incineration
Infectious or potentially infectious waste	Items contaminated by body fluids from a patient known, or thought, to be suffering from an infectious disease	Can be disposed of at a licensed alternative plant or through inceneration
Offensive/hygiene waste, waste, non-infectious	Soiled gloves or dressings, from a non-infectious patient	Landfill
Domestic waste	Uncontaminated packaging and rubbish, including gloves that are not visibly soiled	Landfill

potentially lead to illness being transmitted. This would include the bodily fluids of a patient known to be suffering from an infectious disease.

- Offensive/hygiene waste: Non-infectious waste, from human healthcare. Likely to include items contaminated by bodily fluids, but where the patient is known not to be suffering from an infectious illness.
- Domestic waste: This form of waste presents no risk to human health and is similar to the domestic waste you would produce at home. Most of the packaging for healthcare products, gloves without visible signs of soiling, and wipes that have been used to clean a patient's finger for a blood glucose reading that is not visibly soiled can all be disposed of this way.

Table 6.3 provides examples of typical waste arising from pre-hospital care service activity.

Storing and Handling Healthcare Waste

All waste should be stored in appropriate receptacles, in line with your organisation's procedures. At times it may be necessary to transport full bags of waste. If doing this you should ensure that all bags or containers are sealed and stored safely in the vehicle.

When handling healthcare waste consider the risks it poses and protect yourself appropriately by using PPE. At minimum when handling infectious or offensive waste bags, or containers, wear gloves and also use other appropriate PPE if you anticipate any leakage of waste contained within.

Always label and sign items as appropriate. Note that sharps bins have labels on them which should be completed.

Decontamination Process

Decontamination is a key principle of infection prevention and control. It prevents both healthcare workers and patients from contracting infectious diseases that could be avoided, preventing patient death and patient discomfort as well as reducing costs.

Decontamination is divided into three separate processes:

- Cleaning is defined as the process that removes physical dirt or visible contamination from surfaces, but without necessarily destroying potentially infectious microorganisms (SWAST, 2013).
- Decontamination or disinfection refers to the destruction of microorganisms so that they no longer represent a danger of initiating infection, or other harmful response (HSE, 2015b).
- Sterilisation is the process that removes all viable microorganisms including viruses.

Cleaning, decontamination and sterilisation may not all be required; it depends on the item.

Table 6.3 Types of waste arising from pre-hospital care activity

Activity	Waste type	Receptacle/bag	Justification	Disposal route
Injections	Contaminated sharps or syringes with medicine residue	Yellow lidded sharps receptacle (Figure 6.4)	Potentially contaminated with medicinal products	Incineration
Items/equipment for treating patients	Contaminated packaging, gloves, aprons, other PPE, dressings, airways, suction liners, laryngoscope blades	Infectious waste in orange waste receptacles	Due to lack of patient records/ screening, unlikely to be able to classify as non-infectious	Alternative treatment or incineration
Items/equipment for treating patients	Uncontaminated aprons, other PPE, non-medicated intravenous bags, non-infectious urine, faeces, vomit and their containers	Offensive/ unhygienic waste disposed of in yellow and black striped ('tiger') bags	Risk assessment to determine no possible contamination and non-infectious	Non-hazardous municipal incineration/ energy from waste or landfill **Note:** Liquids (including body fluids) are banned from landfill
Waste packaging as a result of treating patients	Contaminated packaging: plastic and cardboard	Infectious after use, disposed of in orange bag	Due to lack of patient records/ screening, unlikely to be able to classify as non-infectious	Alternative treatment or incineration
Refuse/rubbish	Uncontaminated packaging and refuse/rubbish	Non-infectious, black or clear bag	Used packaging, while patient treatment is being carried out in the vehicle, will usually not be infectious/ clinical waste	Non-hazardous municipal incineration/ energy from waste materials, recycling facilities or landfill

Remember back to the chain of infection: decontamination is all about trying to break the transmission of potentially infective processes from reaching a new susceptible host.

Decontamination Process

It is likely that your organisation will have a cleaning schedule, which will cover things like the buildings you work in, the vehicles you work on, and the equipment you use at work. The schedules should detail how often things need to be cleaned, what procedure to use and with what products.

Refer to your organisation's infection prevention and control policy for further details. An example of a cleaning schedule is included in Table 6.4.

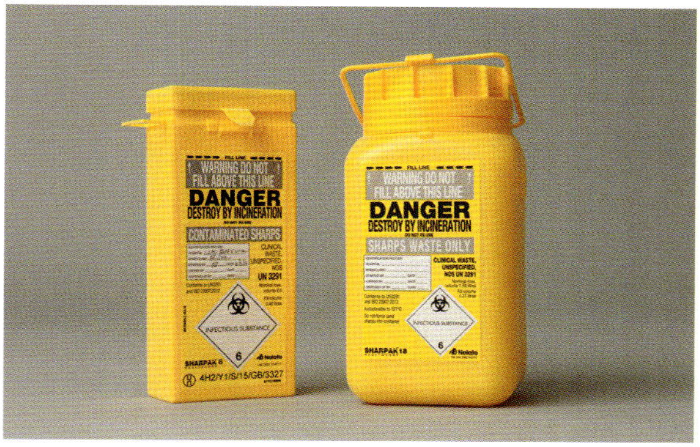

Figure 6.4 *Sharps bins come in different shapes and sizes.*

Cleaning schedules are designed to protect both healthcare workers and patients. Following the schedules is essential for maintaining a clean environment that reduces the chances of both you and your patients becoming unwell from contact with harmful microorganisms.

National Cleaning Colour Code

The national colour coding of hospital cleaning materials was introduced by the National Patient Safety Agency (2007a) as a unified way of identifying which cleaning equipment should be used in different settings. The purpose behind this was to reduce the risk of cross-infection from cleaning equipment being used in a variety of different settings throughout hospitals and therefore increasing the likelihood of cross-contamination.

The colours used are:

RED: Bathrooms, washrooms, showers, toilets, basins and bathroom floors	**BLUE:** General areas, including departments, offices and basins in public areas
GREEN: Kitchen and dining areas	**YELLOW:** Isolation areas, including inside of ambulances

When cleaning the different areas you should be sure to use the appropriate equipment for that area. In your place of work, equipment should be clearly segregated and colour coded to help with this.

Decontamination Procedure

Cleaning

Cleaning is the first step of effective decontamination and refers to removing visible dirt, including organic matter, and reducing the presence of microorganisms. Cleaning should include the use of detergent and hot water to remove all visible contamination and then be allowed to thoroughly dry (SWAST, 2013).

Table 6.4 Cleaning schedules

Item to be cleaned	When it should be cleaned	How to clean
Diagnostic equipment	After each patient contact	Use combined detergent and disinfectant wipes
Ambulance floor	Whenever visibly dirty and at least once per shift	Sweep/mop and bucket using an appropriate detergent or chlorine-based solution as directed locally
Outside of ambulance	Whenever visibly dirty and at least once per shift	Wash with warm water and vehicle detergent as supplied
Ambulance internal surfaces, within patient reach	After every patient contact	Clean with water and detergent unless visibly soiled in which case combined detergent and disinfectant wipes should be used

Decontaminating (disinfecting)

This should be carried out after a detergent clean and uses a range of products to reduce the number of viable microorganisms still remaining. A general principle is that disinfection should be minimised and instead single use equipment used wherever possible (SWAST, 2013).

Depending on what you are trying to clean you may use different products, but one product you are likely to have available is some form of sanitising wipes. Clinell® combined detergent and disinfectant wipes are found widely in healthcare settings for decontaminating solid items and surfaces; instructions for their use are shown in Figure 6.5.

Storage of Cleaning Equipment

It is likely that your place of work will have a dedicated place for the storage of cleaning agents and equipment. As detailed above, cleaning equipment should be stored in a colour-coded manner and cleaning agents and chemicals are subject to specific rules under the Control of Substances Hazardous to Health (COSHH) Regulations detailing how they should be stored and what to do in the case of a spill.

PPE for Decontamination

A number of chemicals involved in the procedure of decontamination can be harmful to health if you are exposed to them inappropriately or in high doses. Whenever you are decontaminating you should protect yourself from coming into direct contact with chemicals or any microorganisms that you may be attempting to clean. Be sure to use the appropriate PPE; this is likely to include:

- Gloves
- Apron
- Sleeve Protector
- FFP3 face mask protection – if you are having to scrub something to clean it then there is a high possibility the liquid will become aerosoled, meaning you could inhale associated microorganisms.

Dealing with a Biological Spillage

Biological spillage refers to the accidental or malicious spilling of bodily fluids, including blood, urine, vomit and faeces. In your place of work you should have a spill pack immediately available to use.

Although there may be slight differences based on the type of kit, it is likely the procedure for their use will follow the below procedure (SWAST, 2013):

1. Isolate the area where the spill has occurred
2. Select and apply appropriate PPE (gloves, apron and potentially sleeve protectors and face mask)
3. Place an absorbent pad or granules on the spill
4. Allow fluid to be soaked up into the absorbent material
5. Remove pad or granules and dispose into the appropriate waste container or bag

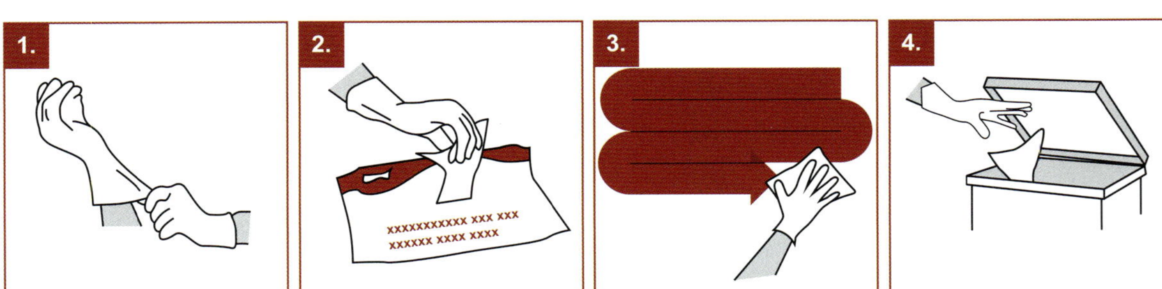

1. Wear recommended PPE.
2. Remove one wipe from the pack.
3. Working from clean to dirty, wipe in an 'S' shaped pattern, taking care not to go over the same area twice.
4. Change wipe if it becomes dry or soiled and discard. Allow to air dry.

Figure 6.5 *Instructions for using Clinell wipes™.*

6. Using a disinfectant wipe in the manner described above, clean the areas covered by the spill
7. If the spill was on a floor, mop, using an appropriate cleaning solution
8. Dispose of all cleaning materials into the appropriate waste bag.

Handling Linen and Laundry

All health providers use a large amount of linen on a daily basis and it is important that it is handled in such a way as to help prevent it from contributing to the spread of infection. Fresh linen should be stored in a neat clean environment where it cannot be exposed to potential infection risks. If working in the pre-hospital setting you should carry a stock of clean linen, but you should not carry too much and ensure that it is neatly stored, away from patient contact, most likely in a cupboard. If linen is visibly dirty then it should not be used but be replaced with fresh linen.

After each patient contact replace the linen, after you have cleaned, ensuring that you follow the procedures below for disposing of the old used linen.

When dealing with used linen, you must segregate and store it according to how it has been used (HSE, 2015e).

Used Linen

Most used linen will be placed into a linen bag at hospital or a white plastic bag that can be sealed ready for collection.

Infectious and Visibly Soiled Linen

Linen that has been used by a patient with a known infection or has been visibly soiled with body fluids should be treated as infectious and placed into a red alginate bag, before being placed into a red linen bag plastic sack. This signifies that the linen is infected and will be handled and washed in a specific manner to reduce the risk of cross-infection.

Storing Linen

You should be aware of the procedures for storing used linen and make sure it is stored in such a way that it does not present a cross-infection risk to healthcare workers or patients.

Also be careful when moving linen as full bags can be heavy. Apply safe movement principles to reduce the risk of being injured by the manual handling procedures (see Chapter 7: Manual Handling).

Sharps Injury

If handled correctly, there should be minimal risk of a sharps injury occurring; however, accidents do happen, so you should be aware of the action to undertake if you are injured by a sharp object while at work. You should take particular care with any 'used sharps' as these present a risk for transmitting infection. To reduce the risk of sharps injury you should:

- Keep sharps covered whenever possible
- Immediately dispose of used sharps into approved containers
- Know where your sharps are stored and check the integrity of packaging frequently
- Ensure that others around you are aware when you are using a sharp item.

If you do receive a sharps injury, then you should (HSE, 2015c):

- Encourage the wound to gently bleed, ideally holding it under running water
- Wash the wound using running water and plenty of soap
- Don't scrub the wound while you are washing it
- Don't suck the wound
- Dry the wound and cover with a waterproof plaster or dressing
- Seek urgent medical attention as prophylaxis may be required
- Report the injury.

Sharps injuries from needles and cannulation equipment are considered to be high risk and can potentially spread infections of blood-borne viruses, including:

- Hepatitis B
- Hepatitis C
- Human immunodeficiency virus (HIV).

You should seek expert medical help as soon as possible after a sharps injury. Your employing organisation will most likely have a procedure in place for doing this, which you should be aware of.

Splash Contamination

There is a risk of diseases being transmitted if blood or other bodily fluids are splashed onto healthcare staff in a location where they can easily enter the body. These locations include:

- Open cuts or wounds
- Mucosal membranes including the eyes and mouth.

If this happens you should immediately irrigate the area with copious amounts of tap water.

Following this, you should attend an ED or MIU so that a risk assessment can be undertaken and post exposure prophylaxis administered if it is thought to be necessary, along with gathering blood samples (SWAST, 2013).

Occupational Health

Healthcare is a potentially stressful and physical environment and the hard work, combined with rota shifts, can, in some circumstances, be detrimental to your health. However, your occupational health team is there to help keep you well at work, both physically and mentally (NHSHWN, 2015).

If you become unwell through work, or suffer from a work-related condition, it is likely that you will be assessed and receive support from your occupational health team who can refer you for appropriate treatment or make suggestions for reasonable adjustments to be made in order for you to do your job safely and successfully. An example of reasonable adjustments might be the purchasing and supply of different gloves to help with recurrent contact dermatitis, or supply a different, customised chair for office workers with back problems.

The occupational health team can also support you if you are exposed to infectious diseases at work. For example, if you receive a sharps injury from a hepatitis positive patient, your occupational health team can arrange for appropriate treatment and tests to be undertaken.

It is likely you will be given details of the services your occupational health team provides and how you can contact them when you join your employing organisation.

Reporting Incidents

Any incidents relating to infection prevention and control should be recorded through the usual incident reporting system in place within your organisation.

Stress

Learning Objectives

By the end of this section you will be able to:

- Describe common signs and indicators of stress.
- List strategies for managing stress.

Introduction

Stress is the adverse reaction people have to excessive pressures or other types of demand placed on them. There is a clear distinction between pressure, which can create a 'buzz' and be a motivating factor, and stress, which can occur when this pressure becomes excessive (HSE, 2007).

Six broad areas have been highlighted as being the primary sources of stress at work (HSE, 2007):

- Demands: This includes issues such as workload, work patterns and the work environment
- Control: How much say the person has in the way they do their work
- Support: This includes the encouragement, sponsorship and resources provided by the organisation, line management and colleagues
- Relationships: This includes promoting positive working to avoid conflict and dealing with unacceptable behaviour
- Role: Whether people understand their role within the organisation and whether the organisation ensures they do not have conflicting roles
- Change: How organisational change (large or small) is managed and communicated in the organisation.

Signs of Stress

Stress can cause changes in those experiencing it, making it important for everyone to look out for changes in a person's or a group's behaviour, particularly in emergency services, where half of employees experience work-related stress (PIE, 2014). However, in many cases, only you will notice the changes that occur as a result of the stress you experience (HSE, 2008a).

Stress can show itself in many different ways and people will exhibit different signs and symptoms. Some of the well-known signs and symptoms of stress include (HSE, 2014a):

Behaviour Change

- Difficulty sleeping
- Altered eating habits
- Smoking and/or drinking more
- Avoiding friends and family
- Sexual problems

Physical

- Tiredness
- Indigestion and nausea
- Headaches
- Aching muscles
- Palpitations

Mental

- Increased indecision
- Difficulty in concentrating
- Poor memory
- Feeling inadequate
- Low self-esteem

Emotional

- Mood swings, becoming irritable or angry
- Increased anxiety
- Feeling numb
- Hypersensitivity
- Feeling drained and listless.

Managing Stress

Although stress is not an illness, it can cause serious illness if not identified and managed. The success of coping strategies to help reduce the effects of stress will vary from person to person. Consider some of the strategies that have been recommended (NHS Choices, 2014a).

Take action to help relieve stress:

- If you're not sure about the trigger for your stress, keep a diary of stressful episodes for 2–4 weeks
- Exercise: Physical activity can help remove some of the emotional intensity of stress
- Eat and drink healthily: Eat a balanced diet and avoid excessive amounts of caffeine and alcohol
- Take control: This can be easier said than done, but identify problems and think about possible solutions. Having a suggestion adopted by an organisation to help in your daily work, particularly when it is benefiting patients, is very satisfying (Pilbery, 2013)
- Talk to someone: Sharing work troubles can help ease the stress as well as provide an opportunity for others to understand how you are feeling and help you see things a different way
- Avoid unhealthy habits: Don't rely on alcohol, smoking and caffeine as a method of coping. The temporary relief they provide can lead to long-term health problems
- Accept the things you can't change: There are inevitably going to be aspects of the job that you cannot change. Accept those and focus on areas where you can have an impact and take control.

For further information on looking after your own mental well-being and that of your colleagues, refer to the end of Chapter 20: Mental Health later in the book.

Chapter 7

Manual Handling

Musculoskeletal Anatomy and Physiology

Learning Objective

By the end of this section you will be able to:

- Identify and describe the anatomy and physiology of the musculoskeletal system and its relation to safe moving and handling.

Introduction

Although often considered together, the skeleton is usually regarded as a system, whereas skeletal muscle (as opposed to smooth muscle found in blood vessels, for example) is a tissue and not a system. However, both are closely related as can be seen by their respective functions.

The skeletal system serves six basic functions (Tortora, 2008):

- **Support**: It is the structural framework for the body, supporting soft tissues and providing points of attachment for tendons and the majority of the skeletal muscles.
- **Protection**: Many of the most important internal organs are protected by the skeleton, for example the brain, heart, lungs and spinal cord.
- **Movement**: Since the majority of skeletal muscles attach to bones, when they contract, bones are made to move.
- **Mineral storage**: Bones store a number of minerals, mostly calcium and phosphorus, which can be released as required.
- **Blood cell production**: Some bones contain red bone marrow, which produces red and white blood cells, and platelets.
- **Energy storage**: Bone containing yellow bone marrow, which is mostly made up of fat, provides an energy reserve.

Skeletal muscle performs a range of functions, either through sustained contraction, or by alternating contraction and relaxation (Marieb, 2013):

- **Body movement**: This is not just a function of muscles on their own, but an integrated process of bones, muscles and joints.
- **Stability of body position**: Skeletal muscle contractions stabilise joints and maintain body posture, such as sitting upright, or keeping the head upright.
- **Generating heat**: Contracting muscular tissue generates heat, known as thermogenesis. Involuntary skeletal muscle contraction to generate heat is better known as shivering.

Anatomical Terms

In order to be able to accurately describe the location of an organ or a wound, or the movement that resulted in an injury, it is necessary to be able to use terms that describe position and direction.

These always relate to the standard anatomical position (Figure 7.1). When referring to left and right, it is always the patient's right and left, not yours.

Terms of Position and Direction

Common terms used to describe position and direction include (Kapit, 2001; Tortora, 2008):

- **Superior**: Also referred to as cranial or rostral. Towards the head or upper part of a structure or the body; above. For example, the head is superior to the abdomen.
- **Inferior**: Away from the head or towards the lower part of a structure or the body; below. For example, the abdomen is inferior to the head.
- **Anterior**: Towards or at the front of the body. For example, the sternum is anterior to the spine.
- **Posterior**: Sometimes also called dorsal. Towards or at the back of the body; behind. For example, the heart is posterior to the sternum.
- **Medial**: Towards or at the midline of the body. For example, the heart is medial to the lungs.
- **Lateral**: Away from the midline of the body. For example, the arms are lateral to the chest.
- **Proximal**: Closer to the point of attachment of a limb to the torso. For example, the elbow is proximal to the hand.
- **Distal**: Further from the point of attachment of a limb. For example, the knee is distal to the hip.
- **Superficial**: Towards or at the body surface. For example, the skin is superficial to the skeletal muscles.
- **Deep**: Away from the body surface. For example, the lungs are deep to the skin.

Terms of Motion

Common terms used to refer to motion of the body and/or limbs include (Kapit, 2001):

- **Extension**: Normally, straightening of a joint. Extreme (abnormal) extension is called

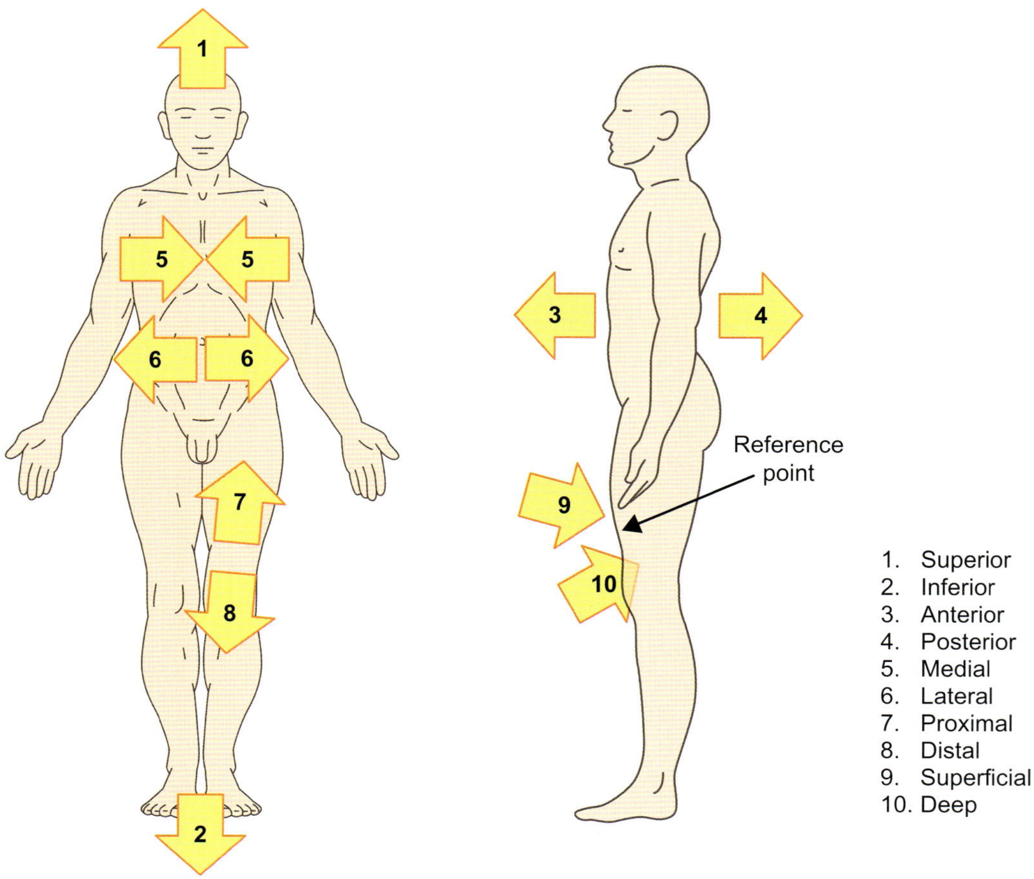

Figure 7.1 *Anatomical terms of position and direction.*

hyperextension. At the ankle and wrist, extension is called dorsiflexion.

- **Flexion**: Bending a joint, or reducing the angle between the bones of a joint. Flexion of the ankle joint is called plantar flexion.
- **Abduction**: Movement of a joint that results in a bone moving away from the midline.
- **Adduction**: Movement of a joint that results in a bone moving towards the midline.

Joints

Since bones do not bend without getting damaged, connective tissues form joints that keep the bones together, while allowing some degree of movement (usually). There are three basic types (Tortora, 2008; Kapit, 2001):

- **Fibrous**: These joints have limited or no movement, such as the sutures that hold the bones of the skull together.
- **Cartilaginous**: As with fibrous joints, these permit little or no movement. An example of this type of joint is the intervertebral disc.
- **Synovial**: These are freely moveable joints that contain a cavity between the articulating bones. The ends of the bones within the joint are covered in a smooth, slippery articular cartilage, which reduces friction and helps to absorb shocks.

Synovial Joints

There are different types of synovial joint. Table 7.1 describes four of these and gives examples of where they can be found in the body (Kapit, 2001).

The Skeletal System

There are 206 bones in the adult human skeleton and they are generally split into two groups: the axial and appendicular skeleton (Figure 7.2). The axial skeleton consists of 80 bones, including the skull, vertebrae, sternum and ribs. The appendicular skeleton consists of the remaining 126 bones, including the shoulder and pelvic girdles and bones of the arms, wrists, hands, thighs, legs and feet (Kapit, 2001).

Breaks in bones (fractures) are more common in the appendicular skeleton, but tend to be more serious if they occur in the axial skeleton (Tortora, 2008).

Types of Bones

Virtually all of the bones in the human body can be classified by their shape (Table 7.2) (Tortora, 2008).

Skull

The skull is made up of 22 bones, with 8 forming the cranial cavity, and the remainder, the facial bones, forming the face (Figure 7.3). Regions of the brain, which are located within the cranial bones, are generally named after the cranial bone, which is located superficially, for example the front and temporal lobes.

Vertebral Column

The vertebral column (spine) is made up of 33 irregular bones known as vertebrae (Figure 7.4) (Kapit, 2001):

- 7 cervical
- 12 thoracic
- 5 lumbar
- 5 sacral – although these usually fuse into a single bone, the sacrum
- 4 coccygeal – again, these normally fuse to form the coccyx.

It functions as a strong, flexible rod that allows for a range of movements, while supporting the head, protecting the spinal cord and providing points of attachment for the ribs, pelvis and back muscles.

Table 7.1 Types of synovial joint

Joint name	Movement	Example location
Ball and socket	All directions	Hip and shoulder
Hinge	One direction; flexion, extension	Elbow
Pivot	Rotation	1st and 2nd cervical vertebrae
Gliding	Gliding movements over two flat articulating surfaces	Acromioclavicular joint

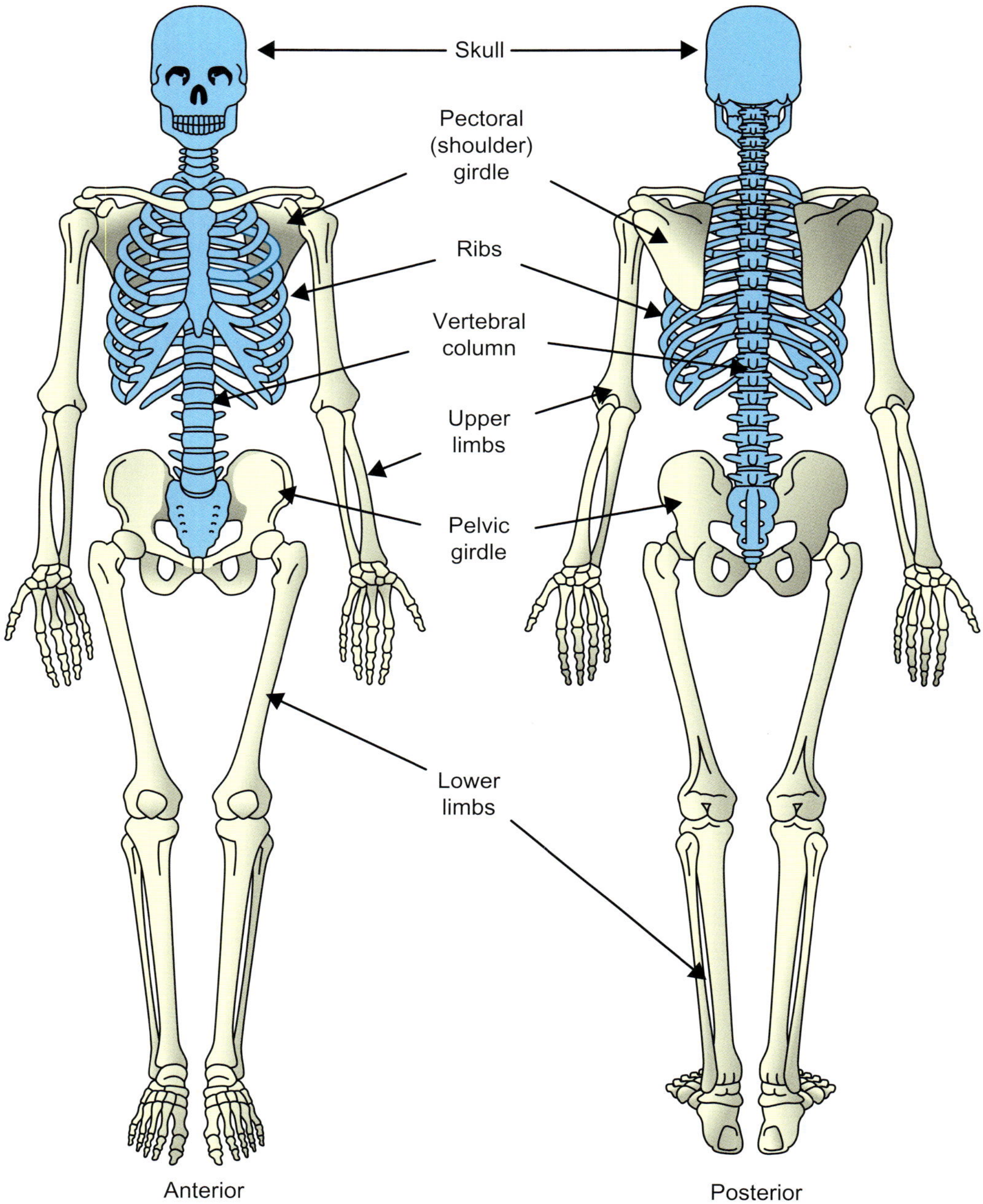

Figure 7.2 *Axial and appendicular skeleton. The axial skeleton is in blue.*

In between the vertebrae are intervertebral discs; these form strong joints, allowing for a range of movements while absorbing vertical forces. When compressed, the discs flatten, but in some cases they can bulge or protrude, leading to compression of spinal nerve roots. In this case, they are said to be herniated (or slipped) discs (Tortora, 2008).

Thoracic Cage

The thoracic cage is the bony part of the thorax, which is usually used to refer to the whole chest. It encloses the organs and vessels within the thoracic cavity and is made up of the sternum, costal cartilages, ribs and thoracic vertebrae (Figure 7.5) (Tortora, 2008).

Table 7.2 Types of bones

Bone type	Description	Example
Long	As their name suggests, these bones are longer than they are wide. They are made up of a shaft (diaphysis) and a variable number of ends (epiphyses) and are slightly curved to increase their strength.	Humerus (upper arm)
Short	These are more cube-like bones of almost equal length and width, and make up many of the bones in the wrist and ankle.	Trapezoid (wrist)
Flat	These bones provide protection for underlying organs and a point of attachment for muscles. Examples include the skull and sternum.	Sternum
Sesamoid	These develop in tendons that are subject to high levels of friction, tension and stress, such as the palms of the hand and soles of the feet. They do not develop in everyone, with the exception of the patella (kneecap), which virtually everyone possesses.	Patella (kneecap)
Irregular	Bones are considered irregular if they have a complex shape that does not fit in any of the other categories. Examples include the vertebrae and hip bones.	Vertebra

There are 12 pairs of ribs, with the first 7 known as true ribs as they physically connect with the sternum thanks to a strip of costal cartilage. The remaining pairs of ribs are called false ribs as they do not directly connect with the sternum, or (as in the case of the 11th and 12th pairs of ribs) do not connect with the sternum at all (Marieb, 2013).

Upper Limbs

Each of the upper limbs consists of 30 bones (Figure 7.6) (Kapit, 2001):

- 1 in the upper arm (humerus)
- 2 in the lower arm (radius and ulna)
- 8 in the wrist (carpal bones)
- 5 in the palm (metacarpals)
- 14 in the fingers (phalanges).

The Hand

The bones and muscles of the hand, in conjunction with the forearm, are capable of a wide range of movements that allow for fine dexterity and are essential for many activities. Thus, injuries to the hand can have a major impact on the patient.

The bones of the hand consist of five metacarpal bones that articulate proximally with the distal four carpal bones, and distally with the five phalanges. The metacarpals are the main structure of the palm of the hand. The phalanges, or fingers, are formed by three separate phalanxes, which are referred to as proximal, middle and distal (Figure 7.7).

Pelvic Girdle

The pelvic girdle comprises two hip bones (sometimes called coxal bones), which themselves are composed of three bones, which have fused by the time adulthood is reached (Figure 7.8): ilium, ischium and pubis. Anteriorly, the hip bones meet at the pubic symphysis joint, and posteriorly, with the sacrum at the sacroiliac joints. Together, these bones form a bowl-like structure known as the bony pelvis (Tortora, 2008).

Lower Limbs

Each of the lower limbs consists of 30 bones (Figure 7.9) (Tortora, 2008):

- 1 femur (thigh)
- 1 patella (kneecap)
- 1 tibia and 1 fibula (lower leg)
- 7 tarsals (ankle)
- 5 metatarsals and 14 phalanges (foot).

The Knee

The knee is the largest synovial joint in the body and consists of the weightbearing articulation between the femur and tibia and the non-weightbearing articulation of the patella and the femur (Figure 7.10).

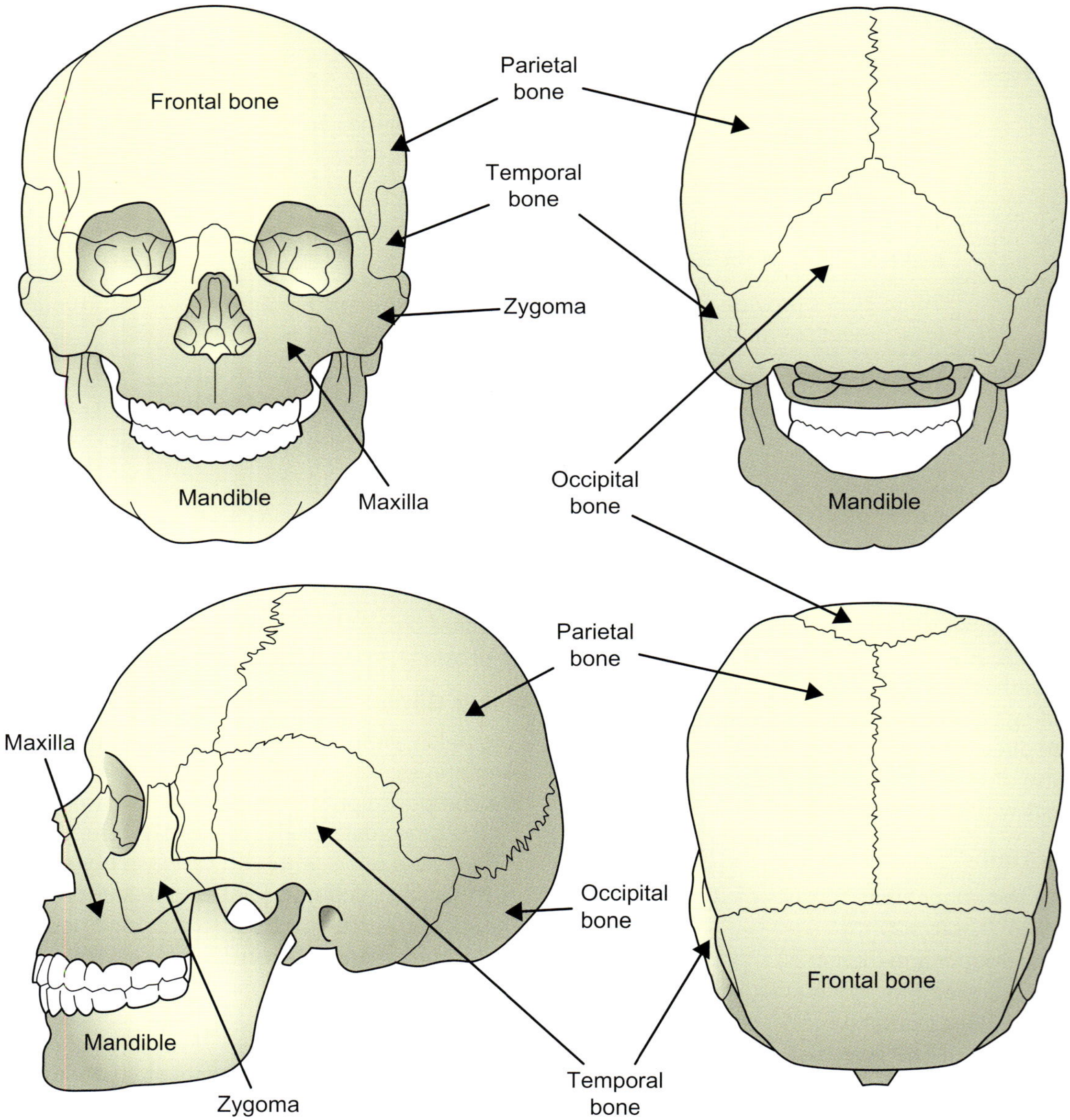

Figure 7.3 *View of the skull.*

The knee is basically a hinge joint, although it does allow for a small amount of rotation. It is strengthened by the collateral ligaments, located on either side of the joint, as well as the two cruciate ligaments, which join the adjacent ends of the femur and tibia, resisting anterior and posterior movement of the joint. Other soft tissues, such as the muscles and the menisci, also serve to stabilise the joint. The knee also has an efficient locking mechanism, which reduces the amount of muscle energy required to keep the joint extended when standing (Drake, 2005).

The Foot

The foot is a mobile structure and functions to support bodyweight and transmit power for walking, running etc. It is shaped like an arch, with the heel and metatarsal heads making contact with

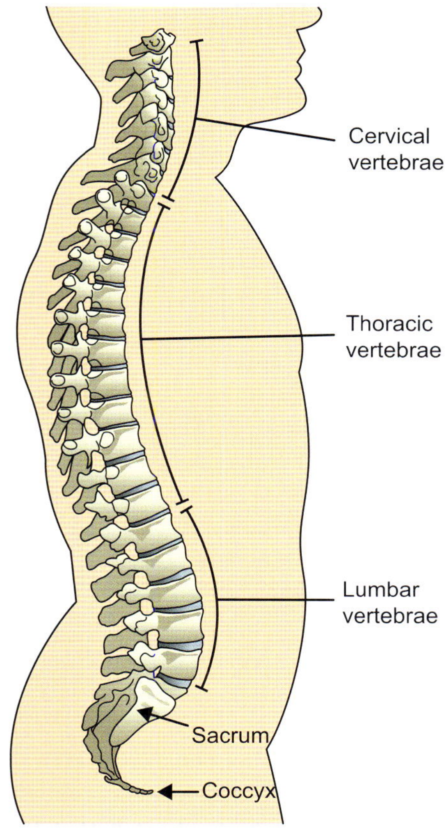

Figure 7.4 *The vertebral column.*

the ground. This helps to absorb and distribute downward forces from the body when standing and moving across various terrains. There are 26 bones in the foot and they are shown in Figure 7.11.

Skeletal Muscles

Skeletal muscles produce movement by exerting a force on tendons, which pull on bones or other structures. They do this by contracting, and since the two articulating bones do not generally move equally, the point of attachment of the muscle tendon to the bone that initiates the movement is called the origin. The point of attachment to the other bone is called the insertion (Tortora, 2008). Figures 7.12 and 7.13 highlight a number of skeletal muscles; you do not need to know the names of all of the muscles, but being familiar with some of the main ones, especially those you can feel when examining the patient, can be helpful.

Mechanics of Movement

To produce movement, bones act as levers and joints as the fulcrum – the fixed point around which the lever (bone) can move. A lever is affected by two forces: the effort, which causes movement

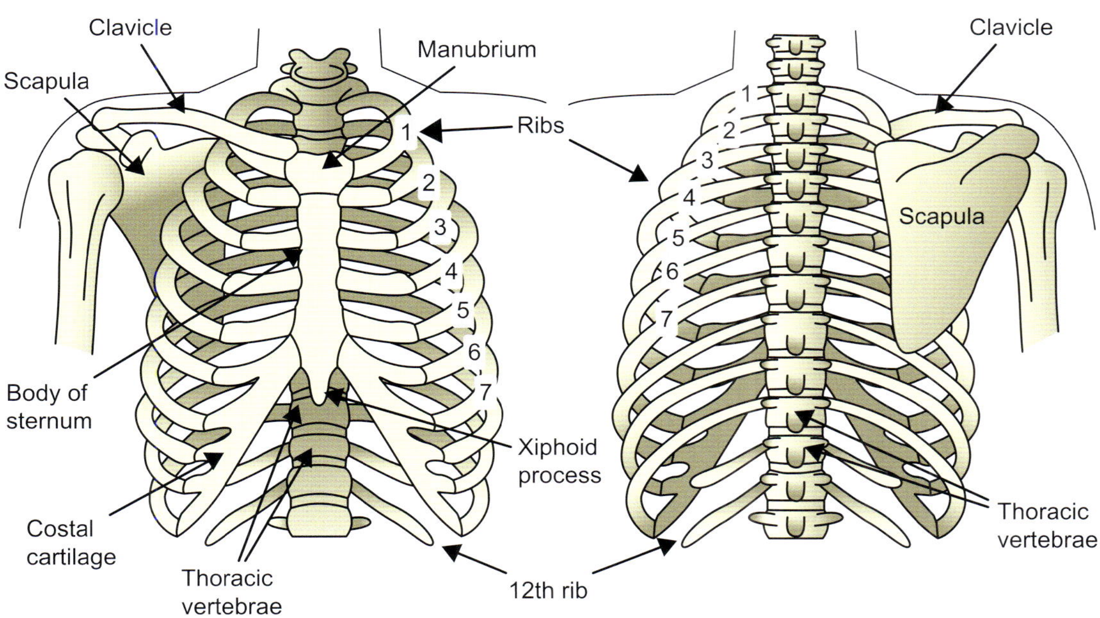

Figure 7.5 *The anterior (left) and posterior (right) thorax.*

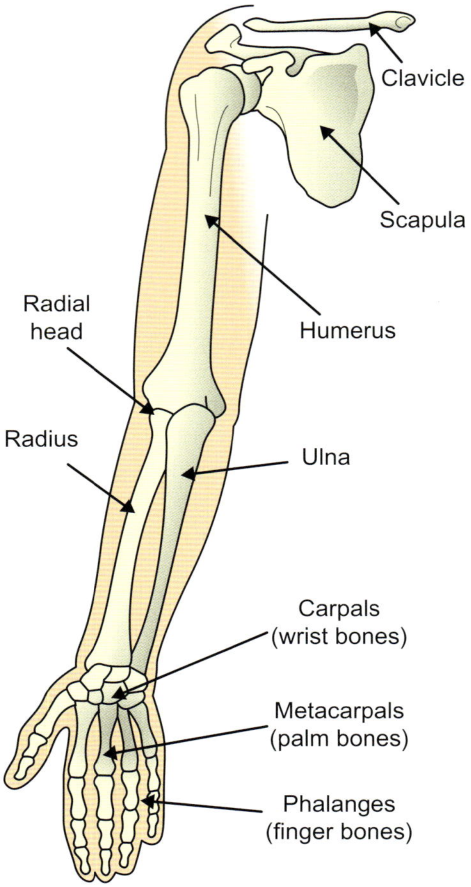

Figure 7.6 *The upper limb – anterior view.*

(i.e. the muscles), and the load, or resistance, which acts in opposition to the effort (Tortora, 2008).

A lever allows a given effort to move a heavier load, or move it further or faster, than it could without the lever (Marieb, 2013). If the load is close to the fulcrum and the effort applied is far away, a small effort over the large distance will move a heavier object over a small distance. This lever is said to operate at a mechanical advantage. Conversely, if the load is far from the fulcrum and the effort applied is near, the effort required must be greater than the load for movement to occur. This lever is said to operate at a mechanical disadvantage. This is because this lever can move a small load rapidly over a large distance (Tortora, 2008). There are three types of levers, determined by the position of the fulcrum (F), effort (E) and load (L), as shown in Table 7.3.

Principles of Manual Handling

Learning Objectives

By the end of this section you will be able to:

- Define manual handling.
- Explain principles for safe moving and handling.
- Describe what action should be taken if an individual's wishes conflict with their plan of care in relation to health and safety and their risk assessment.

Introduction

Manual handling injuries are an issue that all emergency service staff face, due to the greater risks from having to perform moving and handling tasks in emergency situations, where risk mitigation may not be possible at the same level as other activities performed in a more controlled environment.

Moving and handling injuries are the most common cause of all injuries sustained by operational firefighters (Scottish Fire and Rescue, 2015). As an emergency medical responder, it is inevitable you will need to move or support the moving of both equipment and patients. By having a good understanding of the risks associated with moving and handling and how to reduce those risks, you can best prepare yourself and avoid injury.

Definitions

The Health and Safety Executive (HSE, 2016) define manual handling operations as any transporting or supporting of a load (including the lifting, putting down, pushing, pulling, carrying or moving thereof) by hand or bodily force.

A load is defined as a discrete moveable object and may include packages, such as your medical equipment, or patients, whether it be helping them to sit in a chair, guiding them by the arm when they feel unsteady on their feet, or carrying them on a stretcher to an ambulance trolley.

Consequences of Poor Manual Handling

As an emergency medical responder, it is inevitable that occasionally you will need to perform some moving and handling tasks. It is well known that

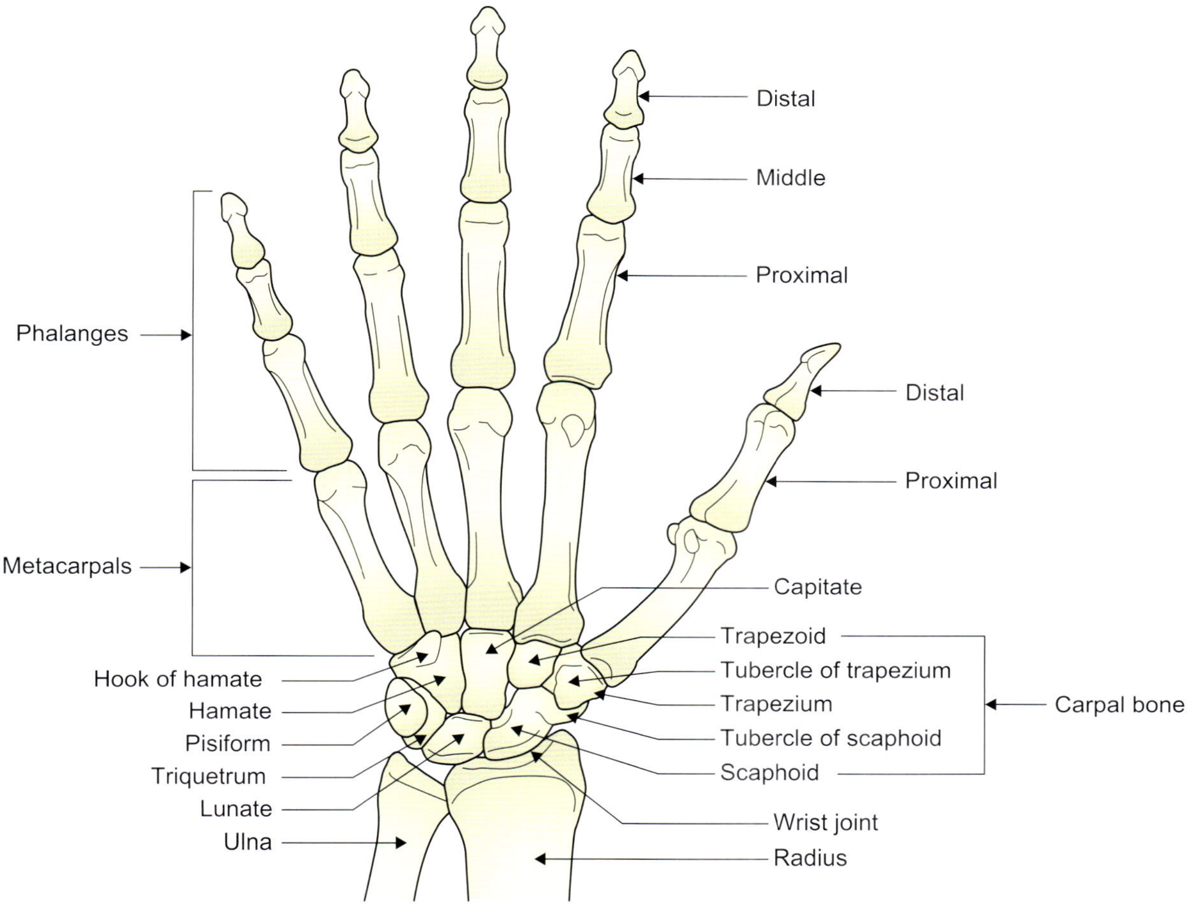

Figure 7.7 *The bones of the hand.*

poor moving and handling techniques, as well as repetitive tasks, significantly increase the risk of musculoskeletal injuries, particularly in the back.

One of the most common injuries is a 'slipped disc', also known as a herniated disc.

Herniated Disc

In the anatomy and physiology section, we looked at how the spinal column is constructed of vertebrae, with intervertebral discs in between. These discs, which are designed to help take the load through the spine and to cushion the vertebrae, can be damaged by repetitive action or sudden movements, causing the outer layer (the annulus fibrosis) to rupture and protrude out beyond the normal diameter of the vertebrae (Figure 7.14).

When this happens it pinches on the nerves, causing significant pain and even potential nerve damage (Nellist, 2013). Most commonly, due to the natural curvature and the increased weight in this area, this occurs in the lumbar region, meaning that the nerves involved often include the sciatic nerve and lead to sciatic leg and back pain, which is very uncomfortable (Figure 7.15).

Consequences to Others

You should also consider that it would not be just you who can be injured by poor or inappropriate techniques. It is likely that any inappropriate technique will also lead to injury of your colleagues and even potentially your patient.

It is unavoidable that sometimes you will need to undertake moving and handling procedures in

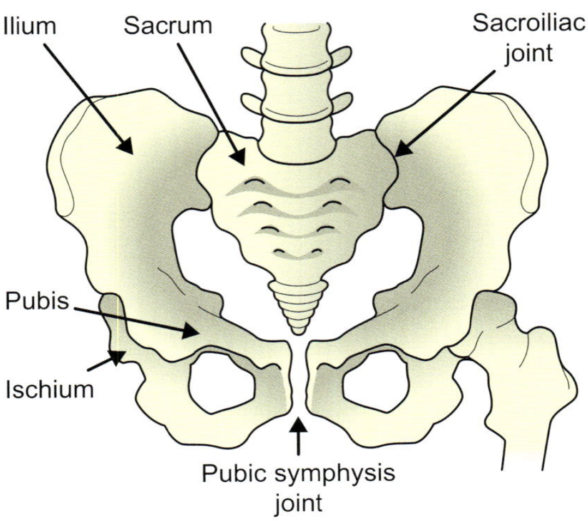

Figure 7.8 *The pelvic girdle.*

high-pressure emergency environments, but even then you should continue to apply good principles of moving and handling to ensure that nobody is injured by such actions.

Risk Assessment

In Chapter 6: Health and Safety, you learned about risk assessment, and manual handling is a perfect example of a set of actions that need a risk assessment to be undertaken **before** taking action. The difficulty in emergency situations is that the time available to make this risk assessment may be short.

There are five steps to risk assessment (HSE, 2006):

- Identify the hazards.
- Decide who might be harmed and how.
- Evaluate the risk and decide on precautions.
- Record your findings and implement them.
- Review your assessment and update if necessary.

This is not very user-friendly or specific to manual handling, and so these steps can be encapsulated in the TILEE acronym (HSE, 2011; Gregory, 2010b):

- **T**ask: Consider whether the lift involves:
  - holding the load away from the body
  - long distances
  - strenuous effort or twisting.
- **I**ndividual: Consider whether the lift:
  - requires specialist training
  - presents a hazard
  - is able to be performed by you and your colleagues.

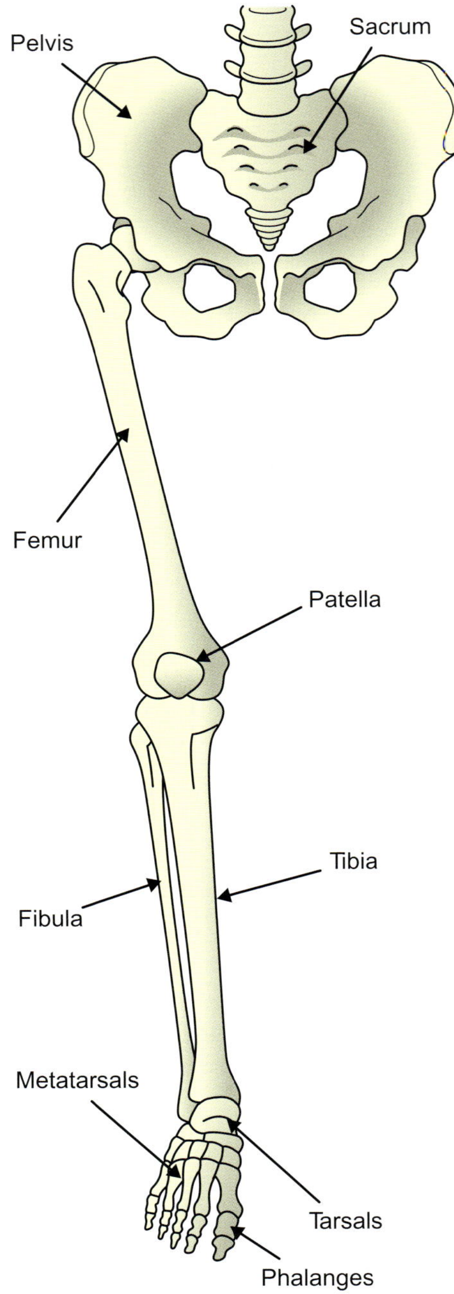

Figure 7.9 *The lower limb.*

- **L**oad: Is the load:
  - heavy
  - difficult to get hold of
  - unstable
  - unpredictable

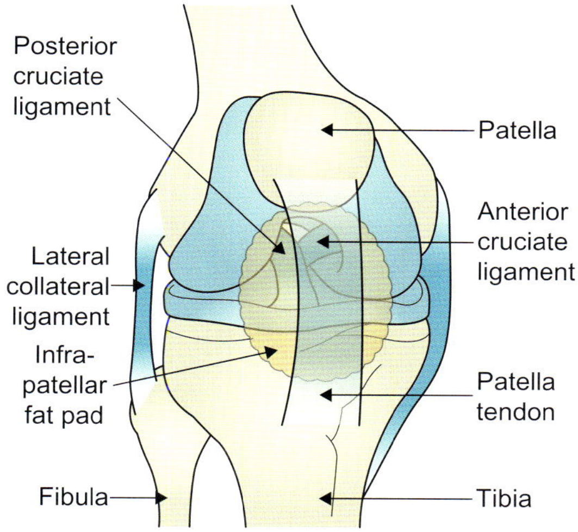

Figure 7.10 *The knee joint.*

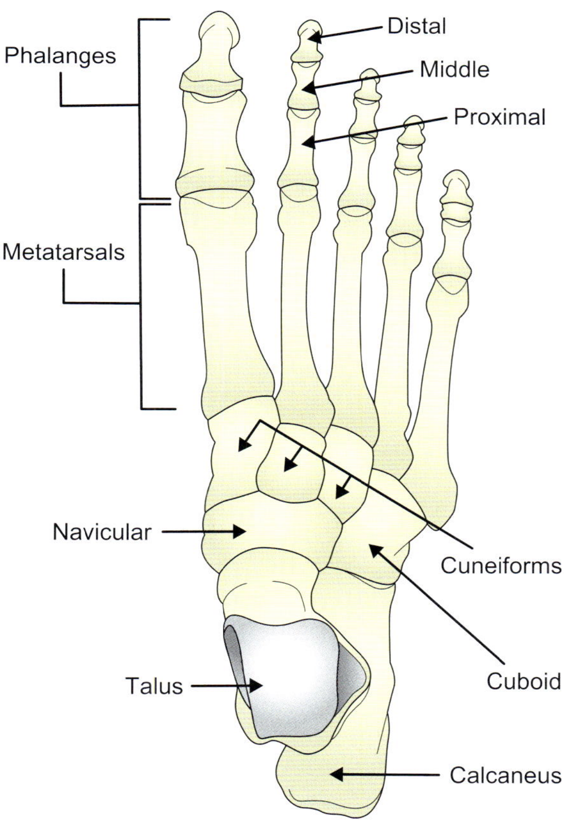

Figure 7.11 *The bones of the foot.*

- o harmful
- o likely to grab out when alarmed at being carried down the stairs.

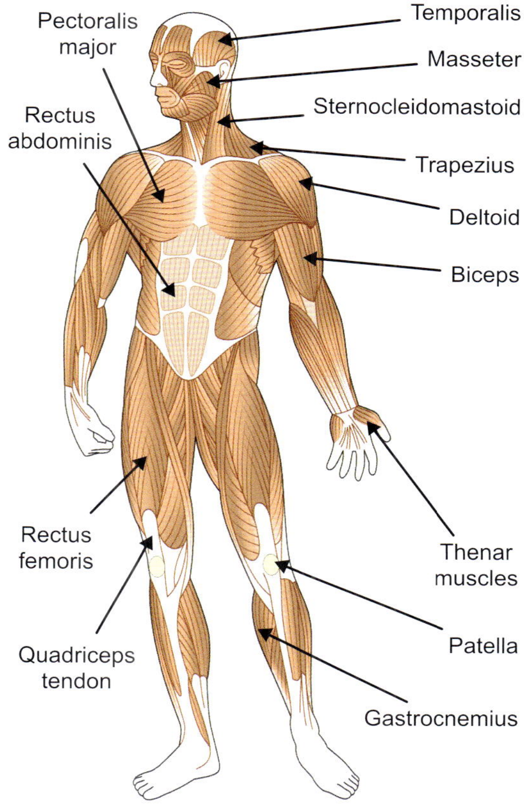

Figure 7.12 *Anterior view of superficial muscles.*

- **E**nvironment: Determine the presence of:
  - o constraints on posture, e.g. low ceiling, confined spaces
  - o poor, uneven flooring
  - o hot/cold/wet weather
  - o poor lighting
  - o noise.
- **E**quipment: Consider whether you:
  - o have the right equipment
  - o have the correct training
  - o can request additional equipment.

Reducing Risk

Legal Responsibility

The Manual Handling Operations Regulations 1992 (HSE, 2016) bring together European Directive 90/269/EEC on the manual handling of loads, general duties placed on employers by the Health and Safety at Work etc. Act 1974 and the requirements of the Management of Health

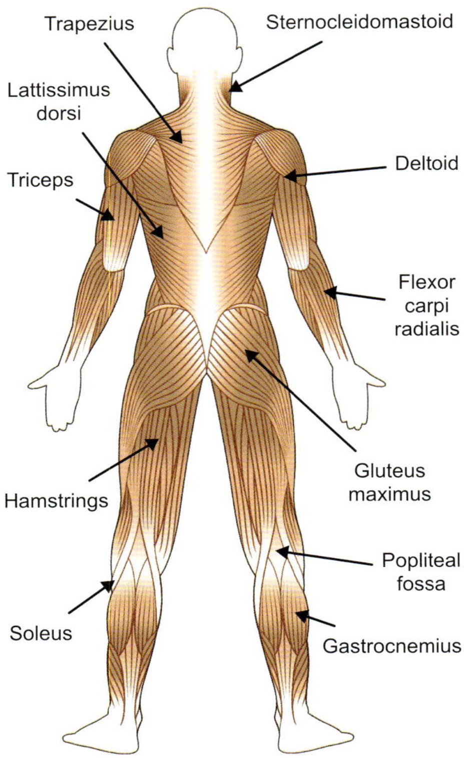

Figure 7.13 *Posterior view of superficial muscles.*

and Safety at Work Regulations 1999 to detail how employers should reduce the risk from moving and handling injury so far as is reasonably practicable.

This should be done by assessing the risk, reducing the risk so far as is practicable and then regularly reviewing the risk to see if further controls are required.

An example of this is the introduction of the Mangar ELK, which we will look at in more detail later in this chapter. The ELK is used to lift people from the floor, safely and with minimal strain to you as an emergency medical responder. Before the ELK was introduced, responders had to lift the patient themselves, which was far more dangerous for responders and patients alike.

Reducing the Load in Practice

Once you have identified a risk relating to manual handling, you will need to determine how best to manage it. Strategies for managing risk are best considered in advance, for example during your training, or by consulting manuals or guidance provided by your service and the Health and Safety Executive. When you are at the patient's side, however, these approaches are not suitable. You will seldom work alone, so ask colleagues for advice and don't be afraid to request additional help if your risk assessment suggests this would be beneficial. This is especially true for larger patients or where manoeuvres will be difficult due to limited access.

You should not use equipment you are not familiar with, but some equipment does come with a manual or simple diagrams printed on its surface, which you can use to remind yourself about the correct way it should be used, or the sequence of actions required. Don't forget that other manual handling equipment may be available in your location, such as hoists, which can help reduce the risk to you and the patient. However, this will usually rely on a trained member of staff being available to help you.

Biomechanics

Biomechanics is the application of the physical laws of mechanics to the human body. In order to reduce the risk of injury and facilitate manual handling, it is important to be aware of the following mechanical principles (Smith, 2011b):

- force
- gravity and equilibrium
- friction
- stress and strain
- pressure
- levers
- moment of force or turning force
- stability and equilibrium.

General Principles

You are going to learn about specific moving and handling equipment and techniques in the next section, but it is helpful to know the basic principles to adopt when approaching a manual handling task (HSE, 2003).

Procedure

1. **Think before handling**. Plan the manoeuvre. Can handling aids be used? Where is the load going to be placed? Will help be needed with the load? Remove obstructions, such as

discarded wrapping materials. Can you reduce the moving and handling manoeuvre? For a long lift, consider resting the load midway on a table or bench to change grip.

2. **Prepare the load**. Whatever your load may be, prepare it so that it is as safe as possible to move. This may include securing items if carrying a load of medical stores, or warning a patient what is going to happen and not to grab out with their hands when on a chair.
3. **Adopt a stable position**. The feet should be apart with one leg slightly forward to maintain balance (alongside the load, if it is on the ground). The worker should be prepared to move their feet during the lift to maintain their stability. Avoid tight clothing or unsuitable footwear, which may make this difficult.
4. **Start in a good posture**. At the start of the lift, slight bending of the back, hips and knees is preferable to fully flexing the back (stooping) or fully flexing the hips and knees (squatting). **Don't flex the back any further while lifting**. This can happen if the legs begin to straighten before starting to raise the load.
5. **Keep the load close to the waist**. Keep the load close to the body for as long as possible while lifting. Keep the heaviest side of the load next to the body. If a close approach to the load is not possible, try to slide it towards the body before attempting to lift it.
6. **Avoid twisting the back or leaning sideways**, especially while the back is bent. Shoulders should be kept level and facing in the same direction as the hips. Turning by moving the feet is better than twisting and lifting at the same time.
7. **Keep the head up when handling**. Look ahead, not down at the load, once it is held securely. **Move smoothly**. The load should not be jerked or snatched as this can make it harder to keep control and can increase the risk of injury. **Don't lift or handle more than can be easily managed**. There is a difference between what people can lift and what they can safely lift. If in doubt, seek advice or get help.
8. **Put down, then adjust**. If precise positioning of the load is necessary, put it down first, then slide it into the desired position.

There is no such thing as completely 'safe' handling, but try to keep to the maximum weights for lifting and lowering in the zones shown in Figure 7.16. If you are twisting, reduce weights by 10% if you are required to twist beyond 45°, and by 20% if you must twist beyond 90° (HSE, 2016).

Handling Aids

Your employer should provide aids to assist in manual handling. As part of patient handling, this may include:

- handling belts
- slide sheets
- transfer (banana) boards
- turntables
- lifting cushions
- powered ambulance stretcher
- tail lifts on the back of the ambulance.

As an emergency medical responder, you may not have all of these tools available to you all the time, and you should limit your moving and handling to only that which is immediately required and that which you can perform safely.

The ambulance staff that will be backing you up will have been trained extensively in moving and handling patients and may have additional aids for reducing the risk, so you should wait for this where possible.

Moving and Handling Equipment and Techniques

Learning Objectives

By the end of this section you will be able to:

- Describe the aids and equipment that may be used for moving and positioning.
- Describe the impact of specific conditions on the correct movement and positioning of an individual.

Introduction

This section provides guidance on different techniques that can be utilised for moving and handling patients. As an emergency medical responder you may not be trained in all of these

Table 7.3 Classes of lever

Class of lever	Mechanism	Examples
First	Effort and load opposite each other with the fulcrum in the middle.	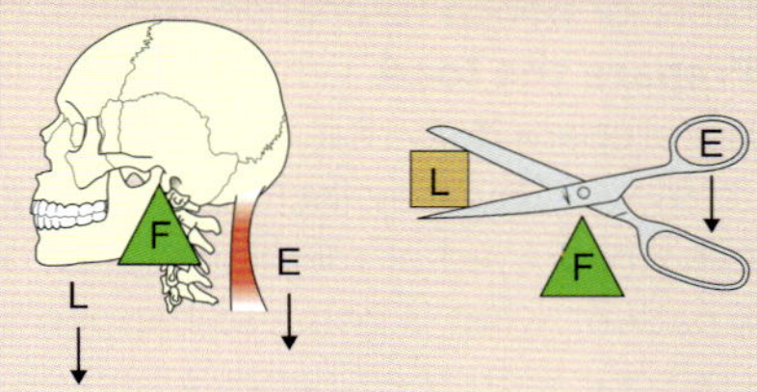
Second	Effort applied at one end, with fulcrum at the other end and load in the middle. Uncommon in the human body.	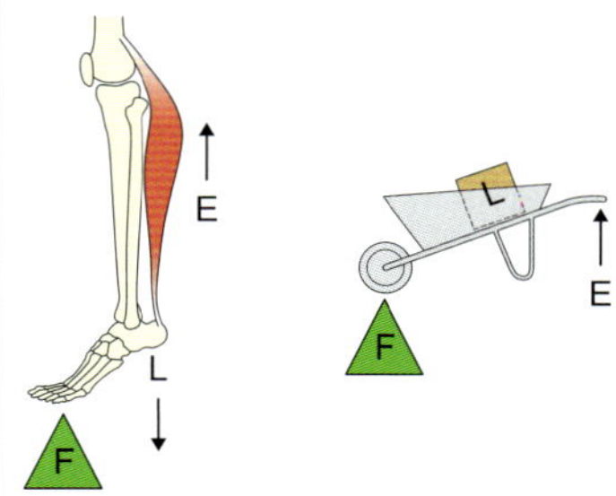
Third	Effort between load and fulcrum. Allows for rapid and extensive movements, such as throwing.	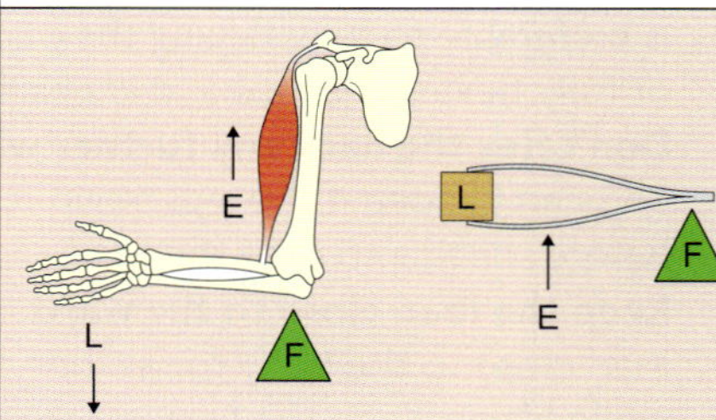

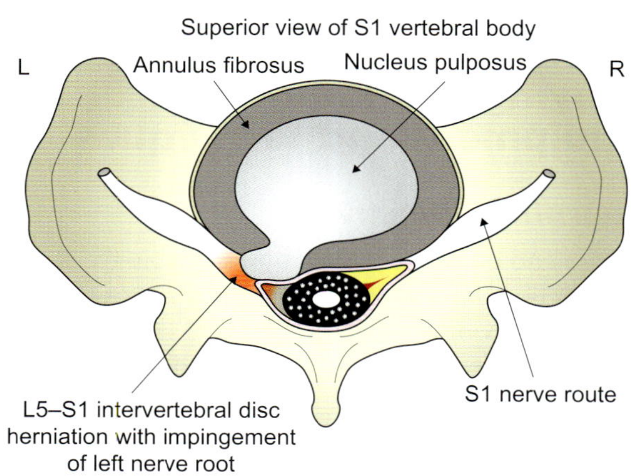

Figure 7.14 *Herniated disc.*

techniques by your service, and should only perform those that you have been trained in, can safely undertake on your own and that cannot wait until additional help arrives.

Patients on the Floor

The usual advice from a call handler in response to a 999 call is to advise the caller not to move the patient. Usually this will be the case for you as an emergency medical responder as well, and where possible you should avoid moving the patient until they have been assessed by a suitable person, unless you have had additional training to undertake this assessment.

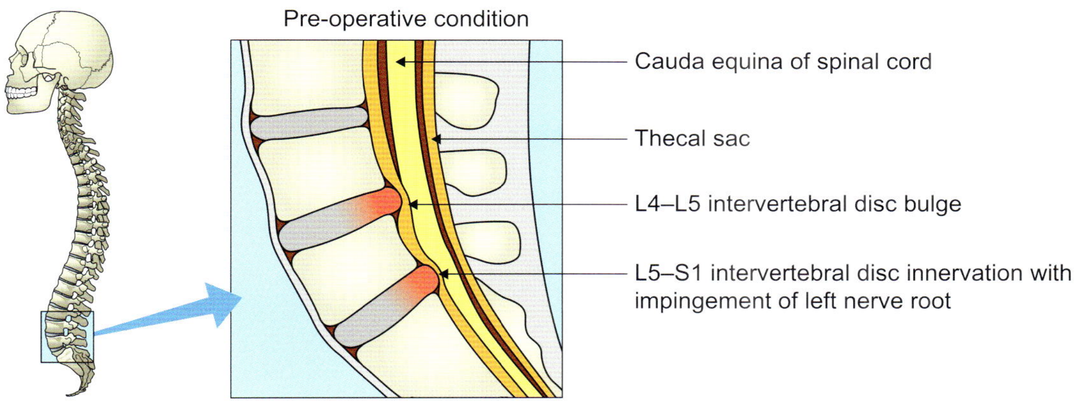

Figure 7.15 Lumbar spine herniation.

There are several techniques for helping a patient to get from the floor to seated in a chair by themselves and these have been included below; however, as discussed above, you should normally not move a patient until they have been clinically assessed. Follow your local policy on this.

For patients who are unable to get themselves up from the floor, it is likely a lifting device, such as a lifting cushion, will be required. You should be aware of such equipment being carried by your service or other services that may be able to assist you.

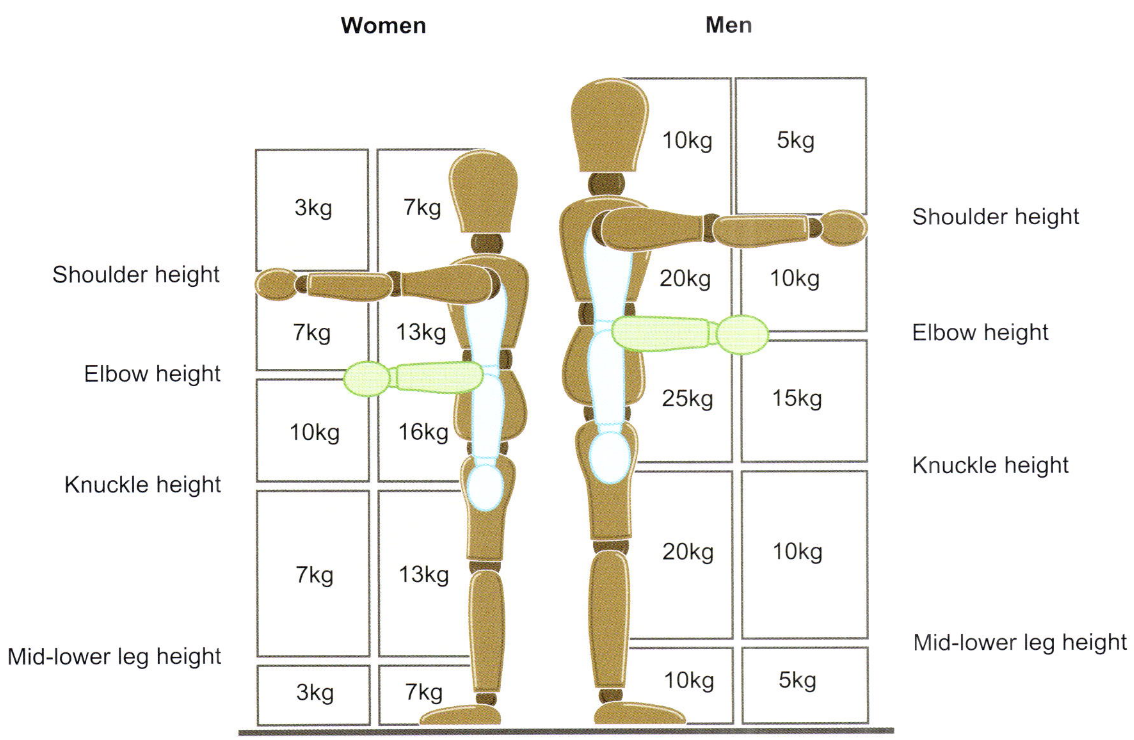

Figure 7.16 Guideline weights for lifting and lowering.

Instructing a Patient to Get Off the Floor – One-Chair Method

Procedure

In order to undertake this procedure, the patient needs to be able to roll on to their side and be able to kneel, so it may not be suitable for patients with knee and hip problems.

Take the following steps to instruct a patient to get off the floor using a single chair (Smith, 2011b):

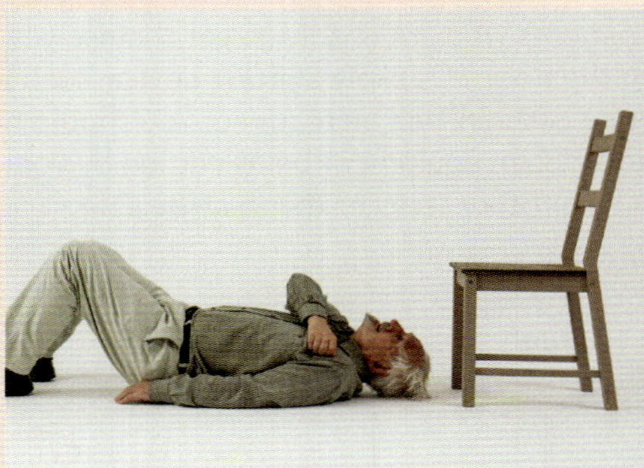

1. Position a chair at the head end of the fallen patient. Instruct them to bend their knees up and to bring one arm across their chest.

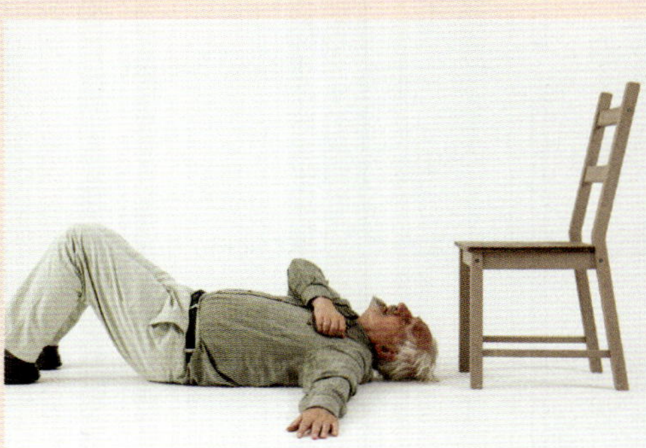

2. Instruct the patient to move their other arm away from the body.

Procedure – *cont*

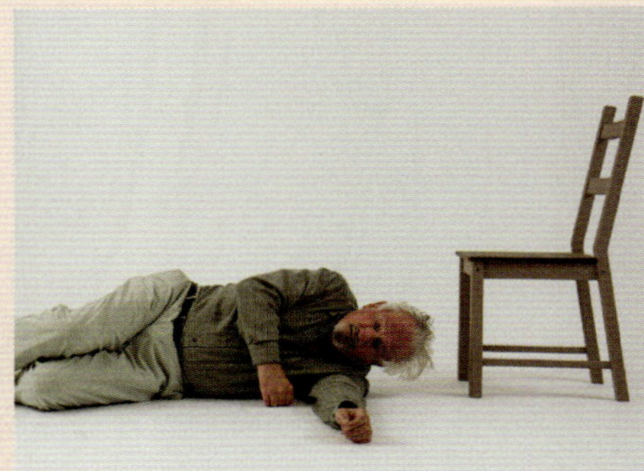

3. Instruct the patient to roll onto their side and bring their arm over their body so that it is flat on the floor.

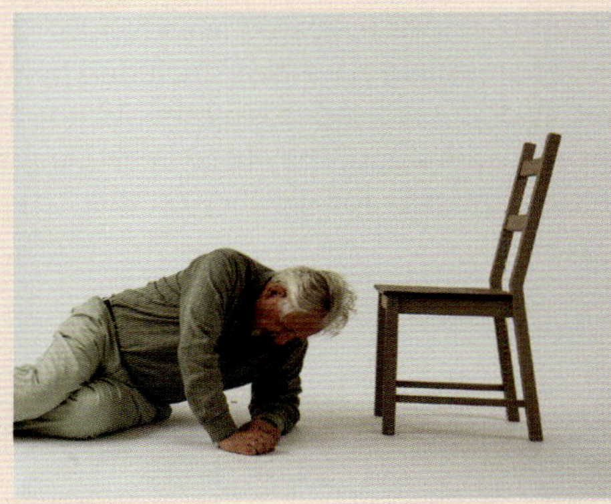

4. Instruct the patient to push up on their hand and at the same time push up on their forearm that is resting on the floor, until they are half-sitting.

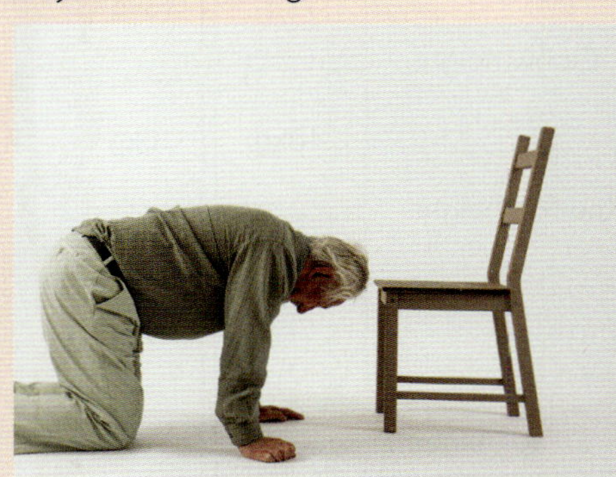

5. Continue to verbally support the patient as they continue to push upwards, until they end up on all fours facing the chair.

Procedure – *cont*

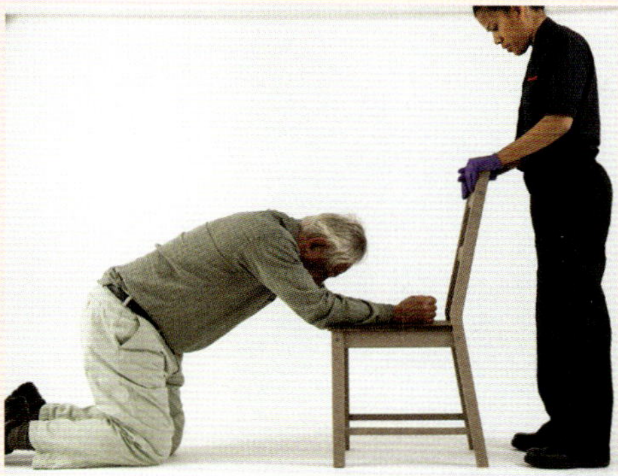

6. While holding the chair steady, instruct the patient to lower their arms onto the chair seat and lean on it.

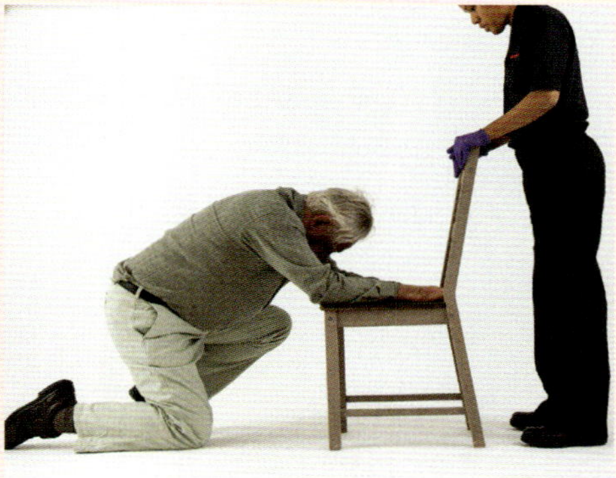

7. Instruct the patient to raise their stronger leg and place the foot of that leg on the floor.

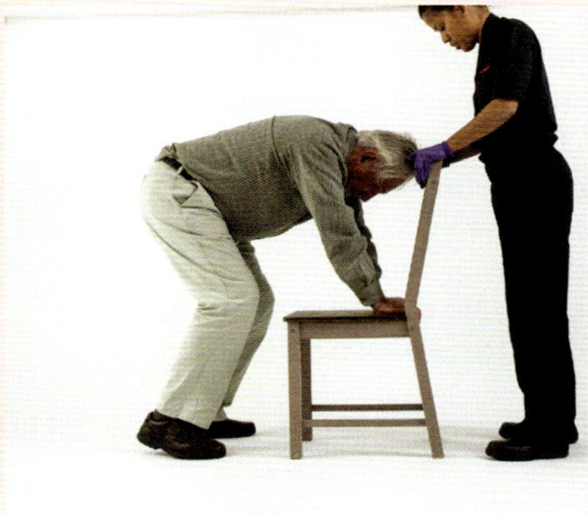

8. Instruct the patient to push up and straighten their legs.

Procedure – *cont*

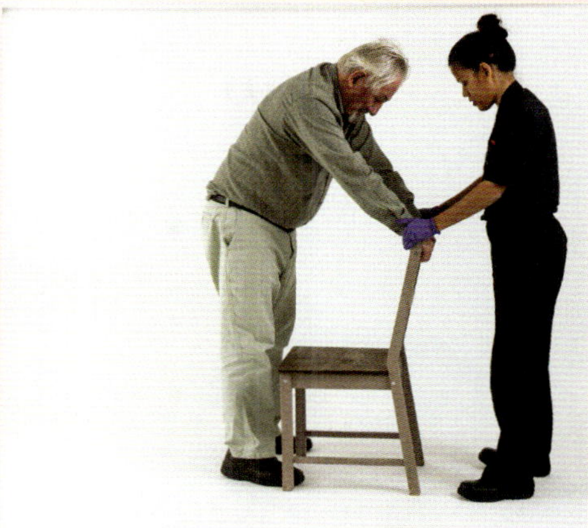

9. Allow the patient time to stabilise themselves and stand up straight, placing their hands on the back of the chair.

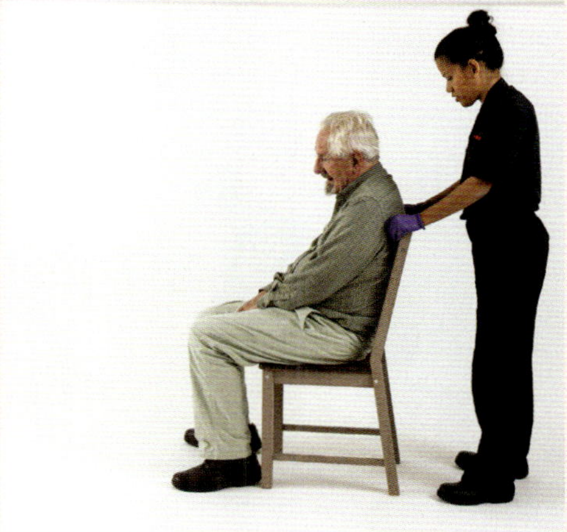

10. Instruct the patient to carefully turn and sit on the chair

Instructing a Patient to Get Off the Floor – Two-Chair Method

Procedure

This procedure is preferred when the patient cannot kneel and requires no physical intervention by the ambulance crew member.

Procedure – *cont*

Take the following steps to instruct a patient to get off the floor using two chairs (Smith, 2011b):

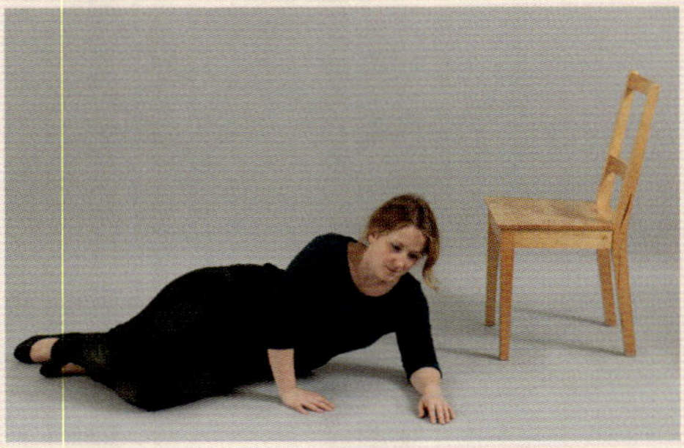

1. Position a chair at the head end of the fallen patient. Instruct them to bend their knees up and roll into side lying. They should then bring one arm over the chest until their hand is flat on the floor. Instruct them to push up with one hand and their lower arm into a side sitting position as in the one-chair method.

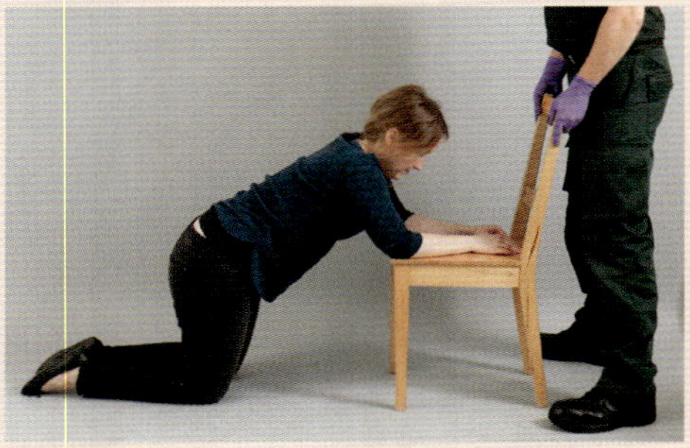

2. Instruct the patient to face the chair and place their forearms on the seat.

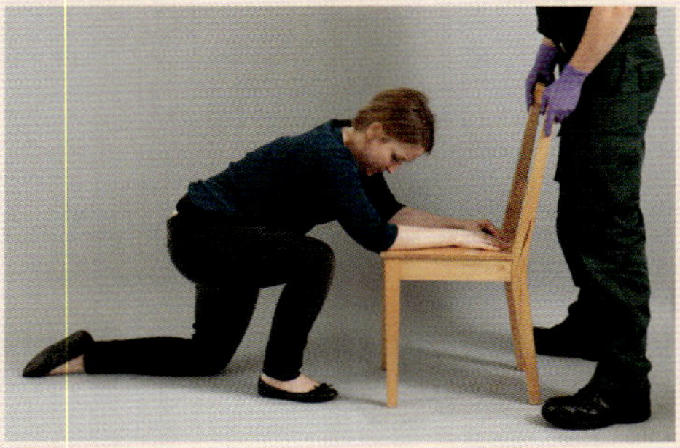

3. Instruct the patient to bend one knee and place the foot of that leg onto the floor, while at the same time pushing up on their forearms and hands.

Procedure – *cont*

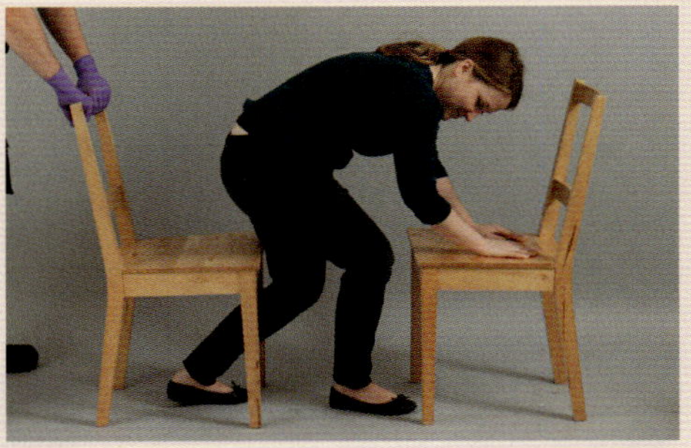

4. Place a second chair behind the patient, ensuring it is under their hips.

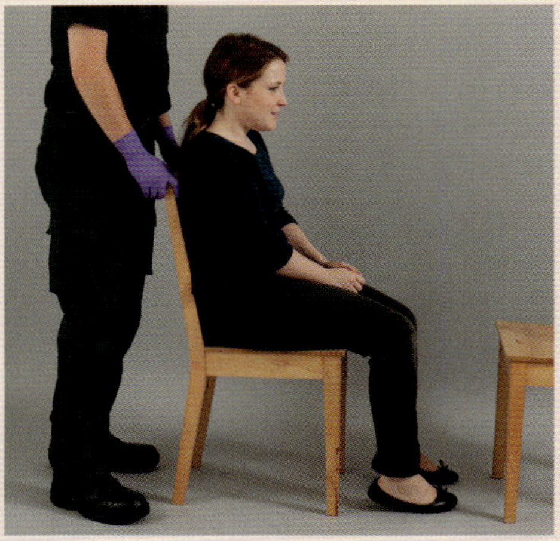

5. Instruct the patient to sit backwards onto the chair.

Lifting Cushion

If a patient cannot get themselves off the floor using the one- or two-chair method, a lifting cushion (Figure 7.17) may be helpful. The patient needs to be able to partly assist with a transfer, for example, by shuffling/rolling onto the cushion. They also need to have sitting balance if using a cushion with no back (Smith, 2011b).

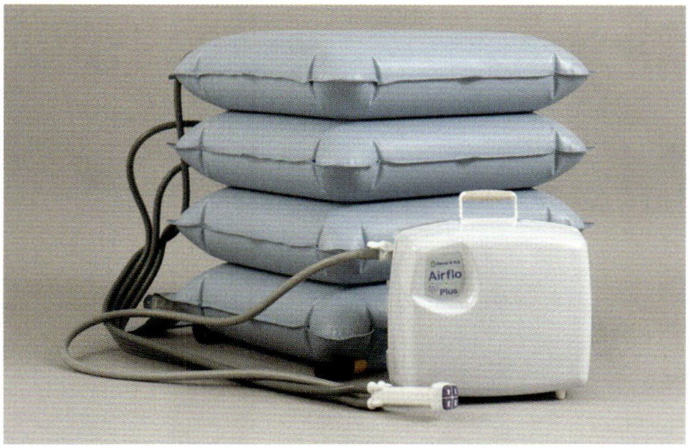

Figure 7.17 *The Mangar ELK lifting cushion.*

Procedure

Take the following steps to assist a patient from the floor using the Mangar ELK (Mangar International, 2012; Smith, 2011b):

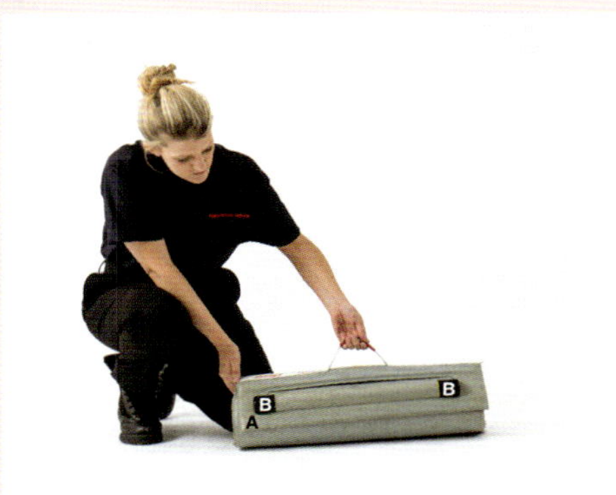

1. Unroll the ELK by unclipping the flap (A) from the ends of the stability bar (B).

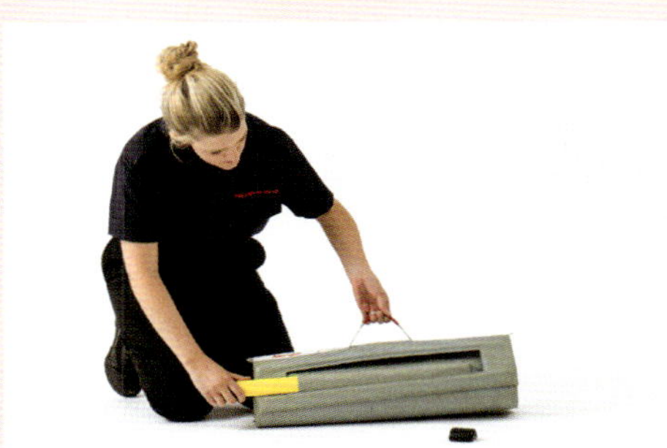

2. Remove the end cap and then the stability bar from its pocket (B) in order to provide a more comfortable transfer for the patient.

Procedure – *cont*

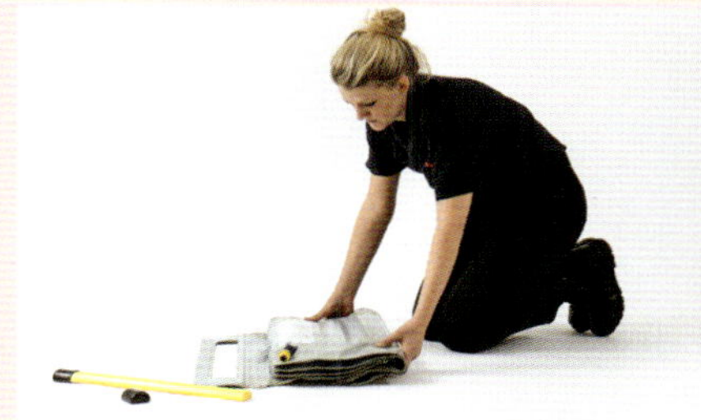

3. Fold the edge of the ELK underneath itself by folding along the line of the stability bar pocket.

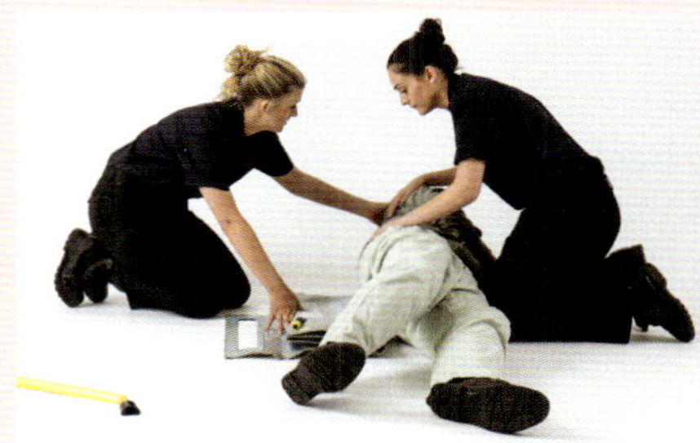

4. One crew member should roll the patient onto their side. A second crew member should position the ELK so that its 'upper' edge is approximately level with and tight up against the patient's waistband. If the patient cannot sit up on their own, consider inserting a handling sling level with their shoulder blades, so you can assist them to sit up. **Note**: Place a blanket, groundsheet, towel or similar under the ELK if using it on a rough surface.

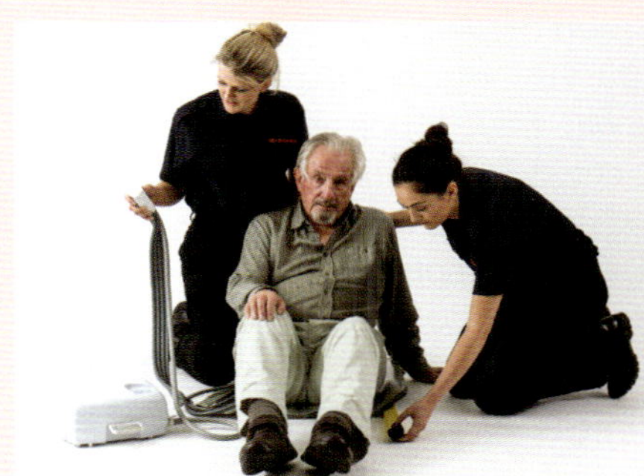

5. Roll the patient over onto the ELK until they are lying fully and squarely on the cushion. Unfurl the edge of the ELK, replace the stability bar and fit the end cap.

Procedure – *cont*

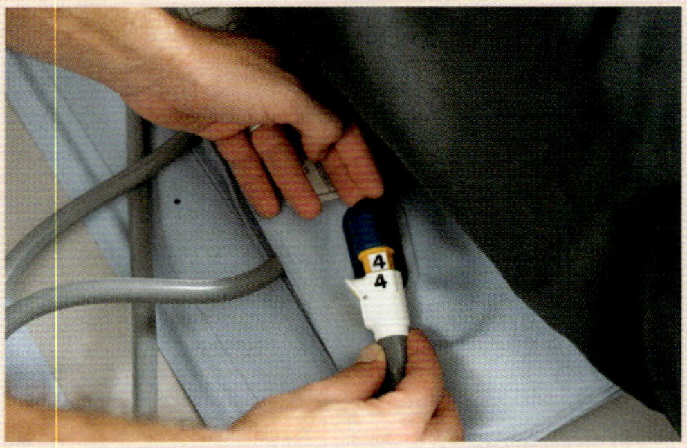

6. If not already completed, connect the four distribution hoses from the 4-way hand control to the four connectors on the ELK. The ends of the hoses are colour coded and numbered to match the corresponding ELK connectors (No. 4 is the top compartment; No. 1 the bottom). **Note**: If the fallen person is very large, it is recommended to connect the compressor and the hand control before the person is rolled onto the ELK.

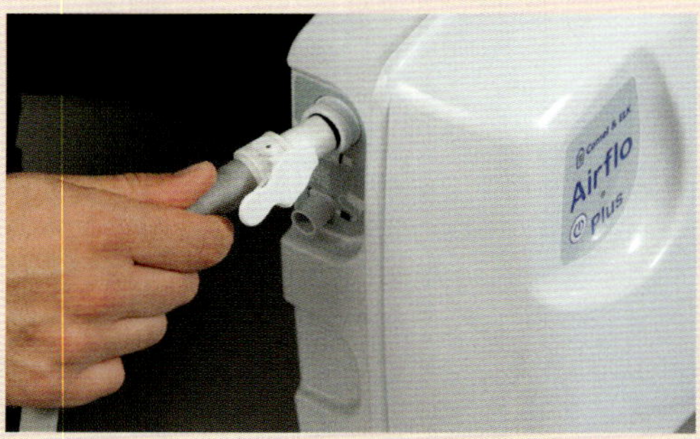

7. Position the Airflo compressor at the side of the ELK, ensuring that it will not be in the way while lifting and supporting the patient. Connect the hose from the 4-way hand control to the air outlet socket on the Airflo compressor and select the AUTO function on the Airflo compressor by pressing the power button until the LED light comes on.

Procedure – *cont*

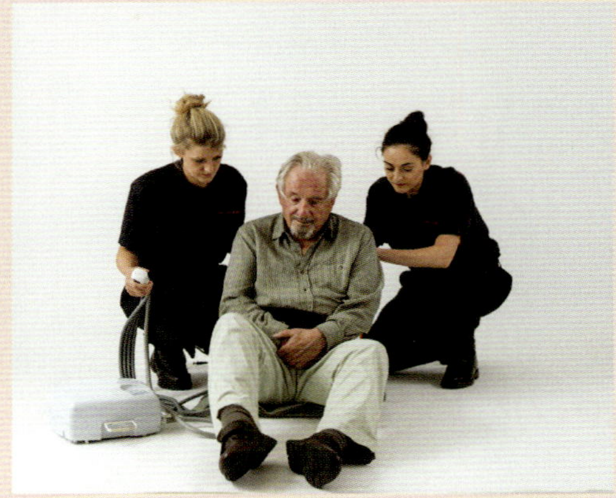

8. Kneeling beside the patient, place them in a seated position on the ELK. If necessary, place a transfer belt (with looped handles) around the patient's chest and adjust to fit. Explain to the patient what to expect when the ELK elevates.

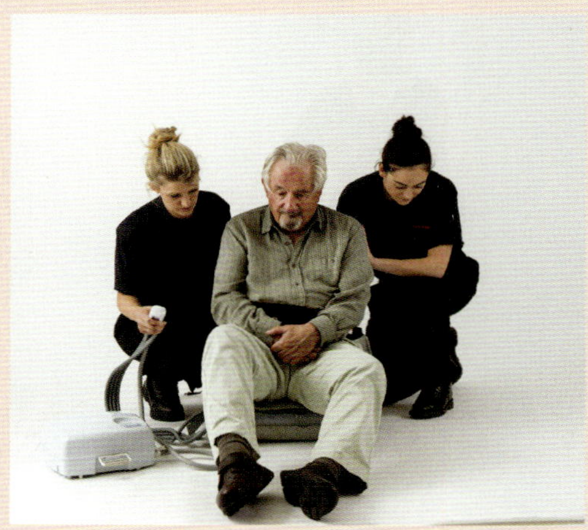

9. Press the number 1 button on the 4-way hand control. Steady the patient as the ELK lifts. Stop inflation when the first (bottom) compartment becomes hard. The compressor will automatically stop as each compartment becomes fully inflated.

Procedure – *cont.*

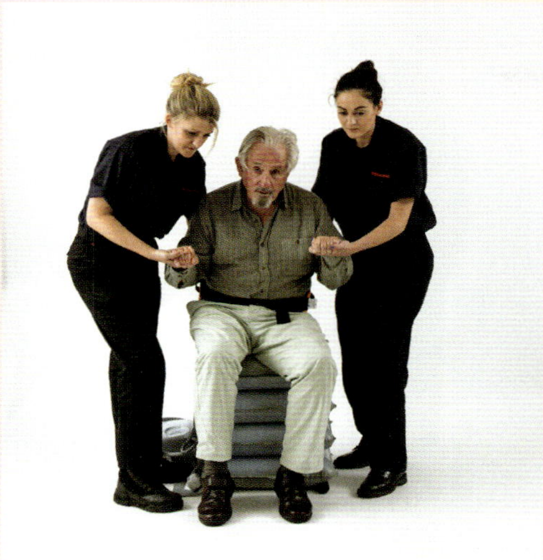

10. Continue to operate buttons 2, 3 and 4, in sequence, in exactly the same manner. Support the patient at all times. Always inflate the ELK sections from the bottom up. When all four compartments are inflated, the patient may be helped to stand or to transfer.

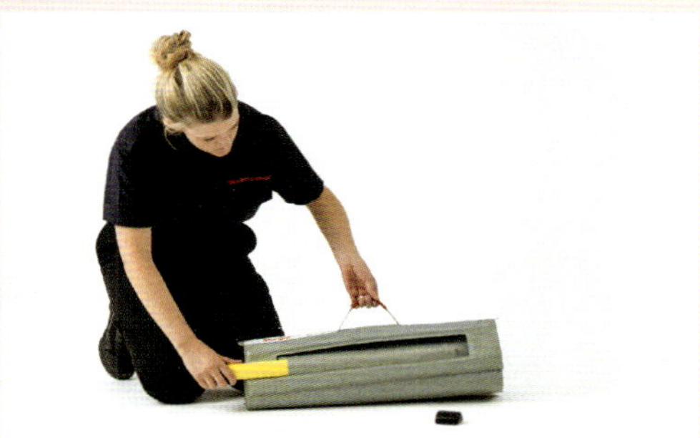

11. To deflate, disconnect each of the air hoses from the ELK. After use, roll the ELK up with the 4-way hand control and re-secure the flap around the ends of the stability bar.

Seated Patients

Many patients will be seated, on the toilet, a chair or their bed, when you need to either assist them to stand or transfer them onto a carry chair or ambulance trolley. As before, you should see what the patient is capable of as they may be able to stand with no or minimal assistance.

Sitting to Sitting Transfer

A transfer board (also called a banana board, on account of the curved shape and yellow colour of some boards) can enable the patient to transfer from a chair or bed onto the carry chair or vice versa. In order to use this technique, the patient must be able to (Smith, 2011b):

- flex forward and transfer their weight laterally
- place their feet on the floor
- place their arm towards the end of the board

and assist with movement across it.

A crew member can assist by bringing the patient's feet around and helping to transfer the patient's weight laterally. However, if the patient requires help with their feet and support to sit, then a second crew member should be used, preferably with a handling belt applied.

Procedure

Take the following steps to assist a patient to use a transfer board (Smith, 2011b; EEAST, 2014):

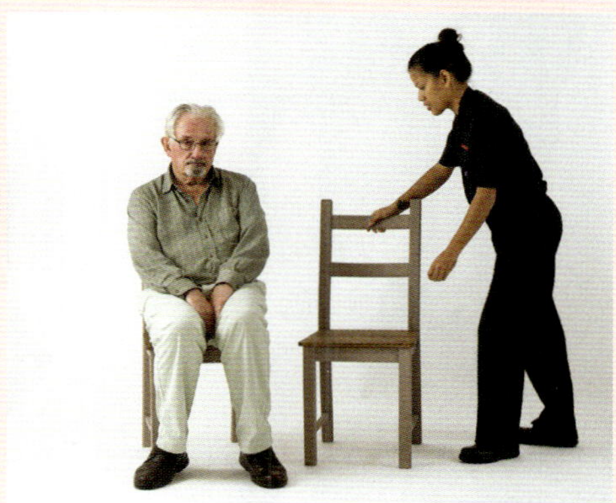

1. Explain the procedure to the patient and ensure they have suitable footwear. Place the destination chair at the correct angle (this will vary depending on the board used).

Procedure – *cont*

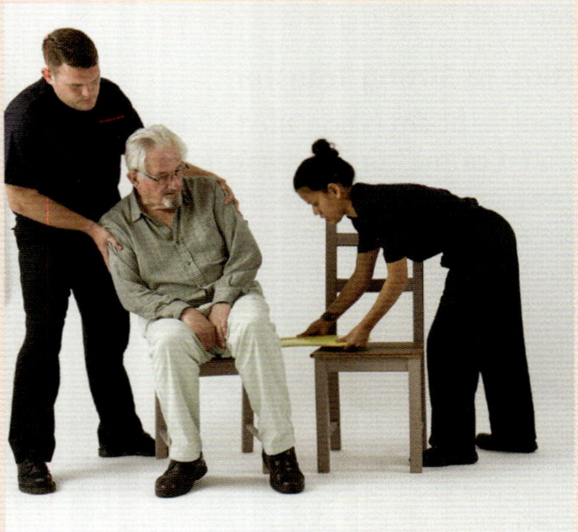

2. Ask the patient to lean away from the transfer side and insert about a third of the board under the patient's buttock. Ensure that a third of the board rests on the destination chair. Ensure the board is level.

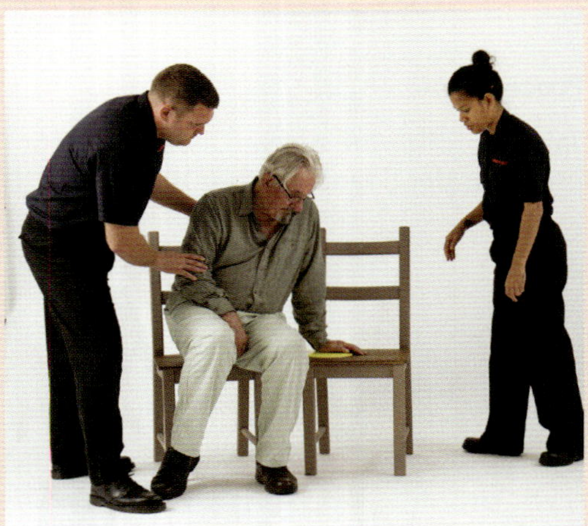

3. Instruct the patient to place their hand towards the far end of the board and lean towards it. Ensure the patient's fingers are not under the board.

Procedure – *cont*

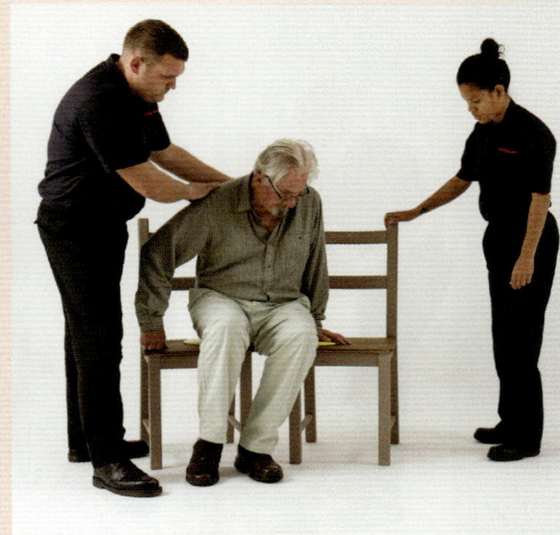

4. The patient should now shuffle across the board, using their other hand and feet to push. If they have reduced ability to push through their legs, use a turntable.

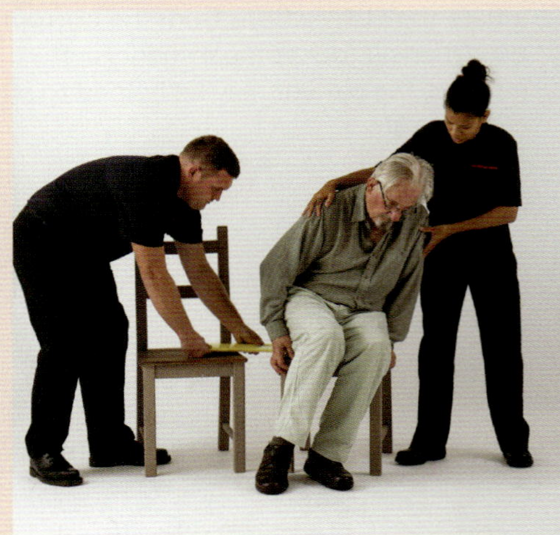

5. Once the patient has transferred onto the destination chair, they should be instructed to lean away from the board to allow its removal. Remove the turntable if used.

Sitting to Standing Transfer

Standing up out of a chair can be a challenge for some patients, even though they may be able to walk once they are upright.

Procedure

Take the following steps to assist a patient to transfer from a sitting position to standing (Smith, 2011b; EEAST, 2014):

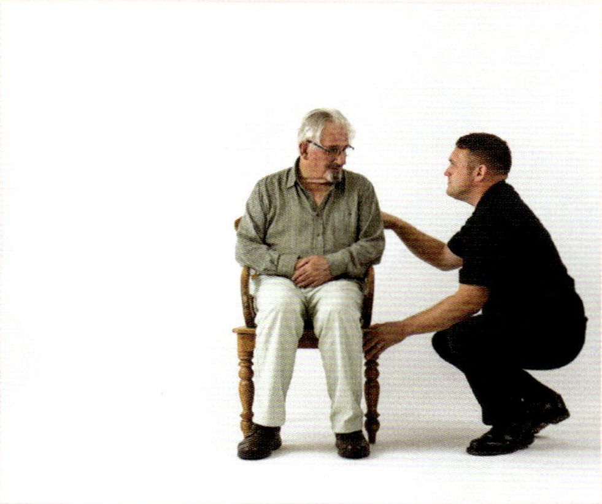

1. Explain the procedure to the patient and ensure they have suitable footwear. Instruct the patient to lean forward so that their back is off the back of the chair. Then instruct them to shuffle their bottom towards the front of the chair/edge of the bed and ensure that both of their feet are firmly on the floor.

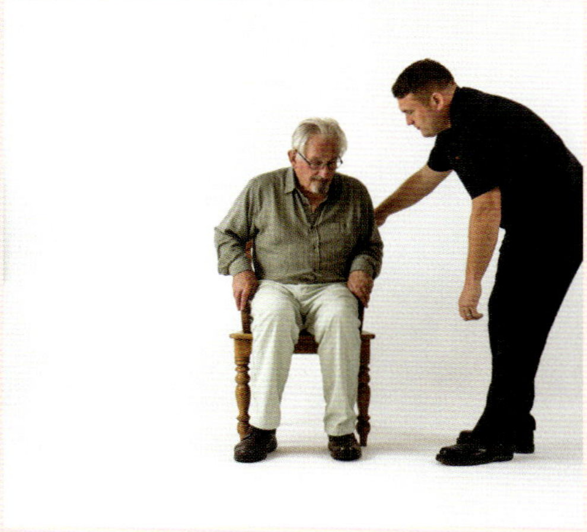

2. Instruct the patient to place their hands on the arms of the chair, or the mattress if on

Procedure – *cont*

a bed, or crew member's hands. Instruct the patient to lean forward so that their chin is over their knees and encourage them to look up and not at the floor. Instruct them that you will give the command 'Ready, steady, stand', and on 'stand', the patient should push up on the arms of the chair/mattress/crew member.

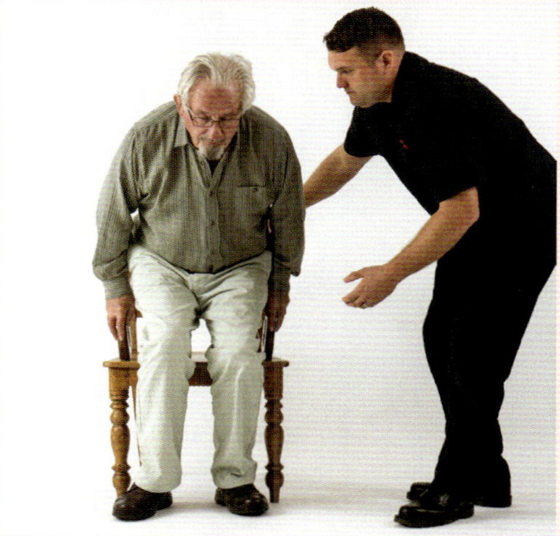

3. Alternatively, if there are no arms on the chair or the patient requires additional assistance, place a handling belt around the patient. Position yourself and another crew member either side of the patient, with your inside hand taking hold of the handling belt and your outer hand in a palm-to-palm hold (Figure 7.18). Instruct the patient as in Step 2.

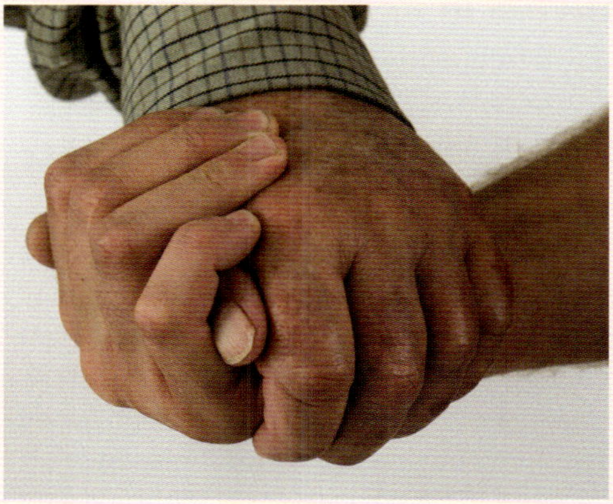

Figure 7.18 *Palm-to-palm hold.*

Procedure – *cont*

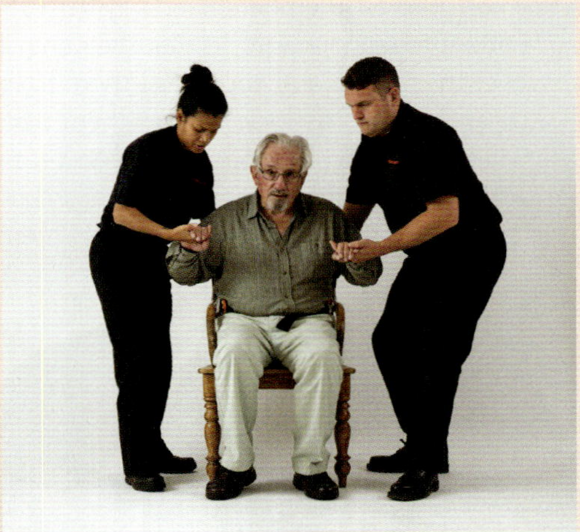

4. Give the command 'Ready, steady, stand'. If you are assisting the patient, a gentle rocking motion can help, and then on 'stand', move forward and then upwards with the patient as they stand.

5a. If the patient normally walks with a frame, provide this for them. It may help the patient's confidence if you walk slightly behind and to one side, with your hands just above their hips.

5b. Alternatively, two crew members can walk with the patient, taking care not to impede the patient's natural step and allowing them to move their feet in their own time.

Patients in Bed

You will frequently encounter patients in bed or on a hospital trolley who require transferring either from bed to ambulance trolley or bed to chair.

Patient Transfer Board

A patient transfer board is often available in hospitals and nursing homes to enable the transfer from bed to ambulance trolley and vice versa. An alternative is to use a hoist, if available and patient condition allows. As an emergency medical responder, it is likely you will be asked to assist in this procedure, though you should follow the instructions of those qualified in the use of the equipment.

Procedure

Take the following steps to transfer a patient from bed to trolley using a patient transfer board (NEAS, 2014):

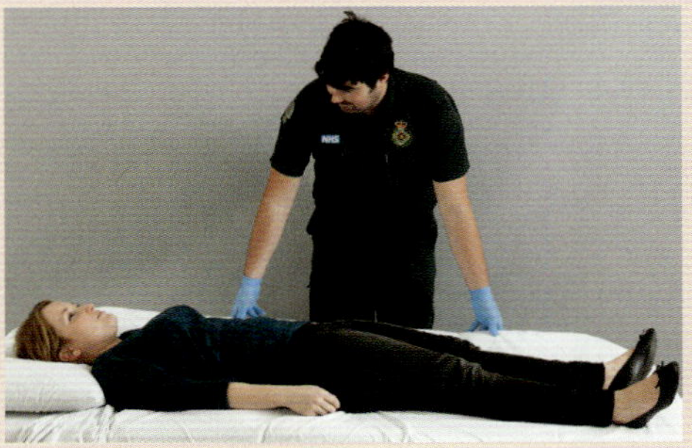

1. Explain the procedure to the patient and gain consent where possible. Place the ambulance trolley next to the bed.

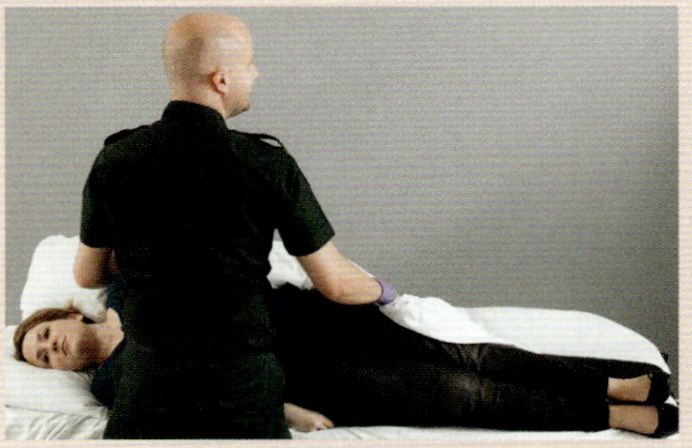

2. Using the sheet on the bed/trolley, one crew member should grip the sheet at the level of the patient's shoulders and roll the patient towards them.

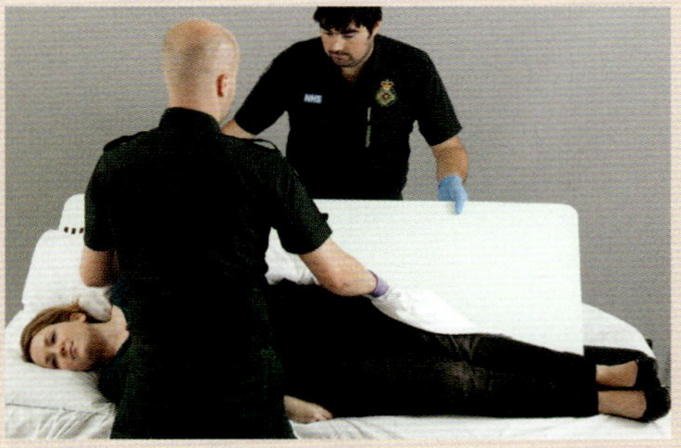

3. A second crew member can then position the board between the patient and the trolley.

Procedure – *cont*

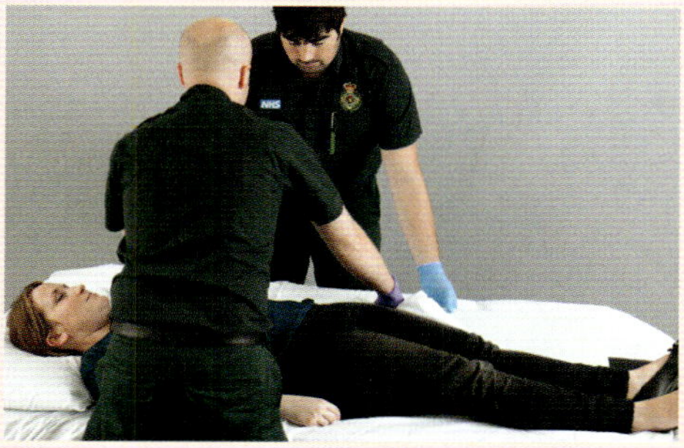

4. The first crew member lowers the patient onto their back, while the second maintains the position of the board. The patient's feet should be on the lower end of the sheet.

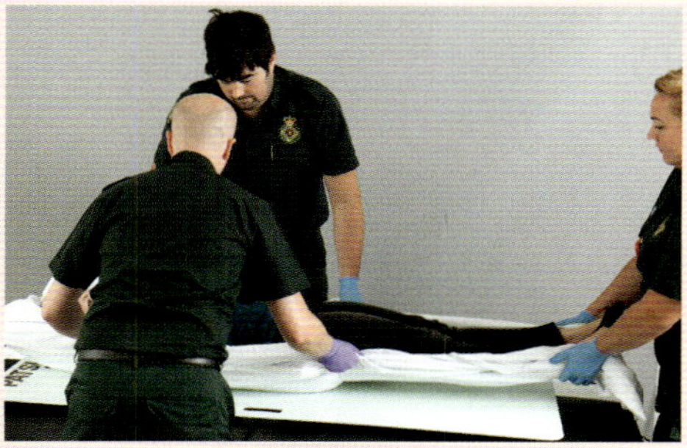

5. With both crew members gripping the sheet at the patient's shoulder and hip, slide the patient across the board and onto the trolley. Additional crew members are helpful to ensure that the patient's legs and feet transfer smoothly.

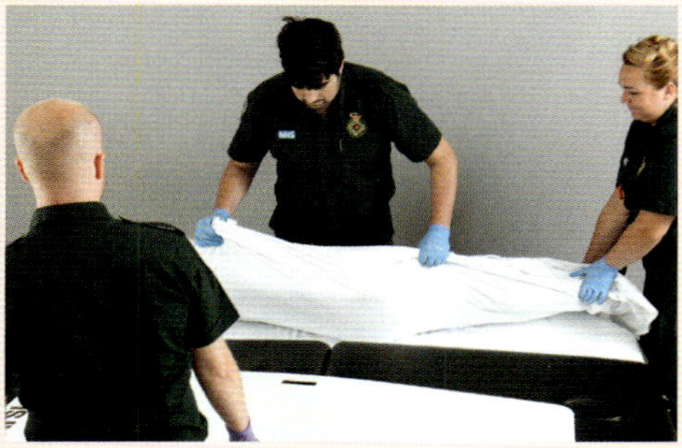

6. After ensuring the patient is centrally positioned, roll them to one side and remove the board.

Procedure – *cont*

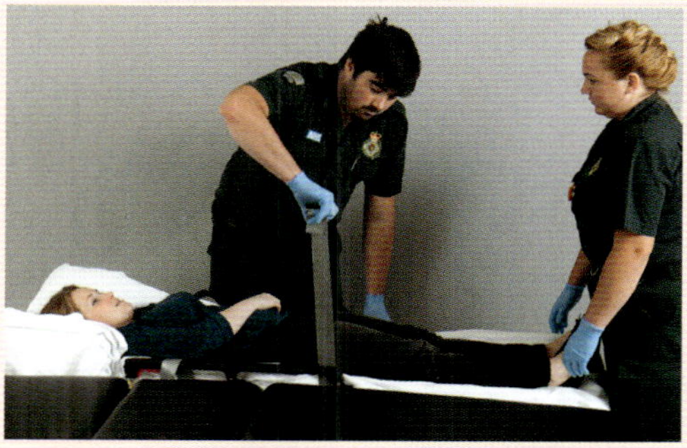

7. Roll the patient onto their back and secure them to the trolley. Don't forget to clean the board.

Carry Chair

The carry chair is an important manual handling aid, used by ambulance services as the primary method for transporting patients up and down stairs and into the ambulance. However, it is associated with a high risk of lower back injury when used to lift patients (Ferreira, 2005). In addition, the carry chair is not a wheelchair, so plan movements to keep the distance to be travelled to a minimum.

It is likely that you will be asked to assist the ambulance service in moving a patient who has been placed on a carry chair. Information on the use of the carry chair is included here, but you must remember to only use equipment you are familiar with, have been trained to use and are confident in.

Ferno Compact 2 Carry Chair

The procedure below relates to the Ferno Compact 2 carry chair, commonly found on ambulances. However, there are many models, including those with tracks to assist with descending stairs, so ensure you are appropriately trained, particularly in the lifting techniques required for these chairs, as they are not covered here.

Procedure

Take the following steps to prepare and transport a patient on the Ferno Compact 2 carry chair (EEAST, 2014):

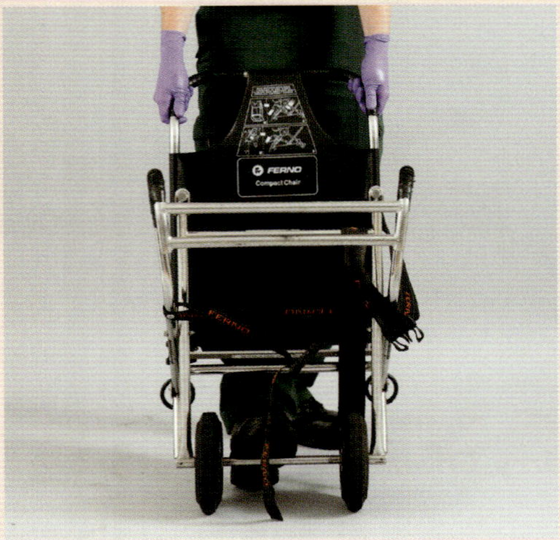

1. Unroll the carry chair by placing it on the ground. With your foot on the chair's foot bar, lift the back up and rearward.

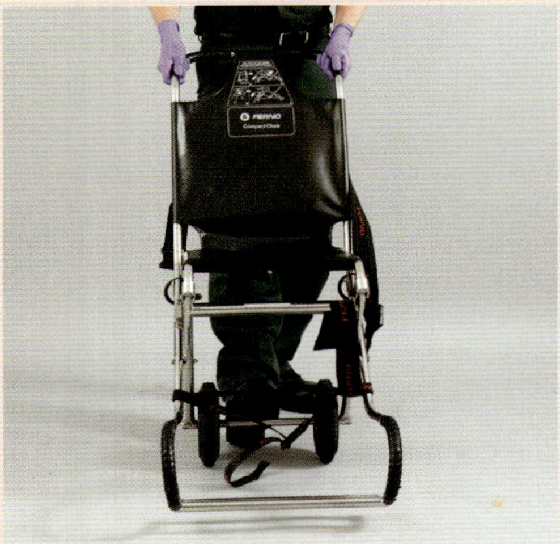

2. Completely unfold by firmly pushing up the back until a click is heard.

Procedure – *cont*

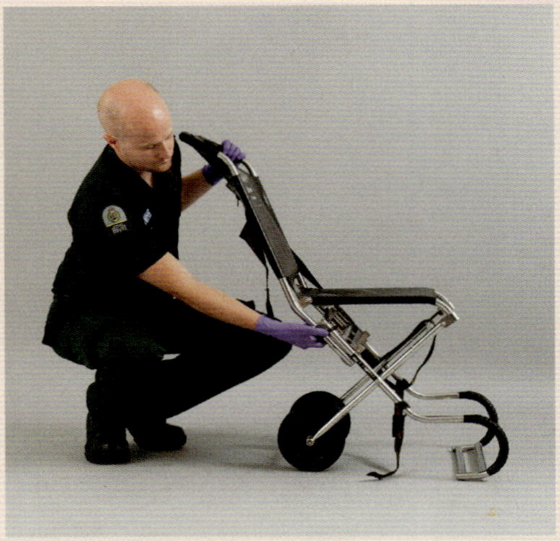

3. Once the chair is locked, move both of the safety rings down over the hinge brackets.

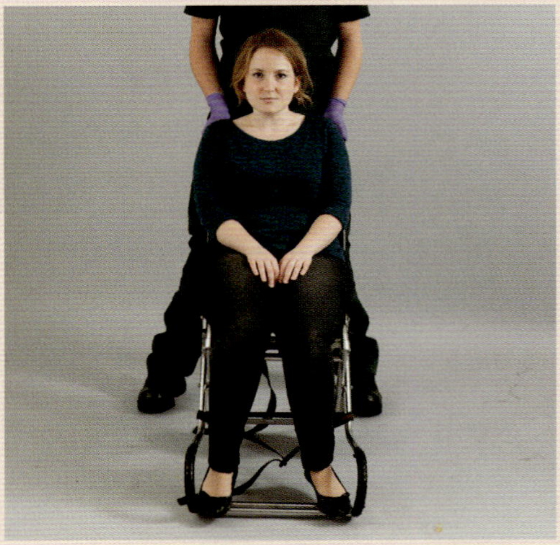

4. When a patient is on the carry chair, ensure that one crew member has a firm grip on the back of the chair at ALL times.

Procedure – *cont*

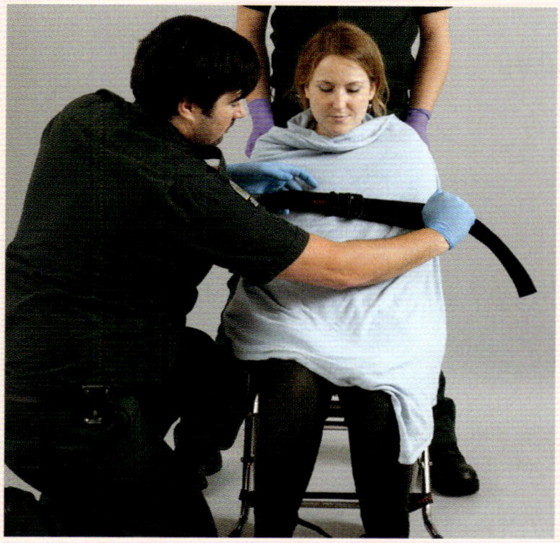

5. Secure the patient on the chair using the chest restraint. A leg restraint is also provided, which can be used if deemed necessary. Blankets can be used with the chair and are helpful for improving patient comfort, but ensure that they are kept clear of moving parts.

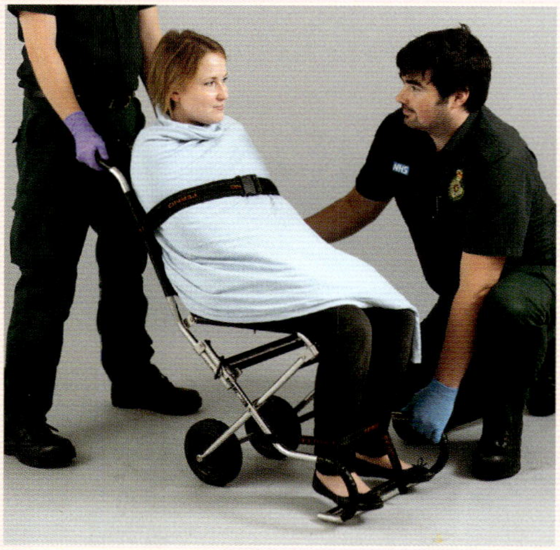

6. Once the patient is secured on the chair, crew members need to position themselves at the back and front of the chair. Instruct the patient not to grab out with their arms during the manoeuvre.

Procedure – *cont*

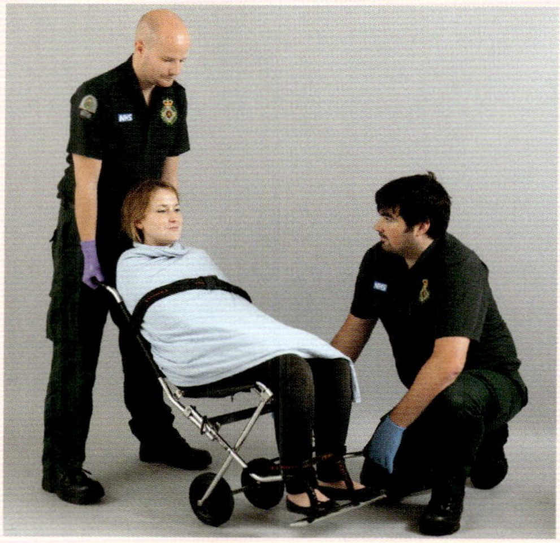

7. Explain to the patient that you are about to tip them backwards, but reassure them that they will not fall. The crew member at the back of the chair then tilts the chair backwards, until the weight of the chair and patient are balanced on the wheels. The chair can be rolled without lifting, but uneven terrain is likely to require the assistance of one or more additional crew members to ensure the chair does not tip over.

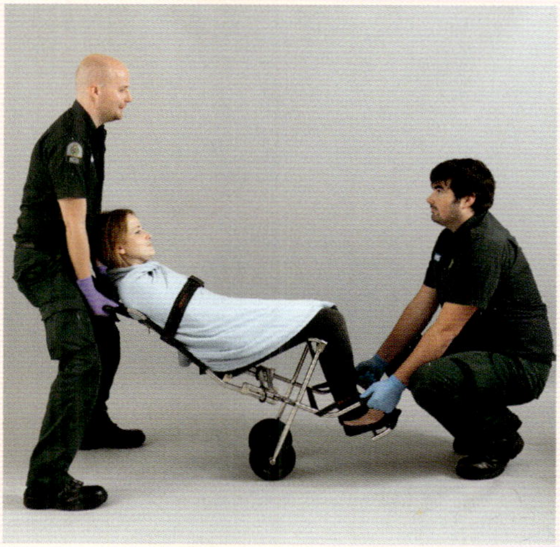

8. To carry the chair, it should be tilted backwards as before, and then crew members should grasp the front and back carrying handles and lift simultaneously.

Blanketing on a Carry Chair

Moving patients in a carry chair is very frequent in the pre-hospital setting and something you are likely to be asked to assist with. For patients, this can be a scary experience, as a carry chair feels unstable; if you have never been in one, try it out as part of your training.

One way to make the experience more pleasant is to securely wrap the patient up in blankets before moving them. This is particularly beneficial in cold or wet weather and the patient can stay wrapped in blankets all the way from their house to the emergency department, keeping them warm and comfortable.

Procedure

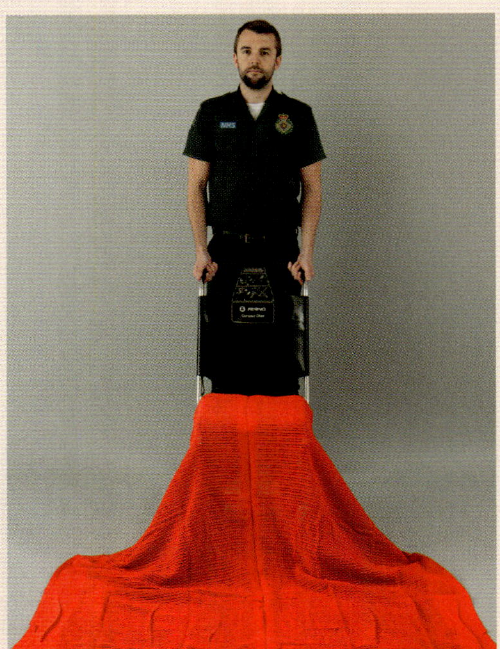

1. Setup the carry chair and get two blankets and a bed sheet. Place the first blanket on the bottom half of the chair with the longest edge of the blanket running vertically in line with the chair.

Procedure – *cont*

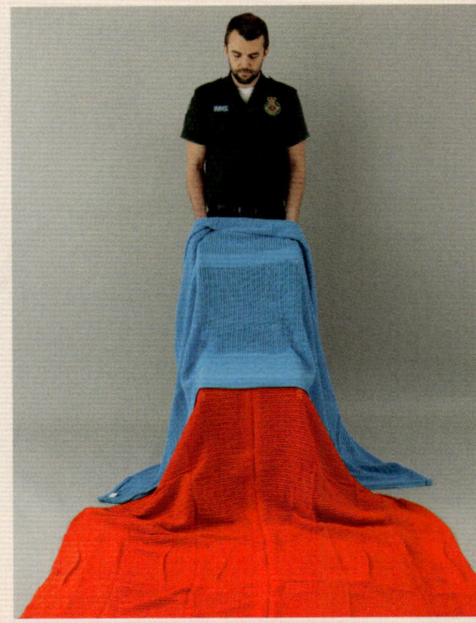

2. Place the next blanket across the top half of the chair with the longest edge running horizontally. The blanket should be slightly to one side so there is a shorter and a longer edge when wrapping around the front of the patient.

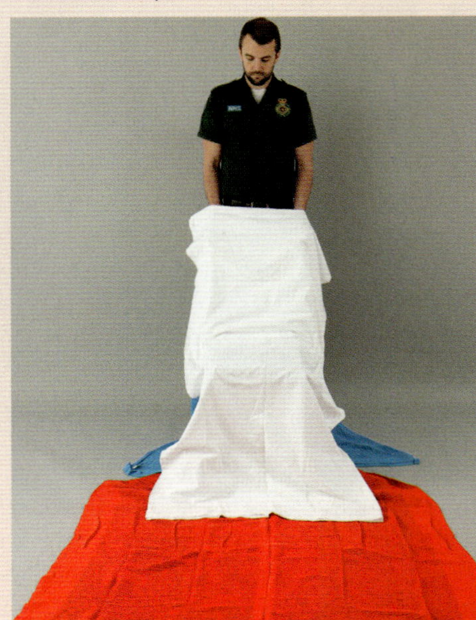

3. Place a bed sheet on top of the blankets.

Procedure – *cont*

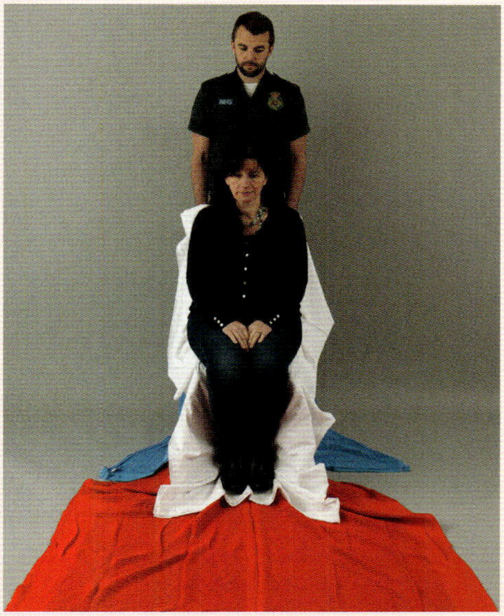

4. Assist the patient to sit in the chair. Make sure someone is holding the top of the chair whenever a patient is sitting in it.

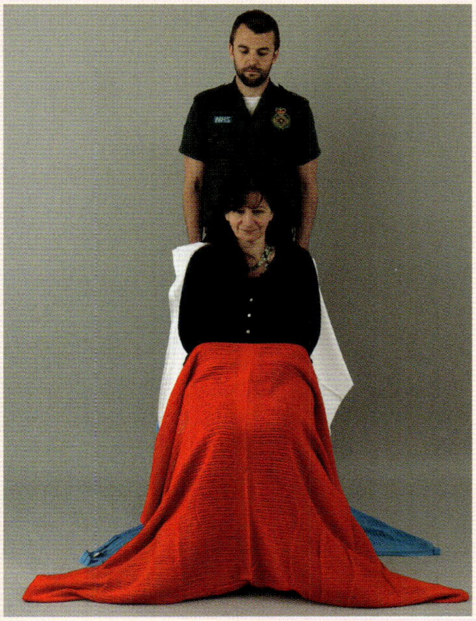

5. Fold the blanket up and over the patient's legs and onto their lap.

Procedure – *cont*

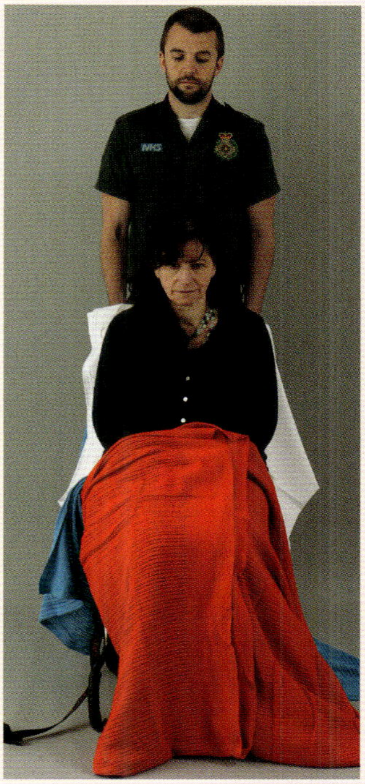

6. Fold the sides of the blanket neatly up into the middle. Make sure no excess blanket is left hanging loose as this can become trapped in the wheels when the patient is moved.

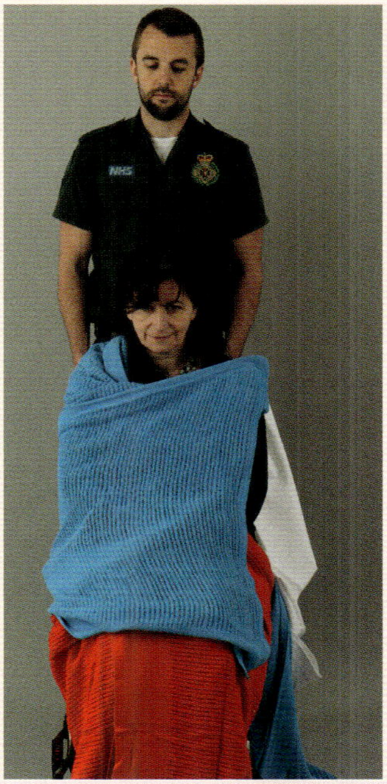

7. Once both sides of the lower blanket have been folded up, cross the upper blanket across the chest of the patient, starting with the shorter edge first.

Procedure – *cont*

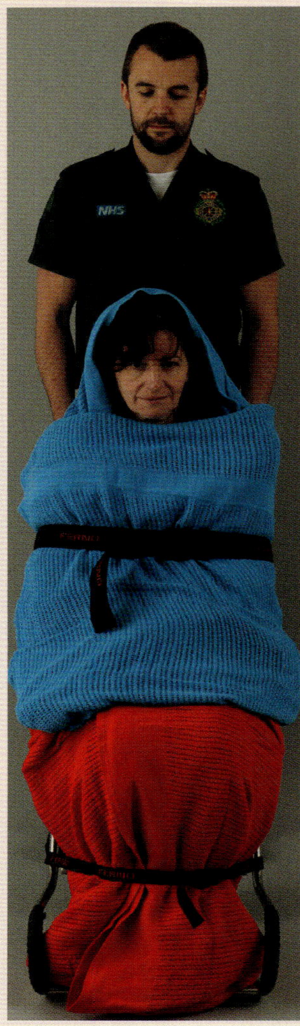

8. There should be enough blanket behind the patient's head to create a hood if needed. Remember to strap the patient in using both the chest and leg straps.

Ambulance Trolley

In your role, you may be asked to assist the ambulance service in moving a patient on an ambulance trolley or placing a patient on one and making them comfortable and secure. There are a wide range of ambulance trolleys available; in your area you may become familiar with those used by your local ambulance crews. Basic pre-shift checks common to most trolleys include the following (EEAST, 2014):

- Check that the mattress and restraining system (seat belts) are properly installed and functioning. Damaged mattresses present an infection control risk and should be replaced.
- Check that the trolley sides can be raised, lowered and locked in position.
- Check that the trolley can be raised and lowered satisfactorily.
- Check that the wheels and brakes of the trolley are effective.
- Ensure that the trolley locks properly into the ambulance locking device.
- If the trolley has push/pull handles, check their operation and stow them away.
- If the trolley has a headrest, check that it locks in position when attached to the trolley.

Trolley Positioning

Ambulance trolleys can be placed in a range of positions to improve patient comfort and clinical condition. The positions may need to be adopted and changed quickly as the patient's condition changes, so ensure you are familiar with how to place the trolley into and out of these positions.

Trolley Positions

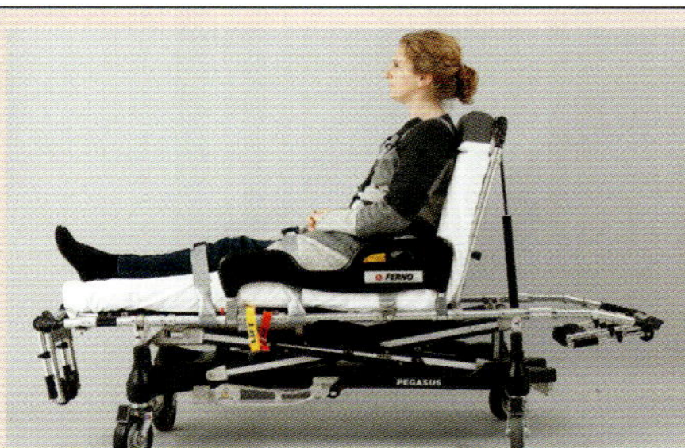	**Upright position**. This is preferred for patients with breathing problems.

<table>
<tr><td>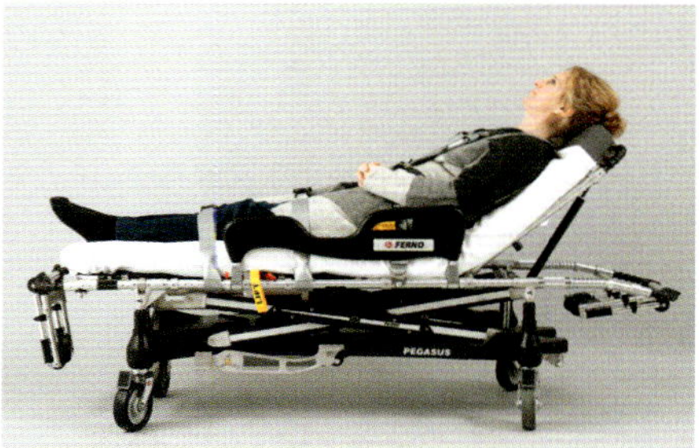</td><td>Semi-recumbent position. This consists of placing the patient's head and torso at an angle of 45°.</td></tr>
<tr><td>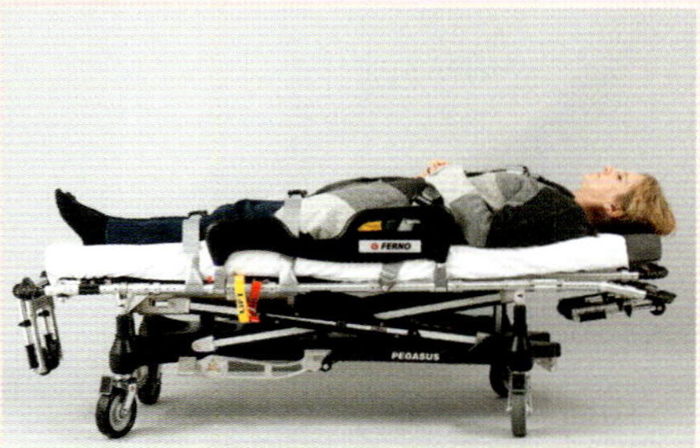</td><td>Recumbent position. This is the preferred position for patients with suspected spinal injuries and/or shock.</td></tr>
<tr><td>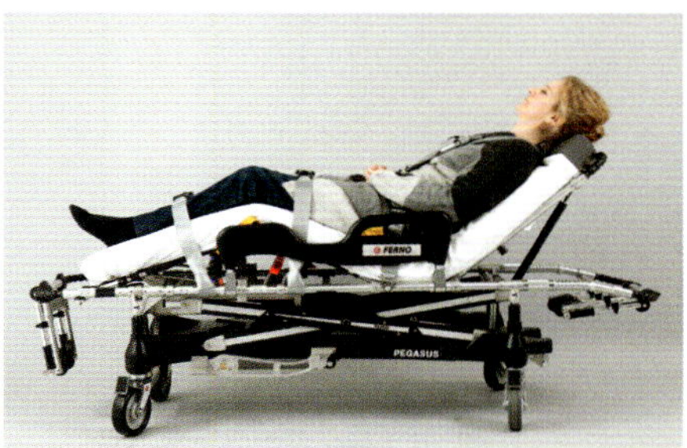</td><td>Fowler position. This position can help relieve tension on abdominal muscles, which may make abdominal illness and injuries less painful.</td></tr>
<tr><td>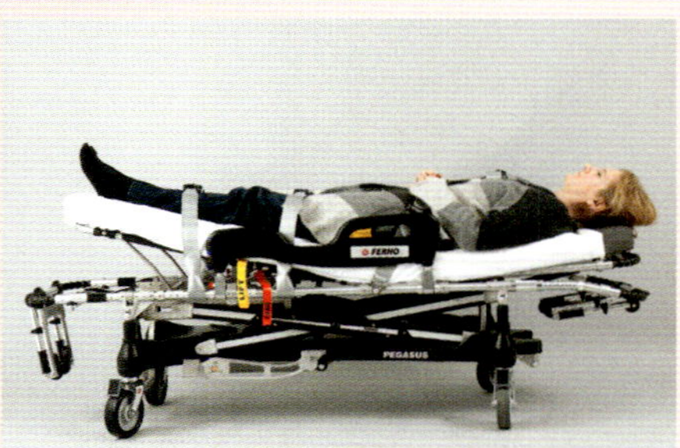</td><td>Lower limbs raised. This is helpful for controlling bleeding in lower leg injuries, and will increase cardiac output for several minutes in hypovolaemia (Geerts, 2012).</td></tr>
<tr><td>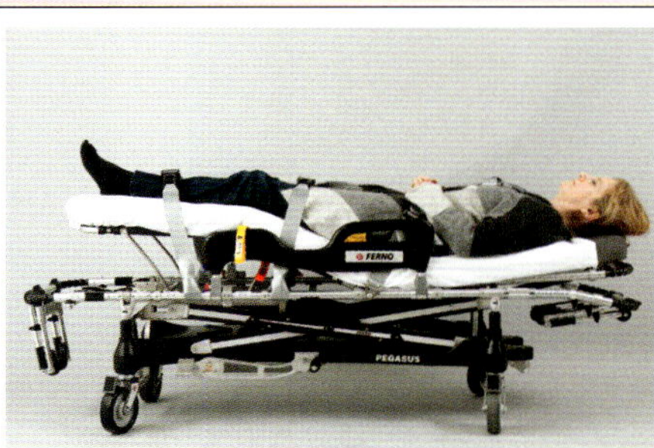</td><td>Trendelenburg. This position is frequently taught but has been found to have a temporary effect on blood pressure and no effect on cardiac output. In addition, this position may aggravate an already impaired ventilatory function due to the weight of the abdominal contents resting on the diaphragm. It may also increase intracranial pressure in patients with a traumatic brain injury (NAEMT, 2014; Peña, 2012; Johnson, 2004).</td></tr>
</table>

Chapter 8

Drug Administration

Drug Legislation and Guidelines

Learning Objectives

By the end of this section you will be able to:

- Identify relevant legislation and clinical guidelines relating to the administration of medication.
- List several routes of administration for medication.
- Explain your role in the checking and administering of medication.

Introduction

You will frequently administer drugs to patients in your role as an emergency medical responder, particularly oxygen. It is important to remember that any drugs you do administer must be done so in accordance with the policies and procedures set out by the service medical director. However, you have a responsibility to ensure that the necessary checks are carried out prior to drug administration.

Legislation and Guidelines

The two key pieces of legislation relating to the administration of medicines are:

- Medicines Act 1968
- Misuse of Drugs Act 1971.

Both have been amended since their introduction. However, other legislation also relevant when discussing medicines includes the Control of Substances Hazardous to Health Regulations 2002 and the Health and Safety at Work etc. Act 1974, but these are not explored further here.

Medicines Act 1968

Under this Act, medicines are classified into three types (Pilbery, 2013):

- General Sales List medicines (GSL): These can be sold to the public and do not require a prescription or the supervision of a pharmacist
- Pharmacy medicines (P): These can only be sold under the supervision of a pharmacist
- Prescription-only medicines (POM): These medicines require a prescription from an appropriate practitioner, such as a doctor or non-medical prescriber.

It is likely that some of the drugs (medicines) that you are authorised to administer fall into the POM category. However, certain drugs can be administered in emergency situations, such as adrenaline (JRCALC, 2016).

Routes of Administration

Drugs can be administered to patients via a number of routes. These are typically divided into two types: parenteral and non-parenteral.

Parenteral routes require the skin or mucous membranes to be breached, such as by an intravenous, intramuscular, intraosseous or subcutaneous injection. Non-parenteral routes rely on passive absorption of the drug, such as by inhalation, nebulisation, oral, rectal, sublingual, buccal, transdermal or intranasal administration (JRCALC, 2016).

Drug Administration

Prior to the administration of any drug, check the following (JRCALC, 2016; Pilbery, 2013):

- The patient is not **allergic** to the drug about to be administered
- It is the **correct** drug
- The **dose** of the drug required
- The **presentation** of the drug, including its concentration (e.g. 4 mg in 2 ml) and the container it comes in (e.g. ampoule, tablet, prefilled syringe)
- Whether the **packaging** is intact
- If it is a fluid, the **clarity** (except for intravenous diazepam, which comes as a milky-white emulsion)
- The **expiry** date.

Administering Medication to Patients

Learning Objectives

By the end of this section you will be able to:

- Explain the procedure to prepare and administer medication by the following routes:
    - Oral
    - Sublingual
    - Nebuliser.

Administering Oral Medication

The majority of your patients' medication at home will be taken orally. Oral medication comes in a variety of forms including tablets, capsules, lozenges and syrups.

Procedure

Take the following steps to administer oral medication (Pilbery, 2013; Gregory, 2010b):

1. Take standard precautions
2. Ensure consent has been obtained
3. Check the drug:
    - Correct drug
    - Correct dose
    - In date
    - Intact packaging
4. Check that the patient is not allergic to the drug
5. Avoid touching the medication, unless the patient is not capable of self-administering. Ensure you are wearing gloves in this case
6. Present it to the patient with clear instructions:
    - Most oral medication can be swallowed, except aspirin, which should be chewed or dissolved first
7. Provide water, if indicated and permitted
8. Ensure the administration is documented.

Administering Sublingual Medication

If you are authorised to administer drugs via the sublingual route, follow the procedure outlined below.

Procedure

Take the following steps to administer sublingual medication (Pilbery, 2013):

1. Take standard precautions
2. Ensure consent has been obtained
3. Check the drug:
    - Correct drug
    - Correct dose
    - In date
    - Intact packaging
4. Check that the patient is not allergic to the drug
5. Explain the procedure to the patient
6. Ask the patient to place the tip of their tongue on the roof of their mouth and hold their breath
7. Hold the drug container close to the patient's mouth (your thumb should be almost touching the patient's chin) and aim the spray at the underside of their tongue
8. Press down on the top of the drug container once
9. Ask the patient to close their mouth and not to inhale the spray
10. After a few seconds remind the patient to breathe freely again
11. Ensure the administration is documented.

Administering Nebulised Drugs

Nebulisers enable drugs to be inhaled. In the ambulance service, this will usually be salbutamol and ipratropium for patients suffering from asthma, chronic obstructive pulmonary disease and expiratory wheeze due to allergy, anaphylaxis or smoke inhalation, for example (JRCALC, 2016).

Procedure

Take the following steps to administer drugs via a nebuliser (Pilbery, 2013; Gregory, 2010b):

1. Take standard precautions
2. Obtain consent if possible
3. Check the medication:
   - Correct drug
   - Correct dose
   - Expiry date
   - Integrity of packaging
4. Add medication into the chamber. This may involve unscrewing the two parts of the nebuliser (figure 8.1)

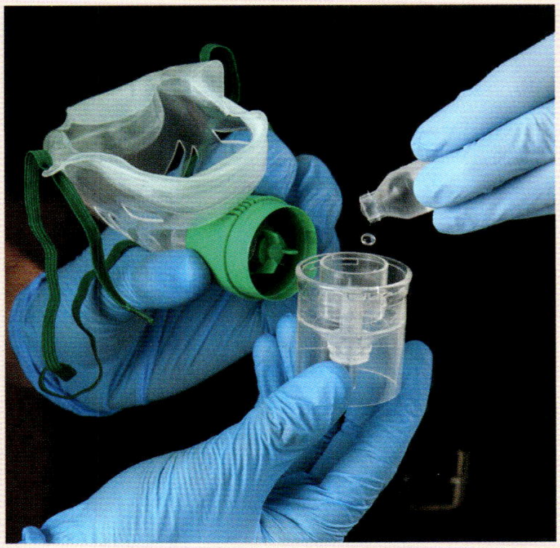

Figure 8.1 *Adding medication to the nebuliser chamber*

Procedure – *cont*

5. Connect the nebuliser to the oxygen source and set the flow rate to 6–8 l/min. A fine mist should be generated
6. Place the mask over the patient's face and adjust the elastic to make a good seal
7. Coach the patient's breathing. They should breathe in slowly and deeply and aim to hold their breath for 3–5 seconds before breathing out again
8. Ensure the administration is documented.

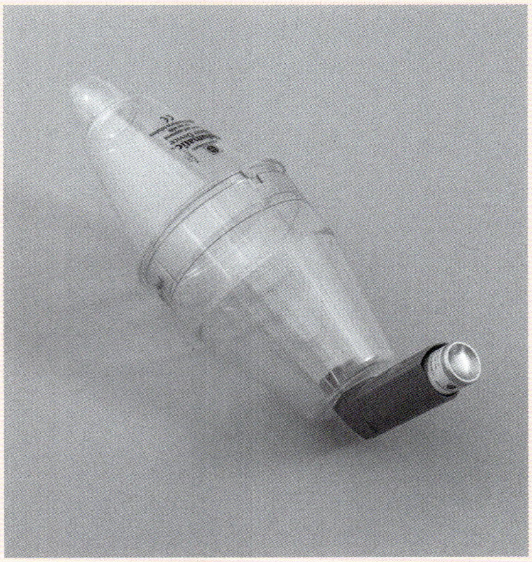

Figure 8.2 *An inhaler and spacer.*

Note that the administration of drugs such as salbutamol with the patient's own inhaler is as effective as a nebuliser if they use a spacer (Figure 8.2). This is particularly true of children (BTS/SIGN, 2016).

Chapter 9

Scene Assessment

Scene Assessment and Safety

Learning Objectives

By the end of this section you will be able to:

- Outline and explain the parts of an initial scene assessment when acting in a casualty care role.
- Explain the importance of ensuring scene safety prior to approaching any incident for:
    - patients
    - yourself
    - your colleagues
    - bystanders.

Introduction

As a firefighter, you will already be very experienced at assessing and managing dangerous scenes, and those skills are not going to be repeated here. Your service will have multiple policies and procedures in place for the assessment and management of scenes based on your fire and rescue role. However, as a casualty carer, you may also have additional responsibilities.

The assessment of the scene from a casualty care perspective may include different elements, and you should be aware of what your colleagues from the ambulance service and other pre-hospital emergency care services may be considering so you can work with them effectively.

This chapter outlines the assessment and management of a scene with emphasis on casualty care, but at an actual incident you may have to mix this with your firefighter role, depending on how you are deployed.

To help you cover the essential aspects of a scene assessment, consider using the SCENE mnemonic (JRCALC, 2016):

- **S**: safety
- **C**: cause including the nature of illness (NOI) or mechanism of injury (MOI)
- **E**: environment
- **N**: number of patients
- **E**: extra resources needed.

Safety

You should consider how you will maximise safety at scene for you, the casualty and others present. Sometimes this may mean that casualty care must be delayed ensuring that further injuries are not sustained by those attempting to help.

To reduce risks, you should undertake a dynamic risk assessment (DRA), which is something you should be familiar with already. DRA underpins subsequent decision making and is focused on thinking before you act, and not the other way around (Asbury, 2014). See Figure 9.1 for an example of a DRA model.

Cause

Although you are likely to have been given some details about the incident or call you are attending, you should not be completely led by this. Establishing the presenting complaint from the patient's perspective will come later in the assessment process, but you may be able to determine what has happened from the scene, particularly in trauma cases, such as when viewing the wreckage of two cars that have collided. However, it is important to keep an open mind even at this stage. For example, although you are attending a road traffic collision, your patient may have suffered from a medical problem, such as a cardiac arrest, which led to their losing control of the car. Conversely, a medical-sounding call, such as a patient with low blood sugar, may also have a traumatic component if, for example, they fell and injured themselves as a result (Pilbery, 2013).

In trauma cases, find out about the mechanism of injury (MOI), which you will cover in Chapter 17: Trauma Emergencies. Knowledge of the MOI can assist in determining what injuries may have been sustained. Equally, for medical patients, establishing the nature of illness (NOI) can assist with the diagnosis, particularly in cases where bystander and/or patient information is limited (for example if the patient was discovered unresponsive). Clues from the scene, for example medical equipment

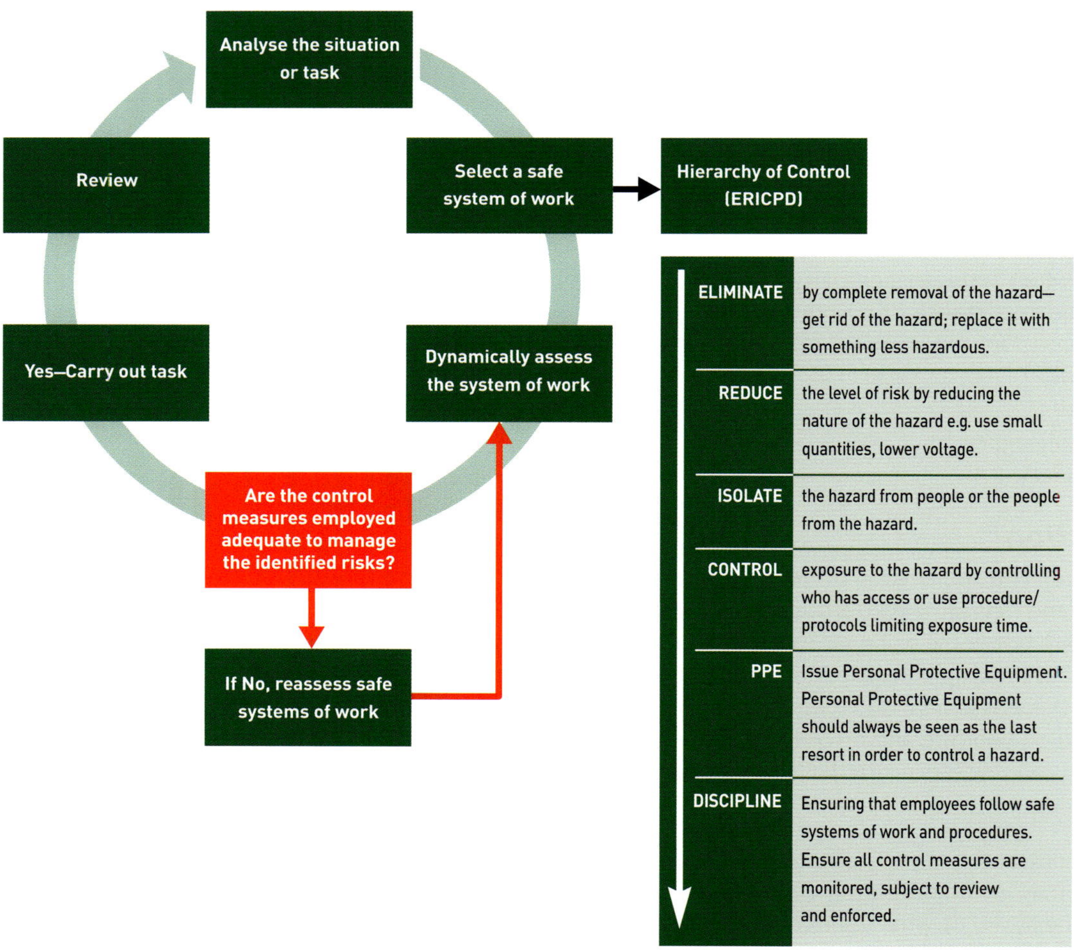

Figure 9.1 *Dynamic risk assessment model.*
Source: National Ambulance Resilience Unit (NARU), National Ambulance Service Command and Control Guidance (October 2015)

such as home oxygen or hoists, medication and/or care notes, may provide clues as to the underlying problem (Bledsoe, 2014).

Environment

Consider whether there are any environmental factors that need to be taken into account. These may complicate your extrication by affecting access to and from the scene and/or increase the risk of harm to the patient due to the development of hypothermia, for example. Incidents involving water can be hazardous for patient and crew alike. Terrain may be an issue, particularly if the patient is located well away from roads that are suitable for an ambulance. In these cases, helicopters and/or mountain rescue teams can prove useful.

Other risky environments include confined spaces, where there may be a risk of low levels of oxygen and/or the presence of toxic/explosive substances or, in the case of buildings or other structures, further collapse. These require specialist equipment and rescue knowledge. This additional support may come from fire service urban search and rescue teams (USAR) or ambulance hazardous area response teams (HART) (Bledsoe, 2014). Where possible it should be a mixture of both working collaboratively.

Number of Patients

Determine the number of patients early on in your assessment to help you decide whether you can manage the scene on your own. It may also help to identify patients who have either wandered off from the scene or who have been ejected from a vehicle, for example, and are currently hidden from view.

In addition, since most acts of terrorism are covert (i.e. there is often no prior knowledge of the time, location or nature of the attack), it is possible that you could be responding first to the aftermath of a terrorist attack. In these cases, the number of patients involved may provide the most important indication that a chemical, biological, radiological, nuclear, explosive (CBRNE) event has occurred (Pilbery, 2013). In these cases, you should use the STEP 1-2-3 Plus method (JESIP, 2013):

Step 1: One casualty and no obvious reason. Approach using normal procedures.

Step 2: Two casualties and no obvious reason. Approach with caution, consider all options. Provide a report on arrival to the emergency operations centre (EOC).

Step 3: Three or more casualties in close proximity and no obvious reason. Use caution and follow Plus, the Joint Emergency Services Interoperability Principles (JESIP) first responder flowchart.

Extra Resources

Depending on the number of patients, the severity of their injuries and the nature of the incident, you may need additional help and/or equipment from other emergency services. For example, you may require the police to keep a scene safe, or additional ambulances, including the air ambulance, for patient transport. Don't forget others, such as the coastguard, mountain rescue, utility and public transport companies. Request help early, as it may take time for messages to be passed on and the relevant staff to arrive on scene.

Major Incidents

Learning Objectives

By the end of this section you will be able to:

- Explain the term 'emergency preparedness, resilience and response'.
- Define the terms 'major incident' and 'interoperability'.
- Describe the following EPRR models:
  - the Joint Decision Model
  - the Dynamic Risk Assessment.
- State the ambulance service responsibilities with regard to a major incident.
- State who can declare a major incident.
- Describe the potential roles for ambulance officers on scene.
- State the role of strategic, tactical and operational commanders.
- Explain the principles of triage sieve and sort.

Introduction

Emergency

According to the Civil Contingencies Act 2004 an emergency is defined as:

- an event or situation which threatens serious damage to human welfare in a place in the UK
- an event or situation which threatens serious damage to the environment of a place in the UK
- war, or terrorism, which threatens serious damage to the security of the UK.

To distinguish the latter definition of emergency from the regular emergency work of the ambulance service, the term used most often is 'major incident'.

Fire and rescue services and National Health Service (NHS) ambulance services are both classed as category 1 (primary) responders under the Civil Contingencies Act 2004. As such, these organisations are expected to have plans in place to prevent emergencies, and to reduce, control and mitigate emergencies once they occur (NARU, 2015). In addition, business continuity arrangements also need to be in place to ensure services are maintained to patients even in the event of disruptions, such as severe weather or an IT failure, for example. Collectively, all these activities fall under the umbrella term emergency preparedness, resilience and response (EPRR) (NHS England, 2015).

Interoperability and JESIP

Introduction to Interoperability

Interoperability is the extent to which organisations can work together effectively to achieve a joint aim. This requires planning that anticipates emergency management and incident response contingencies and challenges, but is essential if emergency service personnel are to work effectively with colleagues within their own and other services (NARU, 2015).

To support this, in 2012 the Joint Emergency Services Interoperability Principles (JESIP) was launched to improve the way emergency services work together at multi-agency incidents (JESIP, 2017).

The JESIP Principles

Under the interoperability framework, there are five main working principles of improving interoperability, which are (JESIP, 2017):

- **Co-locate**: Commanders of each service should be brought together to a single, safe and easily identified location near the scene.
- **Communicate**: Clear communication in plain English (avoiding jargon and service specific terms).
- **Co-ordinate**: Commanders need to agree on the lead service, identify priorities, resources and capabilities in order to mount an effective response to the incident.
- **Jointly understand risk**: Share information about the likelihood and impact of threats and hazards and agree measures to control risk.
- **Shared situational awareness**: Use tools such as the joint decision model and METHANE.

The Joint Decision Model

The joint decision model is a standard decision-making process used by commanders from different agencies to bring together available information, reconcile objectives and make effective decisions (Figure 9.2).

METHANE Communication Model

Historically, different services have used different models to communicate key information at the scene of a major incident, but now, under the

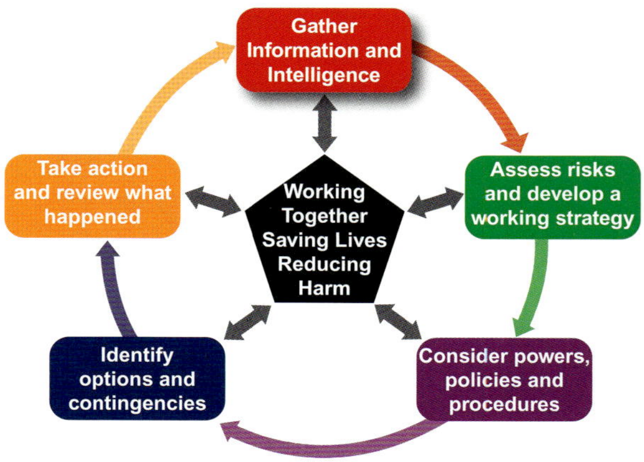
Gather Information and Intelligence
Assess risks and develop a working strategy
Consider powers, policies and procedures
Identify options and contingencies
Take action and review what happened
Working Together Saving Lives Reducing Harm

Figure 9.2 *JESIP joint decision-making model.*
Source: National Ambulance Resilience Unit (NARU), National Ambulance Service Command and Control Guidance (October 2015)

doctrine of joint working established by JESIP, all emergency personnel are encouraged to use the same communication model: METHANE (JESIP, 2017).

The mnemonic METHANE is designed to provide the initial communication surrounding details of the major incident. It consists of (NARU, 2015):

- **Major incident declared or standby**: The person making the report should be explicit whether this is a major incident declaration or a standby in anticipation of the occurrence of a major incident.
- **Exact location of the incident**: Where possible the grid reference or GPS co-ordinates should be included, along with any landmarks or iconic sites.
- **Type of incident**: What is the exact nature of the incident? For example, rail, chemical, road or terrorist.
- **Hazards**: What hazards are known to be present or could potentially manifest themselves?
- **Access and egress**: What are the agreed or best routes to and from the scene?
- **Number of casualties**: How many casualties are there and, if possible to determine, what are the level and severity of injuries?
- **Emergency services**: Which emergency services are present and which are required? Include specialist resource request if known.

Classification of Incidents

Major, Mass and Catastrophic Incidents

NHS organisations and ambulance services are required to develop emergency preparedness arrangements for three levels of incident involving casualties (DoH, 2007a):

- **Major**: Involving tens of patients and handled by individual trusts. An example is the London Bridge Attack on 3 June, 2017.
- **Mass**: Involving hundreds of patients and requiring mutual aid response from neighbouring trusts. An example would be the 7 July, 2005 London bombings.
- **Catastrophic**: Involving thousands of patients and severely disrupting health and social care and other support functions. An example would be the Great East Japan Earthquake on 11 March, 2011.

Types of Incident

Major incidents are often divided into a number of types (SWAST, 2014a; EEAST, 2013):

- **Big bang**: A serious transport accident, explosion or series of smaller incidents.
- **Rising tide**: A developing infectious disease epidemic, or a capacity/staffing crisis.
- **Cloud on the horizon**: A serious threat, such as a major chemical or nuclear release, developing elsewhere and needing preparatory action.
- **Headline news**: Public or media alarm about a personal threat.
- **Internal incidents**: Fire, breakdown of utilities, major equipment failure, hospital acquired infections, violent crime and internal security issues.
- **Deliberate**: Release of chemical, biological, radiological, nuclear and explosive (CBRNE) materials.
- **Mass casualties**
- **Pre-planned major events** that require planning: Demonstrations, sports fixtures, air shows.

Role of the Ambulance Service

NHS ambulance trusts have the responsibility for alerting, mobilising and co-ordinating the medical response to short notice or sudden impact emergencies. This includes (NARU, 2015):

- initiating and maintaining a Command and Control System to provide appropriate support and guidance to all NHS responders and other agencies
- co-ordinating all NHS communications on scene
- managing the health, safety and welfare of all NHS responders
- providing casualty triage, treatment and transport, including the selection of appropriate receiving hospitals
- provision of specialist incident response capabilities, including hazardous area working, decontamination of casualties and active shooter incidents.

During a major incident, the response of the ambulance service revolves around seven key principles (Mackway-Jones, 2012):

- **Command and control**: Each emergency service on scene has an incident commander, but the police usually take overall command.

- **Safety**: Personal safety is paramount and the appropriate personal protective equipment (PPE) must be worn. This does not always happen when crews are faced with a major incident. Of particular concern are hazardous materials or CBRNE incidents.
- **Communication**: This is the most common failing at major incidents (Mackway-Jones, 2012; JCO, 2010a). The terrestrial trunk radio (TETRA) network should in theory alleviate some of the problems that have occurred in the past, but the use of runners should be considered if required.
- **Assessment**: A rapid initial assessment of the scene can provide an estimate of the number of those injured and the severity of their injuries. This can be refined as the incident unfolds.
- **Triage**: The dynamic process by which casualties are sorted into priorities for treatment. It needs to be repeated frequently.
- **Treatment**: 'Do the most for the most' is the standard mantra. This depends on skills of the providers, severity of injuries and time on scene. The nature of the environment and casualty load may restrict the ability of the providers to give 'gold standard' care.
- **Transport**: Most patients will probably be transported to hospital by ambulance, but alternative methods of transport can be used. The aim is to get the right patient to the right place at the right time.

Incident Command and Control

The ambulance service employs a three-tier command system comprising a strategic commander, tactical commander and an operational commander. This is a hierarchical system whereby individuals are empowered through their role within the structure, providing them with specific authority over others for the duration of the event (NARU, 2012).

Strategic

The strategic commander is in overall charge of each service, responsible for formulating the strategy for the incident. Each strategic commander has overall command of the resources of their own organisation, but delegates tactical decisions to their respective tactical commander(s) (LESLP, 2015).

Tactical

The tactical commander works at the tactical level and is also known as the ambulance incident commander (AIC). Their responsibilities include relaying information between the strategic and operational commander and providing the support and resources that the operational commander requires. They may formulate the response plan and pass this to the operational commander to implement.

Operational

The operational commander has responsibility for the activities undertaken at the scene. They are usually located at the incident scene, ideally alongside the operational commanders of the other responding agencies at the forward command post (SWAST, 2014a).

Additional Roles

A key principle of any command system is limiting how much responsibility a single person has to contend with. In order to achieve this at a major incident, commanders will often delegate responsibilities for tasks to others. There are a number of roles and responsibilities that can be delegated by operational commanders of ambulance services; these are shown in Figure 9.3 and explained in further detail below.

Additional support roles are not always required and/or may be undertaken by a single officer, depending on workload. They include (NARU, 2015):

- **Safety officer**: Responsible for the health and safety of all NHS responders entering and working within the cordons of the incident.
- **Parking officer**: Responsible for creating and maintaining a clear and functional parking area. They will ensure vehicles and crews are logged into the area and direct resources to the casualty clearing station (CCS) when casualties need removing from the incident.
- **Loading officer**: Responsible for keeping a log of the number and destinations of casualties transported from the CCS.
- **Primary triage officer**: Responsible for co-ordinating the triage of all casualties at the incident.
- **Casualty clearing officer (CCO)**: Responsible for the management of the CCS. Works closely with

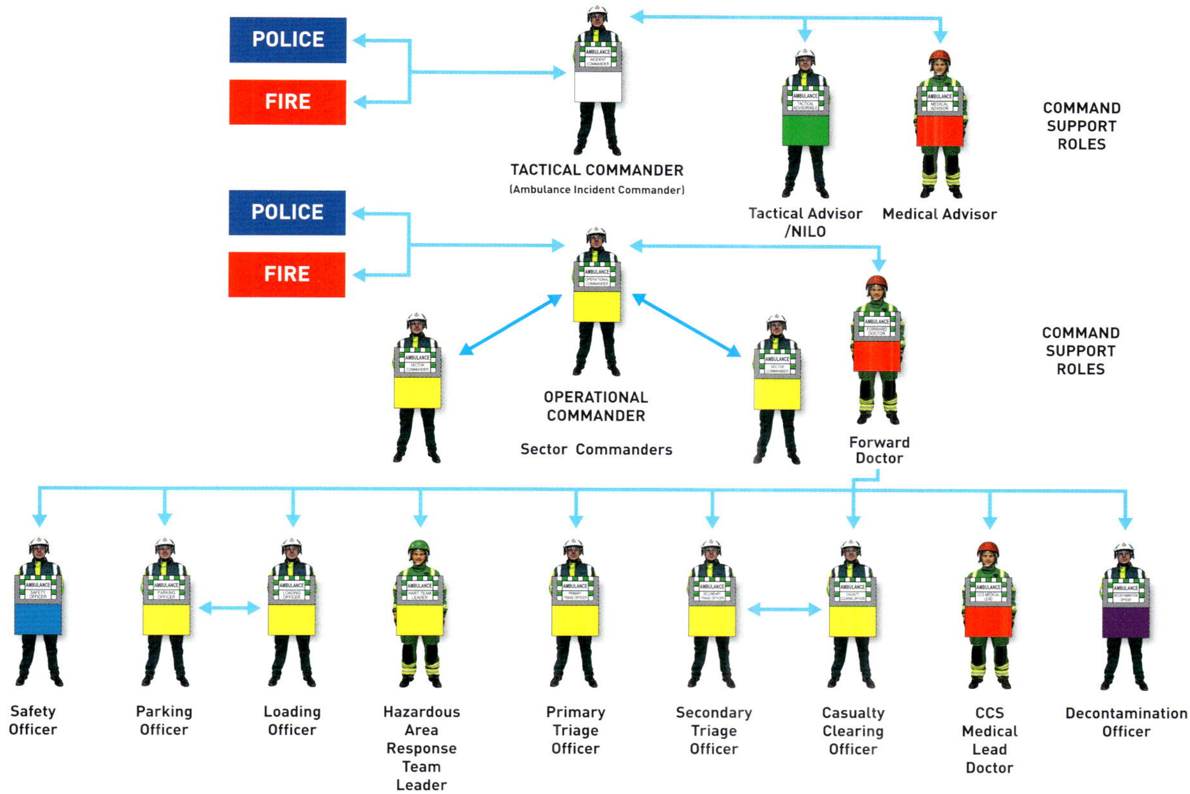

Figure 9.3 *An incident command structure for an NHS ambulance service.*
Source: National Ambulance Resilience Unit (NARU), National Ambulance Service Command and Control Guidance (October 2015)

the triage, parking and loading officers to ensure an efficient triage and treatment of all casualties and the appropriate use of available transport resources.

- **Equipment officer**: Responsible for ensuring the supply and re-supply of equipment to all responding NHS resources.
- **Hazardous area response team (HART) leader**: Provides direct line management for all HART resources.

Triage

The aim of triage is to do the most for the most, and it should be used whenever the number of casualties exceeds the number of skilled rescuers. It is a dynamic process and therefore needs to be repeated many times during the care of each casualty.

Triage Sieve and Sort

There are two phases to triage. The first, the triage sieve (Figure 9.4), takes place where the casualty is found (NASMeD, 2013). This is a fast, physiological assessment of the casualty.

The second, more in-depth assessment is called the triage sort and generally takes place at the casualty clearing station. As a casualty carer, it is unlikely you would normally be involved in triage sort unless assisting a qualified health professional, in which case you follow their instructions at the time.

Over- and Under-Triaging

A key aspect of triaging is not under- or over-triaging, i.e. making sure that the right priority is identified for any casualty. An example of over-triage would be a patient who is not breathing,

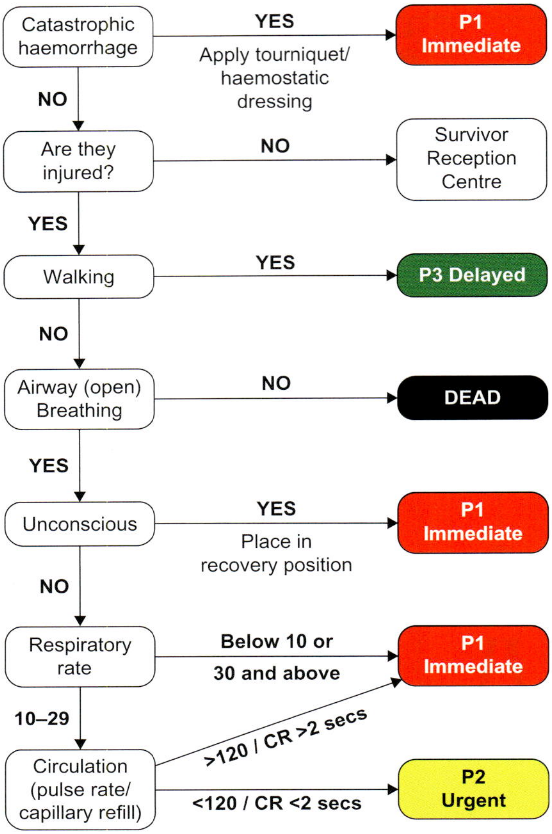

Figure 9.4 *The triage sieve.*
Source: National Ambulance Resilience Unit (NARU), National Ambulance Service Command and Control Guidance (October 2015)

even with airway opened, but has a pulse. This patient should be triaged as dead, but this can be difficult to reconcile with casualty carers, who ordinarily would attempt to resuscitate this patient (JCO, 2010b; Kilner, 2002).

Over-triage is dangerous, as it puts pressure on already scarce resources and has been adversely linked to critical mortality (the number of deaths in critically injured survivors) (Frykberg, 1988).

Under-triage can occur when triaging casualties with normal physiological observations (i.e. respiratory rate of 10–29 breaths per minute and heart rate less than 120 beats per minute or capillary refill time less than two seconds) but who are unable to walk. The triage sieve makes no allowance for patients who cannot normally walk, for example casualties who require a wheelchair to mobilise or babies who have not yet learned how to walk.

Under-triage can also occur when the casualty has a normal respiratory rate and is triaged without consideration given to their pulse rate or capillary refill time, which are abnormal. This results in the casualty being triaged as 'urgent' instead of the correct category, 'immediate' (Kilner, 2002).

Treating and Triaging

Only very basic treatment interventions undertaken during the sieve, such as the insertion of basic airway adjuncts or turning an unconscious patient into the recovery position, can be justified. Catastrophic haemorrhage should also be controlled (SWAST, 2014a).

Recording Your Findings

There are various triage tagging systems in use. The simplest are 'slapper bands', which are in use by several ambulance services in the UK. More commonly, you will find triage labels, with space to allow the recording of findings and to provide a means to identify the patient (Figure 9.5). It doesn't matter which system your service uses as long as you know where the tags are and how to use them.

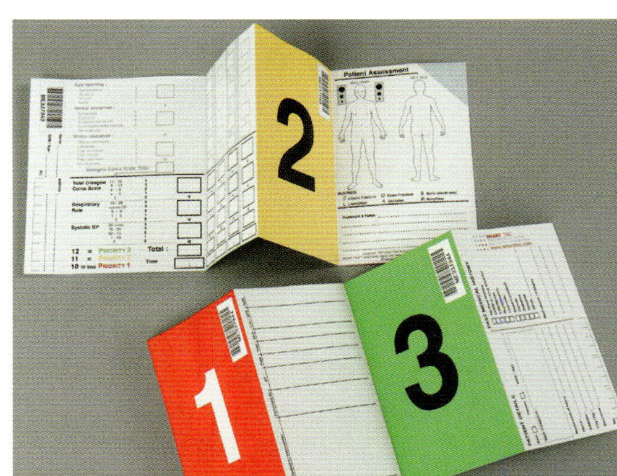

Figure 9.5 *Triage labels.*

Chapter 10

Patient Assessment

Learning Objectives

By the end of this chapter you will be able to:

- State the components of the patient assessment process.
- Describe the CABCDE approach to initial patient assessment, including:
  - catastrophic haemorrhage
  - airway
  - breathing
  - circulation
  - disability
  - exposure/environment.
- State the components of the tool AVPU to assess level of consciousness.
- Outline how to obtain a patient history using the acronyms SAMPLE and SOCRATES.
- Describe the steps in a 'head-to-toe' assessment.

Introduction

Once you have completed your scene assessment, the next step is to conduct a patient assessment. This chapter will break down the patient assessment process into its separate parts so you can explore them further. Figure 10.1 shows the patient assessment process from start to finish. This chapter and some of the subsequent chapters are going to cover this in some detail, so for now just concentrate on the order of the assessment process, rather than on what it is you are expected to do during each stage (Pilbery, 2013; JRCALC, 2016).

Primary Survey

The primary survey (Figure 10.2) is a swift patient assessment and management process, which can be completed within 60–90 seconds. It is designed to be a step-wise approach, meaning that any abnormalities identified in one step should be addressed before moving on to the next. Patients who have suffered traumatic injuries should be checked for life-threatening (or catastrophic) haemorrhage, before the airway is checked. In addition, you should give consideration to the trauma patient's cervical spine and avoid unnecessary movement of the head and neck. This is covered in more detail in Chapter 17: Trauma Emergencies.

General Impression

The general impression is your first and immediate assessment of the patient and their current location, which will give you an early indication as to how sick and/or injured your patient is. Some of this information you will have already gathered from your scene assessment. However, now your focus is specifically on the patient. Note the patient's approximate age, gender and ethnicity, as your management and expectations of what the patient can do will vary. For example, a 1-year-old child will not present in the same way as an adult. In addition, patient positioning can give you early clues. Is the patient sitting up and interacting with you (Figure 10.3a) or are they lying apparently lifeless on the floor (Figure 10.3b)? This step relies heavily on experience and intuition, and can be challenging (NAEMT, 2011).

Primary Survey

General impression
Catastrophic haemorrhage
Airway (consider c-spine)
Breathing
Circulation
Disability
Exposure/Environment

↓

History Taking

Presenting complaint
SAMPLE history

↓

Secondary Survey

Vital signs
'Head-to-toe' assessment

↓

Reassessment

Primary survey
Vital signs
Presenting complaint
Review treatment
Monitor patient condition

Figure 10.1 *The patient assessment process.*

Primary Survey

General impression
Catastrophic haemorrhage
Airway (consider c-spine)
Breathing
Circulation
Disability
Exposure/Environment

Figure 10.2 *The primary survey.*

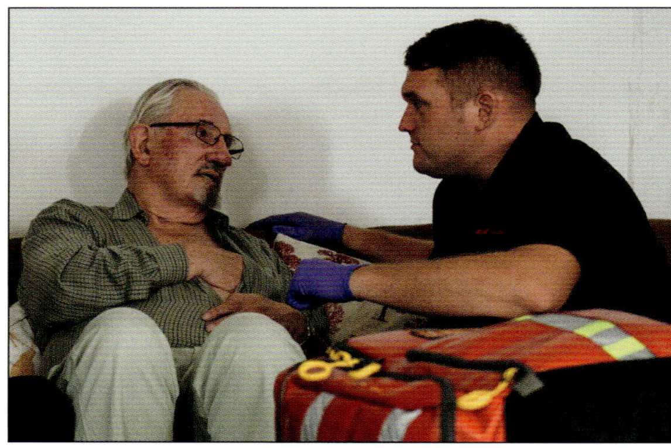

Figure 10.3a *General impression. Compare this patient to the one in Figure 10.3b.*

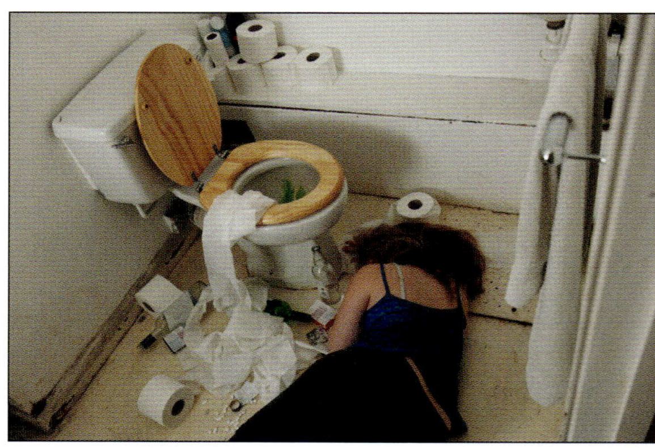

Figure 10.3b *General impression.*

This is also your chance to assess how responsive the patient is. If the patient is awake, introduce yourself with 'Hello, my name is . . .', and identify yourself as being an emergency medical responder from the fire service. Ask how they would prefer to be addressed.

If the patient appears not to be awake or is unconscious, check for responsiveness by asking them if they are all right, or try giving them a command like 'Open your eyes'. If they do not respond, gently shake the patient's shoulders. Patients who fail to respond are critically ill until proven otherwise (Nolan, 2012).

Catastrophic Haemorrhage

Bleeding that is likely to cause death in minutes is referred to as catastrophic haemorrhage. This bleeding needs to be stopped, even before assessing the airway, to prevent the patient from bleeding to death. This is covered in Chapter 17: Trauma Emergencies.

Airway

Assessment of the airway involves three steps:

- **Look** for signs of airway obstruction.
- **Listen** for noisy or absent breathing.
- **Feel** for air movement as the patient breathes.

Remember, the primary assessment proceeds in a step-wise manner. Any signs of obstruction, such as snoring or gurgling sounds, need to be addressed now before moving on to breathing. You will learn how to deal with airway problems in Chapter 11: Airway.

Breathing

Once you have a patent (open) airway, you are ready to move on to breathing. As with the airway assessment, you will adopt a look, listen, feel approach.

The first question you should ask is whether the patient is breathing. If they aren't, you must start chest compressions as part of providing basic life support (covered in Chapter 18: Cardiac Arrest). If they are breathing, you need to decide whether this is adequate. You can start with the respiratory rate and depth of breathing (indicated by chest movement).

Circulation

In medical patients, circulation is the next step following airway and breathing. You can obtain a good idea of the patient's circulation by looking at the colour of their limbs (usually the hands as they are most accessible and normally visible). Feeling for a pulse is covered in Chapter 13: Circulation; the pulse can tell you the heart rate and adequacy of the cardiac output, particularly if distal pulses (such as that in the wrist) are absent when a central pulse (such as that found in the neck) is palpable. A patient who does not have a central pulse needs basic life support immediately, followed by prompt attaching of an automated external defibrillator (AED).

Disability

Disability in the primary assessment refers to the patient's level of consciousness, or how awake they are. There are many causes of unconsciousness and these are covered in Chapter 14: Disability. During the primary assessment, you will need to check three things to assess the patient's disability (JRCALC, 2016; Pilbery, 2013):

- level of consciousness
- pupils
- blood sugar.

Level of Consciousness

A rapid assessment of the patient's level of consciousness (LOC) can be undertaken using the acronym AVPU:

A: alert
V: responds to verbal stimulus
P: responds to pain
U: unresponsive.

Pupils

When looking at a patient's pupils, notice whether they are of equal size and if they react to light. There are a number of reasons why this may not be the case and you'll find out about these in the Disability chapter later on.

Blood Sugar

Hypoglycaemia, or low blood sugar, is a cause of reduced level of consciousness, which can usually be corrected by the administration of glucose, either orally (by mouth) or intravenously. In addition, there are drugs that can mobilise the body's own glucose stores and you'll learn about these in Chapter 16: Medical Emergencies.

Exposure/Environment

You will undertake a full 'head-to-toe' assessment later on in the patient assessment process, but a quick look early on will provide you with clues to any obvious illness/injury that needs to be managed quickly. For example, some types of rashes (e.g. non-blanching) signal serious illness such as sepsis or anaphylaxis. This quick check also provides a chance to identify sites of hidden bleeding that you did not pick up on earlier on in your assessment.

Working out-of-hospital, however, you do need to be mindful about maintenance of patient privacy by not unnecessarily exposing them, as well as ensuring that they do not lose body heat.

History Taking

Presenting Complaint

The presenting complaint is usually the reason you have been called to the patient (Figure 10.4). Most presenting complaints fall into the categories of pain, discomfort and/or abnormal body function. Sometimes this is explicit ('I have terrible chest pain'), but can be vague, particularly in the elderly ('I just don't feel right today') (Gregory, 2010b; Pilbery, 2013). Avoid using words like 'problem' or 'complaint' when finding out the reason for the emergency call.

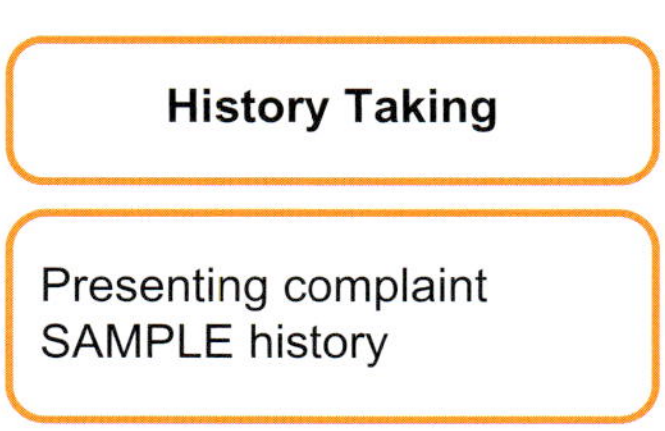

Figure 10.4 *History taking.*

SAMPLE History

Once you know the presenting complaint, you will need to ask further questions. At the bare minimum, this should include the parts of the SAMPLE acronym (Pilbery, 2013):

S: Signs and symptoms of the presenting complaint.
A: Allergies (particularly to medication, although food allergies might be relevant).
M: Medications.
P: Past medical history.
L: Last oral intake.
E: Events that led to the current illness or injury.

Signs and Symptoms of the Presenting Complaint

To help you organise the signs and symptoms of the presenting complaint, you can use the acronym, SOCRATES. This was originally designed with assessment of pain in mind, but can be helpful for other presenting complaints:

S: Site. Where is the symptom located?
O: Onset. When did it (the presenting complaint) start?
C: Character. How does the patient describe their symptom, particularly pain? Is it sharp or dull, for example?
R: Radiation. In the case of pain, does it stay in one place (can the patient point to it with one finger) or does it go elsewhere (i.e. radiate)?
A: Association. Are there any other signs and symptoms associated with the presenting complaint?
T: Timing. How long has the patient had the symptom, and if it has resolved, what time was this? In the case of pain, also consider whether the pain is intermittent (comes and goes).
E: Exacerbating/relieving factors. What makes the symptom worse/better? Include self-treatment, such as taking analgesia.
S: Severity. On a scale of 0 to 10, where 0 is no pain and 10 is the worst pain imaginable, what score does the patient give it now?

Allergies and Medication

Allergies

The range of drugs that you can administer is limited, but there is still scope for patient harm if administered inappropriately. You should always ask the patient about any allergic reactions to medication they have received in the past. It is also a good idea to ask about other allergies, such as those caused by food, animals, pollen or metal (Douglas, 2005).

Medication

Ask if the patient's medication can be made available for the ambulance crew when they arrive. It is also a good idea to ask about any over-the-counter medicines (i.e. those not prescribed by a doctor, but obtained from a pharmacist or supermarket), as well as herbal and homeopathic remedies (Pilbery, 2013).

Past Medical History

You will probably cover some of the patient's medical history while obtaining the history of the presenting complaint, but the following questions will help you uncover other medical illnesses or surgery that may prove helpful (Douglas, 2005; Gregory, 2010b):

- Have you had any illnesses that you saw your GP about?
- Have you had to take any time off work because of ill health?
- Have you had any operations?
- Have you been admitted to hospital, and if so, why?
- Have you suffered any injuries?

Last Oral Intake and Events Leading to Illness/Injury

Last Oral Intake

Find out when the patient last had anything to eat or drink. This information is useful for patients who are unconscious or who may require surgery, as patients with a full stomach are at risk of aspiration. Also, you may be able to identify the onset of food poisoning and/or food allergies (Gregory, 2010b).

Events Leading to the Illness or Injury

This is also known as the history of the presenting complaint, and if you have used the SOCRATES acronyms, you will have already obtained most of the information required.

Additional information that is useful to obtain includes (Gregory, 2010b):

- Associated symptoms: For example, does the patient have shortness of breath and nausea with their chest pain?
- Previous episodes: Find out what happened last time, including any diagnoses made or hospital admissions.
- Effect on daily living: Does the presenting complaint interfere with getting to the toilet or making a cup of tea, for example?

Secondary Survey

The secondary survey is often tailored to your findings from the primary survey and history (Figure 10.5). For example, if the presenting complaint is shortness of breath, then you must ensure that you obtain a respiratory rate and oxygen saturations, and auscultate the lungs.

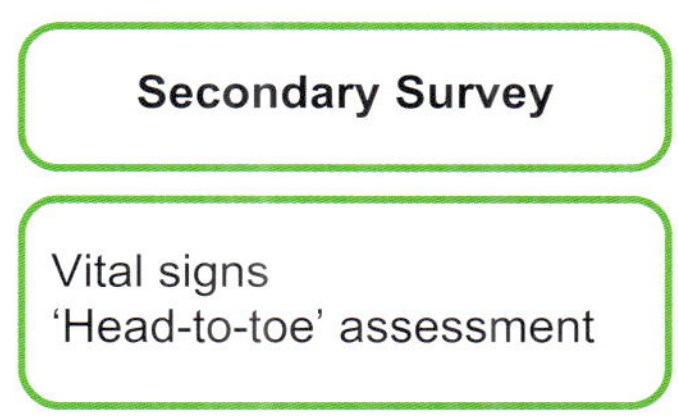

Figure 10.5 *The secondary survey.*

Vital Signs

If you have not already done so, now is the time to obtain some physiological observations from the patient, or obtain vital signs. Your service may have a specified minimum set of observations to obtain, but this will generally include:

- respiratory rate
- oxygen saturations
- pulse rate
- blood pressure
- level of consciousness (AVPU)
- pain score
- blood sugar
- temperature
- National Early Warning Score (NEWS).

Being able to record vital signs accurately is a fundamental skill, and these will be explored in depth in the relevant chapters as you progress through the book.

National Early Warning Score

In order to standardise the initial assessment of an acute illness, the Royal College of Physicians, in conjunction with other healthcare professions, has developed the National Early Warning Score (NEWS, now in its second revision and known as NEWS2) (Figure 10.6). It is aimed at improving (RCP, 2015):

- the assessment of acute illness
- the detection of clinical deterioration
- initiation of a timely and competent clinical response.

Note: NEWS2 is not suitable for children under 16 years or women who are pregnant, as physiological responses to acute illness are different in these groups (RCP, 2015).

Once you have recorded the patient's clinical observations, simply add up the score awarded to each of the physiological parameters. For example, consider a patient with the following observations:

- Respiratory rate: 10 breaths/min
- Oxygen saturations: 93%
- Air or oxygen: Air
- Systolic blood pressure: 108 mmHg
- Pulse: 110 beats/min
- Consciousness: Alert
- Temperature: 38.1°C

When calculating the NEWS2 score, use the SpO_2 Scale 1, unless directed to use Scale 2 by a clinician

National Early Warning Score (NEWS2)

Physiological parameter	Score 3	2	1	0	1	2	3
Respiration rate (per minute)	≤8		9–11	12–20		21–24	≥25
SpO_2 Scale 1(%)	≤91	92–93	94–95	≥96			
SpO_2 Scale 2(%)	≤83	84–85	86–87	88–92 ≥93 on air	93–94 on oxygen	95–96 on oxygen	≥97 on oxygen
Air or oxygen?		Oxygen		Air			
Systolic blood pressure (mmHg)	≤90	91–100	101–110	111–219			≥220
Pulse (per minute)	≤40		41–50	51–90	91–110	111–130	≥131
Consciousness				Alert			CVPU
Temperature (°C)	≤35.0		35.1–36.0	36.1–38.0	38.1–39.0	≥39.1	

Figure 10.6 *National Early Warning Score version 2.*
Available at: https://tfinews.ocbmedia.com/media/news_score-3.pdf

or local policy. Under consciousness, there is an additional 'C', which stands for a new onset of confusion, disorientation or reduction in level of consciousness.

In this case, the patient's NEWS2 score would be calculated as: 1 + 2 + 0 + 1 + 1 + 0 + 1 = 6.

Trigger Scores

Patients are categorised into three broad groups:

- Low score: NEWS 1–4.
- Medium score: NEWS 5–6 or a single RED score (i.e. physiological parameter that scores a 3).
- High score: NEWS of 7 or more.

Follow local guidance as to the appropriate actions to be taken with patients who have low, medium and high scores. Always pass on the NEWS of a patient to the ambulance crew when they arrive on scene.

'Head-to-Toe' Assessment

It is not always appropriate to perform a 'head-to-toe' or full-body examination for every patient, but in cases of multiple injury, or in cases when the patient is found collapsed and the history is limited or non-existent, it can be helpful to identify signs of injury, or illness. The assessment outlined here is a rapid full-body assessment, which should take around 60–90 seconds to complete. Clinicians that you work with are likely to perform more thorough assessments on specific areas of the body depending on the presenting complaint.

Procedure

Take the following steps to perform a 'head-to-toe' assessment (Pilbery, 2013):

1. Look at the face for obvious injuries, such as lacerations, bruising and deformities.
2. Inspect the area around the eyes and eyelids.
3. Check the eyes for redness and the presence of contact lenses.
4. Assess the pupils with a pen torch, to ensure that they react to light.
5. Look behind the ears for bruising and in the ear for signs of fluid or blood leaking out.
6. Look for bruising, lacerations and deformity around the head, and then gently feel for tenderness and depressions of the skull.
7. Feel the cheekbones for tenderness, symmetry and instability.
8. Feel the maxilla (the bone just below the nose).
9. Check the nose for blood and fluid leaking out.
10. Feel the jaw.
11. Assess the mouth and nose for cyanosis (blue-tinged skin), foreign bodies (including loose teeth and/or dentures), bleeding, lacerations and deformities.
12. Smell the patient's breath for specific odours (such as pear-drops, which can be present in some diabetic patients).
13. Look at the neck and note any obvious lacerations, bruises and/or deformity. Look for bulging veins in the neck and feel the trachea to ensure it is centrally located.
14. Feel the back of the neck for tenderness and deformity.
15. Look at the chest for any obvious injury, and watch the chest rise and fall as the patient breathes.
16. Gently feel the ribs to ensure they are intact and to identify if they are tender. Do not press over any obvious bruising or fractures.
17. Check the abdomen and pelvis for obvious injury, and gently feel the abdomen, which should be soft and non-tender.
18. Look at the pelvis for signs of injury, then gently feel the iliac crests for signs of instability, tenderness or crepitus. Do not compress the pelvis (sometimes called 'springing').
19. Check the extremities (arms and legs) for lacerations, bruises, swelling, deformities and the presence of medical bracelets. Feel for distal pulses and check motor and sensory function. Compare the right and left sides.

Reassessment

The first thing you will probably notice about the reassessment section is that it contains many of the things you have already undertaken as part of the patient assessment process (Figure 10.7). As with scene safety, a patient's clinical condition is dynamic and frequently changes, either due to the illness and/or injury they have acquired, or as a result of an intervention you have performed, such as defibrillation. Frequent reassessment will mean that you will not miss these changes. Trends in vital signs, for example, are important to note, so ensure that you record vital signs, along with the time they were recorded, on the patient care record.

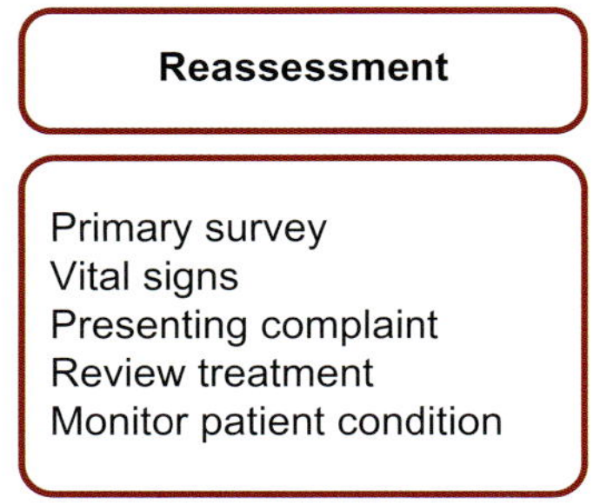

Figure 10.7 *Reassessment.*

Chapter 11
Airway

Airway Anatomy

Learning Objective

By the end of this section you will be able to:

- Identify and describe the structures of the upper and lower airway.

Introduction

The respiratory system is made up of a number of structures (Figure 11.1):

- nose
- mouth
- pharynx (throat)
- larynx (voicebox)
- trachea (windpipe)
- bronchi
- lungs.

Structurally, the respiratory system is split into two halves: the upper and lower respiratory systems. The upper consists of everything above the cricoid cartilage, and the lower, the cricoid cartilage and lower structures.

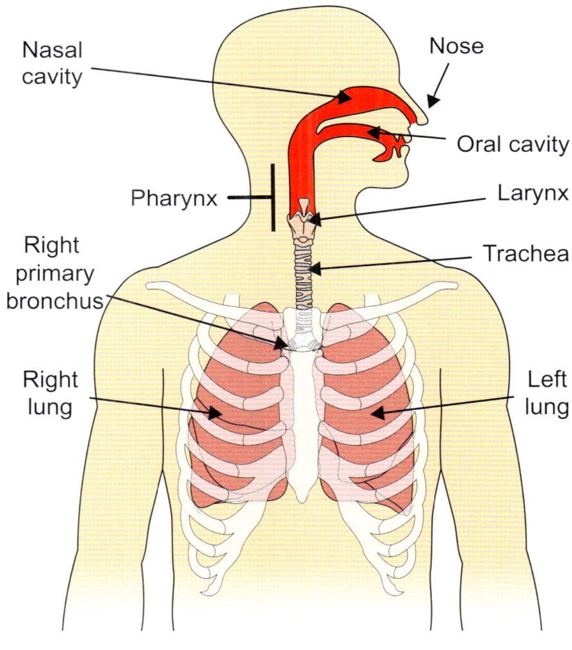

Figure 11.1 *The structures of the respiratory system.*

Nose

This is mostly constructed from cartilage, and is external to the skull. Its orifices (nostrils, or nares) open into the nasal cavity of the skull, and are divided by the nasal septum. The nasal cavity contains the superior, middle and inferior turbinates (Figure 11.2), which increase the internal surface area of the nasal cavity, which in turn increases

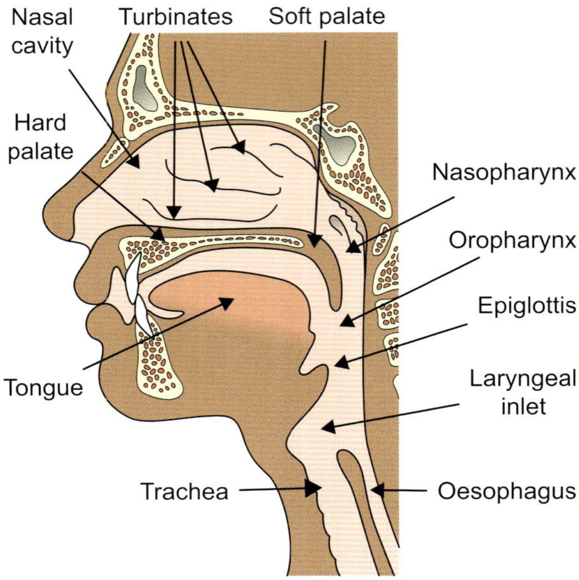

Figure 11.2 *The upper airway.*

the temperature and humidity of air that passes through during breathing (Drake, 2005).

Mouth

The mouth (or oral cavity) starts at the lips and is continuous with the oropharynx posteriorly. The roof of the mouth is made up of the hard and soft palates, with the floor made up of mostly soft tissue, including the tongue. The tongue is a muscular, non-compressible tissue that attaches to the mandible, stylohyoid process and hyoid bone. The tongue, in the past, has been accused of being the most common cause of obstruction. However, research conducted on adult anaesthetised patients has demonstrated that it is usually the soft palate and epiglottis that cause obstruction of the airway, not the tongue (Nolan, 2012).

Pharynx

The pharynx is a funnel-shaped tube extending from the back of the nasal cavity to the top of the oesophagus. Although a continuous structure, it is typically divided into three sections anatomically (Figure 11.3):

- nasopharynx
- oropharynx
- laryngopharynx.

Nasopharynx

This is the area at the back of the nasal cavity above the level of the soft palate. It is bordered by the sloping base of the skull above, and mostly skeletal muscle on either side, forming a domed vault at the top of the pharyngeal cavity.

Elevation of the soft palate during swallowing helps to ensure that food does not rise up into

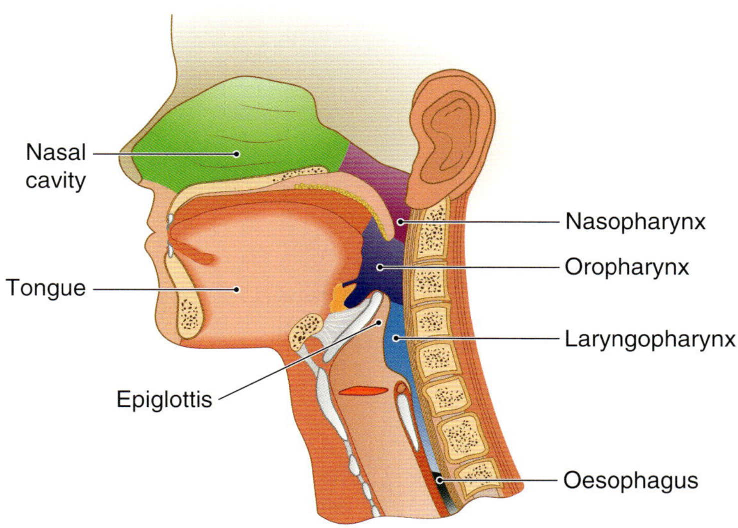

Figure 11.3 *The pharynx.*

the nasal cavity. The tissues that cover the top of the nasopharynx contain the pharyngeal tonsil.

Oropharynx

This is the area posterior to the oral cavity, below the level of the soft palate but continuous with the nasopharynx, and above the margin of the epiglottis (which marks the start of the laryngopharynx).

Laryngopharynx

This is continuous with the oropharynx, running from the superior margins of the epiglottis to the top of the oesophagus around the level of the sixth cervical vertebra (spinal bone) in adults.

Larynx

The larynx is a hollow structure made up of muscles and ligaments. In adults, it is cylindrical in shape, with the narrowest part of the airway at the level of the vocal cords. It is continuous with the trachea below and opens into the laryngopharynx posteriorly.

The larynx is suspended from the hyoid bone above, and trachea below, by a series of membranes and ligaments, which makes it very mobile within the neck (Figure 11.4). During swallowing, it moves upwards and forwards causing the epiglottis to swing downwards, effectively closing the laryngeal inlet while at the same time opening the oesophagus.

As well as acting as a valve to close off the respiratory tract during swallowing, the larynx also produces sound for speech, singing etc.

Trachea

The trachea extends from the cricoid cartilage to the level of the sixth thoracic vertebra, where it splits into the left main bronchus and right main bronchus (together, the bronchi) at the carina (Figure 11.5). In an adult, the trachea is approximately 12–15 cm long and consists of C-shaped cartilages, which are completed posteriorly by the trachealis muscle (Kovacs, 2011).

Bronchi

The trachea divides into the left main bronchus and right main bronchus (together, the bronchi) at the carina (Figure 11.5). These bronchi split into secondary bronchi, tertiary bronchi, the bronchioles, and finally the terminal bronchioles. The right main bronchus is more vertical, wider and shorter than the left, which explains why objects

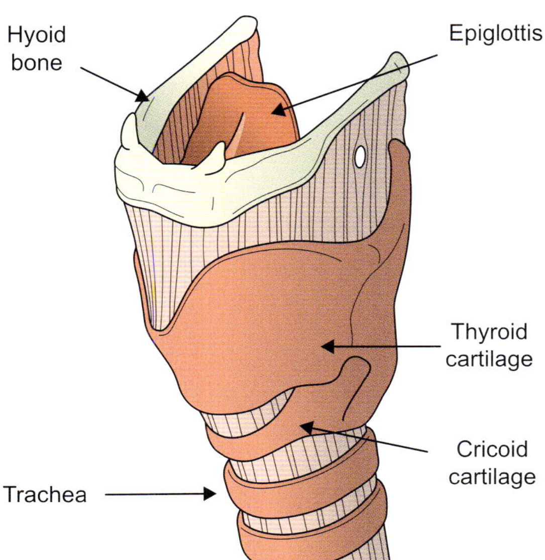

Figure 11.4 *The larynx.*

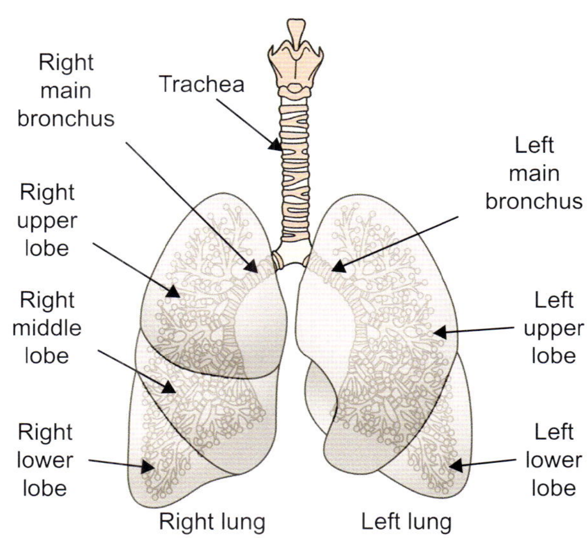

Figure 11.5 *The lower airway.*

that are inhaled (foreign bodies) tend to end up here. In a similar design to the trachea, the main bronchi are incomplete rings of cartilage.

Lungs

The lungs are a pair of spongy, cone-shaped organs located in the thoracic (chest) cavity. They are separated by the mediastinum, a region in the thoracic cavity that contains the heart, major vessels, oesophagus and trachea, among others. This means that if one lung collapses, due to air entering the thoracic cavity after a traumatic injury, for example, the other lung may remain inflated.

The lungs are covered by the pleura, which consists of two layers: the parietal pleura, which covers the wall of the thoracic cavity, and the visceral pleura, which covers the lungs. In between is the pleural cavity, a potential space filled with a fluid to prevent friction and allow the pleura to slide over each other during breathing. It also helps the membranes stick together due to the surface tension of the fluid, in a similar way that a glass with a wet bottom lifts the coaster it was sitting on.

The lungs extend from the diaphragm to just above the clavicles. The left lung is smaller than the right due to the space taken up by the heart. It also has only two lobes, the upper and lower, whereas the right lung has three, the upper, lower and middle lobes (Tortora, 2008).

Assessing and Managing the Airway

Learning Objectives

By the end of this section you will be able to:

- Identify clinical signs that indicate a need to manage the airway.
- Explain factors that affect airway patency and the step-wise approach to airway management.
- Explain how to perform a range of manual airway manoeuvres.
- Describe the equipment required for suction and its safe use.

Introduction

More often than not, your patient will be conscious and able to talk, scream or cry, indicating that they have a patent airway. For some, however, you will need to assist them in opening and maintaining their airway. Basic manoeuvres with nothing more than your hands are often enough to open and keep open a patient's airway, but things can change and it is important that you frequently reassess airway patency, i.e. perform a dynamic airway assessment.

In this section, clinical signs of airway compromise and the step-wise approach to airway management that is recommended by pre-hospital practice guidelines to address them will be reviewed (JRCALC, 2016):

- head tilt–chin lift
- jaw thrust
- jaw thrust with head tilt
- recovery position.

Once the manual manoeuvres have been covered, the following more advanced procedures will be described:

- suction
- oropharyngeal airways
- nasopharyngeal airways
- supraglottic airway devices.

Children and infants have a chapter all to themselves (Chapter 19), since the management of a child's airway requires modification based on their age.

Assessing the Airway

In Chapter 10: Patient Assessment, you were introduced to the three-step approach to airway assessment:

- **Look**: As you approach the patient, note their position as it can give you an indication of the patency of the airway. Conscious patients who have adopted a tripod position (Figure 11.6) or who are showing other signs of increased work of breathing may have a partially obstructed airway.

- **Listen**: Even without a stethoscope, you can sometimes hear sounds that indicate a potential airway obstruction. High-pitched inspiratory (although sometimes can be expiratory too) sounds can be a sign of upper airway narrowing (known as stridor). Lower-pitch sounds usually heard on expiration (wheeze) are a sign of lower airway partial obstruction, particularly in acute exacerbations of conditions such as asthma. Other sounds include snoring, typically due to the soft tissues of the pharynx relaxing, and gurgling, due to fluid, secretions or vomit etc. Snoring can usually be remedied with manual airway manoeuvres or an adjunct such as an oropharyngeal airway, whereas gurgling is an indication that the patient's airway requires suction.
- **Feel**: You will not always need to place your ear close enough to your patient's mouth to feel their breath on your cheek. However, in unresponsive patients it is important to determine if there is airflow and not just rely on chest movement. The chest can move even in complete airway obstruction, and is sometimes associated with a see-saw, paradoxical movement of the abdomen with the chest. So, as the chest expands, the abdomen sinks and vice versa.

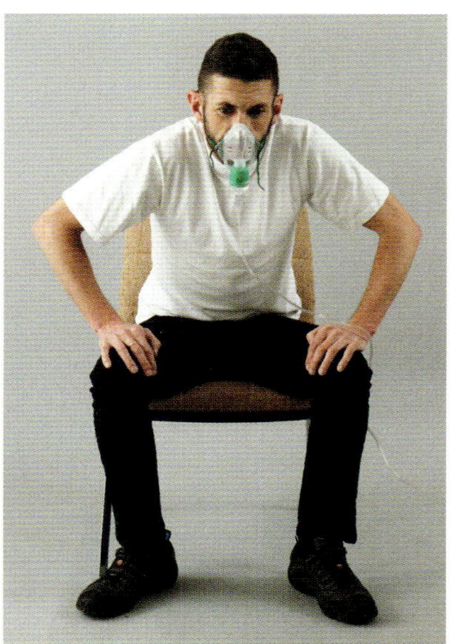

Figure 11.6 *A patient in the tripod position.*

Step-Wise Approach to the Airway

In general, you will start with basic manoeuvres, such as the head tilt–chin lift or recovery position for patients who have an obstructed airway. Depending on the patient's condition and potential threats to their airway, you may elect to escalate their management to include airway adjuncts, such as oropharyngeal airways (OPAs) and nasopharyngeal airways (NPAs). If these are insufficient, you may elect to insert a supraglottic airway device (SAD) instead. Finally, if you are working with senior clinicians, they may decide to intubate the patient. Depending on the patient's condition, it may be necessary to rapidly escalate airway management. Figure 11.7 shows a recommended step-wise approach to the airway (JRCALC, 2016).

Manual Airway Manoeuvres

Manual airway manoeuvres can be achieved with just your (or a colleague's) hands. They are great for the initial management of the airway, and in some cases may be all that is required.

Head Tilt–Chin Lift

When to do it (indication):

- An unresponsive patient who has an airway obstruction caused by loss of pharyngeal muscle tone.

When not to do it (contra-indication):

- If the patient has a suspected spinal injury.

Advantages:

- No equipment is required.
- Technique is simple and non-invasive.

Disadvantages:

- Does not protect the airway from aspiration.
- Not suitable for patients with cervical spinal injury.

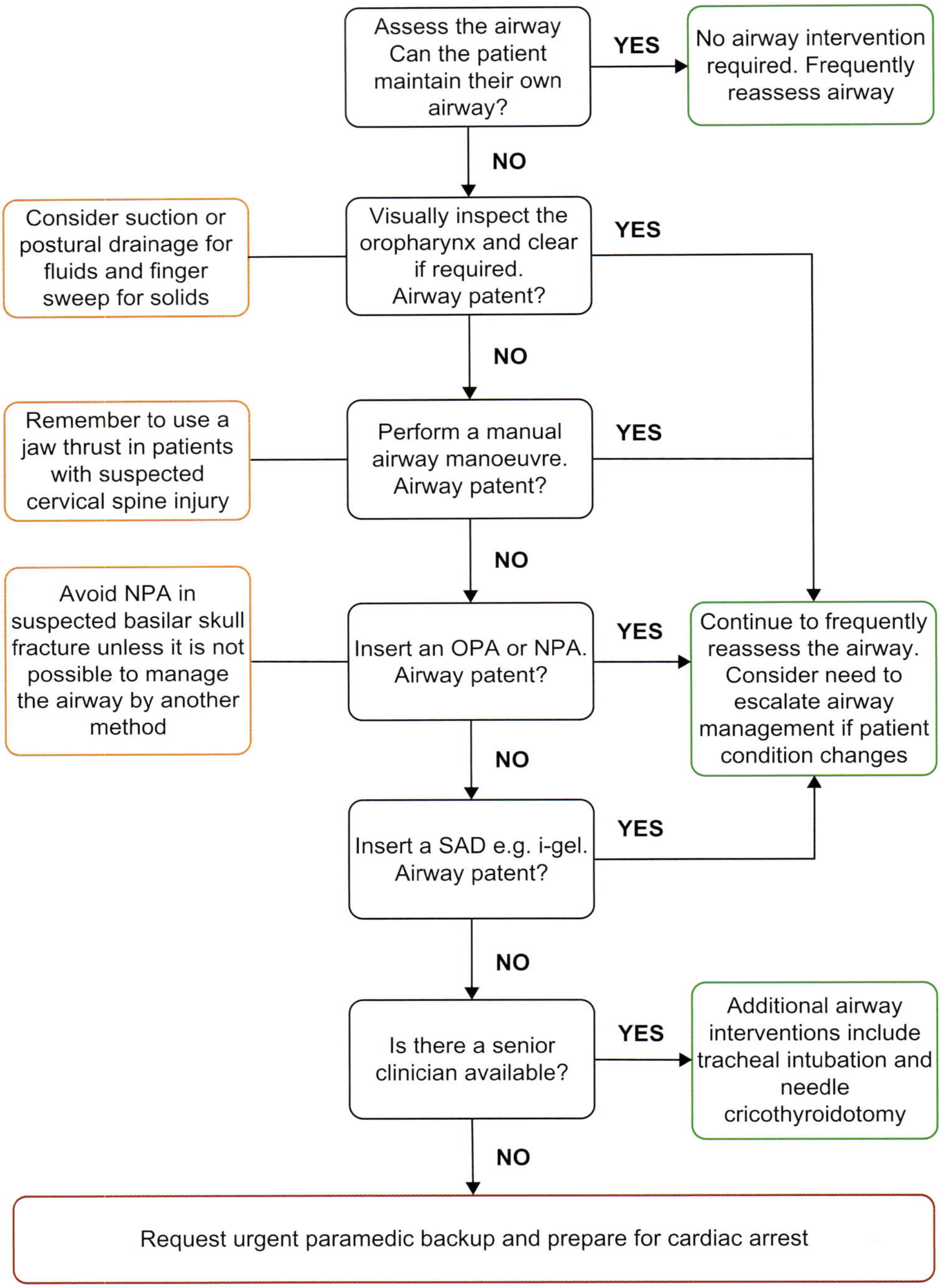

Figure 11.7 *Step-wise approach to airway assessment and management.*

Procedure

Take the following steps to perform a head tilt–chin lift (Pilbery, 2013; Nolan, 2012):

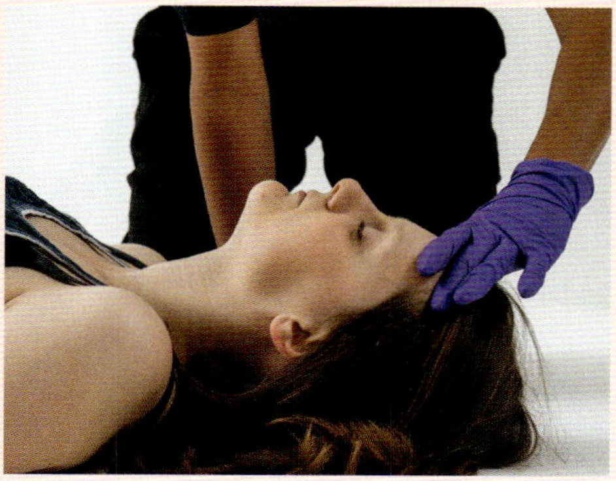

1. With your patient lying on their back (supine), position yourself at the patient's side. Place the hand closer to the patient's head on their forehead and gently tilt the head backwards.

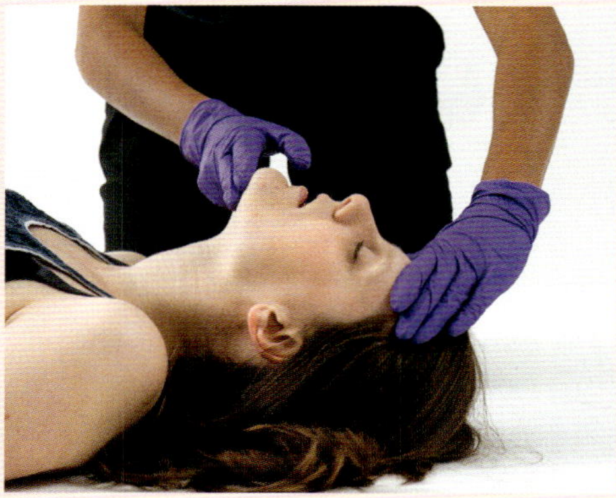

2. Place two fingers on the bony part of the chin and gently lift upwards.

Jaw thrust

When to do it (indication):

- An unresponsive patient who has an airway obstruction caused by loss of pharyngeal muscle tone.

When not to do it (contra-indication):

- A responsive patient unless they have a fractured jaw.

Advantages:

- No equipment is required.
- Technique is simple and non-invasive.
- Maintains neutral alignment of the head when cervical spinal injury suspected.

Disadvantages:

- Does not protect the airway from aspiration.
- Difficult to maintain for prolonged periods.
- Requires second person to provide ventilations, if required.

Procedure

Take the following steps to perform a jaw thrust (Pilbery, 2013; Nolan, 2012):

- With your patient lying on their back (supine), position yourself at the patient's head.
- Identify the angle of the mandible.
- Place your fingers behind the mandible and lift in an upwards and forwards direction (Figure 11.8).
- Using your thumbs, open the patient's mouth.

Jaw Thrust with Head Tilt

When to do it (indication):

- An unresponsive patient who has an airway obstruction caused by loss of pharyngeal muscle tone and jaw thrust alone is not sufficient to open the airway.

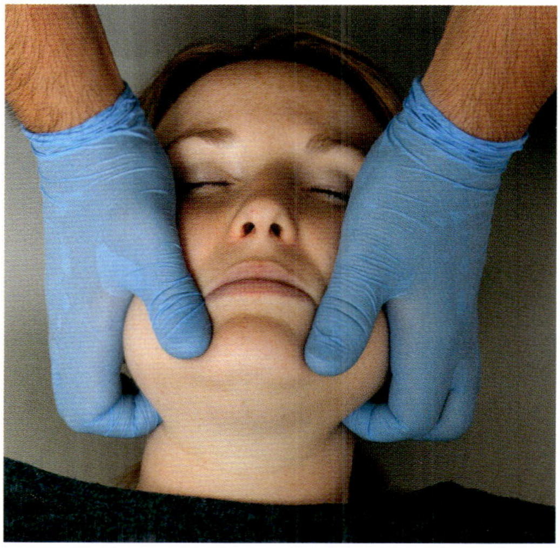

Figure 11.8 *Lifting the mandible.*

When not to do it (contra-indication):

- A responsive patient.

Advantages:

- No equipment is required.
- Technique is simple and non-invasive.

Disadvantages:

- Does not protect the airway from aspiration.
- Difficult to maintain for prolonged periods.
- Requires second person to provide ventilations, if required.

Procedure

Take the following steps to perform a jaw thrust with head tilt (Pilbery, 2013):

- With your patient lying on their back (supine), position yourself at the patient's head.
- Identify the angle of the mandible.
- Place your fingers behind the mandible and lift in an upwards and forwards direction.
- Using your thumbs, open the patient's mouth.
- Tilt the head backwards.

Recovery Position

When to do it (indication):

- A spontaneously breathing but unconscious patient who does not have a spinal injury.

When not to do it (contra-indications):

- Patients with spinal injuries.
- Patients who require assisted ventilation or insertion of an advanced airway.

Advantages:

- Simple and quick to perform, even for a single rescuer.
- Does not require equipment.
- Encourages postural drainage of secretions or vomit from the patient's mouth.

Disadvantages:

- Not a definitive airway, i.e. does not guarantee that the patient will not aspirate.
- Sometimes difficult to assess patient's breathing.

Procedure

There are several variations of the recovery position. This is the method that the European Resuscitation Council recommend (Zideman, 2015):

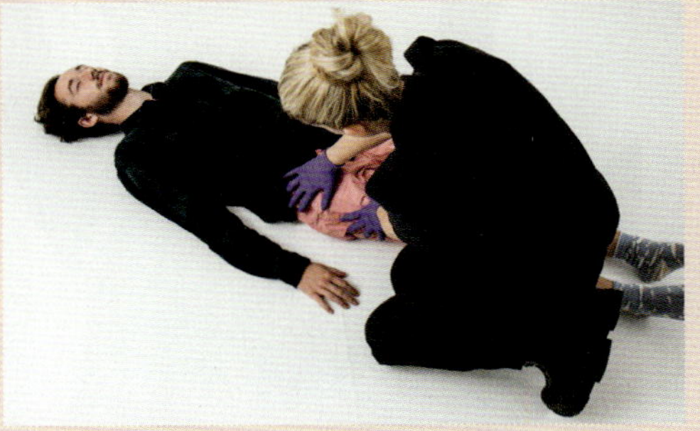

1. Kneel beside the patient and straighten both of their legs. Quickly check if they have any items in their pockets that should be removed before rolling them over.

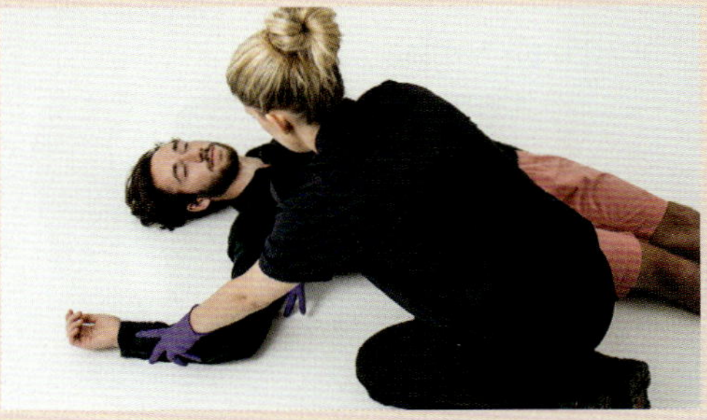

2. Place the arm nearer to you at right angles to their body, with the arm bent at the elbow and palm of the hand facing upwards.

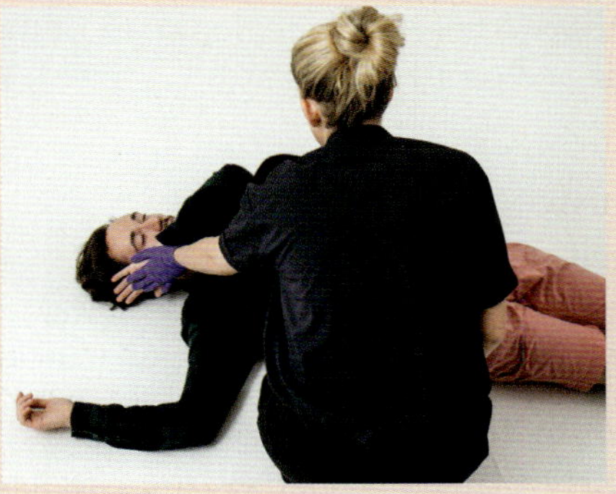

3. Bring the other arm across the chest and hold the back of their hand against the cheek that is nearer to you. Don't let go.

Procedure – *cont*

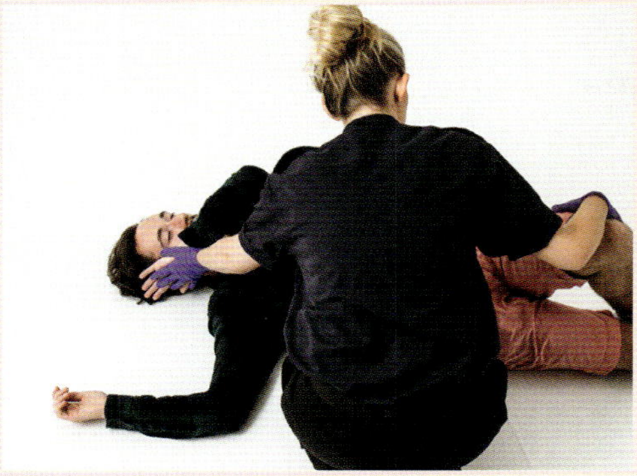

4. With your other hand, grasp the leg further away from you just above the knee and lift upwards so the leg flexes. Keep the foot on the ground.

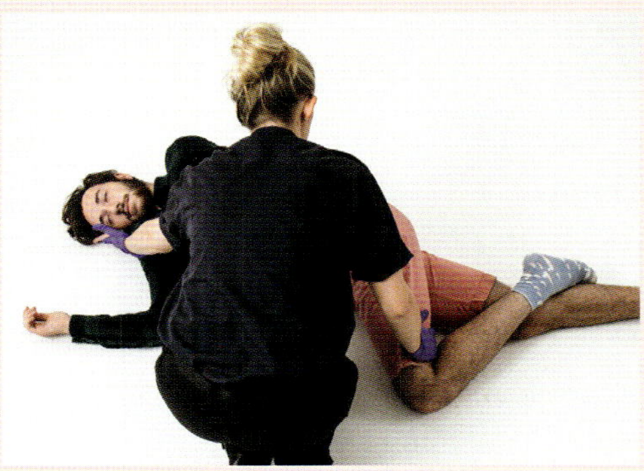

5. While supporting the head, pull the leg towards you, so that the patient rolls to face you.

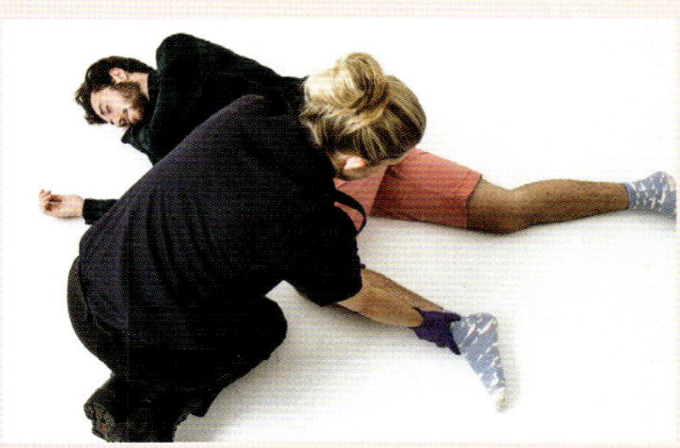

6. Adjust the uppermost leg so that the patient's hip and knee are bent at right angles.

Procedure – *cont*

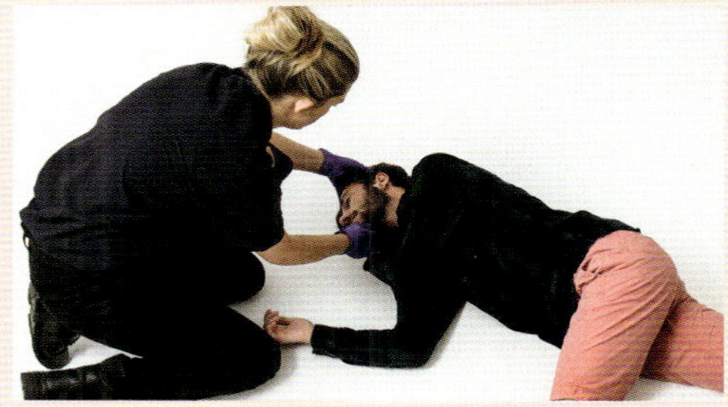

7. Tilt the head back to ensure the airway remains open. Adjust the patient's hand that is under their cheek, if required, to maintain head tilt and keep the patient facing slightly downwards, to allow free drainage of secretions from the mouth. Reassess frequently.

Suction

If you can hear gurgling in the airway, then you should think about suction. Suctioning an airway involves removing vomit, blood and secretions with suctioning equipment. As part of your equipment, you will usually have a mains-operated/battery-powered suction unit (Figure 11.9) and a hand-operated device

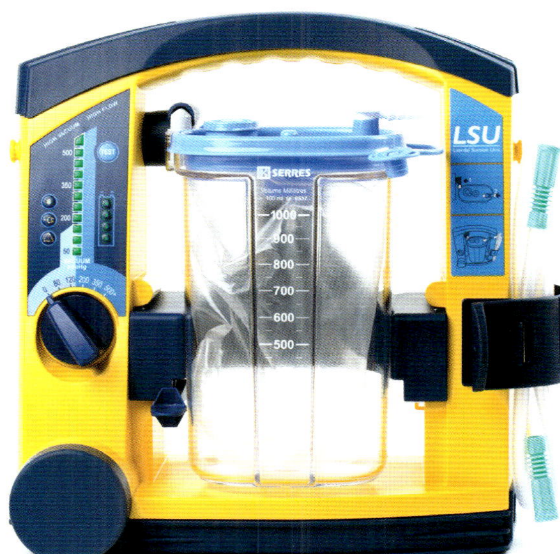

Figure 11.9 *Mechanical suction device reproduced by the kind permission of Laerdal Medical.*

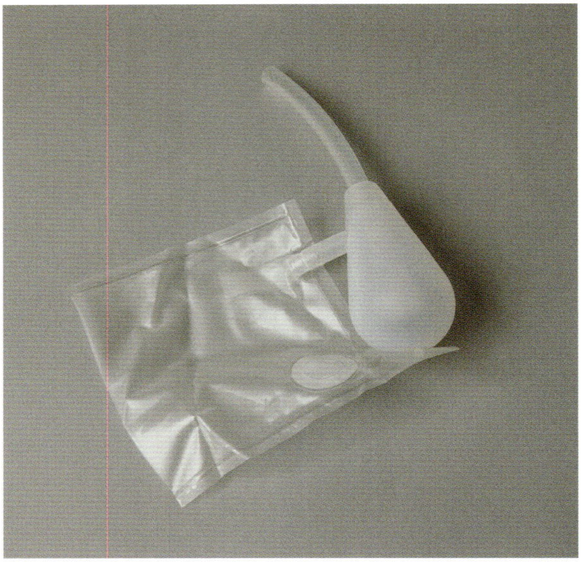

Figure 11.10 *Hand-operated suction device.*

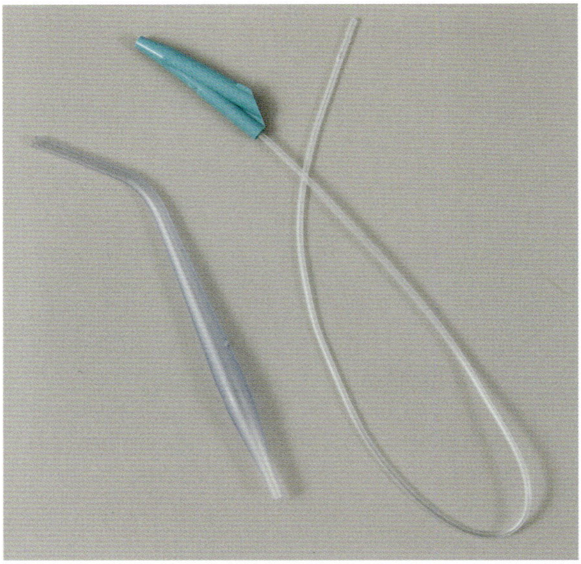

Figure 11.11 *Suction catheters. Rigid, wide-bore (left) and flexible (right).*

(Figure 11.10). Make sure you are familiar with the operating instructions for the devices you carry.

Suction Catheters

You are likely to have two types of suction catheters: a rigid, wide-bore catheter (sometimes called a Yankauer) and a smaller, flexible catheter that can fit down an oropharyngeal or nasopharyngeal airway, but is limited by its small size and is unsuitable for blood and vomit (Figure 11.11).

When to do it (indication):

- In patients who cannot maintain and clear their own airway and in whom vomit, blood or secretions are at risk of entering the lower respiratory tract.

When not to do it (contra-indication):

- In patients who can maintain and clear their own airway.

Advantage:

- Prevents aspiration of vomit, blood or secretions.

Disadvantage:

- Suctioning removes air as well as secretions. Keep suction times short.

Procedure

Take the following steps to perform suction using a mechanical suction device (Randle, 2009; Roberts, 2014):

1. Prepare your equipment. You will need:
   - suction unit
   - Yankauer and soft-tip catheters and suction tubing
   - gloves
   - protective eyewear
   - oxygen.
2. Explain the procedure to the patient and obtain consent if conscious.
3. Pre-oxygenate if possible.
4. Put on gloves and eyewear.
5. Attach suction tubing and catheter and switch on suction unit if using a mechanical device.
6. Open the patient's mouth and insert the catheter into their mouth without suctioning. Make sure you can visualise the end of the suction catheter at all times.
7. Apply suction by occluding the control vent on the catheter (mechanical device) or squeezing the handle (hand-operated device) and gently

withdraw the catheter. Suction for no more than 15 seconds.

8. Re-oxygenate the patient and reassess the airway. Further suction attempts may be required.

Notes:
There is no clear guidance on suction pressures for the emergency management of patients. If you only need to clear small amounts of saliva, then a suction pressure of 150–200 mmHg is sufficient (Randle, 2009). However, in cases where there is a large amount of blood or vomit, turn the suction up to maximum initially and adjust downwards, as required (NAEMT, 2014).

In cases of severe bleeding or active vomiting, positioning the patient to allow for postural drainage is more important: for example, turning a patient onto their side when they are immobilised on an orthopaedic stretcher (Nutbeam, 2013).

Although prolonged suctioning will cause hypoxia (which is why suctioning for no more than 15 seconds is suggested), an airway obstructed by blood or vomit will not allow any air exchange and is likely to result in aspiration. In this case, patient positioning and aggressive suctioning will be required until the airway is at least partially clear. Re-oxygenation can then be performed and suctioning repeated as required. Follow the guidance of the senior clinician on scene (NAEMT, 2014).

Airway Adjuncts

Airway adjuncts are devices that assist in airway management. Probably the most commonly used airway adjunct is the oropharyngeal airway (Figure 11.12), but there are others including the nasopharyngeal airway.

Oropharyngeal Airway (OPA)

When to do it (indication):

- An unresponsive patient with an absent gag reflex.

When not to do it (contra-indication):

- Any patient who has a gag reflex.

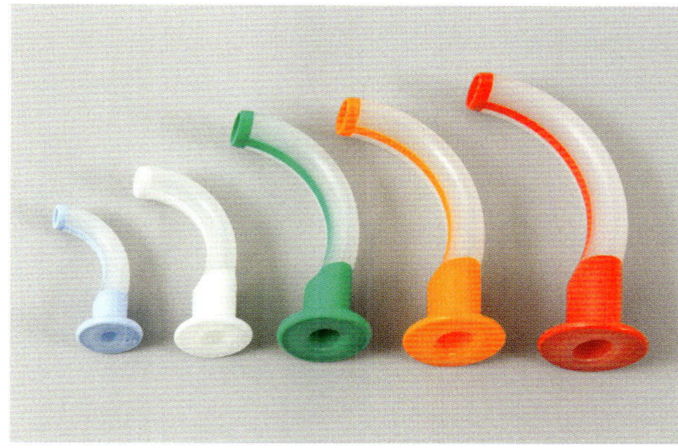

Figure 11.12 *A collection of oropharyngeal airways.*

Advantages:

- Easy to place.
- Technique is simple and non-invasive.

Disadvantages:

- Tongue can be pushed back during insertion, making obstruction worse.
- Does not protect against vomiting.

Procedure

Take the following steps to insert an oropharyngeal airway (Nolan, 2012):

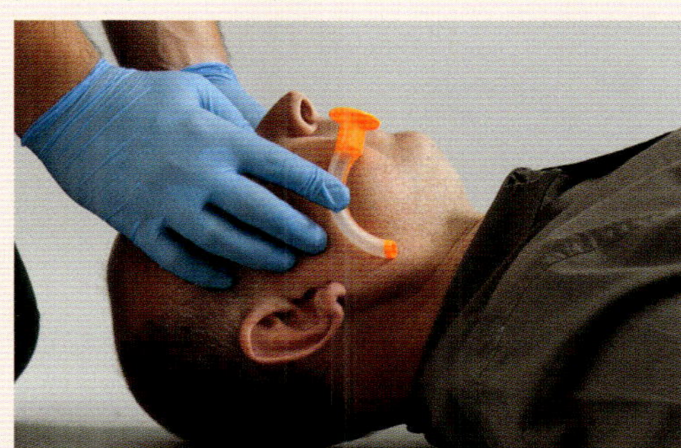

1. Select the correct size OPA by measuring the vertical distance between the patient's incisors and the angle of the jaw.

(continued)

Procedure – *cont*

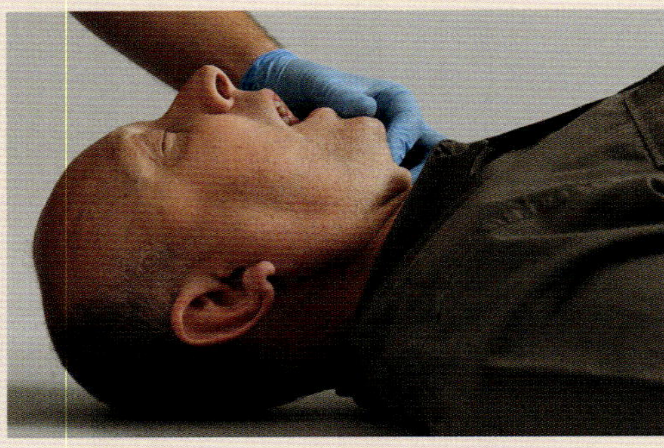

2. Open the patient's mouth and check it is clear of foreign bodies, vomit, blood or secretions. Suction if required.

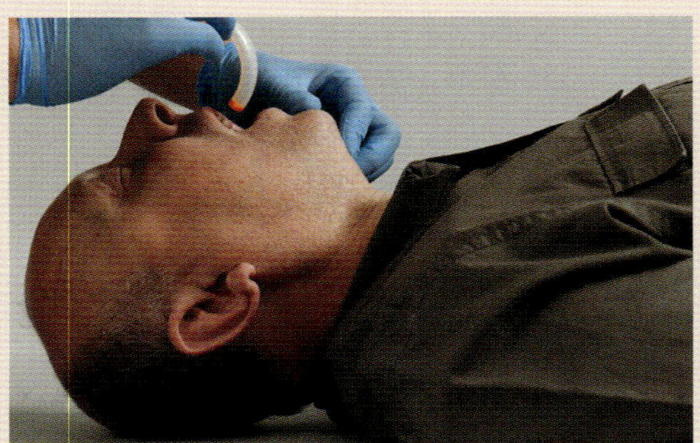

3. Insert the airway 'upside down' along the roof of the mouth until it reaches the soft palate.

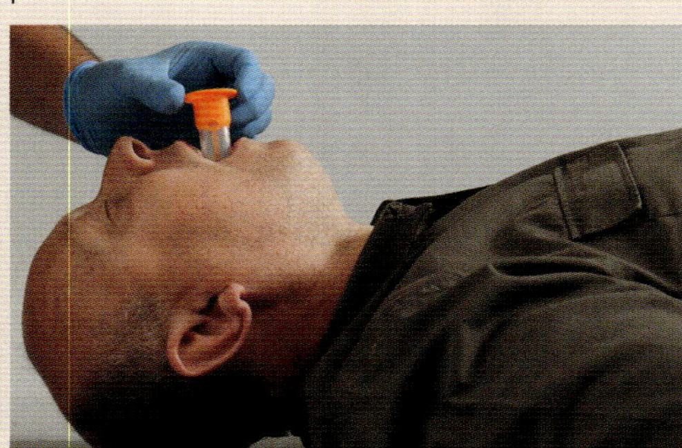

4. Rotate the OPA through 180°.

Procedure – *cont*

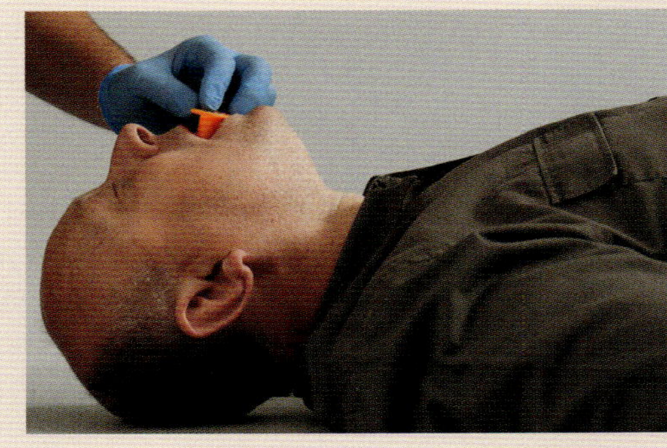

5. Advance the OPA until it rests in the pharynx. Remove immediately if the patient gags. Continue to provide manual manoeuvres such as head tilt–chin lift or jaw thrust as appropriate.

Nasopharyngeal Airway (NPA)

When to do it (indication):

- An unresponsive patient, or a patient with a reduced level of consciousness who has an intact gag reflex.

When not to do it (contra-indication):

- Patients who do not tolerate the procedure.

Cautions:

- Patients who have a basal skull fracture.
- Patients with nasal polyps.

Advantages:

- Can be suctioned through.
- Can be tolerated by patients who are not unconscious.
- Does not require the mouth to open.

Disadvantages:

- Poor technique can cause bleeding.
- Does not protect against aspiration.

Procedure

Take the following steps to insert a nasopharyngeal airway (NPA) (Nolan, 2012; Pilbery, 2013; Gregory, 2010b):

1. Adopt standard precautions.
2. Prepare equipment. You will need the following:

   - an appropriately sized NPA, which is generally considered to be a 7.0 for an average adult male and 6.0 for an average adult female
   - water-soluble gel
   - suction.
3. If the NPA you are using comes with a safety pin, insert it through the non-bevelled end to avoid accidentally inserting the NPA too far.
4. Lubricate the NPA ensuring that the gel does not go over the open ends of the airway.
5. The NPA will be inserted with the bevel facing the nasal septum. This means that the right nostril is usually used, although if the left is clearly larger, then this can be used. In this instance, the NPA will be initially inserted 'upside down' and then rotated through 180° once it enters the nasopharynx (Figure 11.13).
6. Confirm position by listening for breath sounds and ensuring the chest rises and falls.
7. Check for blanching of the patient's nostrils. If this occurs, the NPA should be removed and a smaller diameter NPA inserted instead.
8. Correct technique will minimise the risk of bleeding, but if this occurs, have suction ready.

Supraglottic Airway Device (SAD)

Supraglottic airway devices (SADs) have been used by anaesthetists in operating theatres for over 20 years and have proven to be safe and reliable. SADs generally lead to better ventilation and less air entering the stomach than bag-valve-mask

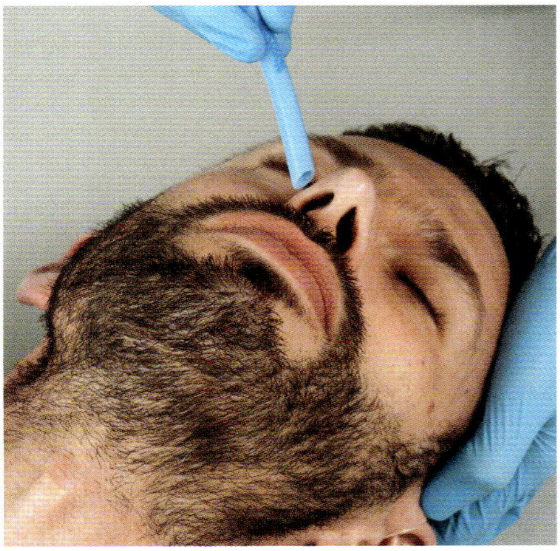

Figure 11.13 *Insertion of the NPA into the right nostril.*

(BVM) ventilation, particularly in the hands of the inexperienced (Nolan, 2012).

The use of SADs is an extended skill and may not be available to every fire and rescue emergency medical responder. As discussed elsewhere, you should always act within your training and scope of practice.

When to do it (indications):
- When BVM ventilation is not effective, is unable to be performed by an experienced person and/or prolonged ventilation is required.
- When intubation fails and BVM ventilation is not possible (can't intubate, can't ventilate).

When not to do it (contra-indications):
- Any patient who has a gag reflex.
- Any patient who is not deeply unconscious.

Advantages:
- Better oxygenation than BVM with an oropharyngeal airway (OPA) (Cook, 2006; Dixon, 2009).
- No need to maintain continuous manual airway seal.
- Easier than endotracheal intubation and does not require laryngoscopy.
- Provides protection from airway secretions.

Disadvantages:
- Does not protect against vomiting.
- May leak when high ventilatory pressures are required, such as in obese or asthmatic patients.

A common SAD in pre-hospital use is the i-gel and the technique for insertion is described here. However, there are others in use and you should be familiar with the devices relevant to your service.

i-gel Insertion Technique

When to do it (indications):
- An unresponsive patient with an absent gag reflex in whom more basic airway manoeuvres are inadequate.
- Airway of choice in cardiac arrest as it is easy to insert.

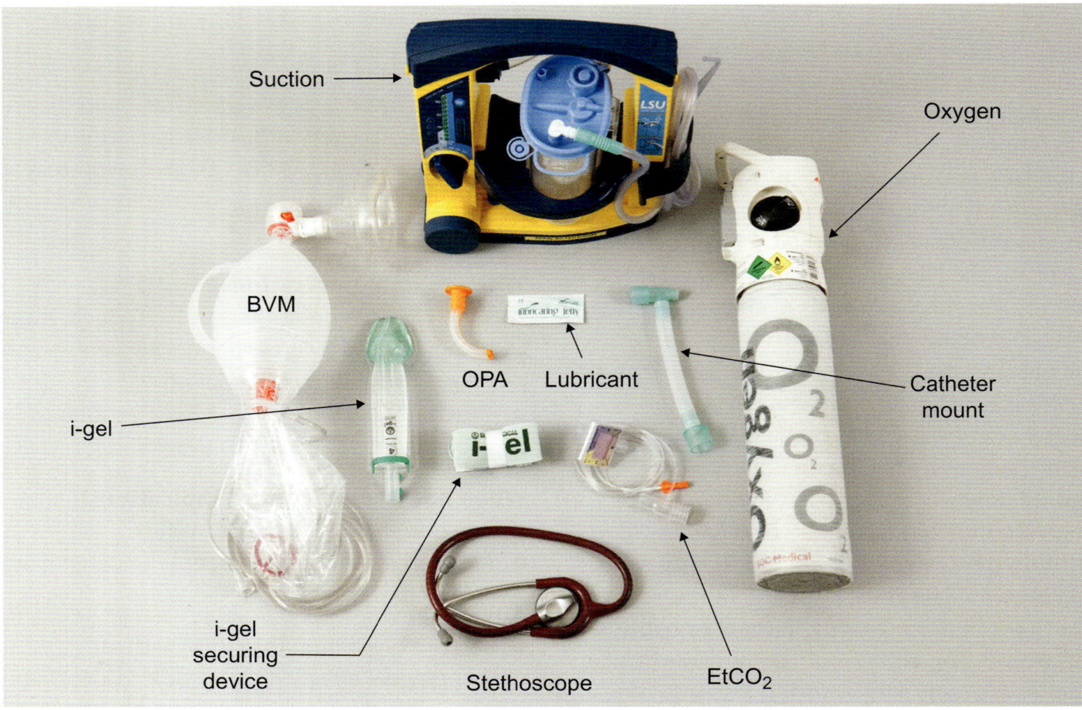

Figure 11.14 *Equipment for i-gel insertion.*

When not to do it (contra-indications):

- Trismus.
- Patients with limited mouth opening.

Advantages:

- Easy to place.
- Straightforward insertion without needing to interrupt chest compressions.
- Small suction catheter can be placed down side-port to drain oesophageal secretions.

Disadvantages:

- May leak, particularly if high inflation pressures are required.
- Does not protect against vomiting.

Equipment

Figure 11.14 shows the equipment you will require in order to insert an i-gel.

Procedure

Take the following steps to insert an i-gel (EEAST, 2014):

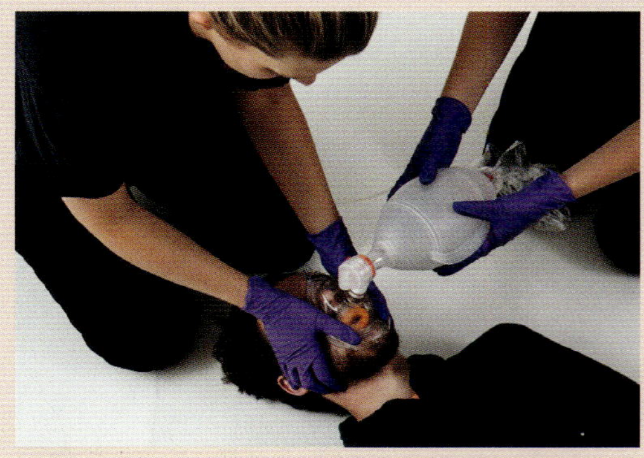

1. Pre-oxygenate the patient while preparing your equipment.

Procedure – *cont*

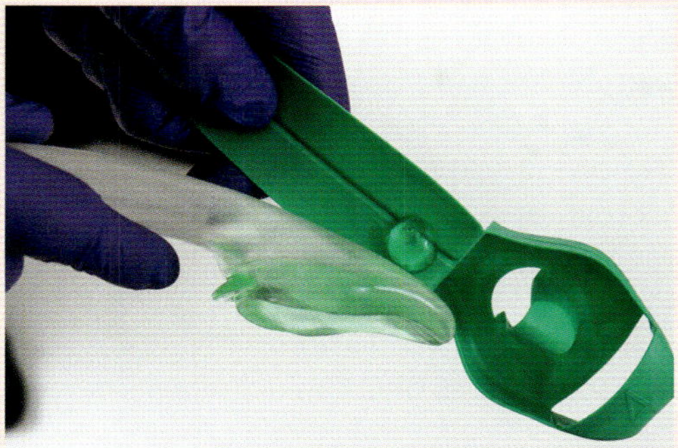

2. Choose the correct size i-gel: 3 for small adults, 4 for medium adults and 5 for large adults. Weight ranges are provided on the i-gel. Open the packaging and remove the device. Place a small amount of water-based lubricant onto the inner and outer rim of the device.

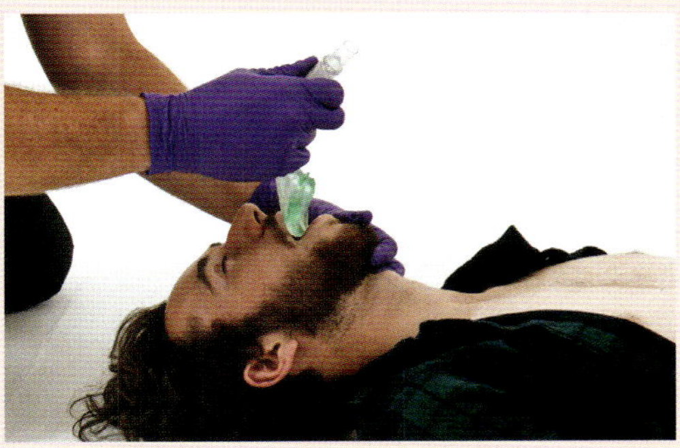

3. With the patient in the 'sniffing the morning air' position, hold the i-gel by the integrated bite block and introduce the green tip into the patient's mouth, directed at the hard palate.

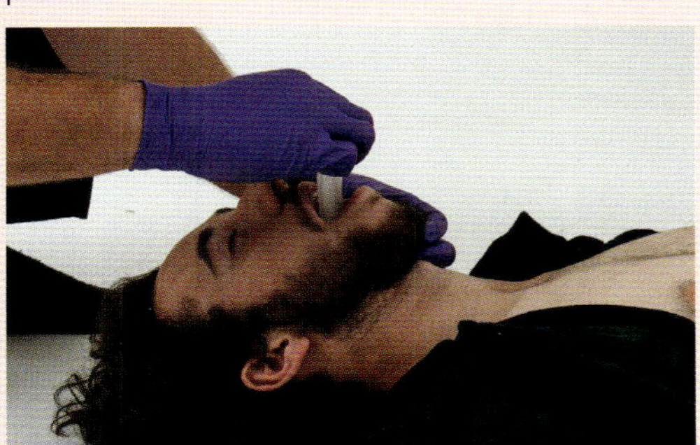

Procedure – *cont*

4. Glide the device downwards and backwards along the hard palate with a continuous but gentle push until a definitive resistance is felt. As a rough guide, the bite block should end up at the level of the incisors.

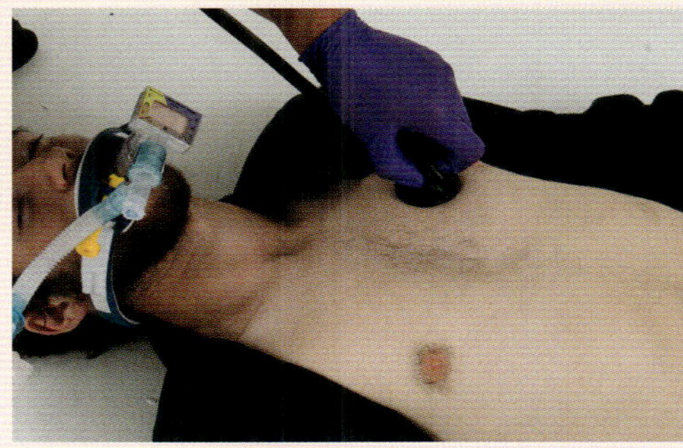

5. Connect the i-gel to your capnography detector, catheter mount and bag-valve-mask. Check for end-tidal carbon dioxide and bilateral chest air entry and movement on ventilating the patient. Once you are confident with the placement, secure/tighten the securing device.

Removal of Foreign Bodies in Adults

For unconscious patients with a definite history of airway obstruction, in addition to performing chest compressions and ventilations at a rate of 30:2, if you are trained to do so, attempt to remove the obstruction under direct vision.

When to do it (indication):

- To facilitate removal of foreign bodies located in the opening of the mouth in the unconscious patient.

When not to do it (contra-indications):

- Any patient who has an effective cough.
- Any patient who is not unconscious.
- Any patient where the obstruction is further back than the opening of the mouth.

Advantage:

- May be more effective at removing foreign bodies than positioning alone.

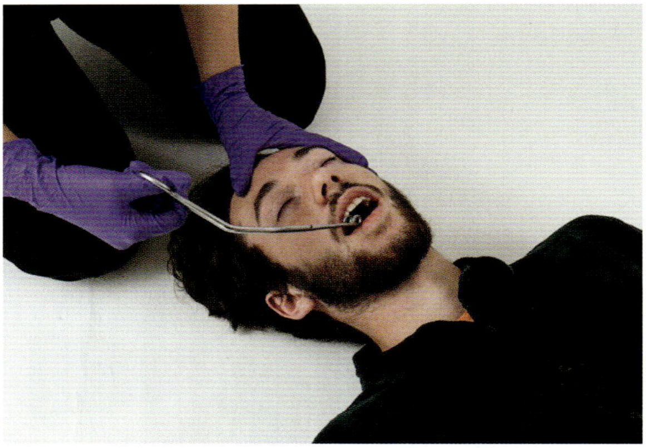

Figure 11.15 *Removal of foreign body using McGill forceps.*

Disadvantages:

- Manipulating a foreign body can cause a partial obstruction to become a complete obstruction.

Procedure

1. Prepare equipment. You will need:
    - suction, to include a rigid and soft suction catheter
    - set of McGills forceps
    - oxygen and non-rebreather face mask.
2. Hold the McGill forceps in your dominant hand. Control the patient's head and airway by placing your left hand on the top of their head (Figure 11.15).
3. Carefully place the forceps either side of the obstruction and tighten the grip.
4. Remove the foreign body and place to one side.
5. Check the airway for further obstruction and suction if required.
6. Once the airway is clear, apply oxygen while you conduct the remainder of the primary survey.

Tracheostomies

Learning Objectives

By the end of this section you will be able to:

- Explain the difference between laryngectomy and tracheostomy.
- Describe how to manage the airway of a patient with a laryngectomy or a tracheostomy.

Introduction

A tracheostomy is an artificial opening made into the trachea through the neck (Figure 11.16a). Patients have them inserted for a number of reasons including (Feber, 2006; Bowers, 2007):

- following trauma or surgery to the head and neck that leads to an airway obstruction
- bypassing a tumour that obstructs the upper airway
- for prolonged ventilation
- for some types of chronic disease where minimising the anatomical dead space is beneficial
- to provide access to chest secretions in the event of respiratory insufficiency
- to protect from aspiration in the event of impaired swallow reflex (for example, neuromuscular disorders).

As the name suggests, a laryngectomy is the removal of the larynx. This is typically due to involvement of the larynx in oral, pharyngeal and laryngeal cancers. If the patient requires a total laryngectomy, the larynx is removed and the trachea cut and stitched to the front of the neck (NTSP, 2014). This is important for subsequent management, because these patients cannot be ventilated from the mouth and/or nose (Figure 11.16b).

Tracheostomy Tubes

There are a wide variety of tracheostomy tubes, which can seem rather overwhelming. However,

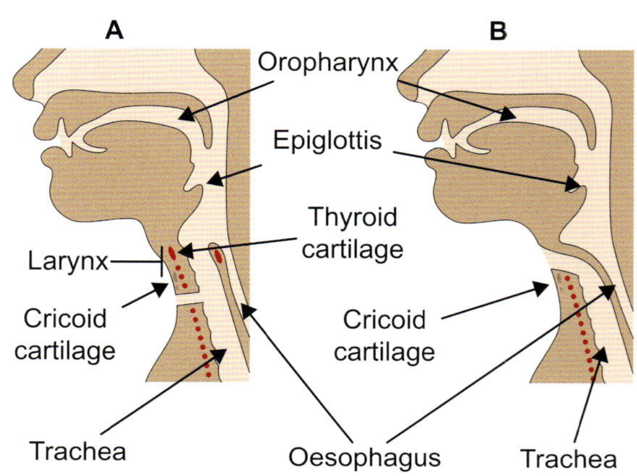

Figure 11.16 *The anatomical differences between a) tracheostomy and b) laryngectomy.*

tubes are broadly classified into the following categories (NTSP, 2014):

- cuffed/uncuffed
- with/without inner cannula
- fenestrated/unfenestrated.

Cuffed/Uncuffed Tubes

A cuffed tracheostomy tube has a soft balloon around the distal end, which is inflated by injecting air into the pilot balloon via the injection port (Figure 11.17). These are used when patients require positive pressure ventilation (PPV) and/or when the patient cannot protect their own airway from secretions. Note that if the cuffed tube is inflated and the lumen becomes blocked or occluded, the patient will not be able to breathe.

Uncuffed tubes tend to be used in longer-term patients, but since they lack the cuff, it is important that these patients have an effective cough and gag reflex to minimise the chance of aspiration. These tubes are not suitable for positive pressure ventilation.

Inner Cannulas

Tracheostomy tubes with an inner cannula (sometimes called double-cannula or double-lumen tubes) consist of an outer tube or cannula which maintains airway patency, and an inner cannula, which can be removed for cleaning and/or disposed of and replaced (Figure 11.18). Uncuffed, double-cannula tracheostomy tubes are the safest type to use in the community (NTSP, 2014).

Fenestrated Tubes

These tracheostomy tubes have an opening in the outer cannula that allows air to pass through the patient's oropharynx and nasopharynx. This is helpful because it allows the patient to talk and produce an effective cough. However, fenestrations increase the risk of aspiration and prevent positive pressure ventilation unless a non-fenestrated inner cannula is used. Non-fenestrated inner cannulas should also be used if the patient requires suction (Figure 11.18).

Management of the Tracheostomy Patient

Patients with tracheostomies have a potentially patent upper airway, since the upper airway and trachea are anatomically connected. However,

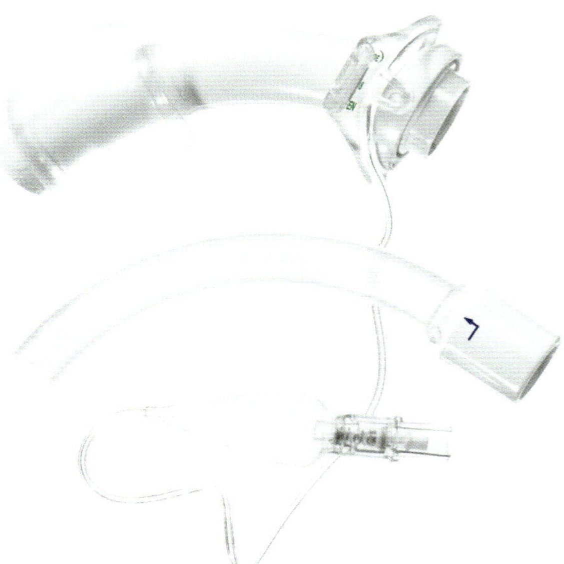

Figure 11.17 *A cuffed, unfenestrated tracheostomy tube (top). Inner cannula with no fenestrations (middle). Pilot balloon and inflation valve for tracheostomy cuff (bottom).*

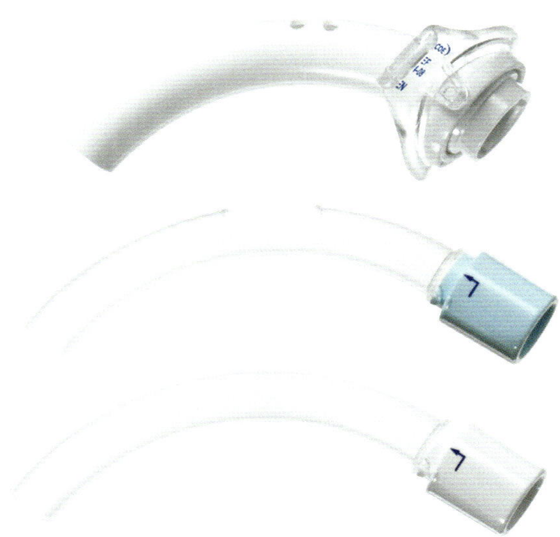

Figure 11.18 *An uncuffed, fenestrated tracheostomy tube (top). Inner cannula with opening for fenestrations (middle). Inner cannula with no fenestrations (bottom).*

it is quite possible that the reason the patient had a tracheostomy in the first place is that their upper airway is difficult or impossible to manage (McGrath, 2012).

Help and Equipment

You will not be able to manage on your own and assistance is vital. If a relative or carer is present, it is quite possible that they know more about tracheostomy management than you do, so listen to their advice and encourage them to help.

Patients may well have equipment to hand, such as replacement tubes, but you can manage with the equipment from your vehicle:

- Airway adjuncts such as oropharyngeal and nasopharyngeal airways.
- Bag-valve-mask.
- Supraglottic airway devices.

Airway and Breathing

Check and open the upper airway as normal. Look, listen and feel for breathing at the face and tracheostomy site for no more than 10 seconds. Apply waveform capnography to the tracheostomy tube as soon as possible (Whitaker, 2011).

If the patient is breathing, apply high-flow oxygen to both face and tracheostomy. If the patient is not breathing, making agonal gasps or there are no signs of life, start chest compressions and follow the basic life support (BLS) algorithm while continuing to troubleshoot the tracheostomy, since this may be the cause of the cardiac arrest (Perkins, 2015).

Tracheostomy Patency

Start by checking for and removing the following:

- Decannulation caps (used when removing tracheostomies) block the end of the tracheostomy.
- Obturators (inserted inside the tracheostomy when first inserting a tube into the patient).
- Speaking valves, which should not be used with an inflated cuffed tube.
- Blocked humidification devices, such as Swedish noses.

If the tracheostomy tube is a double-cannula design, remove the inner cannula, but remember that with some types of tubes the connector required for bag-mask ventilation is mounted on the inner cannula. Pass a suction catheter through the tube and into the trachea to check patency. It should pass easily through the tube. If the suction catheter passes through the tube, suction the tube and attempt to ventilate the patient. If this fails and the tube has a cuff, deflate it and reassess the patient using the same look, listen and feel technique as before at both the face and the stoma site.

Next Steps

If everything attempted thus far has failed to improve the patient's condition, remove the tube. Reassess the patient again and hopefully they will be breathing. If the patient is in cardiac arrest continue with BLS. Attempt to oxygenate the patient via the oral route, but don't forget to cover the stoma site with swabs or a gloved hand. Use standard airway adjuncts to achieve effective ventilation. Alternatively, a paediatric face-mask or supraglottic airway device (SAD) can be placed over the stoma and the patient ventilated. If there is a large air leak from the mouth and/or nose, occlude them both during PPV.

If it is not possible to effectively ventilate the patient, then a suitable clinician will need to attempt endotracheal intubation. This may be possible via the oral route, although they should expect it to be difficult.

In patients with an established tracheostomy or who have a known upper airway problem that is going to make intubation difficult, it can actually be more straightforward to simply insert another, smaller diameter tracheostomy or endotracheal tube into the stoma. (Whitaker, 2011; Kodali, 2013); for this you will need senior clinical support.

Management of the Laryngectomy Patient

Unlike patients with a tracheostomy, laryngectomy patients do not have any connection between the upper airway and their lungs. Do not attempt to ventilate via the mouth/nose. Laryngectomy patients do not normally have tracheostomy tubes either, but may have a tracheo-oesophageal puncture (TEP) valve fitted to allow for speech.

This may be visible inside the stoma, but should not be removed. They are usually fitted with a one-way valve to prevent aspiration (NTSP, 2014).

Since these patients have, in effect, no upper airway, it cannot be obstructed by an inappropriate head position, and due to the reduction in anatomical dead space, chest compressions typically generate sufficient tidal volume to negate the need for PPV if this proves difficult to administer. Instead, just provide a supply of high-flow oxygen to the stoma site.

Tracheostomies are ten times more commonly performed than laryngectomies, so in the event that there is any uncertainty about whether the stoma is a laryngectomy or tracheostomy site, it is better to apply oxygen to both face and stoma.

Help and Equipment

As with tracheostomy patients, these are not patients that you can manage alone, and assistance is vital. If a relative or carer is present, it is quite possible that they know more about laryngectomy management than you do, so listen to their advice and encourage them to help.

Patients may well have equipment to hand such as replacement tubes, but you can manage with the equipment from your vehicle:

- Bag-valve-mask.
- Supraglottic airway devices.

Airway and Breathing

Check and open the upper airway as normal. Look, listen and feel for breathing at the stoma site for no more than 10 seconds. If the patient is breathing, apply high-flow oxygen to the stoma site. If the patient is not breathing, making agonal gasps or there are no signs of life, start chest compressions and follow the BLS algorithm while continuing to troubleshoot the laryngectomy stoma, since this may be the cause of the cardiac arrest.

Laryngectomy Stoma Patency

Most patients will not have a tube in place, but you should remove any stoma cover (sometimes called a 'button') if in place. If a tracheostomy tube is in place and is of a double-cannula design, remove the inner cannula, but remember with some types of tubes the connector required for bag-mask ventilation is mounted on the inner cannula.

Pass a suction catheter through the stoma and into the trachea to check patency. It should pass easily into the trachea. If it does, the stoma is patent, so suction the trachea and attempt to ventilate the patient if they are not breathing. If this fails and there is a cuffed tracheostomy tube in place, deflate it and reassess the patient, preferably with capnography.

Next Steps

If everything attempted thus far has failed to improve the patient's condition, remove any tracheostomy tubes, if present. Reassess the patient again and hopefully they will be breathing. If the patient is in cardiac arrest continue with BLS.

Attempt to ventilate the patient using a paediatric face-mask or SAD placed over the stoma. If this fails, a suitably qualified clinician will need to intubate the stoma with either a smaller diameter tracheostomy or endotracheal tube.

Choking in Adults

Learning Objectives

By the end of this section you will be able to:

- Define choking and list some common causes.
- State the signs that an adult is choking.
- Describe the procedure for managing the choking adult.

Introduction

Choking is a mechanical obstruction of the airway occurring anywhere between the mouth and carina (where the left and right bronchi split from the trachea). Common causes include (Walls, 2012):

- foreign bodies
- blood
- secretions
- teeth
- vomit.

It is not known how common choking is in adults. Death from choking is thankfully rare, mostly because choking episodes are witnessed (Perkins, 2015). In England and Wales, around 370 people die each year as a result of a foreign body in the respiratory tract. Most of these are over 65 years of age (ONS, 2013).

Recognition

The signs of choking in an adult depend on the severity of the airway obstruction that has occurred. Typically, the episode will have occurred while eating, and if the patient is still conscious, they may clutch their neck (Figure 11.19).

In the case of a mild airway obstruction, if you ask the patient if they are choking, they will still be able to speak and confirm that this is the case. They will also be able to breathe and cough.

However, in cases of severe airway obstruction, the patient will be unable to speak, so may only be able to respond to you by nodding their head in response to your question about whether they are choking. Any attempts at coughing will be silent, and if this continues the patient will lose consciousness, possibly before your arrival (Nolan, 2012).

Management

Start by determining the severity of the obstruction. In adults, this is typically determined by the patient's response to the question 'Are you choking?'

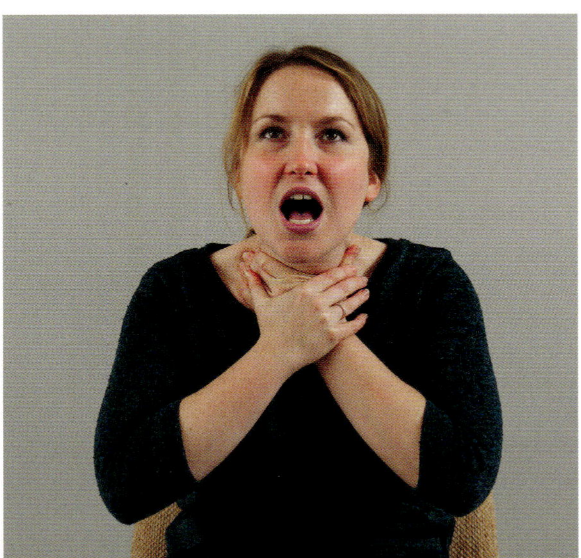

Figure 11.19 *A choking victim clutching her neck.*

A patient who can reply 'Yes' (i.e. can speak, cough and breathe) is classified as mild, whereas the patient who is clutching their throat, is unable to speak and who cannot breathe falls into the severe category.

Conscious and Choking

If the patient is coughing, do not perform any interventions other than encouraging the patient to continue coughing.

If the cough is ineffective, administer up to five back blows, by standing just to the side and slightly behind the patient, leaning them forward, and then administering sharp blows between the shoulder blades with the heel of one hand.

If this fails, move on to abdominal thrusts. Position yourself behind the patient and place a clenched fist just under the xiphisternum. Grasp the fist with your other hand and pull sharply upwards and inwards up to five times.

Repeat the back blows/abdominal thrusts until the obstruction is relieved, or the patient becomes unconscious (Nolan, 2012).

Unconscious and Choking

Lay the patient on their back and start chest compressions and ventilations at a rate of 30:2. Before each set of ventilations, check the mouth to see whether the chest compressions have expelled the foreign body, enabling you to remove it.

Adult Choking Management Algorithm

Figure 11.20 shows the choking management algorithm, which summarises the explanation provided in the previous section.

Choking in the Paediatric Patient

Learning Objective

By the end of this section you will be able to:

- Demonstrate how to manage a choking paediatric patient.

Introduction

It is estimated that around 20 children aged 0–14 years of age per 100,000 population will experience at least one food-related choking episode each

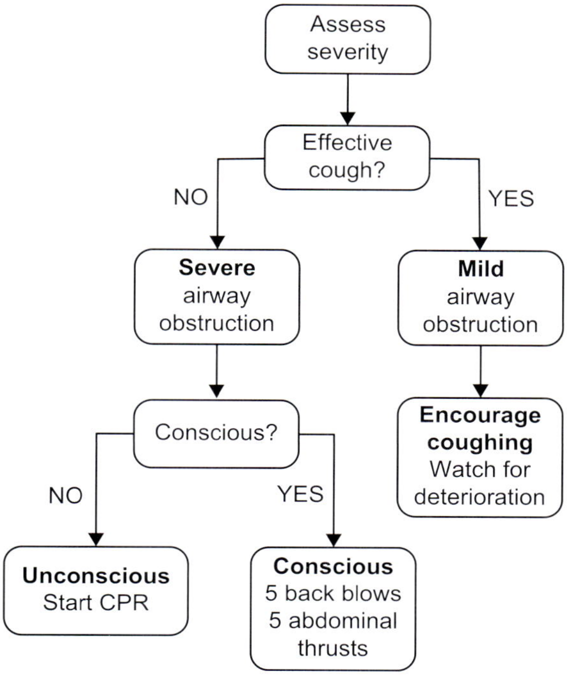

Figure 11.20 *The choking algorithm for adults.*

year. It is more common in boys and children under one year of age (Chapin, 2013). Since most choking episodes involving infants and children are witnessed by an adult, intervention can commence straight away, as long as the adult knows the correct action to take (Skellett, 2016).

The Paediatric Airway

Children's airways more readily obstruct than those of adults, and are particularly sensitive to soft tissue swelling. With a tracheal diameter of around 4 mm in infants compared with 8 mm in the adult, small amounts of swelling dramatically increase airflow resistance and the work of breathing required to maintain adequate ventilation.

The most dramatic differences are found in infants. By the age of 10–12 years, children have mostly adult anatomy, albeit smaller in size (Walls, 2012; Benger, 2009). Other differences include (ALSG, 2010; Fuchs, 2012; AAP, 2013):

- Infants have a large, prominent occiput, which results in neck flexion if they are laid supine on a flat surface. Use padding under the torso to maintain a neutral alignment.
- The glottic opening is at the level of the 1st cervical vertebra (C1) in infants, descending to C3–C4 by the age of 5, resulting in a high, anterior larynx.
- The epiglottis is horseshoe (or omega) shaped, floppy and proportionally larger than that of an adult.
- The tongue is proportionally larger than that of adults, occupying more of the mouth.
- Children possess a small cricothyroid membrane, and in children under 3–4 years of age it is virtually non-existent, making needle cricothyroidotomy very difficult.
- The narrowest portion of the airway in children is at the level of the cricoid ring due to their funnel-shaped larynx compared to the more cylindrical shape of the adult larynx.

Recognition

Major choking episodes in children and infants usually occur during feeding or playing and are often witnessed by a carer. However, remember to ask about any recent history of playing with or eating small objects and consider choking in any child with a sudden onset of breathing problems.

The severity of the obstruction can be determined by the effectiveness of the patient's ability to cough. An effective cough is better than external manoeuvres, so an actively coughing child should be encouraged to continue to do so. Other signs of a mild obstruction include (Maconochie, 2015):

- crying/verbal response to questions
- long cough
- able to take breaths before coughing
- fully alert.

Contrast this with signs of a severe airway obstruction and an ineffective cough:

- unable to verbalise
- quiet/silent cough
- unable to breathe
- cyanosis
- decreasing level of consciousness.

Management

The management of the choking paediatric patient depends on their ability to effectively cough and on whether they are conscious or unconscious (Figure 11.21) (Skellett, 2016).

Conscious and Choking

Infants

Start with back blows. If your patient is an infant, sit on a chair or kneel on the floor and place the infant across your lap in a prone (face-down) position. Support their head with the thumb and fingers of one hand at the angle of their jaw, taking care not to compress the soft tissues. Administer up to five sharp blows between their scapulae with the heel of your other hand.

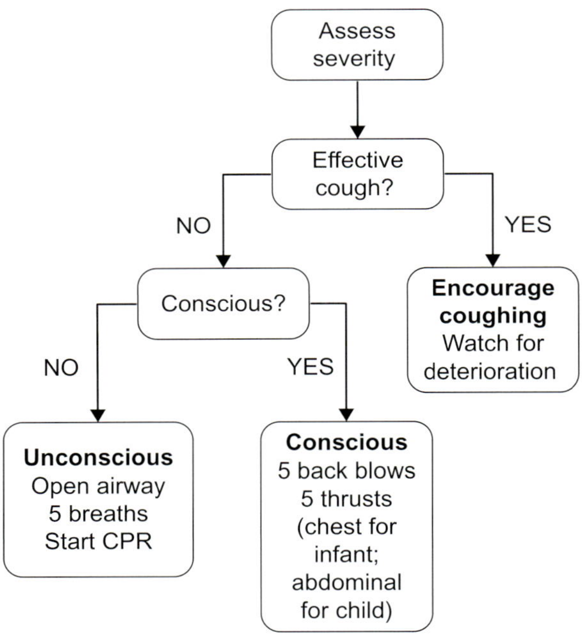

Figure 11.21 *Management of choking in the paediatric patient.*

If these fail, turn the infant onto their back with their head downwards. Locate the landmarks for chest compression (i.e. one finger width above the xiphisternum) and administer up to five chest compressions, making them sharper and slower than those administered during cardiac arrest.

Children (Over One Year of Age)

If the patient is a child, support them in a head-down position and administer up to five inter-scapular blows. If this does not clear the obstruction, administer abdominal thrusts by standing behind the child and leaning them forward. Place a clenched fist midway between the xiphisternum and belly button. Grasp the fist with your other hand and pull inwards and upwards, up to five times.

Frequently reassess and alternate between back blows and chest thrusts in the infant, and back blows and abdominal thrusts in the child.

Unconscious and Choking

If a child or infant becomes, or is, unconscious, place them on their back with appropriate padding to maintain an open airway. Check the mouth for a visible obstruction and make a single attempt to remove it if a foreign body is visible.

Attempt to ventilate, but if this does not cause chest expansion try repositioning the head and try again. If after five attempts you still cannot ventilate the child, move on to chest compressions and alternate with further ventilations using a ratio of 15:2. Don't forget to check the airway for a dislodged foreign body after re-opening the airway prior to ventilating.

Chapter 12

Breathing

Respiratory System Physiology

Learning Objective

By the end of this section you will be able to:

- Describe and explain the function of the respiratory system.

Introduction

In Chapter 11: Airway, you learnt about the structure (or anatomy) of the respiratory system, but it is important to also understand its function (physiology). Functionally, the respiratory system is split into two portions (Tortora, 2008):

- **Conducting portion:** This is made up of the interconnecting cavities and tubes starting at the mouth and nose and ending at the terminal bronchioles. These filter, warm and moisten the air and transfer it to the lungs and out again.
- **Respiratory portion:** This is made up of the tissues inside the lungs which exchange the gas. It consists of the respiratory bronchioles, alveolar ducts and sacs, and the alveoli. This is where gas exchange between the air and blood occurs.

These portions combined enable the respiratory system to perform its functions:

- Gas exchange: Imports oxygen, which is taken up into the blood and delivered to the body's cells. Expires the waste gas carbon dioxide.
- Assists in the regulation of blood acidity levels.
- Removes small amounts of heat and water.
- Filters inspired air, produces vocal sounds and contains receptors providing a sense of smell.

Respiration

Respiration is the process of gas exchange in the body (mainly of oxygen and carbon dioxide). It consists of three steps (Tortora, 2008):

- **Pulmonary ventilation:** The process of moving air into and out of the lungs. It is divided into inspiration (inhalation), when air is moved into the lungs, and expiration (exhalation), when air is moved out of the lungs (Pilbery, 2013).
- **External respiration:** The exchange of gases between the alveoli of the lungs and the blood inside the pulmonary capillaries.
- **Internal respiration:** The exchange of gases between the blood in capillaries around the body and tissue cells.

The Lungs

In order to understand ventilation and external respiration, we need to cover a little more anatomy. Recall from Chapter 11 that the lungs extend from the diaphragm to just above the clavicles. The left lung is smaller than the right due to the space taken up by the heart. It also has only two lobes, the upper and lower, whereas the right lung has three, the upper, lower and middle lobes (Tortora, 2008). Deep grooves known as fissures divide the lobes. Both lungs have an oblique fissure, but the right lung also has a horizontal fissure (Figures 12.1, 12.2 and 12.3).

Lobes, Lobules and Alveoli

Each lobe of the lung has its own secondary branch (bronchus), branching from the right and left primary bronchi (Figure 12.4).

These in turn divide into tertiary bronchi, each supplying a segment of lung called a bronchopulmonary segment. Within these are many much smaller components known as lobules, within which are contained three to five respiratory units, which is where the gas exchange occurs. Respiratory units (or acini) emerge from the terminal bronchioles and consist of several respiratory bronchioles, which subdivide into alveolar ducts and, finally, the alveoli (Patel, 2008).

Alveoli

The alveoli are cup-shaped pouches with very thin walls that enable the exchange of oxygen and carbon dioxide with the pulmonary capillaries that surround them. There are around 140–150 million

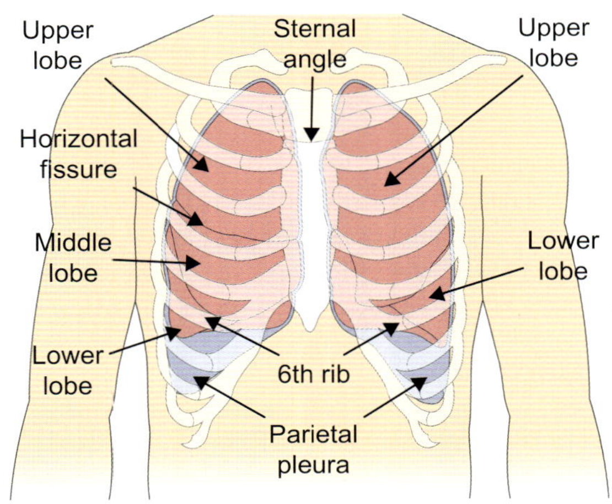

Figure 12.1 *Anterior view of the lungs in relation to surface anatomy.*

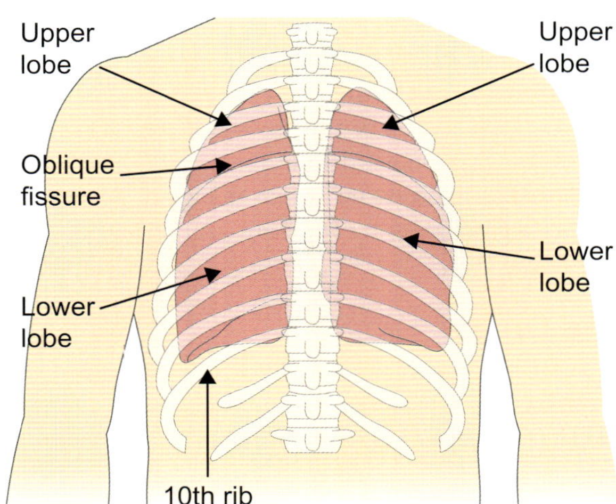

Figure 12.2 *Posterior view of the lungs in relation to surface anatomy.*

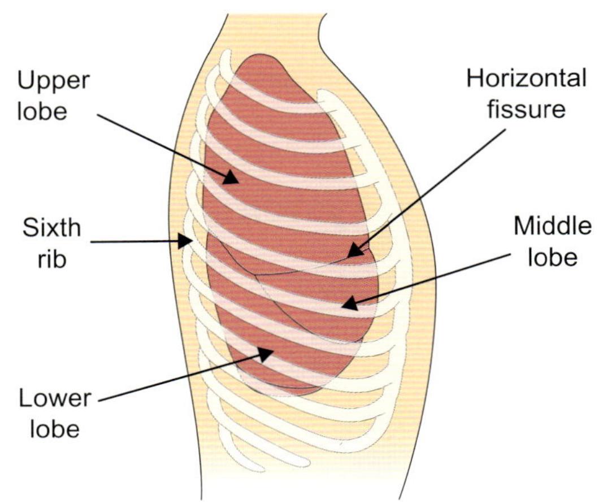

Figure 12.3 *Lateral view of the lungs in relation to surface anatomy.*

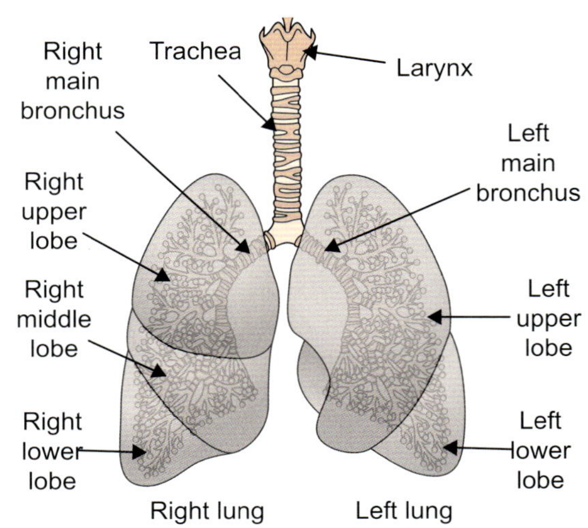

Figure 12.4 *The lower respiratory tract showing the left and right bronchi.*

in each normal lung, creating a surface area for gaseous exchange in the region of two tennis courts (Patel, 2008).

Mechanics of Breathing

Air Pressure

Air moves into and out of the lungs because ventilation changes the pressure inside the alveoli. This is achieved by changing the volume of the thoracic cavity (the contents of the body surrounded by the ribs and diaphragm). As the volume inside this cavity increases, the pressure inside decreases (a relationship known as Boyle's Law). This causes the lungs to expand, increasing their volume and so decreasing the alveolar pressure.

Since air moves from areas of high pressure to low pressure, once the pressure inside the alveoli drops below that outside the body, i.e. atmospheric pressure, air enters the lungs. At the end of inspiration, the volume of the thoracic cavity decreases, and the pressure rises; once it becomes higher than that of atmospheric pressure, air leaves the lungs (Patel, 2008).

Inspiration

During normal, quiet respiration, most of the work of respiration is undertaken by the diaphragm. This is a dome-shaped muscle that seals the thoracic cavity from the abdomen. When it contracts, it flattens and descends, increasing the volume inside the thoracic cavity, and is responsible for about 75% of the air entering the lungs.

The remaining 25% of air entering the lungs is as a result of the external intercostal muscles contracting, which pull the ribs upwards and outwards like a bucket handle (Tortora, 2008).

Expiration

During normal, quiet respiration, breathing out (expiration) is a passive process as no muscles are involved. This is because of elastic recoil, a property of the thoracic wall and the lungs, enabling them to 'spring back' to their original position when they are stretched by the muscles of inspiration.

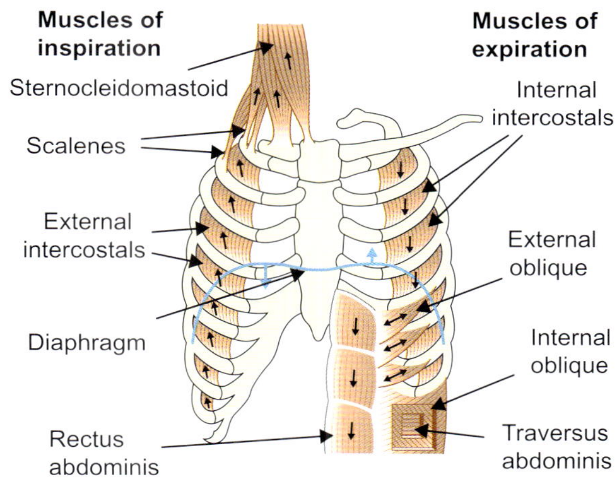

Figure 12.5 *Muscles of inspiration and expiration.*

Forceful Breathing

When exercising and in other instances when the body requires more oxygen, additional, accessory, muscles can be used to aid inspiration and expiration (Figure 12.5). These can often be seen in use by patients in respiratory distress.

Gas Exchange

You have already read that gas moves from areas of high pressure to low, and it turns out that this is the case even for a mixture of gases. Take room air, which you are breathing in. It is made up of the following (percentages are approximate) (Tortora, 2008):

- oxygen (O_2) - 20.9%
- nitrogen (N_2) - 79%
- carbon dioxide (CO_2) - 0.04%
- other gases/water vapour - 0.06%.

The pressure each of the gases exerts to make up the pressure of air is known as the gas's partial pressure. For example, the partial pressure of oxygen (PO_2) in the air is 21 kilopascals (kPa).

Each gas acts independently of the others, so in the alveoli, oxygen moves from an area of higher pressure (the alveoli) to an area of lower oxygen pressure (the pulmonary circulation), by a property known as diffusion.

Diffusion

Diffusion is a process by which molecules (such as oxygen and carbon dioxide) move around. It has two key characteristics (Patel, 2008):

- Diffusion occurs from areas of high concentration to areas of low concentration.
- Diffusion continues until both areas have the same concentration of molecules.

Oxygen diffuses from the alveoli into the pulmonary circulation, whereas carbon dioxide has a higher partial pressure inside the pulmonary circulation so moves across into the alveoli, where it can be expired. In this way, oxygen is taken up by the body and the waste gas, carbon dioxide, is removed (Kapit, 2000).

Control of Breathing

The muscles of respiration are dependent on the nervous system to tell them to contract and relax. This is achieved with two types of nervous system control (Kapit, 2000; Tortora, 2008):

- **Voluntary (or conscious) control:** This originates in the cerebral cortex and is the way you can control your breathing by holding your breath or controlling the flow of air in order to play a wind instrument, for example. In addition, other centres in the brain, such as the hypothalamus and limbic system, can stimulate respiration, allowing laughing and crying to affect the breathing pattern.
- **Automatic control:** These originate from groups of nerve cells (neurons) in the brain stem (mainly the pons and medulla). The neurons in the medulla are responsible for the basic rhythm of breathing and send impulses to the inspiratory muscles via the phrenic and intercostal nerves. Expiratory neurons generally become active only during forceful breathing, such as when exercising.

The respiratory centres containing these inspiratory and expiratory neurons are influenced by sensory input from nerves around the body. For example, stretch receptors prevent the lungs from being overinflated and others are linked to receptors that can detect movement, stimulating the respiratory centres to increase ventilation during exercise.

Breathing is also regulated by the partial pressures of oxygen (PaO_2) and carbon dioxide ($PaCO_2$), and hydrogen ion concentration (pH) in the blood. $PaCO_2$ is the most important and has the most profound effect on respiration. These are detected by special sensory neurons called chemoreceptors that are located close to the medulla (central chemoreceptors) and in the walls of the aortic and carotid arteries (Tortora, 2008).

Note: The extra 'a' in PaO_2 denotes the partial pressure of oxygen in arterial blood.

Using Medical Gases Safely

Learning Objectives

By the end of this section you will be able to:

- Describe dangers of using compressed gas.
- Outline the safe use, storage and handling of medical gases.
- State the guidelines for the use of oxygen therapy including:
    - indications
    - contra-indications.
- Outline the safe use of Entonox including:
    - the properties of Entonox
    - complications of environmental temperature with regards to Entonox
    - the benefits of Entonox therapy
    - indications
    - cautions and contra-indications.
- Explain the use of facial barriers and the bag-valve-mask.

Introduction

The two main medical gases you will use are oxygen and Entonox. These gases are compressed into cylinders of varying sizes (Figure 12.6).

Oxygen behaves differently from air, compressed air, nitrogen and other inert gases. It is very reactive. Pure oxygen, at high pressure, such as from a cylinder, can react violently with common materials such as oil and grease. Other materials may catch fire spontaneously. Nearly all materials including textiles, rubber and even metals will burn vigorously in oxygen (HSE, 2008b).

Even a small increase in the oxygen level in the air to 24% can create a dangerous situation. It becomes easier to start a fire, which will then

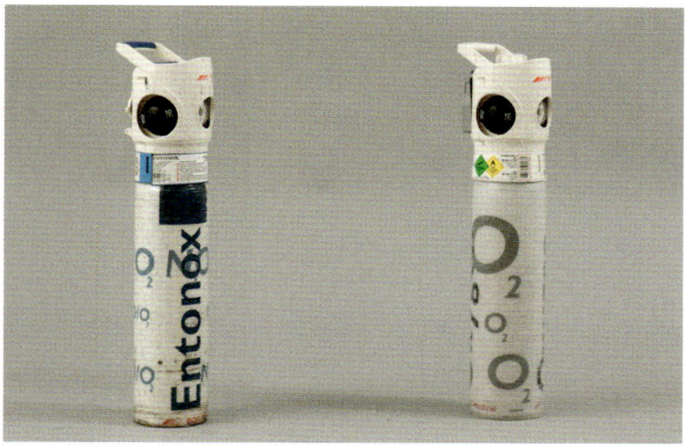

Figure 12.6 *Medical gases. Entonox on the left, oxygen on the right.*

burn hotter and more fiercely than in normal air. It may be almost impossible to put the fire out. A leaking valve or hose in a poorly ventilated room or confined space can quickly increase the oxygen concentration to a dangerous level.

The main causes of fires and explosions when using oxygen are (HSE, 2008b):

- oxygen enrichment from leaking equipment
- use of materials not compatible with oxygen
- use of oxygen in equipment not designed for oxygen service
- incorrect or careless operation of oxygen equipment.

Medical Gas Cylinder Storage

A medical gas cylinder store (Figure 12.7) should meet all of the following requirements (DoH, 2006a):

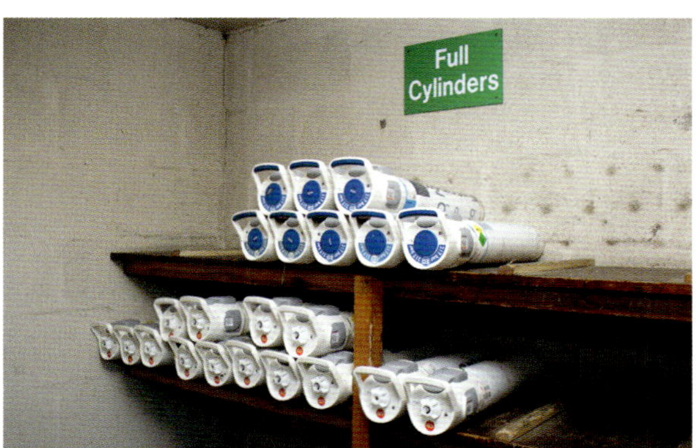

Figure 12.7 *An ambulance station medical gas cylinder store.*

- On ground level, as close as possible to delivery point.
- Clearly identifiable, so it can easily be located in an emergency.
- Not close to any installation that may cause a fire risk (such as the fuel pump).
- Have a level floor, made of concrete or other non-combustible material.
- Well ventilated.
- Only containing medical gases.
- Adequate means of securing large cylinders to prevent falling.
- Clear and separate areas for full and empty cylinders.
- Kept free from naked flames and marked with signage such as 'No Smoking'.
- Not prone to excessively hot or cold temperatures.
- Contain shelving to store smaller cylinders horizontally.
- Secure enough to prevent theft and misuse.

Depending on local arrangements, you may be able to replace your empty oxygen cylinder from this store, or exchange empty cylinders with the ambulance service.

Anatomy of a Medical Gas Cylinder

In this section, the use of integrated valve cylinders (Figure 12.8) is covered, as these are the most commonly utilised. However, you may find that your service still uses the older style of cylinders, which require a regulator head to be fitted before they can be used; you should seek guidance on their use.

There is a British Standard (BS EN 1089-3:2011) relating to the labelling of medical gases to ensure that they are easy to identify and so that inappropriate administration is avoided (BSI, 2011). Medical gases always have a white body, but have different coloured collars to indicate the type of gas. The most commonly encountered gases that you will find on an ambulance are oxygen (black collar), Entonox (blue and white collar) and air (black and white collar).

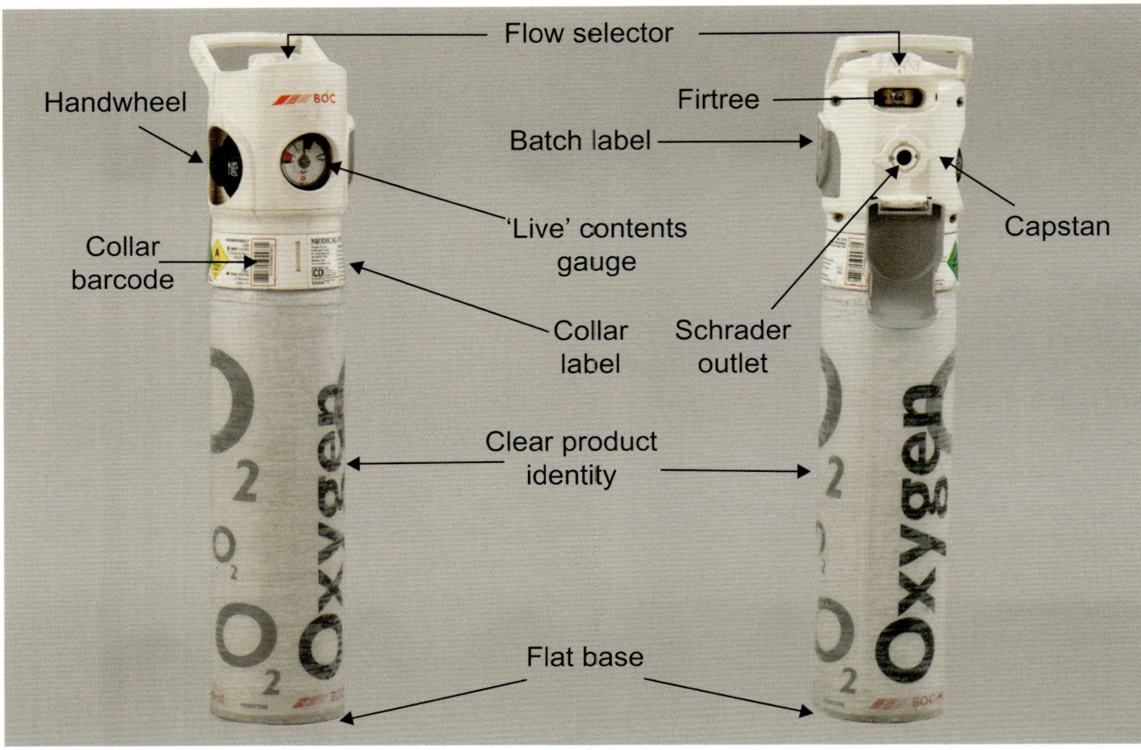

Figure 12.8 *CD-sized integrated valve oxygen cylinder.*

Important components of the cylinder are (BOC, 2013a):

- Flow selector:
  - Desired flow rate can be selected by rotating the dial.
  - Positive 'click' between flow rates to ensure correct setting is chosen.
- 'Live' contents gauge:
  - Shows contents of cylinder, even when turned off.
  - Green = full.
  - Red = low/empty.
- Handwheel:
  - Simple on/off dial. No spanner required.
  - Turn anti-clockwise to open.
  - Turn clockwise to close.
- Clear product identity:
  - Name of gas is written on cylinder collar and body.
- Flat base:
  - Easier to handle.
  - Improves stability.
- Firtree:
  - Attachment point for oxygen tubing.
- Batch label:
  - Located on guard or collar.
  - Shows expiry date.
  - Required when reporting cylinder defect.
- Schrader outlet:
  - Push-fit connector for other methods of administration/connection to artificial ventilators.
  - Gas-specific to avoid inadvertent inappropriate administration.
  - Out sleeve (capstan) can be twisted to release.

Safety First

Prior to using a medical gas, there are a number of safety checks required (BOC, 2013a):

- Make sure your hands are clean. If you have used an alcohol-based hand rub, ensure that it has evaporated completely.
- Check the cylinder to ensure it is clean and free from damage.

- Ensure the cylinder is free from oil and grease, especially around the Schrader and firtree outlets.
- Both oxygen and Entonox are non-flammable, but strongly support combustion. Keep away from naked flames, sources of ignition and combustible materials.

If the medical gas is Entonox, check that it has not been allowed to get too cold. Below -6°C the nitrous oxide will separate from the gas mixture. To prevent this, it should be stored above 10°C for at least 24 hours prior to use. If this is not possible and the bottle is of a portable size, warm the bottle to 10°C and then invert three times prior to use to mix the gases.

Preparing a New Cylinder for Use

The following steps apply to both oxygen and Entonox cylinders (BOC, 2013a; BOC, 2013b):

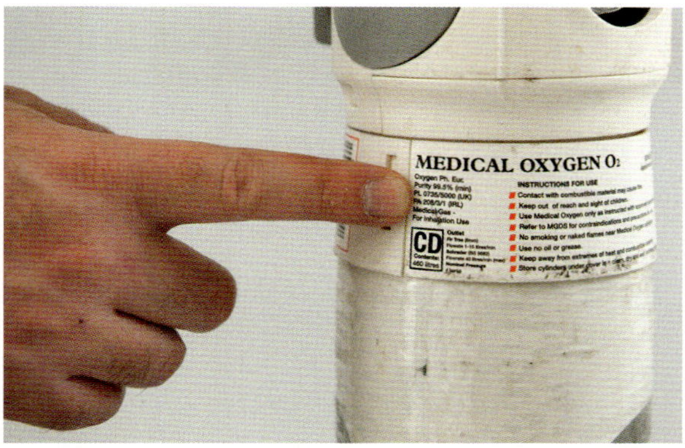

1. Ensure you have the correct medical gas by checking the cylinder label.

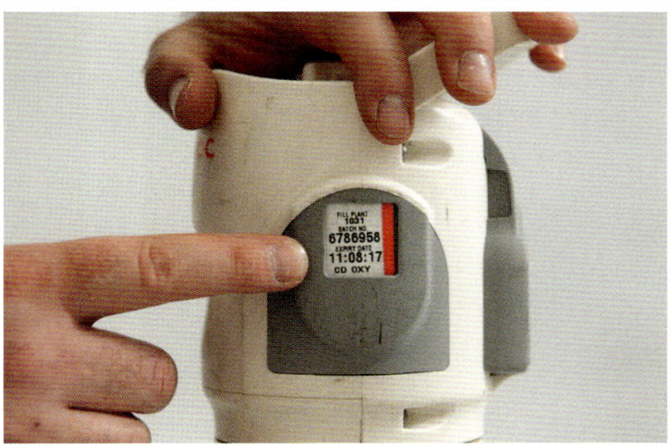

2. Check the expiry date on the batch label fitted to the cylinder.

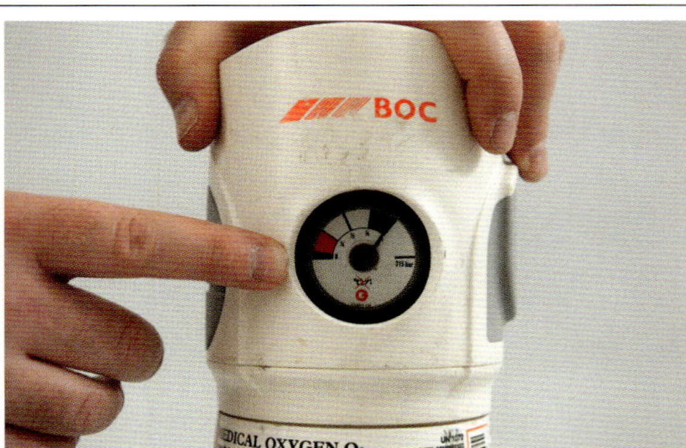

3. Make sure the contents gauge is in the green zone. This indicates that the cylinder is full.

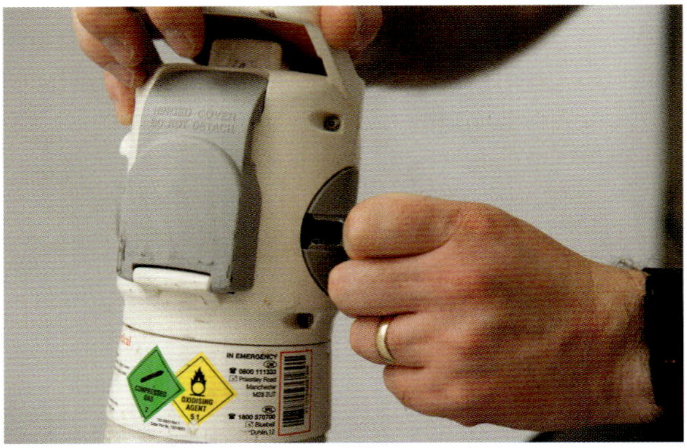

4. Remove the tamper-evident handwheel cover by pulling the tear ring.

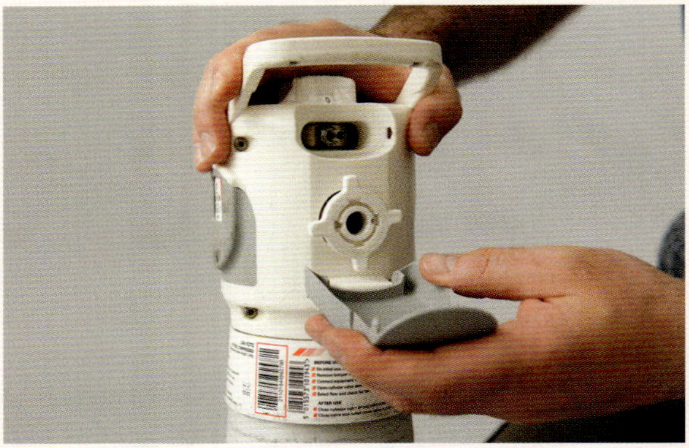

5. Remove the valve outlet cover. Pull the grey cover downwards. It stays attached to the cylinder.

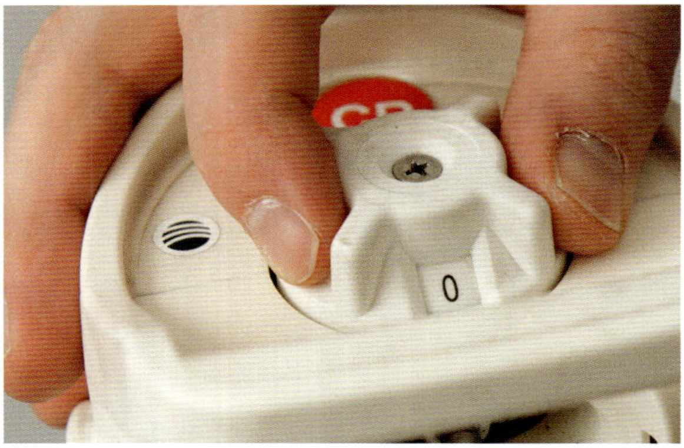

6. Ensure the flow selector on top of the cylinder is set to zero and the handwheel is turned off before connecting equipment.

Oxygen

The most common size of oxygen cylinder that you will be supplied with is the CD size. Table 12.1 shows how long a CD-sized cylinder will supply oxygen for (in minutes) based on the flow rate and gauge level.

Table 12.1 CD-sized oxygen cylinder (460 litres)

Flow rate	Gauge level		
(l/min)	Full (100%)	Half (50%)	Low (25%)
15	30	15	7
10	46	23	11
4	115	57	28

Oxygen Delivery Devices

The firtree connector (Figure 12.9) is used to connect oxygen tubing to the cylinder, which in

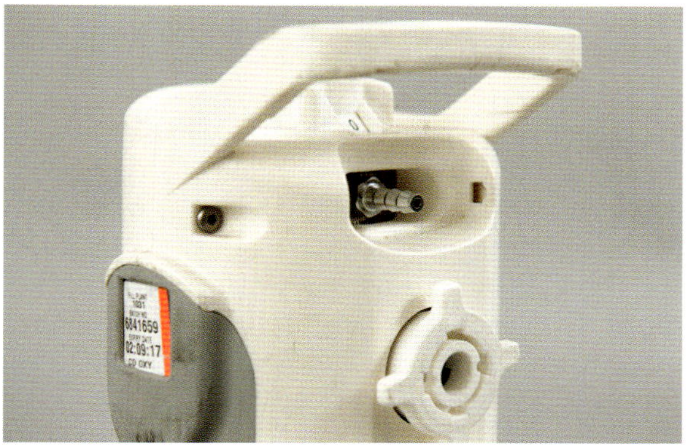

Figure 12.9 *Oxygen firtree connector.*

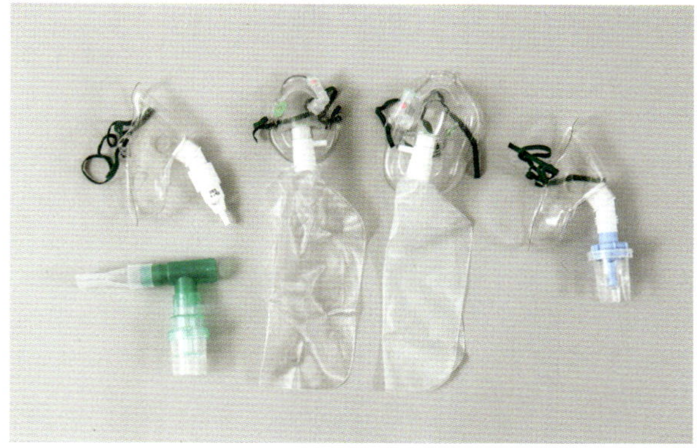

Figure 12.10 *A variety of devices to administer oxygen.*

turn can provide oxygen to a variety of masks and other devices (Figure 12.10).

Note: Oxygen masks and nasal cannulae all require the patient to be spontaneously breathing in order to work. If the patient is not breathing effectively, they require assisted ventilation with a bag-valve-mask or pocket mask.

Procedure

Follow the steps below to provide oxygen to the appropriate oxygen delivery device (BOC, 2013a):

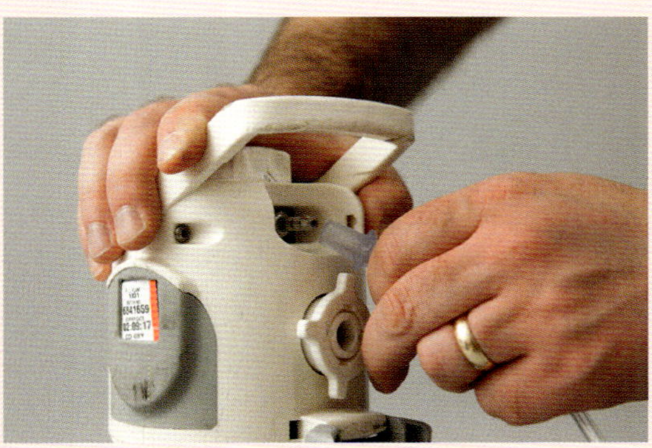

1. Attach tubing from mask or nasal cannulae to the firtree outlet. Ensure the tubing is pushed on securely.

Procedure – *cont*

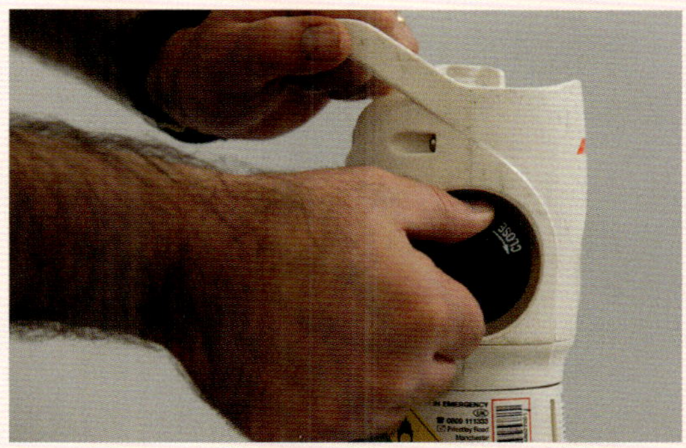

2. Slowly turn on the cylinder by rotating the handwheel anti-clockwise until it comes to a complete stop. Do not use excessive force.

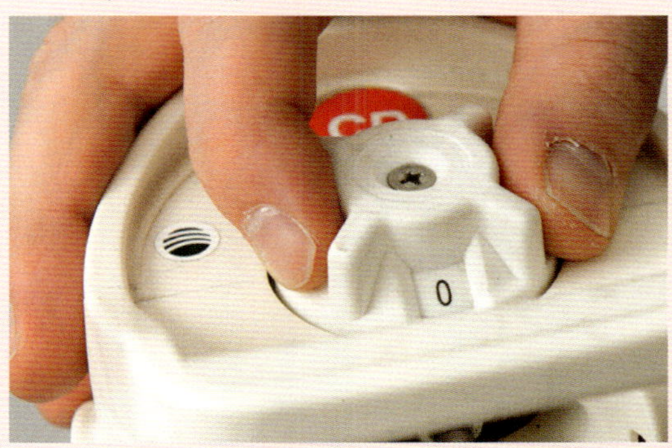

3. Set the prescribed flow by rotating the flow selector dial. Ensure that the correct flow rate number is clearly visible in the flow selector window. Check the gas is flowing.

Supplemental Oxygen Delivery Devices

Non-Rebreathe Mask

This mask is used when the patient requires a high concentration of oxygen (Figure 12.11). At 15 l/min, the mask can deliver up to 85% inspired oxygen. It consists of a mask and reservoir bag that is fitted with a one-way valve, ensuring that the patient can only inhale oxygen from it and not exhale into the bag. The bag must be inflated in order to ensure maximum inspired oxygen.

Medium Concentration Face Mask (Simple Face Mask)

This face mask has ports on either side to allow room air to be drawn inside (Figure 12.12). At 10 l/min, it will deliver around 40% oxygen, but this is variable depending on how well fitting the mask is.

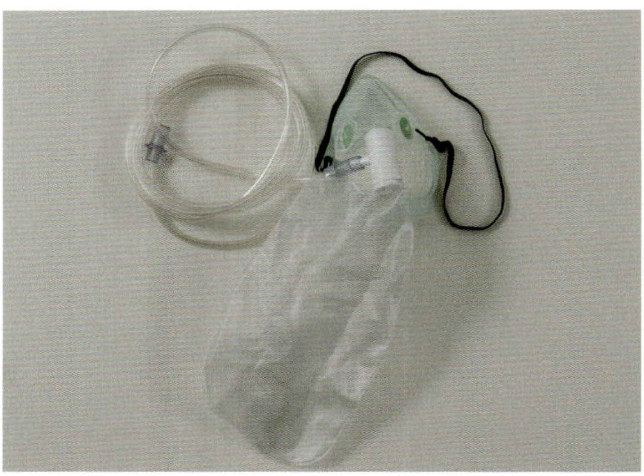

Figure 12.11 *Non-rebreathe mask.*

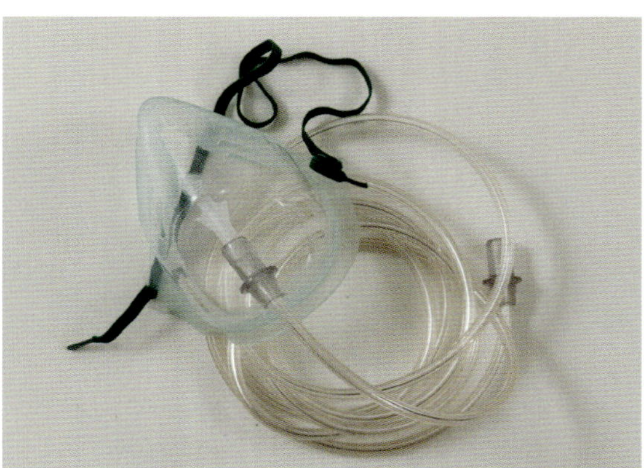

Figure 12.12 *Medium concentration face mask.*

Venturi Mask

This mask also draws in (or entrains) room air, but allows for more accurate oxygen delivery than the medium concentration face mask (Figure 12.13). It comes with a variety of spigots, which are capable of delivering a variety of oxygen concentrations. The percentage of oxygen and flow rate required are usually clearly marked on the spigot. They are particularly useful when providing oxygen to patients with chronic obstructive pulmonary disease (COPD) (see Table 12.4).

Nasal Cannulae

These deliver oxygen via two nasal prongs, which sit just inside the patient's nostrils (Figure 12.14). Oxygen flow rates are typically limited to 1–4 l/min as higher rates lead to irritation of the nasal lining. They are often used by patients on long-term

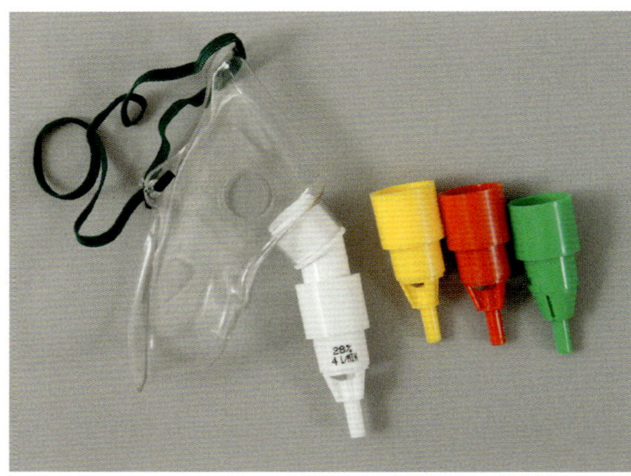

Figure 12.13 *Venturi mask.*

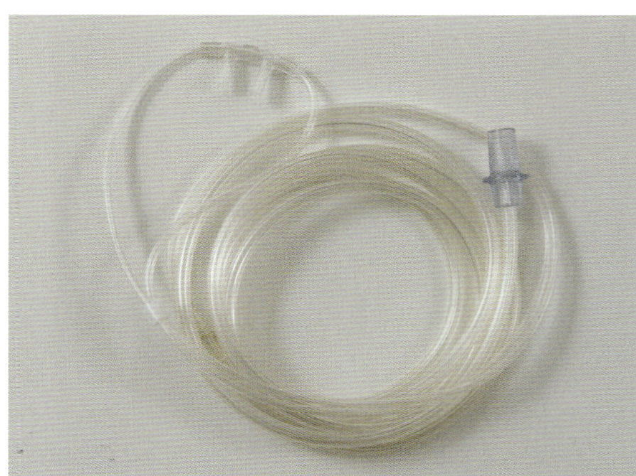

Figure 12.14 *Nasal cannulae.*

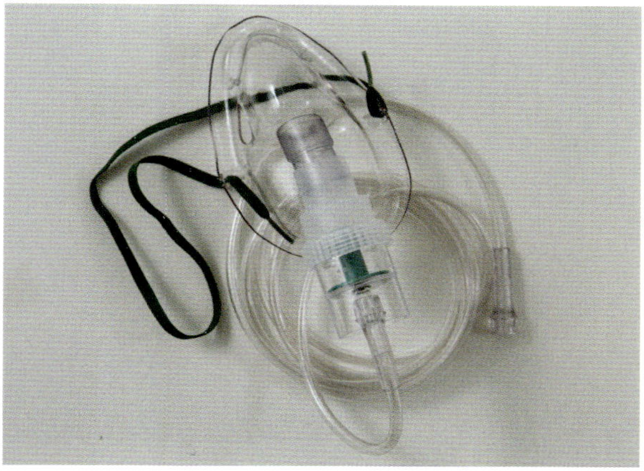

Figure 12.15 *Nebuliser mask.*

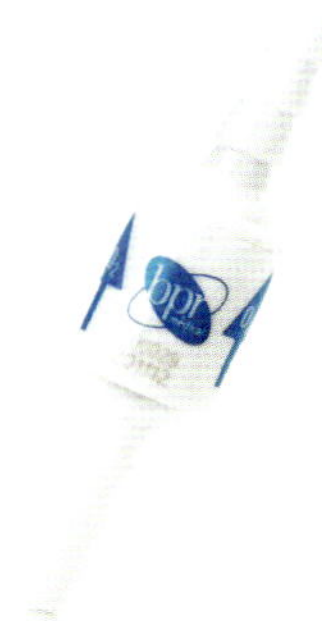

Figure 12.16 *A Firesafe™.*

oxygen therapy and may be preferred by patients who do not tolerate a face mask.

Nebuliser

This is used to deliver aerosolised drugs (Figure 12.15). The pressurised chamber when powered by oxygen turns the liquid drug inside (usually salbutamol or ipratropium) into a mist (i.e. aerosolises the drug), which is then inhaled by the patient. Some nebulisers (particularly if the patient has one at home) are powered using compressed room air.

Firesafe

You may notice a small device inserted into a patient's tubing if they are on home oxygen (Figure 12.16). This is a Firesafe™ – a cannula valve that is designed to cut the oxygen supply to the patient in the event of a fire. It will not affect the oxygen flow to the patient in any other circumstance as long as it is inserted the correct way around (the arrow shows the direction of gas flow).

Assisted Ventilation

Patients who are breathing inadequately, for example because they have a slow respiratory rate or an irregular pattern of respiration, and patients whose breathing is too shallow or who are not breathing at all, require assisted ventilation. Assisted ventilation can be provided with a pocket mask or BVM.

Gastric Distension

In contrast to the normal way we breathe (i.e. the negative pressure inside the chest cavity draws air into the chest), assisted and artificial ventilation requires the use of positive-pressure ventilation, actively blowing air into the lungs. This has some disadvantages as high inflation pressures can result in air going into the stomach instead of the lungs, leading to gastric distension and ultimately vomiting. This is more likely if:

- high inflation pressures are used
- ventilations are performed too fast
- the airway is partially obstructed.

A distended stomach is bad for the patient, as vomit can rise up into the airway and be inhaled (aspirated). It also pushes up the diaphragm, reducing the amount of space for lung expansion (Pilbery, 2013).

Mouth-to-Mouth Ventilation

The most basic ventilation device is your mouth and lungs, using mouth-to-mouth ventilation. However, healthcare professionals and members of the public are sometimes reluctant to perform mouth-to-mouth on people they do not know. In addition, there are risks relating to exposure to blood and other body fluids through direct contact with the patient's mouth and nose. In certain cases, direct mouth-to-mouth contact is not appropriate, such as in cases of poisoning (Nolan, 2010).

Procedure

Take the following steps to perform mouth-to-mouth ventilation (SJA, SAA, BRC, 2014):

1. Place the patient on their back (supine).
2. Open the airway using a head tilt–chin lift, or jaw thrust if cervical spine injury suspected.
3. Pinch the patient's nose to close the nostrils.

4. Take a breath and seal your lips over the patient's mouth.
5. Blow steadily for about 1 second, just enough to make the chest rise.
6. While maintaining the head tilt–chin lift, take your mouth away from the patient and watch the chest fall.
7. Repeat, aiming to provide a breath to an adult every 6 seconds.

Note: If the patient is not breathing and has no signs of life, commence chest compressions, not ventilations (this is covered in Chapter 18: Cardiac Arrest).

Facial Shields

To provide some protection for yourself, a face shield can be used, which provides a plastic barrier between you and the patient. They are also fitted with a filter, which sits over the patient's mouth. As with mouth-to-mouth ventilation, this method does not allow for the administration of supplemental oxygen. The technique is the same as for mouth-to-mouth ventilation.

Mouth-to-Mask Ventilation

Using a pocket mask to provide mouth-to-mask ventilation uses your lungs as before, but does not require direct contact with the patient's mouth. The one-way valve also prevents you coming into contact with blood and secretions from the patient's mouth. You use both hands to hold the mask to the patient's face, which makes it easier to get a good seal and deliver effective ventilations (Figure 12.17) (Pilbery, 2013).

Some pocket masks also have an oxygen port, allowing administration of supplemental oxygen. Even with pocket masks without an oxygen port, oxygen tubing can be placed under one side of the mask.

Procedure

Take the following steps to perform mouth-to-mask ventilation (Nolan, 2012):

1. Place the patient supine with their head in the sniffing position (neck slightly flexed and head extended).
2. Apply the mask to the patient's face using the thumbs of both hands.
3. Grip the jaw and perform a jaw thrust, while pressing down with the thumbs to make a tight seal.
4. Blow gently for 1 second through the valve and watch the chest rise.

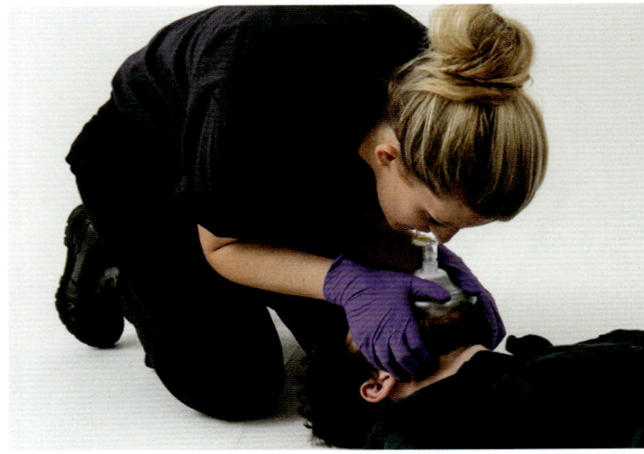

Figure 12.17 *Mouth-to-mask ventilation.*

5. Stop inflation and watch the chest fall.
6. Repeat every 6 seconds or as instructed by the senior clinician.

Leaks between the face and pocket mask can be reduced by increasing the jaw thrust, or changing finger position and pressure being applied. Oxygen, if available, should run at 10 l/min.

Bag-Valve-Mask Ventilation

The bag-valve-mask (BVM) consists of a self-inflating bag, one-way valve and mask. When used without oxygen, it delivers room air (21% oxygen). This can be increased to 45% when high-flow oxygen is attached, but it should generally be used with a reservoir bag attached, as this can result in oxygen concentrations of around 85% (Figure 12.18) with oxygen supplied at 10 l/min (Nolan, 2012).

The BVM can be used by one person, but this requires considerable skill. Where possible, a two-person technique is generally recommended (Monsieurs, 2015).

Procedure – *One-Person Ventilation*

Take the following steps to perform BVM ventilation with one person (EEAST, 2014):

1. Use appropriate personal protective equipment (PPE).
2. Choose the correct mask size, which should rest on the bridge of the nose to the chin.
3. Prepare the BVM, by connecting the mask and high-flow oxygen. Ensure the reservoir bag is inflated.

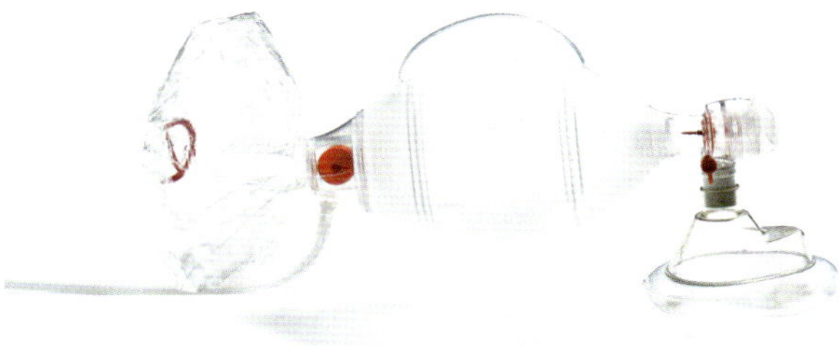

Figure 12.18 Bag-valve-mask with oxygen reservoir bag attached and inflated.

4. Position the mask on the patient's face and ensure an adequate seal.
5. Form a 'C' shape with the thumb and index finger and rest this on top of the mask; place the middle and ring fingers on the ridge of the jaw and the little finger behind the angle of the jaw (Figure 12.19).
6. Gently squeeze the bag just enough to see the chest rise.

Procedure – *Two-Person Ventilation*

This is the same as one-person, with the exception that another person holds the mask to the patient's face using the same method as for the pocket mask (Figure 12.20) (EEAST, 2014).

Oxygen Administration

Oxygen administration for adults is typically divided into four categories, which are outlined here (BTS, 2017). However, you **MUST** follow local instruction about oxygen administration.

Note: Children are not included here. They should always receive high-concentration oxygen if they have a significant illness or injury.

When to administer the drug (Indications):

- Critical illnesses requiring high levels of supplemental oxygen.
- Serious illnesses requiring moderate levels of supplemental oxygen if the patient is hypoxaemic.
- COPD and other conditions requiring controlled or low-dose oxygen therapy.
- Conditions for which patients should be monitored closely but oxygen therapy is not required unless the patient is hypoxaemic.

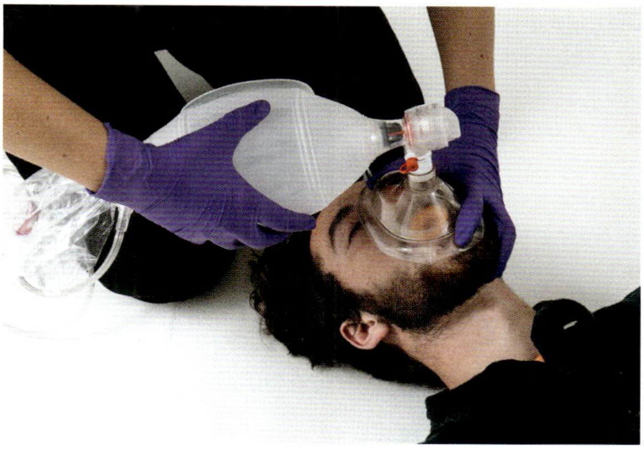

Figure 12.19 Correct hand position for one-person BVM use.

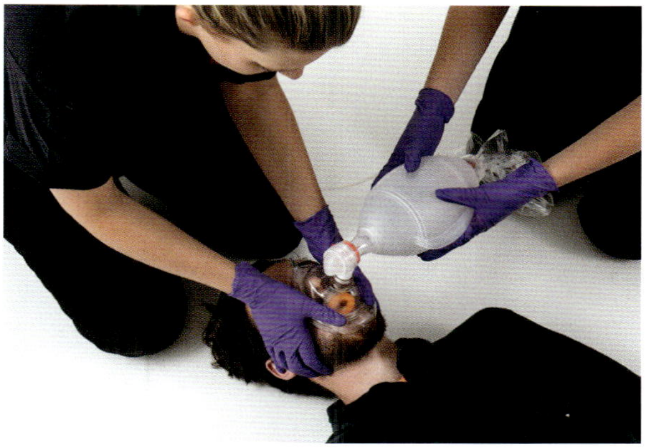

Figure 12.20 Two-person BVM technique.

When not to administer the drug (Contra-indication):

- Explosive environments.

Cautions:

- Oxygen increases the fire hazard at the scene of an incident.
- Defibrillation: ensure pads are firmly applied to reduce spark hazard.

Side effects:

- Non-humidified oxygen is drying and irritating to mucous membranes over a period of time.
- In patients with COPD there is a risk that even moderate doses of inspired oxygen can produce increased carbon dioxide levels, which may cause respiratory depression and this may lead to respiratory arrest.

Dosage and administration:

- Measure oxygen saturation (SpO_2) in all patients using pulse oximetry, where possible.
- For the administration of moderate levels of supplemental oxygen, nasal cannulae are recommended in preference to simple face masks, as they offer a more flexible dose range.
- Administer the initial oxygen dose until a reliable oxygen saturation reading is obtained.
- If the desired oxygen saturation cannot be maintained with a simple face mask, change to a reservoir (non-rebreathe) mask.
- For dosage and administration of supplemental oxygen, refer to Table 12.2 for patients with critical illnesses, Table 12.3 for serious illnesses and Table 12.4 for patients who need controlled or low-dose oxygen therapy.
- For conditions where **NO** supplemental oxygen is required unless the patient is hypoxaemic, refer to Table 12.5.

Table 12.2 High levels of supplemental oxygen for adults with critical illnesses

Condition	Initial dose	Method of administration

• Cardiac arrest or resuscitation:
  • basic life support
  • advanced life support
  • foreign body airway obstruction
  • traumatic cardiac arrest
  • maternal resuscitation
• Carbon monoxide poisoning
Note: Some pulse oximeters cannot differentiate between oxyhaemoglobin and carboxyhaemoglobin. Administer high-concentration oxygen even if oxygen saturations are 94–98%
	15 l/min	Bag-valve-mask (BVM)

• Major trauma:
  • abdominal trauma
  • burns and scalds
  • electrocution
  • head trauma
  • limb trauma
  • neck and back trauma (spinal)
  • pelvic trauma
  • immersion
  • thoracic trauma
  • trauma in pregnancy
• Anaphylaxis
• Major pulmonary haemorrhage
• Sepsis, e.g. meningococcal septicaemia
• Shock
	15 l/min	Non-rebreathe mask

• Active convulsion • Hypothermia	Administer 15 l/min until a reliable SpO_2 measurement can be obtained and then adjust oxygen flow to aim for target saturation within the range of 94–98%	Non-rebreathe mask

Administer the initial oxygen dose until the vital signs are normal, then reduce oxygen dose and aim for target saturation within the range of **94–98%**.

Table 12.3 Moderate levels of supplemental oxygen for adults with serious illnesses if the patient is hypoxaemic

Condition	Initial dose	Method of administration
• Acute hypoxaemia (cause not yet diagnosed) • Deterioration of lung fibrosis or other interstitial lung disease • Acute asthma • Acute heart failure • Pneumonia • Lung cancer • Postoperative breathlessness • Pulmonary embolism • Pleural effusions • Pneumothorax • Severe anaemia • Sickle cell crisis	**SpO_2 < 85%** 10–15 l/min	Non-rebreathe mask
	SpO_2 85–93% 2–6 l/min	Nasal cannulae
	SpO_2 85–93% 5–10 l/min	Simple face mask

Administer the initial oxygen dose until a reliable SpO_2 measurement is available, then adjust oxygen flow to aim for target saturation within the range of **94–98%.**

Table 12.4 Controlled or low-dose supplemental oxygen for adults with COPD and other conditions requiring controlled or low-dose oxygen therapy

Condition	Initial dose	Method of administration
• Chronic obstructive pulmonary disease (COPD) • Exacerbation of cystic fibrosis	4 l/min Increase flow rate to 6 l/min if respiratory rate is > 30 breaths/min (i.e. 50% above minimum specified for the mask)	28% Venturi mask (or patient's own)
• Chronic neuromuscular disorders • Chest wall disorders • Morbid obesity	4 l/min	28% Venturi mask (or patient's own)
Note: If the oxygen saturation remains below 88% change to simple face mask	5–10 l/min	Simple face mask
Note: Critical illness **AND** COPD or other risk factors for hypercapnia	As for Table 12.2	As for Table 12.2

Administer the initial oxygen dose until a reliable SpO_2 measurement is available, then adjust oxygen flow to aim for target saturation within the range of **88–92%** or pre-specified range as detailed on the patient's alert card.

Table 12.5 No supplemental oxygen required for adults with these conditions unless the patient is hypoxaemic but patients should be monitored closely

<table>
<tr><th>Condition</th><th>Initial dose</th><th>Method of administration</th></tr>
<tr><td rowspan="3">• Myocardial infarction and acute coronary syndromes
• Stroke
• Cardiac rhythm disturbance
• Non-traumatic chest pain/discomfort
• Implantable cardioverter defibrillator firing
• Pregnancy and obstetric emergencies:
  • birth imminent
  • haemorrhage during pregnancy
  • pregnancy-induced hypertension
  • vaginal bleeding
• Abdominal pain
• Headache
• Hyperventilation syndrome or dysfunctional breathing
• Most poisonings and drug overdoses (see Table 12.2 for carbon monoxide poisoning, and special cases below for paraquat or bleomycin poisoning)
• Metabolic and renal disorders
• Acute and sub-acute neurological and muscular conditions producing muscle weakness (assess the need for assisted ventilation if $SpO_2 < 94\%$)
• Post-convulsion
• Gastrointestinal bleeds
• Glycaemic emergencies
• Heat exhaustion/heat stroke

SPECIAL CASES
Poisoning with paraquat or bleomycin:
Patients with paraquat or bleomycin poisoning may be harmed by supplemental oxygen so avoid oxygen unless the patient is hypoxaemic.
Target saturation 85–88%.</td><td>$SpO_2 < 85\%$
10–15 l/min</td><td>Non-rebreathe mask</td></tr>
<tr><td>SpO_2 85–93%
2–6 l/min</td><td>Nasal cannulae</td></tr>
<tr><td>SpO_2 85–93%
5–10 l/min</td><td>Simple face mask</td></tr>
</table>

If hypoxaemic ($SpO_2 < 94\%$) administer the initial oxygen dose, then adjust oxygen flow to aim for target saturation within the range of 94–98% as per the table above.

After Use

Procedure

Once you have finished administering oxygen to a patient, take the following steps (BOC, 2013a):

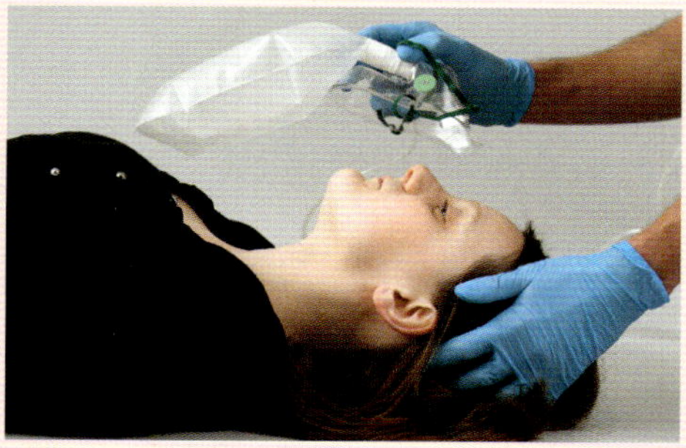

1. Remove the mask or nasal cannulae from the patient.

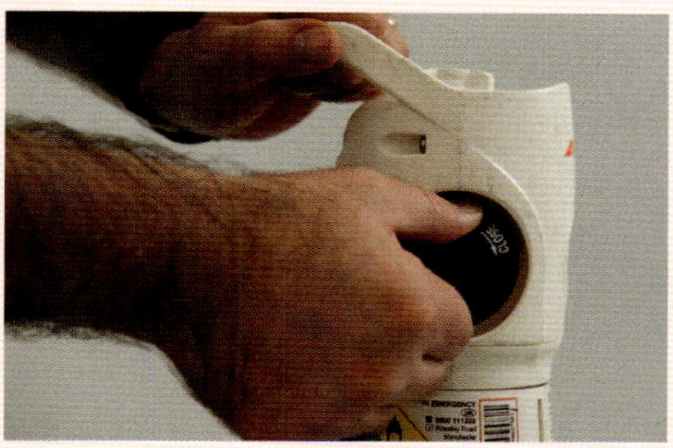

2. Turn off the cylinder by rotating the handwheel clockwise until it comes to a stop. Do not use excessive force.

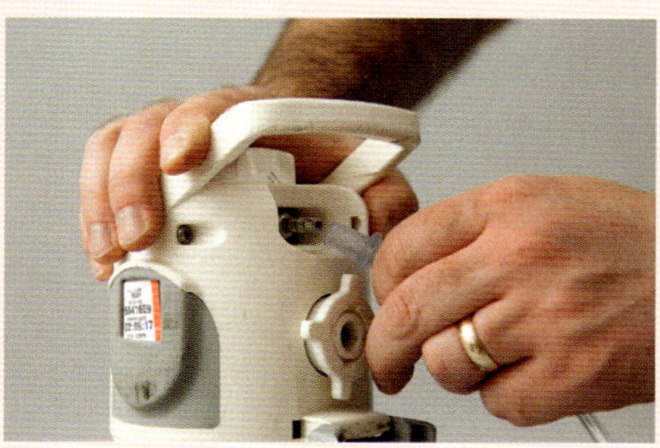

3a. Disconnect equipment. Remove the tubing by firmly pulling the tube while holding the cylinder handle.

Procedure – *cont*

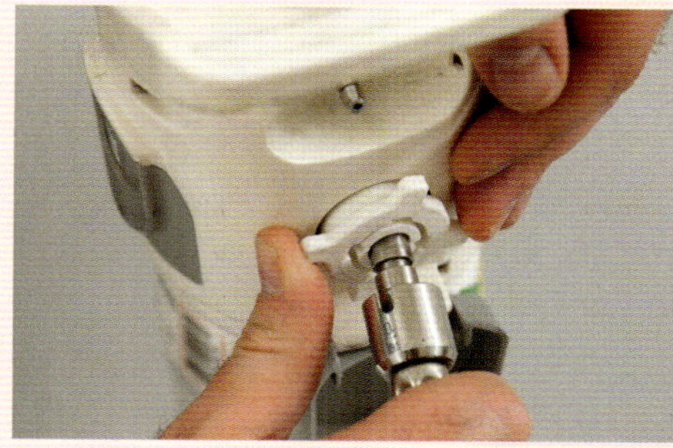

3b. If you have used the Schrader valve, release by twisting the capstan clockwise.

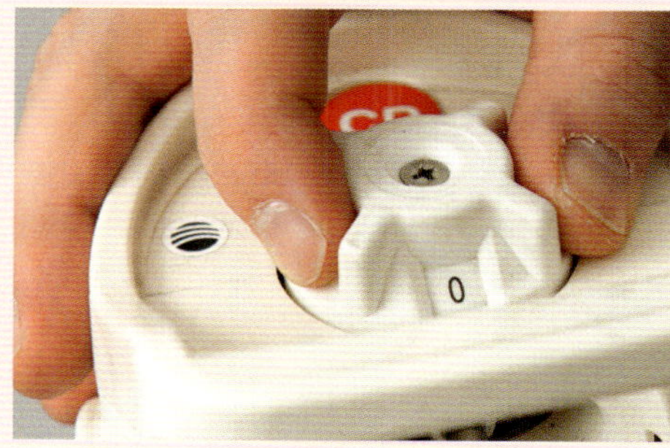

4. Turn the flow selector to zero.

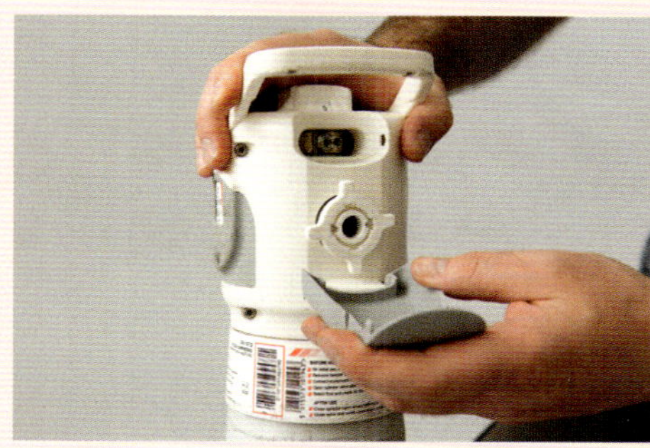

5. Replace the outlet cover by pulling up the hinged grey cover.

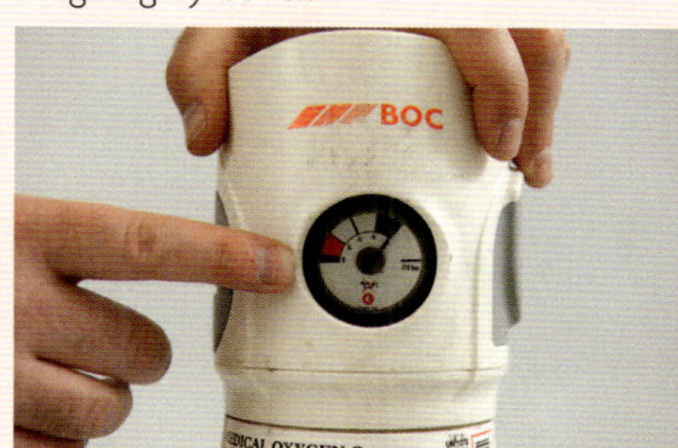

6. Check the cylinder gauge and replace if necessary.

Entonox

Entonox is a combination of 50% nitrous oxide and 50% oxygen. The cylinders that contain Entonox have a blue and white collar (Figure 12.21).

The UK Ambulance Services Clinical Practice Guidelines (JRCALC, 2016) for Entonox administration are as follows:

Indications:

- Moderate to severe pain.
- Labour pains.

Contra-indications:

- Severe head injuries with impaired consciousness.
- Decompression sickness (the bends) where Entonox can cause nitrogen bubbles within the bloodstream to expand, aggravating the problem further. Consider anyone that has been diving within the previous 24 hours to be at risk.
- Violently disturbed psychiatric patients.

Action:

- Inhaled analgesic agent.

Caution:

- Any patient at risk of having a pneumothorax, pneumomediastinum and/or a pneumoperitoneum, e.g. polytrauma, penetrating torso injury.

Side effects:

- Minimal side effects.

Dosage and administration:

- **Adults:**
    - Entonox should be self-administered via a face mask or mouthpiece, after suitable instruction. It takes about 3–5 minutes to be effective, but it may be 5–10 minutes before maximum effect is achieved.
- **Children:**
    - Entonox is effective in children provided they are capable of following the administration instructions and can activate the demand valve.

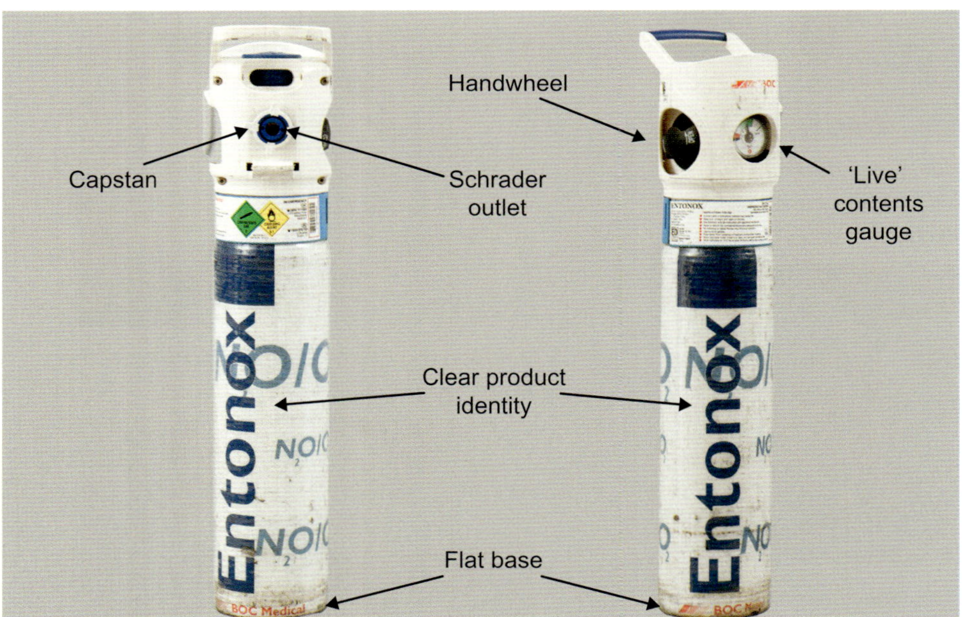

Figure 12.21 *An Entonox cylinder.*

Additional information:

- Administration of Entonox should be in conjunction with pain score monitoring.
- Entonox's advantages include:
  - rapid analgesic effect with minimal side effects
  - no cardiorespiratory depression
  - self-administered
  - analgesic effect rapidly wears off
  - the 50% oxygen concentration is valuable in many medical and trauma conditions.
- Entonox can be administered while preparing to deliver other analgesics.

Preparing Entonox for Administration

Procedure

Take the following steps to prepare Entonox for administration (BOC, 2013b):

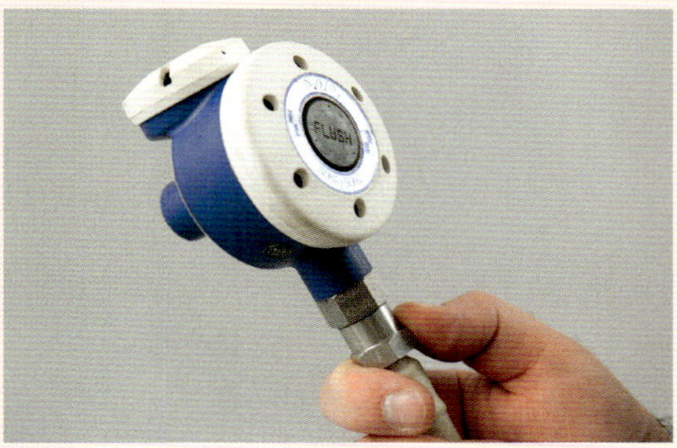

1. Ensure the demand valve is clean and ready for use.

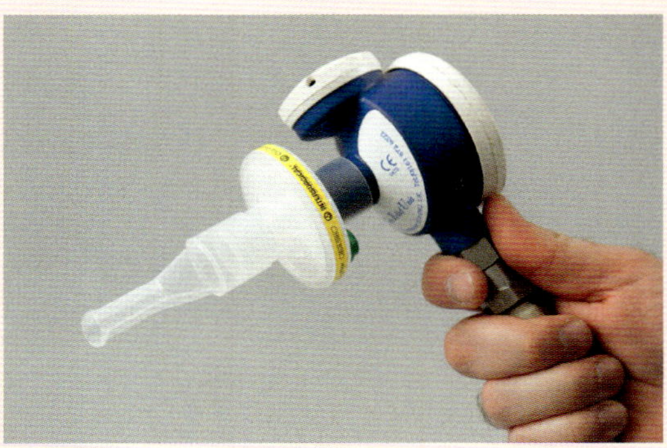

2. Fit a new microbial filter to the demand valve. They are single use.

Procedure – *cont*

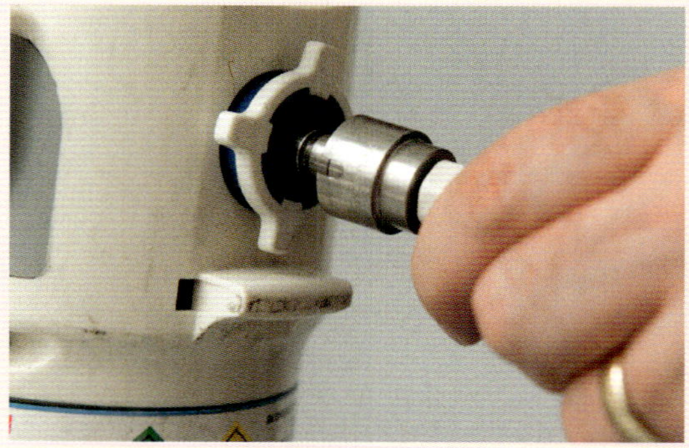

3. Insert the probe on the hose connected to the demand valve into the Schrader outlet on the Entonox cylinder. Push firmly to ensure the probe clicks into place.

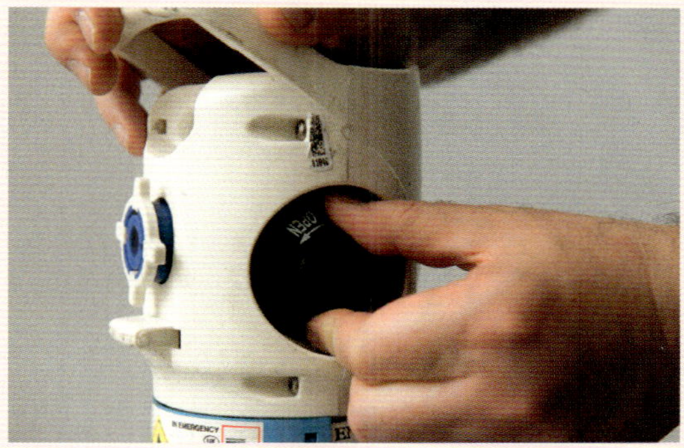

4. Slowly turn the cylinder on by rotating the handwheel anti-clockwise until fully open. Do not use excessive force.

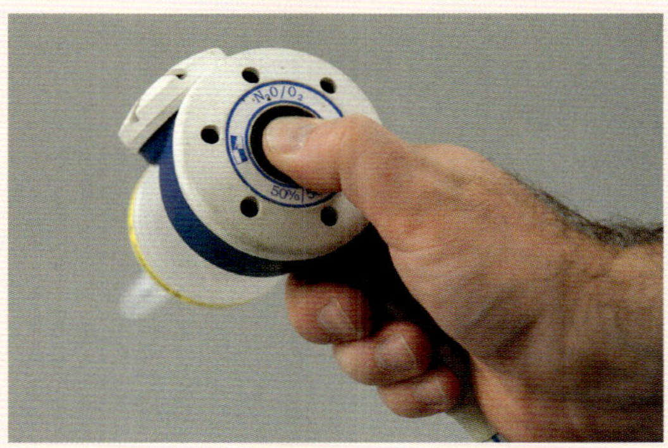

5. Check the demand valve is operative by pushing the 'test button'. You should hear the gas flowing.

(continued)

Procedure – *cont*

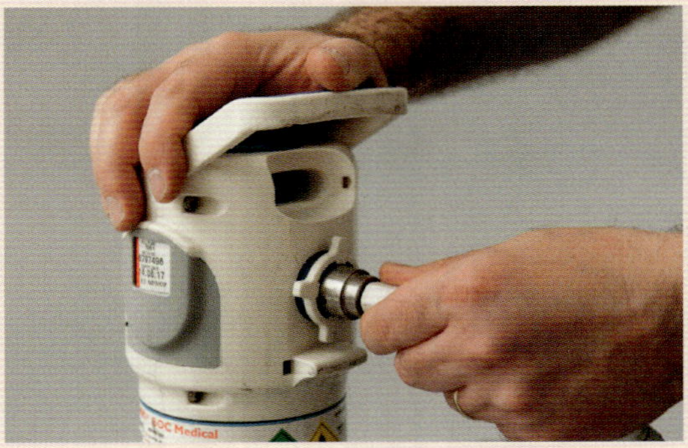

6. Check for leaks, which may be indicated by a hissing sound. If you suspect that you have a leak, turn off the cylinder and check the equipment is properly connected. Turn on the cylinder and re-check for leaks. If the leak continues, turn off and remove the cylinder from service. Report it using your ambulance service equipment defect procedure.

After Use

Procedure

Take the following steps once the patient has finished using the Entonox (BOC, 2013b):

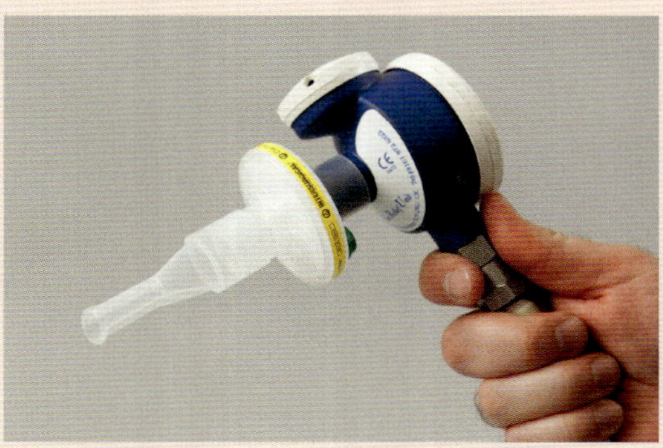

1. Remove the demand valve from the patient. Dispose of the filter and mouthpiece.

Procedure – *cont*

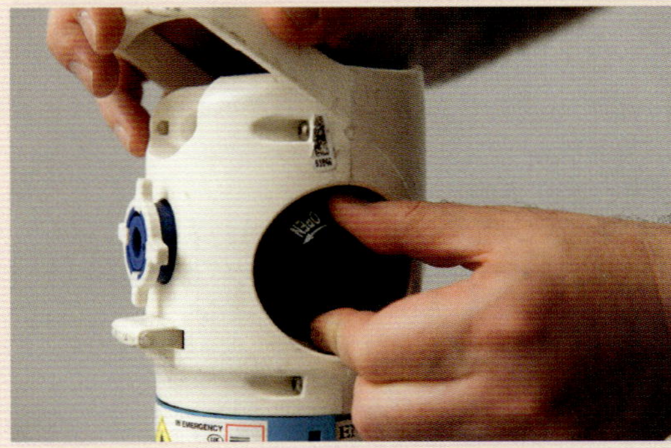

2. Turn off the cylinder by rotating the handwheel clockwise until it comes to a stop. Do not use excessive force.

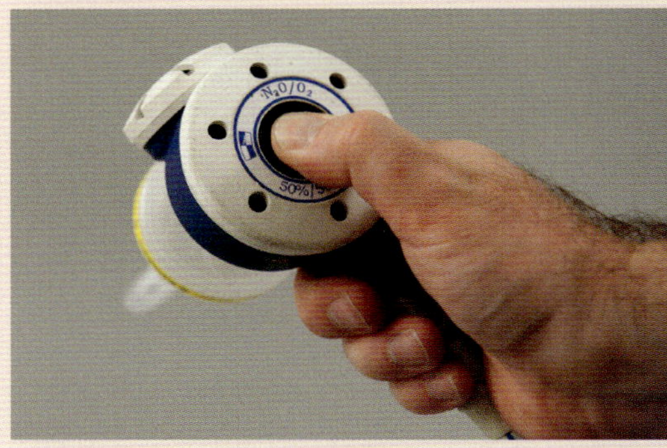

3. Vent any residual gas in the hose by pressing the test button on the demand valve. Keep pressing until the gas has stopped venting.

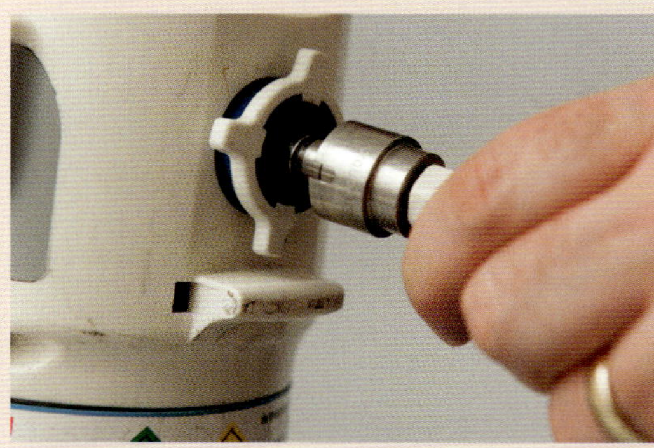

4. Disconnect the probe from the cylinder outlet. Holding the probe, twist the capstan and withdraw the probe from the Schrader outlet.

Procedure – *cont*

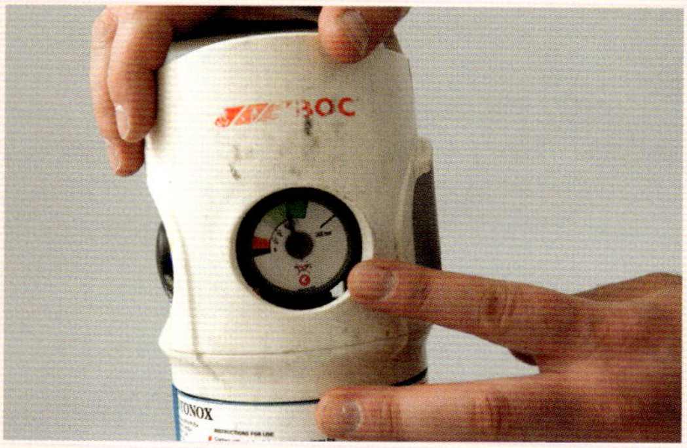

5. Replace the outlet cover by pulling up the hinged grey cover. Check the cylinder gauge and replace if empty.

Assessment of Breathing

Learning Objectives

By the end of this section you will be able to:

- Record the following observations:
  - respiratory rate
  - oxygen saturations.

Respiratory Rate

A normal adult respiratory rate is 12–20 breaths per minute (breaths/min) (Nolan, 2012). The respiratory rate is often overlooked as an important vital sign, but in adults, respiratory rates of 25 breaths/min or more are an indicator of serious illness and a warning that your patient may deteriorate quickly (Smith, 2011a; BTS, 2008). Patients with a respiratory rate of less than 10 breaths/min or more than 30 breaths/min may need assisted ventilation (JRCALC, 2016).

Measuring Respiratory Rate

How fast are you breathing now? Before considering this question, it is likely that you weren't even thinking about your respiratory rate. So it is with patients. Don't tell them that you are going to record their respiratory rate.

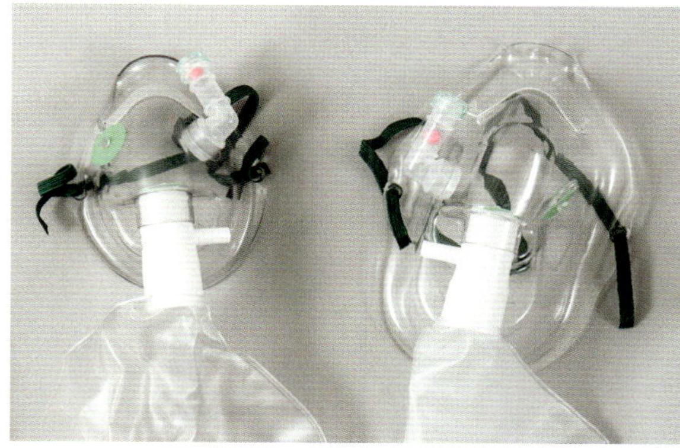

Figure 12.22 *Non-rebreathe masks with integral respiratory rate indicator.*

Ideally, you want to measure your patient's respiratory rate for a full minute using one of the following techniques (Gregory, 2010b):

- watching the chest rise and fall
- using an oxygen mask with an integral respiratory rate indicator (Figure 12.22).

Oxygen Saturations

Oxygen is transported around the body bound to haemoglobin in the blood (oxyhaemoglobin), as it travels from the lungs to the body's tissues. Oxygen saturation is the ratio of oxyhaemoglobin to the total amount of haemoglobin and is usually shown as a percentage (Tortora, 2008).

Oxygen saturations are measured in two ways: invasively and non-invasively. In hospital, it is common for patients to have an arterial blood gas sample taken, whereby a small amount of blood from an artery (often the radial) is taken and the arterial oxygen saturation measured (SaO_2). However, this is not practical to undertake outside of hospital, so oxygen saturations are measured non-invasively using a technique known as pulse oximetry (SpO_2) (Gregory, 2010b).

Pulse Oximetry

Pulse oximetry works by shining red and infrared light through a part of the body that is relatively translucent and has an arterial pulse, such as a finger, toe or earlobe (Figure 12.23). The amount of light

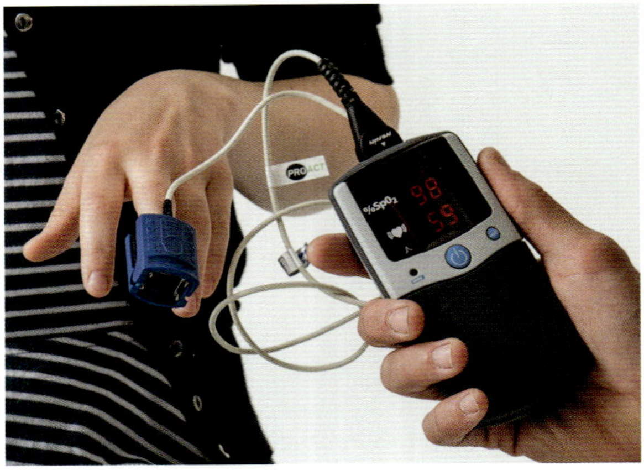

Figure 12.23 *Recording oxygen saturations with a pulse oximeter.*

transmitted through the tissue depends on the amount of oxyhaemoglobin present; this enables the pulse oximeter to calculate the oxygen saturation and will also provide the pulse rate (Pilbery, 2013).

If you refer back to Tables 12.2, 12.3 and 12.4 you will see that the target oxygen saturation for most patients is 94–98%, and in a normal, healthy person oxygen saturations should be 95% and above (Pilbery, 2013).

Indications and Limitations

Indications

Pulse oximetry is useful for (Gregory, 2010b; Walls, 2012):

- assessing the severity of respiratory illness or injury
- providing early warning of a patient who is deteriorating
- providing feedback about the effectiveness of oxygen therapy
- detecting pulses in limbs that have been fractured.

Limitations

Like any tool, the pulse oximeter can produce inaccurate results, particularly in the presence of the following (Pilbery, 2013; Walls, 2012):

- **Bright ambient light**: Simple to solve with a towel over the probe.
- **Excessive patient motion**: Such as shivering, convulsions or a bumpy ambulance ride.
- **Poor perfusion**: Since the pulse oximeter requires an arterial pulse to work, conditions that result in poor peripheral perfusion can lead to problems. Examples include patients in shock, cardiac arrest and who are cold.
- **Nail varnish/polish**: Some dark-coloured nail varnish can affect the accuracy of pulse oximeters, although this is not likely to be too serious. Finger probes can be rotated 90° if this is a worry, but if a reliable and consistent reading is being obtained through nail varnish, then the reading is probably accurate (Chan, 2003; Hinkelbein, 2007).
- **Low blood pressure**: Pulse oximetry becomes more inaccurate as the systolic blood pressure drops below 80 mmHg.
- **Abnormal haemoglobin**: Other molecules can attach themselves to haemoglobin and create an artificially high oxygen saturation reading. Carbon monoxide is probably the best known, so don't be reassured by a high oxygen saturation in a patient who is a victim of smoke inhalation, for example.
- **Response time**: Pulse oximetry is not instantaneous; typically, a reading can take up to 20 seconds depending upon the patient's physiological state. Probes closer to the heart (such as one sited on an earlobe) usually respond faster than probes on fingers and toes.

Recording Oxygen Saturations

Procedure

Take the following steps to record a patient's oxygen saturations (WHO, 2011):

1. Turn the pulse oximeter on.
2. Select the appropriate probe with particular attention to correct sizing and where it will go (usually the finger, toe or ear). If used on a finger or toe, make sure the area is clean. Consider removing nail varnish, or rotate the probe 90°.
3. Connect the probe to the pulse oximeter.
4. Position the probe carefully; make sure it fits easily without being too loose or too tight. If possible, avoid the arm being used for blood pressure monitoring as cuff inflation will interrupt the pulse oximeter signal.

5. Allow several seconds for the pulse oximeter to detect the pulse and calculate the oxygen saturation.
6. Look for the displayed pulse indicator that shows that the machine has detected a pulse. Without a pulse signal, any readings are not reliable.
7. Once the unit has detected a good pulse, the oxygen saturation and pulse rate will be displayed.
8. Like all machines, oximeters may occasionally give a false reading – if in doubt, rely on clinical judgement, rather than the machine.
9. If in doubt, check the pulse oximeter is working properly by placing it on your own finger.

Peak Flow

The measurement of the peak expiratory flow rate (PEFR or PEF), or peak flow, is common in patients with obstructive airways diseases such as asthma and chronic obstructive pulmonary disease (COPD). You should record an asthmatic patient's peak flow before and after treatment, assuming they are capable of undertaking the technique (Figure 12.24) (JRCALC, 2016).

Procedure

Take the following steps to record a peak flow (CCI, 2011; Booker, 2007):

1. Explain the procedure to the patient before starting and ask if they know what their normal or best peak flow value is. You can use the normal value chart (Figure 12.25), but a comparison with the patient's usual value is better.
2. Insert the mouthpiece into the meter (these are single patient use).
3. Ask the patient to hold the peak flow meter with their fingers clear of the scale and slot. Ensure that the holes at the end of the meter are not blocked.
4. With the patient in a standing or upright sitting position, ask them to take a deep breath.
5. Ask them to place the peak flow meter in their mouth and hold horizontally, closing their lips around the mouthpiece before blowing as hard and fast as they can. This should be a short, sharp 'huff'.

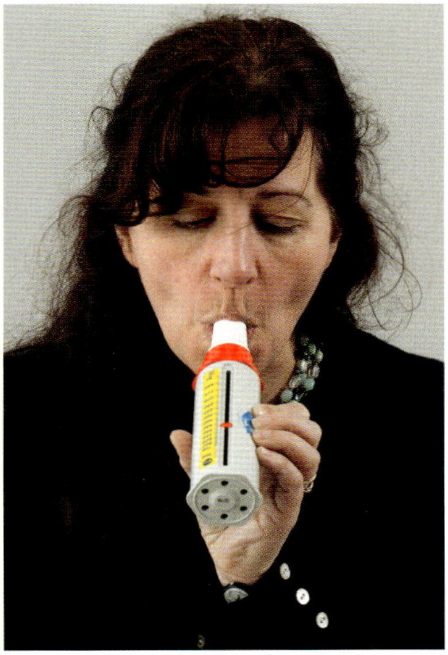

Figure 12.24 *A patient providing a peak flow reading.*

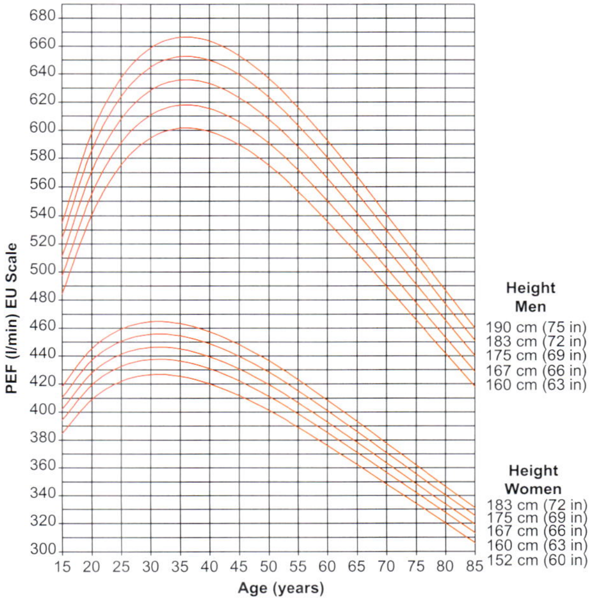

Adapted by Clement Clarke for use with EN13826 / EU scale peak flow meters from Nunn AJ, Gregg I, 1989. New regression equations for predicting peak expiratory flow in adults. *BMJ*, 298, 1068–70.

Figure 12.25 *Normal adult peak flow values.*

6. Note the number on the scale indicated by the pointer.
7. Return the pointer to zero and repeat steps 3–6 twice to obtain three readings.
8. The patient's peak flow is the highest of the three readings.

Common errors in recording a peak flow measurement:

- Failure to take a deep breath.
- The patient holding their breath and not expiring into the flow meter straight away.
- Blocking the mouthpiece with the teeth or tongue.
- Air leaking around the mouthpiece due to blowing the cheeks out, loose-fitting teeth or facial palsy.

Auscultation

Auscultation is the technique of listening to the sounds inside the body, most commonly with the help of a stethoscope.

The Stethoscope

In 1816, René-Théophile-Hyacinthe Laennec (a French doctor) needed to examine the chest of a young woman. Since the technique of listening for breath sounds at the time consisted of placing your ear on the patient's chest, a practice then, as now, generally frowned upon if your patient is a young woman, he rolled up some paper into a tube and discovered that he could hear the woman's heart sounds much more clearly than by direct auscultation (Thadepalli, 2002).

With experimentation, he developed his discovery into a wooden cylinder, which he called a stethoscope. Many of the terms in use today in relation to breath sounds come from Laennec, including pectoriloquy, crepitation (now more commonly called crackles) and rub. Laennec's wooden stethoscope design continued to be used until the mid-19th century, when rubber tubing was developed. However, not until 1925 did the bell and diaphragm design, typically found in modern stethoscopes, come into use after being developed by Bowles and Sprague (Figure 12.26) (Roguin, 2006).

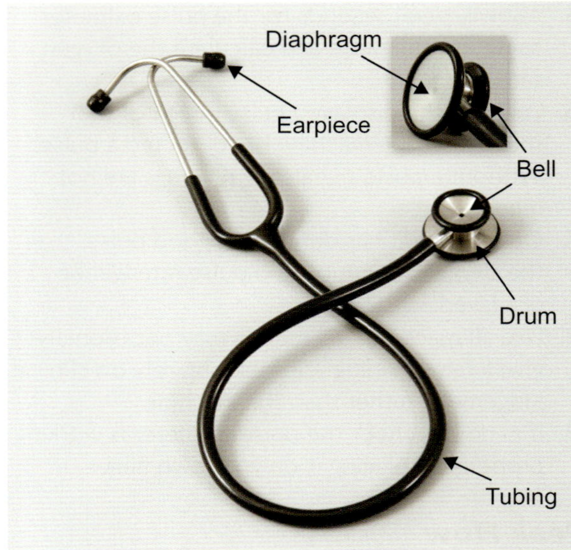

Figure 12.26 *A stethoscope.*

Breath Sounds

There are broadly two types of breath sounds you will hear on auscultation: normal and added (or adventitious).

Normal Breath Sounds

These sounds are caused by turbulent airflow in large airways and are loudest at the trachea at the start of inspiration, and quietest at the end of inspiration, as airflow decreases. If you auscultate elsewhere on the chest, the sound diminishes as it passes through the lung tissue and the chest wall itself (Macleod, 2005). Normal breath sounds are often split into three subtypes:

- **Vesicular**: These are soft and low-pitched and can be heard throughout inspiration and the first third of expiration (Bickley, 2006). They have been described as the sound of wind rustling through leaves (Talley, 2006).
- **Bronchial**: These breath sounds have a high-pitched and hollow or blowing quality, similar to the sound you hear by placing a stethoscope over the trachea. Bronchial breath sounds are similar in duration during both inspiration and expiration, with a gap in between as airflow slows prior to changing direction. These are typically

heard over lung tissue that has been affected by pneumonia (Macleod, 2005).

- **Bronchovesicular**: This is one for the fence sitters, as these breath sounds are louder than vesicular, but quieter than bronchial sounds. Inspiratory and expiratory duration are typically the same, but unlike bronchial sounds, there may not be a gap between the two. These sounds are usually the result of fluid-filled or consolidated lung tissue (Bickley, 2006).

Added (Adventitious) Sounds

There are two types of added sounds: crackles and wheezes.

- **Crackles**: These are interrupted, non-musical sounds, formerly called rales or crepitations (Talley, 2006). Usually, they are caused by the re-opening of collapsed alveoli and small bronchi. The timing and pitch of crackles can provide clues as to the cause. For example, early inspiratory crackles that are rather coarse in quality suggest small airways disease and are common in chronic obstructive pulmonary disease (COPD) (Piirilä, 1995):
  - Fine crackles that occur late in inspiration are typically caused by pulmonary fibrosis, whereas coarser crackles late in inspiration are more suggestive of left-sided heart failure.
  - Crackles can also be heard when air bubbles pass through secretions in the major bronchi, or the dilated bronchi of bronchiectasis. These are usually very coarse, may be heard without a stethoscope and will typically resolve or change location on coughing (Buss, 2010).
- **Wheezes**: These are continuous, musical sounds that are caused by air passing through partially obstructed bronchi and are normally only heard on expiration. They can be localised (e.g. in cancer of the lung) or diffuse, as is typical in asthma. Note that wheeze on inspiration is generally taken to be a significant sign of airway narrowing (Macleod, 2005). Wheezes can be monophasic, that is at a single pitch (which used to be called rhonchi), or polyphonic, i.e. more musical, due to the sound being produced at different pitches:
  - One type of loud monophasic (and usually) inspiratory wheeze that can be heard without a stethoscope is stridor. This is caused by laryngeal spasm and mucosal swelling, which causes vocal cord contraction and airway narrowing (Buss, 2010).

Absent Sounds

Breath sounds are decreased or absent when airflow is limited. This can be due to low inspiratory airflow rates, which generate less turbulent flow required to produce sound. Air or fluid in the pleural space (due to a pneumothorax or pleural effusion, for example) can increase the acoustic impedance and filter or stop transmission of breath sounds to the chest wall. This also occurs at the chest wall itself, if there is an excessive amount of adipose tissue (Buss, 2010).

Auscultating the Chest

Procedure

Ideally, you should expose the patient's chest to perform auscultation, but this will depend on whether you can ensure privacy and adequate environmental heating (such as a warm ambulance). Ensure that you inform the patient about what the procedure involves and obtain consent.

Then take the following steps (Gregory, 2010b):

1. Ask the patient to take deep breaths in and out through their mouth.
2. Place the stethoscope diaphragm on the chest, starting above the clavicle. If the patient is very slim or has a hairy chest, use the bell instead.
3. Listen during inspiration and expiration, before moving the stethoscope to another area of the chest.
4. After each breath, move the stethoscope to the opposite side of the chest to compare each part of the lung fields. Listen to anterior (Figure 12.27), posterior (Figure 12.28) and lateral (Figure 12.29) aspects of the chest for normal and adventitious breath sounds.

Hints

It may be helpful to coach the patient to breathe using 'in... and out'. Avoid long periods of deep breathing as it may cause dizziness. Patients who are short of breath may not be able to comply with your instructions.

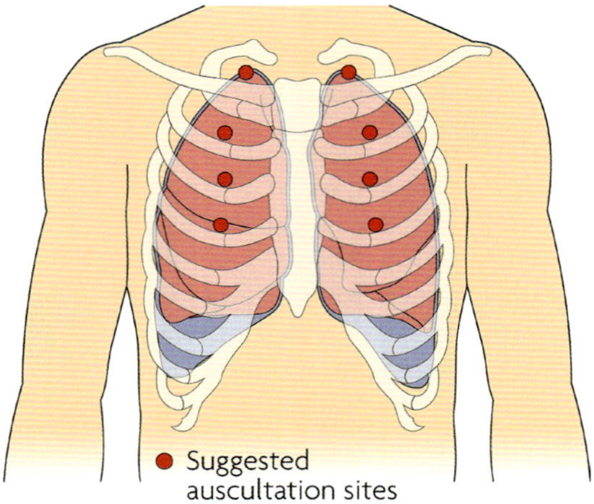

Figure 12.27 *Auscultation sites of the anterior chest.*

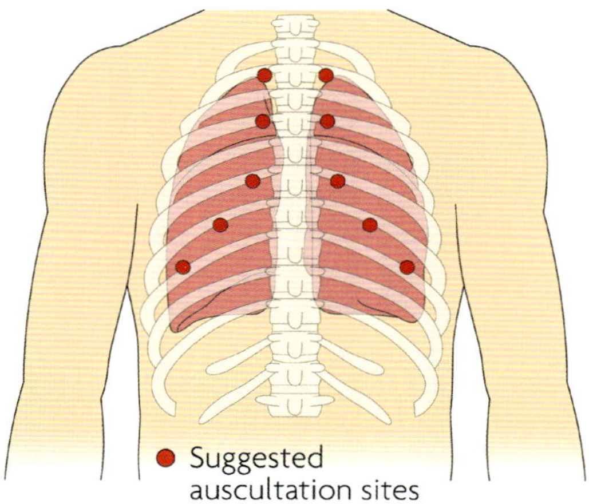

Figure 12.28 *Auscultation sites of the posterior chest.*

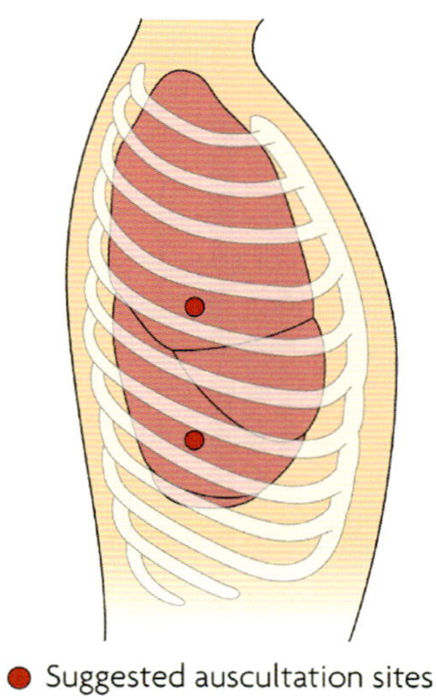

Figure 12.29 *Auscultation sites of the lateral chest.*

Common Respiratory Conditions

Learning Objectives

By the end of this section you will be able to:

- Describe the following conditions of the respiratory system:
  - asthma
  - chronic obstructive pulmonary disease (COPD)
  - pneumonia
  - pulmonary embolism.

Asthma

Definition

Asthma is a condition characterised by intermittent, reversible, airway obstruction (Simon, 2010).

Pathophysiology

Asthma is caused by a chronic inflammation of the bronchi, making them narrower. The muscles around the bronchi become irritated and contract, causing sudden worsening of the symptoms. The inflammation can also cause the mucus glands to produce excessive sputum, which further blocks the air passages.

The obstruction and subsequent wheezing are caused by three factors within the bronchial tree:

- increased production of bronchial mucus
- swelling of the mucosal cells that line the bronchi and bronchioles
- spasm and constriction of bronchial muscles.

These three factors combine to cause blockage and narrowing of the small airways in the lung. Because inspiration is an active process involving the muscles of respiration, the obstruction of the airways is overcome on breathing in. Expiration occurs with muscle relaxation, and is severely delayed by the narrowing of the airways in asthma. This generates the wheezing on expiration that is characteristic of this condition.

Medication

Asthma is managed with a variety of inhaled and tablet medications. Inhalers are divided into two broad categories: preventer and reliever.

Preventer

The preventer inhalers are normally anti-inflammatory drugs and these include steroids and other milder anti-inflammatories, such as Tilade. The common steroid inhalers are beclomethasone (Becotide), budesonide (Pulmicort) and fluticasone (Flixotide). These drugs act on the lung over a period of time to reduce the inflammatory reaction that causes the asthma. Regular use of these inhalers often eradicates all symptoms of asthma and allows for a normal lifestyle.

Reliever

The reliever inhalers include salbutamol (Ventolin), terbutaline (Bricanyl), tiotropium bromide (Spiriva) and ipratropium bromide (Atrovent). These inhalers work rapidly on the lung to relax the smooth muscle spasm when the patient feels wheezy or tight-chested. They are used in conjunction with preventer inhalers. Inhalers are often used through large plastic spacer devices (Figure 12.30). This allows the drug to spread into a larger volume and enables the patient to inhale it more effectively. In mild and moderate asthma attacks some patients may be treated with high doses of 'relievers' through a spacer device. This has been shown to be as effective as giving a salbutamol nebuliser (BTS/SIGN, 2016).

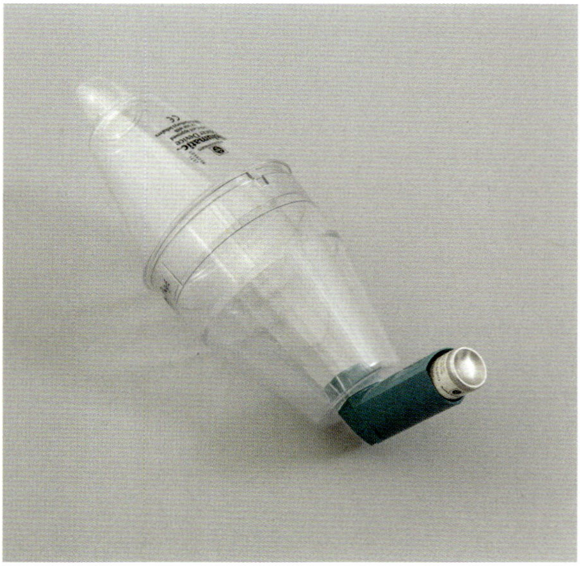

Figure 12.30 *An inhaler with a spacer device.*

Signs and Symptoms

History

Patients will typically tell you about increasing shortness of breath with wheezing over the past 6–48 hours, with increasing inhaler use. The reliever inhalers may also be proving less effective than normal.

Ask specifically about:

- repeated attendances at ED for asthma care in the past year
- previous admissions for asthma
- previous near-fatal asthma, e.g. previously required ventilation/intensive care
- heavy use of reliever inhalers
- brittle asthma.

Assessment of Severity

The signs and symptoms of asthma are organised according to their severity. Table 12.6 shows the broad categories of asthma severity, which in turn will determine the most appropriate interventions for your patient (BTS/SIGN, 2016).

Medication Extended Skill

The indications and contra-indications listed below are taken from the UK Ambulance Services Clinical Practice Guidelines (JRCALC, 2016). However, you should be familiar with your own service guidelines as restrictions on administration may exist.

Salbutamol

Presentation:

- Nebules containing either salbutamol 2.5 mg in 2.5 ml or 5 mg in 2.5 ml.

Actions:

- Salbutamol is a selective beta-2 adrenoreceptor stimulant drug. This has a relaxant effect on the smooth muscle in the medium and smaller airways, which are in spasm in acute asthma attacks. If given by nebuliser, especially if oxygen powered, its smooth muscle-relaxing action, combined with the airway-moistening effect of nebulisation, can relieve the attack rapidly.

Table 12.6 Assessing asthma severity

Moderate	**Severe**	**Life-threatening**
PEF >50–75% of best or predicted	PEF 33–50% of best or predicted	PEF <33% of best or predicted
SpO_2 ≥92%	SpO_2 ≥92%	SpO_2 <92%
Adults: Respiratory Rate <25 breaths/min Heart rate <110 beats/min Able to complete sentences in one breath	**Adults:** Respiratory Rate ≥25 breaths/min Heart rate ≥110 beats/min Inability to complete sentences in one breath	**Adults:** Silent chest Poor respiratory effort Exhaustion Altered consciousness Cyanosis Arrhythmia Hypotension
Children >5 years Able to talk Respiratory rate ≤30 breaths/min Heart rate ≤125 beats/min	**Children >5 years** Too breathless to talk Using accessory neck muscles Respiratory rate >30 breaths/min Heart rate >125 beats/min	**Children >5 years** Silent chest Poor respiratory effort Agitation Altered consciousness Cyanosis
Children 1–5 years Able to talk and feed Respiratory rate ≤40 breaths/min Heart rate ≤140 beats/min	**Children 1–5 years** Too breathless to talk or feed Using accessory neck muscles Respiratory rate >40 breaths/min Heart rate >140 beats/min	**Children 1–5 years** Silent chest Poor respiratory effort Agitation Altered consciousness Cyanosis
Note: Only one sign or symptom is required to qualify a patient for a higher severity. For example, an SpO_2 of 91% would place a patient in the life-threatening column, irrespective of other observations.		

Indications:

- Acute asthma attack where normal inhaler therapy has failed to relieve symptoms.
- Expiratory wheeze associated with allergy, anaphylaxis, smoke inhalation or other lower airway cause.
- Exacerbation of chronic obstructive pulmonary disease (COPD).
- Shortness of breath in patients with severe breathing difficulty due to left ventricular failure.

Contra-indications:

- None in the emergency situation.

Cautions:

- Salbutamol should be used with care in patients with:
  - hypertension
  - angina
  - overactive thyroid
  - late pregnancy (can relax uterus)
  - severe hypertension may occur in patients on beta-blockers and half doses should be used unless there is profound hypotension.
- If COPD is a possibility limit nebulisation to 6 minutes.

Side-effects:

- tremor (shaking)
- tachycardia
- palpitations
- headache
- feeling of tension
- peripheral vasodilatation
- muscle cramps
- rash.

Dosage and administration:

- Nebulise with oxygen running at 6–8 l/min.
- Repeat doses can be administered at 5-minute intervals.
- 6 years and above: 5 mg.
- 1 month to under 6 years: 2.5 mg.
- Birth: not applicable.

Ipratropium Bromide

Presentation:

- Nebules containing ipratropium bromide 250 micrograms in 1 ml or 500 micrograms in 2 ml.

Indications:

- Acute severe or life-threatening asthma.
- Acute asthma unresponsive to salbutamol.
- Exacerbation of chronic obstructive pulmonary disease (COPD), unresponsive to salbutamol.

Actions:

- Ipratropium bromide is an anti-muscarinic bronchodilator drug. It may provide short-term relief in acute asthma, but beta-2 agonists (such as salbutamol) generally work more quickly. Ipratropium is considered of greater benefit in:
    - children suffering from acute asthma
    - adults suffering with COPD.

Contra-indications:

- None in the emergency situation.

Cautions:

- Ipratropium should be used with care in patients:
    - with glaucoma (protect the eyes from mist)
    - who are pregnant or breastfeeding
    - with prostatic hyperplasia.
- If COPD is a possibility limit nebulisation to 6 minutes.

Side effects:

- headache
- nausea and vomiting
- dry mouth (common)
- difficulty in passing urine and/or constipation
- tachycardia/arrhythmia
- paroxysmal tightness of the chest
- allergic reaction.

Dosage and administration:

- Nebulise with oxygen running at 6–8 l/min.
- There is no repeat dose for this drug.
- 12 years and above: 500 mcg.
- 18 months to 11 years: 250 mcg.
- 1 month to under 18 months: 125–250 mcg.
- Birth: not applicable.

Management

The management of asthma depends on the assessment of severity and the patient's response to treatment (Figure 12.31). In some cases, it may be appropriate for a senior clinician to leave patients at home; however, it is vital that the following 'red flags' for identifying higher-risk patients are considered, and that those patients are transported to hospital (BTS/SIGN, 2016; JRCALC, 2016):

- still have significant symptoms
- concerns about compliance
- living alone/socially isolated
- psychological problems
- previous near-fatal or brittle asthma
- exacerbation despite adequate dose of steroid tablets already being taken
- presentation at night (due to circadian variation, most common around 04:00)
- pregnancy.

Chronic Obstructive Pulmonary Disease

Definition

Chronic obstructive pulmonary disease (COPD) is an umbrella term for a range of respiratory diseases that result in airflow obstruction. This obstruction is usually progressive and, unlike asthma, is not fully reversible and does not change markedly over several months (NICE, 2010a).

It is estimated that there are around 3.7 million people with COPD in the United Kingdom (UK), but only 90,000 have been diagnosed. COPD kills about 30,000 people a year in the UK, making it the fifth biggest killer (BLF, 2007).

The two most important respiratory diseases related to COPD are chronic bronchitis and emphysema. Emphysema is a permanent enlargement of the air spaces below the terminal bronchioles as a result of the destruction of the alveolar walls. Chronic bronchitis, on the other

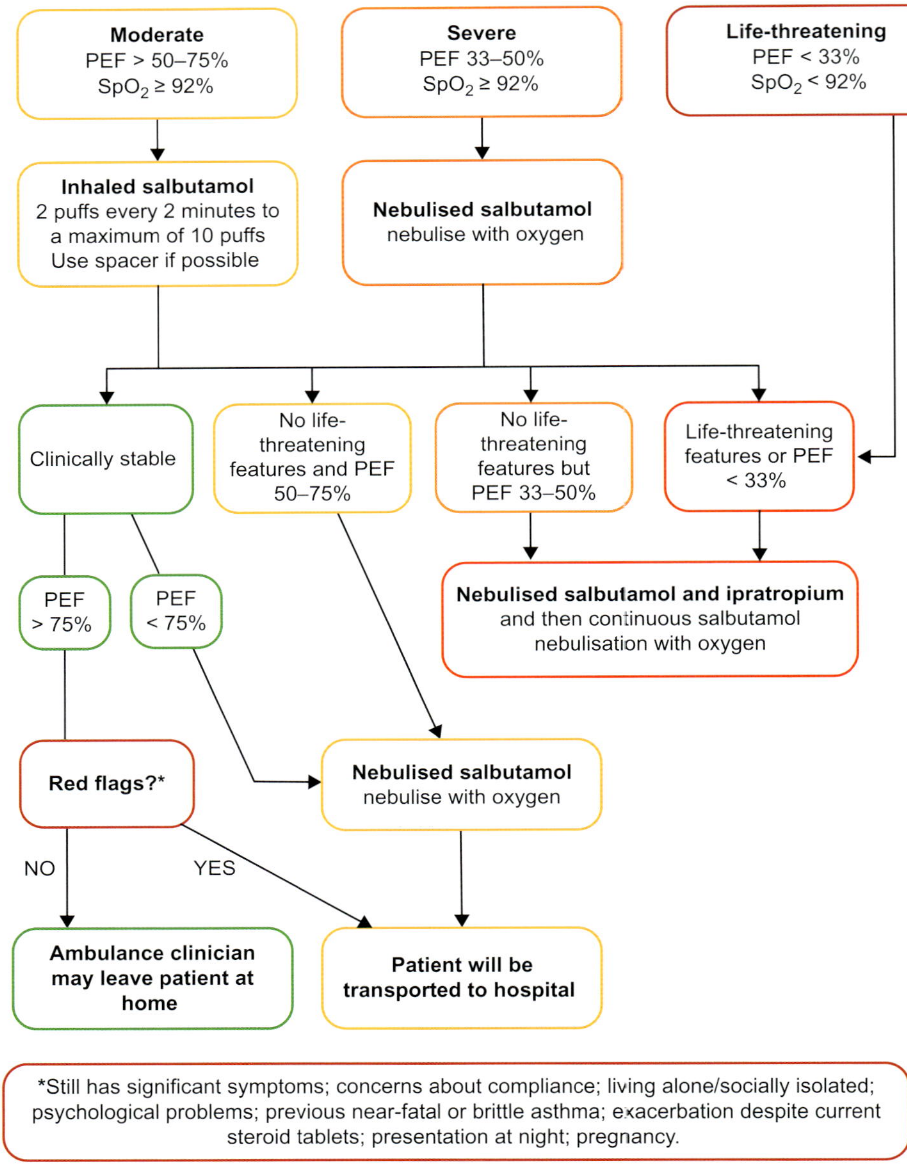

Figure 12.31 *Management algorithm for acute asthma.*

hand, is defined clinically as a persistent cough with sputum production for at least 3 months of the year for two consecutive years (Patel, 2008).

Pathophysiology

COPD

The most important causative factor in chronic bronchitis and emphysema is smoking, although only 15% of smokers develop COPD (Patel, 2008). The general effects of smoking in COPD are:

- Inflammation resulting from activation of inflammatory cells, which release substances that trigger an immune system response. This activates enzymes that can damage lung tissue, although normally these are kept in check. However, in COPD, so many enzymes are produced that they overwhelm the neutralising mechanism, and lung tissue is digested and destroyed. This is thought to be particularly important in the development of emphysema.

- Inflammation as a direct result of inhaling oxidants in the cigarette smoke (you may have heard of free radicals), which damage the cells directly.

Both of these mechanisms lead to alveolar destruction and production of excess mucus, which is made worse by the impairment of the respiratory cilia, hair-like projections that line the airways and move debris and mucus upwards and out of the respiratory tract (Tortora, 2008).

Chronic Bronchitis

Cigarette smoking, occupational exposure and/or recurrent bronchial infections lead to inflammation that narrows the airways, and an increase in mucus secretions coupled with inhibition of the cilia, which leads to an accumulation of secretions and bronchoconstriction due to irritant receptor activation. This also causes the chronic productive cough (Patel, 2008).

Emphysema

In emphysema, the walls of the alveoli are destroyed by enzymes called proteases. These are usually kept under control by another group of enzymes, called anti-proteases. Once the balance is upset (due to smoking, for example) destruction of the alveoli occurs, leading to a collapse of the airways, resulting in obstruction. In addition, as the walls of the alveoli are destroyed, bullae (small, blister-like air pockets) form on the lung. If these bullae form, air can directly enter the pleural cavity, causing a pneumothorax and collapse of the lung on the affected side (Patel, 2008).

Oxygen and COPD

Research studies and audits suggest that over-oxygenation increases mortality and morbidity, but careful pre-hospital titration of oxygen administration to patients with COPD can significantly reduce mortality (Austin, 2010).

The most significant effect of hyperoxia (excessive oxygen) on the respiratory system is hypercapnic respiratory failure in vulnerable populations (such as patients with severe COPD). This can occur even with a partial pressure of arterial oxygen (PaO_2) within normal or near-normal values. It is thought that there are a number of mechanisms that are responsible (O'Driscoll, 2008).

Signs and Symptoms

Patients will usually call for an ambulance during an exacerbation of COPD. Their clinical presentation will depend on which of the two diseases (chronic bronchitis or emphysema) is more dominant. In reality, most patients will have elements of both, but Table 12.7 shows the two ends of the spectrum of illness.

Features of an acute exacerbation of COPD include (JRCALC, 2016):

- increased difficulty breathing (dyspnoea)
- increased sputum production/purulence (containing pus)
- increased cough
- upper airway symptoms, such as cold and sore throat
- increased wheeze
- reduced exercise tolerance
- increased fatigue
- acute confusion.

Table 12.7 Chronic bronchitis vs emphysema

	Chronic bronchitis	**Emphysema**
Also known as:	Blue bloater	Pink puffer
Hyperinflated chest	Yes	Yes
Body size	Obese	Thin
Cyanosis	Yes, centrally	No
Blood levels of CO_2	High	Low

Features that warn of a severe episode of COPD include (JRCALC, 2016):

- marked dyspnoea
- tachypnoea
- purse-lip breathing
- use of accessory muscles
- new-onset cyanosis
- new-onset peripheral oedema
- marked reduction in activities of daily living.

Despite the lists above, it is not always clear that the patient with difficulty breathing has COPD and only 35% of patients will tell you that they have COPD (Durrington, 2005). Therefore, you should consider this as a possibility for any patient who meets the following criteria (BTS, 2017):

- over 50 years of age
- smoker (or ex-smoker)
- has any of:
  - exertional breathlessness
  - chronic cough
  - regular sputum production
  - wheeze
- has no clinical features of asthma.

Management

The management of a patient with COPD depends on the presence of any of the following time-critical features:

- major ABCD problems
- extreme breathing difficulty (compared to normal)
- cyanosis (although peripheral cyanosis can be normal)
- exhaustion
- hypoxia unresponsive to oxygen (in COPD patients hypoxia is considered to be an SpO_2 below 88%).

These patients require a blue-light transfer to the nearest emergency department, so be sure to update the emergency operations centre (JRCALC, 2016).

For patients with no time-critical features, you should ask if they have a treatment plan and follow this, if available. Treatments typically include (JRCALC, 2016):

- **Oxygen**: Target range of 88–92%. Venturi masks are a good choice for delivering accurate percentages of oxygen, although nasal cannulae may be better tolerated by patients.
- **Bronchodilators**: Salbutamol and ipratropium (once only). If the nebuliser is powered by oxygen, nebulisation should be limited to 6 minutes.

Patients may need taking to hospital, but depending on how well they respond to treatment, they may be suitable for referral to their GP, respiratory team or advanced paramedic. The ambulance staff will decide the most appropriate management.

Pneumonia

Definition

Pneumonia is an infection of the terminal bronchioles and alveoli (lung parenchyma) (Patel, 2008). It is more common in the elderly and during the winter months (Simon, 2010).

It is often classified in three main ways, although the first is the most commonly used (Dunn, 2005; Osler, 2012):

- **Setting**: i.e. hospital or community-acquired pneumonia.
- **Anatomy**: Lobar, if the infection is localised to a lobe of the lung, or bronchopneumonia if the infection is more widespread.
- **Organism**: Bacterial, viral, fungal.

Risk Factors for Community-Acquired Pneumonia (CAP)

The following factors undermine the lung's natural defences and so increase the risk of pneumonia (Patel, 2008):

- excessive alcohol
- cigarette smoking
- chronic heart and lung diseases
- bronchial obstruction
- immunosuppression (e.g. due to chemotherapy for cancer)
- drug abuse.

Pathophysiology

This inflammatory process is typically due to a bacterial or viral infection, which has usually entered the lungs having been inhaled from the environment or nasopharynx. Normally, these organisms should be destroyed by the body's lung defences, but if they survive and multiply, infection results. This leads to a build-up of fluid and blood cells (red and white) in the alveoli, known as consolidation (Porth, 2003).

Signs and Symptoms

When taking a history, the following symptoms are suggestive of pneumonia (Johnson, 2012):

- fever with or without rigors
- cough (often productive with green, blood-stained or rusty-coloured sputum)
- pleuritic chest pain
- muscle or joint pain.

When examining a patient you may notice the following signs:

- high temperature (pyrexia)
- increased respiratory rate (tachypnoea)
- increased heart rate (tachycardia).

Management

Not all patients with pneumonia need to go to hospital. However, while waiting for an ambulance, patients who have difficulty breathing should receive oxygen. Don't forget to consider whether the patient may have sepsis.

Pulmonary Embolism

Definition

An embolus is a blood-borne substance (including air) that is transported from one part of the circulation to another, lodging in a vessel that is too small to allow the embolus to pass. When the embolus lodges in the pulmonary vessels, it is termed a pulmonary embolism (PE) (Patel, 2008). Deep vein thrombosis (DVT) and pulmonary embolism represent the spectrum of one disease known as venous thromboembolism (VTE) (Tapson, 2008). Although an embolus can consist of air, fat or amniotic fluid, for example, the most common is a clot from a DVT (Porth, 2003; Torbicki, 2008).

Risk Factors

The risk factors for developing a venous thromboembolism are well known and can help to identify patients who may have a PE (Torbicki, 2008):

- High risk:
  - fracture (hip or leg)
  - major general surgery
  - major trauma
  - spinal cord injury.
- Moderate risk:
  - chronic heart or respiratory failure
  - chemotherapy
  - hormone replacement therapy
  - cancer
  - oral contraceptive therapy
  - paralytic stroke
  - post-partum
  - previous VTE
  - thrombophilia.
- Low risk:
  - bed rest for more than 3 days
  - immobility due to sitting (e.g. prolonged car or air travel)
  - increasing age
  - obesity
  - pregnancy
  - varicose veins.

Pathophysiology

Thrombi (blood clots) most often form in the deep veins of the calf (hence the name, deep vein thrombosis) and can grow to lengths of 30–50 cm (Tapson, 2008). The proximal end of the thrombus can extend into the popliteal vein, where the risk of embolisation is greater. Once the thrombus (or a portion) breaks off, it becomes an embolus, travelling up the femoral vein and into the iliac veins. From there it is free to ascend via the inferior vena cava to the heart. It continues into the right atrium, the ventricle and finally into the lungs via the pulmonary trunk and left and right pulmonary arteries (the only arteries to carry deoxygenated blood), which divide and subdivide until they form capillaries around the alveoli.

In healthy patients, an obstruction of up to 25% of the pulmonary arterial bed will only cause mild respiratory symptoms, such as shortness of breath. Once this increases to 30–50% there will also be cardiovascular compromise, including cardiac arrest. Patients with pre-existing respiratory and/or cardiovascular disease will be symptomatic at much lower percentages (Torbicki, 2008; Wood, 2002).

Signs and Symptoms

Common signs and symptoms of PE include difficulty breathing (dyspnoea) and rapid breathing (tachypnoea). Pleuritic chest pain is the most common symptom (JRCALC, 2016).

Other signs and symptoms include:

- Signs:
  - respiratory rate greater than 20 breaths/min
  - pulse rate greater than 100 beats/min
  - pulse oximeter reading (SpO_2) less than 92% in air
  - signs of a deep vein thrombosis (DVT), which includes pain, swelling and/or tenderness on only one leg, often in the calf (Simon, 2010).
- Symptoms:
  - cough
  - haemoptysis (blood from the respiratory tract, usually coughed up)
  - syncope (faint).

Management

Patients with suspected PE need swift transport to hospital. Treatment is mainly supportive of the ABCs (airway, breathing and circulation). Place the patient in a position of comfort (often sitting up, unless they have low blood pressure), provide oxygen if required, to maintain the SpO_2 in the range 94–98%, and be prepared for cardiac arrest (JRCALC, 2016).

Chapter 13
Circulation

Cardiovascular System Anatomy and Physiology

Learning Objectives

By the end of this section you will be able to:

- State the functions of the cardiovascular system.
- Describe the anatomy and function of the heart.
- State the components of the electrical pathway of the heart.
- Explain the difference between arteries and veins.
- Describe the stages of the cardiac cycle.

Introduction

At the most basic level, the cardiovascular system is composed of blood vessels that transport blood around the body thanks to the work of a pump, the heart (Pilbery, 2013). The heart is actually two pumps (the ventricles), each with its own reservoir (the atria), which normally serve two different circulations. The right side of the heart pumps blood to the pulmonary circulation, which travels around the lungs enabling the blood to take up oxygen and give up carbon dioxide. This blood then returns to the left side of the heart, where it is pumped into the systemic circulation to be transported all around the body via the largest artery in the body, the aorta. Both these pumps operate simultaneously and, thanks to valves in the heart, in one direction.

The main functions of the cardiovascular system are (Evans, 2012):

- transportation of nutrients, such as oxygen, glucose (sugar), fatty acids and water
- removal of waste products from metabolic processes, such as carbon dioxide and urea
- hormonal control, by delivering hormones to their target organs (and secreting some of its own)
- regulation of temperature by controlling heat distribution between the core and skin of the body
- reproduction, by producing penile erection and providing nutrition for the unborn fetus
- host defence, by transporting immune cells and other mediators.

Heart

The heart is relatively small, considering the work it has to do; it is only about the size of your fist. It sits within the mediastinum, a region in the middle of the thoracic cavity that extends from the sternum to the vertebral column, and sits between the lungs. About two-thirds of the heart sits to the left of the body's midline. It is cone-shaped, with the pointed apex orientated anteriorly (to the front), inferiorly (downwards) and to the left, and the flat base directed posteriorly (to the back), superiorly (upwards) and to the right (Tortora, 2008).

Pericardium and Heart Wall

The pericardium is a fibrous sac that surrounds and protects the heart, keeping it fixed within the mediastinum, but allowing for the vigorous contractions required to move blood around the pulmonary and systemic circulations (Tortora, 2008). The outer, parietal, layer is fixed to the fibrous pericardium, whereas the inner, visceral, layer (also called the epicardium) forms the outer layer of the heart wall.

The wall of the heart is made up of three layers:

- **Epicardium**: Also known as the visceral layer of the pericardium.
- **Myocardium**: The heart muscle, which makes up most of the bulk of the heart and is responsible for the pumping action that moves blood around the body.
- **Endocardium**: The smooth inner layer, which also covers the valves of the heart and is continuous with the innermost lining (endothelium) of the blood vessels attached to the heart.

Chambers of the Heart

The heart has four chambers. The two superior chambers are called atria and the two inferior chambers, the ventricles (Figure 13.1) (Tortora, 2008; Kapit, 2001; Evans, 2012).

Right Atrium

The right atrium receives deoxygenated blood from the body, via large veins called the superior and inferior vena cavae, and from the coronary (heart) circulation via the coronary sinus.

It is separated from the left atrium by a thin partition known as the interatrial septum, and from the right ventricle by the tricuspid valve, so called because it is made up of three cusps. This valve is also sometimes referred to as the right atrioventricular valve.

Right Ventricle

The right ventricle makes up most of the anterior surface of the heart and receives blood from the right atrium via the tricuspid valve. To prevent this valve from everting (turning inside out like an umbrella in strong winds) during contraction of the ventricles, the valve is anchored by tendon-like cords known as the chordae tendineae, which

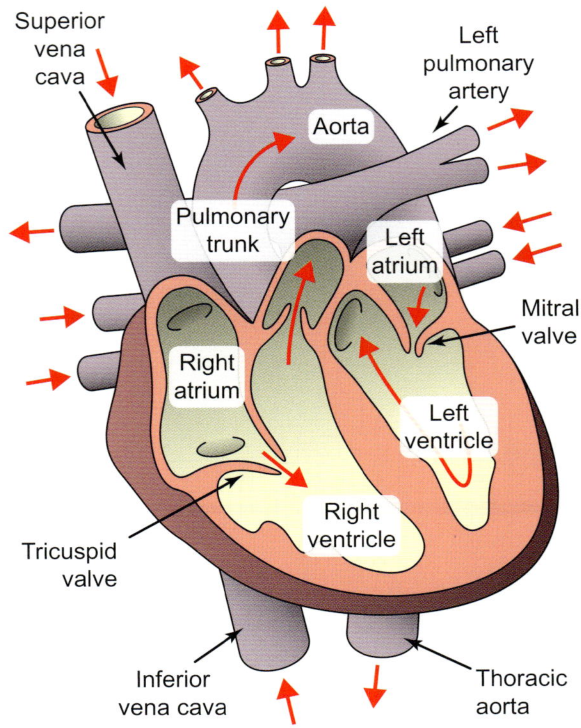

Figure 13.1 *Chambers of the heart and related anatomy.*

connect to papillary muscles. Like the atria, the ventricles are separated by a partition, known as the interventricular septum.

Blood leaves the ventricle via the pulmonary valve, where it enters the pulmonary trunk, which splits into the left and right pulmonary arteries. As you will discover later in the in this chapter, these arteries are unusual because they transport deoxygenated blood.

Left Atrium

The left atrium makes up the majority of the base of the heart. Blood enters the atrium from the lungs via four pulmonary veins and exits through the bicuspid (two cusps) valve. This is also known as the mitral valve (because of the valve's resemblance to a bishop's mitre or hat) and the left atrioventricular valve.

Left Ventricle

This forms the apex of the heart and also contains the chordae tendineae and papillary muscle assembly to secure the mitral valve. Blood exits via the aortic valve where it travels up the ascending aorta. Some blood leaves here and enters the coronary arteries to provide oxygen and nutrients to the heart itself. The remaining blood is transported throughout the body.

The left ventricle is the largest part of the heart as it has to pump the blood all the way around the arterial circulation of the body.

Electrical Conduction Pathway

In order to ensure an effective pumping action of the heart, there is a network of specialised auto-rhythmic (self-excitable) muscle cell fibres that trigger co-ordinated muscle contraction (Figure 13.2), forcing blood around the heart chambers in the direction dictated by the heart valves.

Sino-Atrial Node

The sino-atrial (SA) node is the main pacemaker of the heart and sits within the right atrium. Electrical impulses travel from the SA node across both atria, causing the muscles to contract (depolarise) and forcing blood down into the ventricles below. The electrical signal from the SA node travels down to the atrioventricular (AV) node.

Atrioventricular Node and Bundle of His

The AV node is found in the right atrial wall. Its primary function is to delay the electrical impulse from the SA node long enough for the atria to depolarise, allowing time for atrial muscle contraction to squeeze additional blood into the ventricles (known as the atrial kick). Between the AV node and bundle branches is the bundle of His, which originates in the wall of the right atrium and straddles the interventricular septum. In normal physiology, this is the only way electrical impulses can pass between the atria and ventricles (Garcia, 2004).

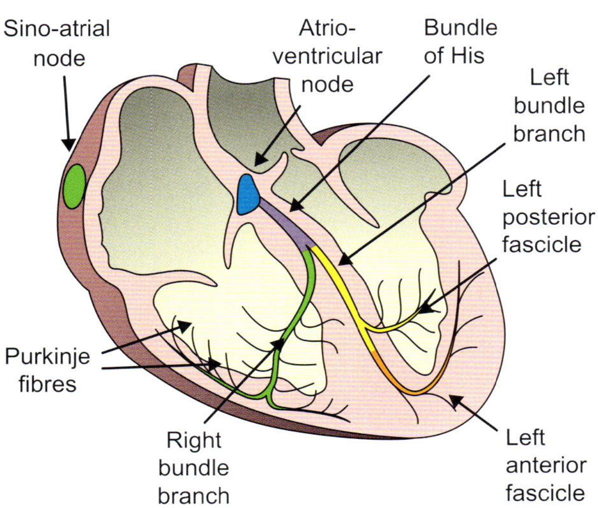

Figure 13.2 *The electrical conduction pathway of the heart.*

Left Bundle Branch

The left bundle branch starts at the end of the bundle of His, travelling through the interventricular septum, providing fibres that innervate the left ventricle and left side of the interventricular septum. It splits into two fascicles (branches): anterior and posterior. The left posterior fascicle is a fan-like structure that provides innervation to the posterior and inferior left ventricle via the Purkinje system. The left anterior fascicle is a single strand, innervating the anterior and superior portions of the left ventricle (Garcia, 2015).

Right Bundle Branch

The right bundle branch also originates from the bundle of His and sprouts fibres that innervate the right ventricle and right face of the interventricular septum, stimulating the Purkinje fibres. These fibres (named after a Czech physiologist, Jan Purkinje) consist of individual cells located just under the endocardium, and directly innervate myocardial (heart muscle) cells causing them to depolarise (contract) (Boyett, 2009).

Coronary Arteries

The heart requires its own blood supply in order to function properly. There are two main arteries that serve the heart, the right and left coronary arteries, which originate at the base of the ascending aorta (Figure 13.3).

Right Coronary Artery

The right coronary artery (RCA) runs down the right side of the heart between the right atrium and ventricle. Most people (around 80%) are right dominant; the RCA gives rise to the posterior descending artery (PDA). In around 8%, this artery arises from the left circumflex (Cx) artery (termed

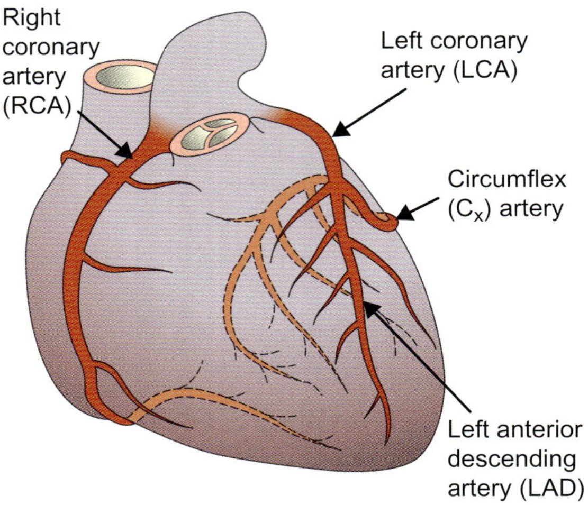

Figure 13.3 *Coronary artery anatomy.*

left dominance), with the remainder being served by both arteries (Goldberg, 2007). The PDA serves the inferior wall of the left ventricle as well as the inferior part of the septum.

Left Coronary Artery

The left coronary artery (LCA) passes behind the pulmonary trunk and splits almost immediately into two branches, the anterior interventricular branch (often referred to as the left anterior descending artery, LAD) and the circumflex artery (Cx). The LAD descends obliquely towards the apex of the heart, supplying the anterior part of the septum and anterior wall of the left ventricle (Drake, 2005).

Blood

Blood is a connective tissue consisting of a liquid (plasma) and cells performing a range of essential functions for the body (Tortora, 2008; Munden, 2002):

- Plasma makes up around 55% of blood; it carries antibodies (an important part of the immune system) and nutrients to the body's tissues, and removes waste products.
- The formed elements make up the remaining 45% and consist of red and white blood cells and platelets.
- Red blood cells (erythrocytes) carry oxygen to the tissues and remove carbon dioxide.
- White blood cells (leukocytes) are an important part of the immune and inflammatory processes.
- Platelets (thrombocytes), along with clotting factors, are an essential component of normal blood clotting, particularly in cases of bleeding (haemorrhage).

Blood Vessels

There are five main types of blood vessels in the body. The largest are the elastic arteries that leave the heart before subdividing into medium-sized muscular arteries. These further subdivide into even smaller arteries known as arterioles. These are important vessels as they control blood flow into the capillaries, which are thin-walled vessels that allow for the exchange of substances between the blood and tissues. The capillaries unite to form small veins, known as venules, which subsequently merge to form larger and larger veins that return blood to the heart (Tortora, 2008).

Vessel Structure

Most blood vessels (except capillaries) are made up of three layers or tunics (Figure 13.4). The internal layer (tunica intima or interna) consists of a smooth inner layer (the endothelium), a basement membrane and, in medium-sized arteries, a layer of elastic tissue that helps to maintain blood pressure. Ordinarily, the endothelial layer is the only one that comes into contact with blood in the lumen of the artery (Kapit, 2001).

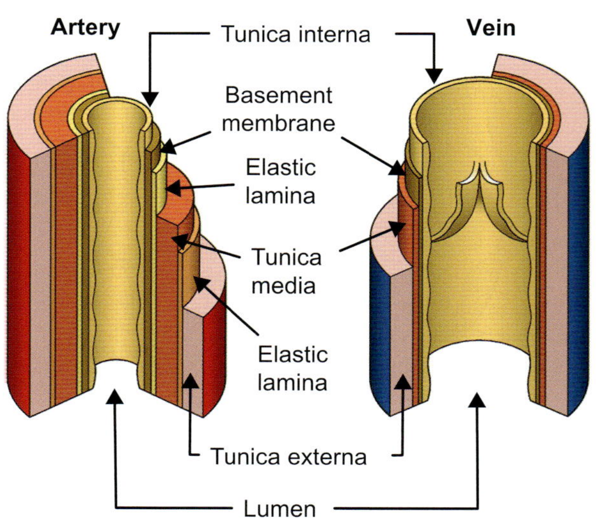

Figure 13.4 *The structure of blood vessels.*

The medium-sized veins have one-way valves formed from the endothelial layer. These are designed to prevent blood flow from travelling in the wrong direction (i.e. away from the heart). They resist gravity-induced pooling, particularly in the lower limbs (i.e. the legs).

The next layer is the tunica media. This is made up of smooth muscle and elastic fibres, and is most developed in the medium-sized arteries and least developed in the veins. In the aorta and other large arteries there is a higher proportion of elastic fibres, making the walls highly compliant and able to stretch easily without tearing when subjected to pressure changes. This is advantageous, because as blood is ejected from the heart, the walls of the aorta stretch, acting as a pressure reservoir, which can ensure blood flow continues, even when the ventricles are relaxed (Tortora, 2008).

The final layer is the tunica externa, which is constructed mostly from elastic and collagen fibres, but is also home to the vasa vasorum (the blood supply to the arteries) and nervi vasorum (motor nerves) (Kapit, 2001).

Arteries

Figure 13.5 shows the main arteries that branch from the aorta. Don't worry about memorising them all.

Veins

Figure 13.6 shows the main veins that are drained by the superior and inferior vena cavae.

Cardiac Cycle

During a single cardiac cycle, both the atria and ventricles take it in turns to contract and relax, forcing blood from an area of high pressure (due to the contracted muscle) to low pressure. The cycle is short, just 0.8 seconds in a person with an average

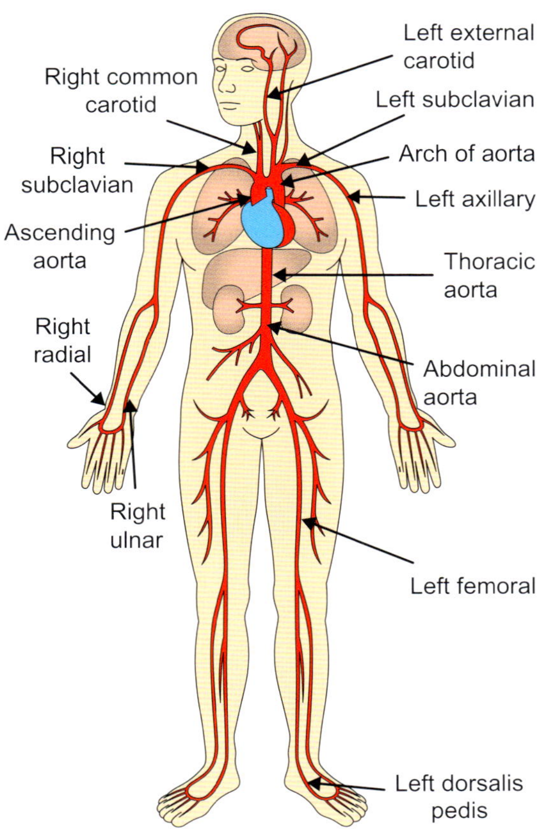

Figure 13.5 *The aorta and its branches.*

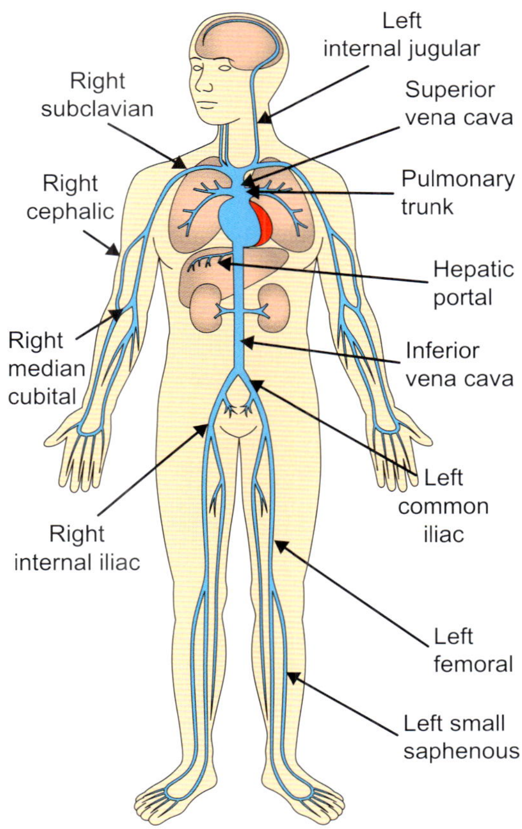

Figure 13.6 *Veins of the body.*

heart rate of 75 beats/min (Tortora, 2008; Garcia, 2015; Kapit, 2000).

Atrial Systole

This takes about 0.1 second. It starts with the sino-atrial (SA) node generating an action potential (electrical signal) when it depolarises (its voltage changes from negative to positive). This in turn causes the depolarisation of the atrial cardiac muscle cells, which contract (atrial systole). Blood is forced out of the atria, through the atrioventricular (AV) valves and into the ventricles, topping them up.

During this period, the electrical impulses from the SA node reach the AV node, pause to allow for atrial muscle contraction, and then continue down the bundle of His, the bundle branches and into the Purkinje fibres, leading to ventricular depolarisation.

Ventricular Systole

This lasts about 0.3 seconds, and during this time the atrial muscle relaxes (atrial diastole). Ventricular depolarisation causes the ventricular muscles to contract, and as the pressure inside the ventricles increases, the AV valves close and there is a brief period where all four valves of the heart are shut. This is known as isovolumetric contraction and lasts 0.05 seconds.

Contraction of the ventricles continues and eventually overcomes the pressure in the pulmonary and systemic circulations, causing the pulmonary and aortic valves (collectively known as the semilunar valves) to open. Blood is ejected into the pulmonary trunk and ascending aorta.

Meanwhile, the cardiac cells reset their voltage from positive (depolarised) to negative, a process known as repolarisation.

Relaxation Period

This is the longest period in a cardiac cycle (around 0.4 seconds) and now both the atria and the ventricles are relaxed. This period is the most shortened when heart rate increases.

Ventricular repolarisation leads to relaxation of the ventricles (ventricular diastole), and as the pressure inside the ventricles falls, the semilunar valves close. As with systole, there is a brief period where all four valves are closed (isovolumetric relaxation). The pressure continues to fall, leading to the AV valves reopening and passive filling of the ventricles begins. By the end of diastole, the ventricles will be 75% full, just in time for another action potential from the SA node to start the process all over again.

Electrocardiograms

The electrical signals that are responsible for the muscle contraction and relaxation during the cardiac cycle can be recorded on an electrocardiogram (ECG) (Figure 13.7). They are useful for determining cardiac rhythm disturbances (arrhythmias) and

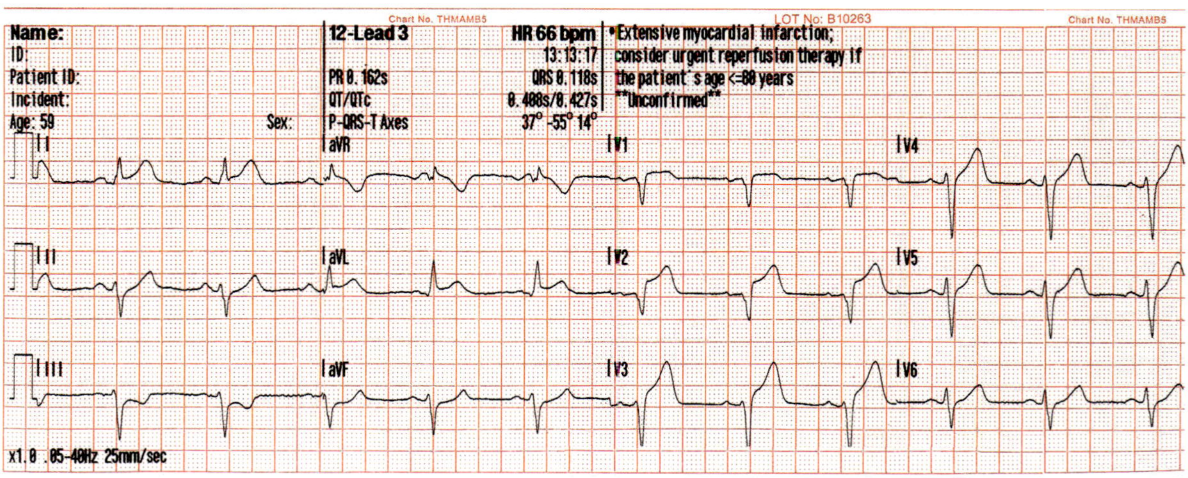

Figure 13.7 An example of a 12-lead ECG.

detecting myocardial injury, such as occurs during a heart attack (myocardial infarction).

As the heart's muscle cells depolarise and repolarise during the cardiac cycle, a potential difference (voltage) is generated, which can be detected on the surface of the body. Each cell generates its own electrical impulse, which has a strength and direction. The sum of all of these vectors is known as the heart's electrical axis and this is recorded on the ECG.

Recording the ECG is achieved with the use of electrodes that are placed in specific locations on the body, to capture the electrical activity of the heart. They are often compared to cameras placed around the heart to build up a three-dimensional picture. In reality, we do not refer to these electrical views as cameras, but as leads, which are not to be confused with the physical leads that the electrodes are attached to. To record a 12-lead ECG, for example, you will only actually place 9 or 10 physical leads on the patient.

The ECG Complex

An ECG complex is made up of a series of waves (a deflection from the baseline), segments and intervals, which represent electrical events in the heart (Figure 13.8) (Garcia, 2015):

- **P wave**: Atrial depolarisation.
- **PR segment**: This is the part of the complex between the end of the P wave and the start of the QRS wave. It should be along the baseline (the line from one TP segment to the next).

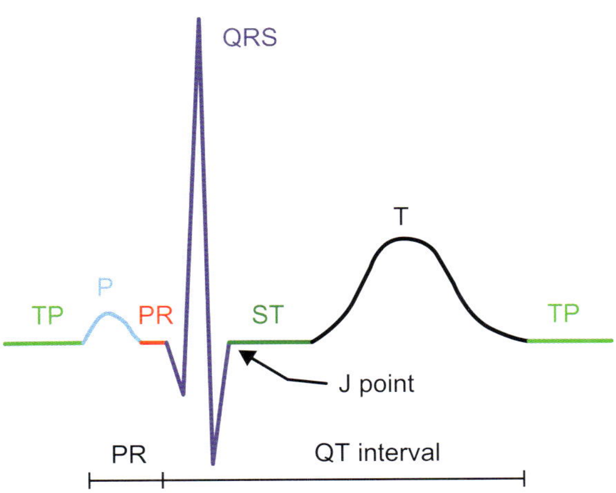

Figure 13.8 *Basic components of an ECG complex.*

- **QRS wave**. It should be 0.12–0.20 seconds (three to five small squares).
- **QRS complex**: This represents ventricular depolarisation and is typically made up of a Q, R and S wave. It should be less than 0.12 seconds or three small squares in duration.
- **ST segment**: This is the part of the complex between the end of the QRS wave and the start of the T wave. The point at which the QRS wave ends and the ST segment begins is known as the J point. The ST segment should be on the baseline.
- **T wave**: This wave represents ventricular repolarisation and is the first deflection (positive or negative) that occurs after the ST segment. It should begin in the same direction as the QRS complex.

Assessment of Circulation

Learning Objectives

By the end of this section you will be able to:

- Describe how to accurately measure the following:
  - pulse
  - capillary refill time
  - blood pressure.

Introduction

If you are asked to assess a patient's pulse, or obtain a manual blood pressure, you have been given a big responsibility, since only you will know how fast, regular and strong the pulse feels, or when you can hear the Korotkoff sounds in your stethoscope as the blood pressure cuff is deflated.

Treatment decisions are made based on clinical observations, so make sure you record observations accurately. In some patients, these observations can be difficult to obtain. If you are struggling, let the ambulance clinician know; they will understand that it can be difficult. You must never estimate or make up observations, as to do so can have a major impact on treatment decisions.

Pulse

The alternating expansion and recoil of the elastic arteries after ventricular systole creates a pressure wave, called a pulse, that can be felt in any artery that lies near the surface of the body and can be compressed against a bone or other firm structure (Tortora, 2008).

Pulses are assessed for two main reasons (Gregory, 2010b):

- to determine the patient's cardiovascular status
- to provide reassurance and gain a bond with patients who may be anxious.

Pulse Locations

Pulses are palpable all over the body, but you should be able to confidently locate the radial, brachial and carotid pulses (Figure 13.9). The other sites are useful for specific conditions, for example, checking that a patient with a leg fracture has a dorsalis pedis pulse.

Radial Pulse

The radial artery can be palpated at the wrist, on the radial side (thumb side) of the palmar (inner)

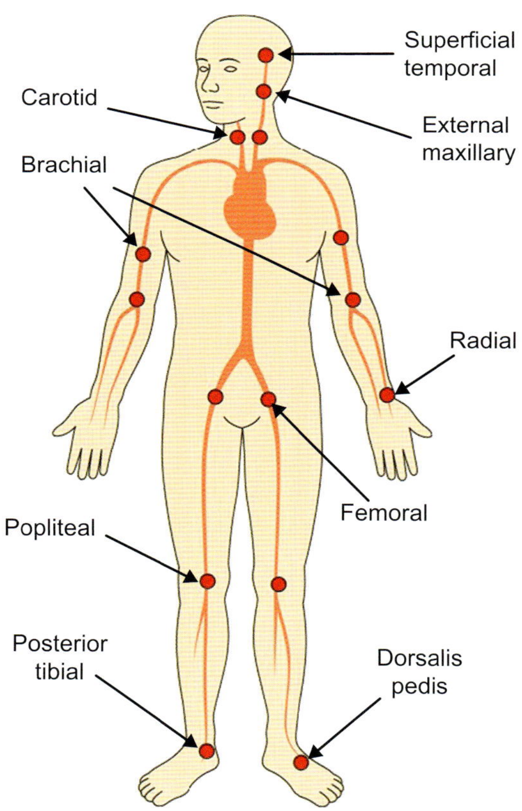

Figure 13.9 *The location of common palpable pulses.*

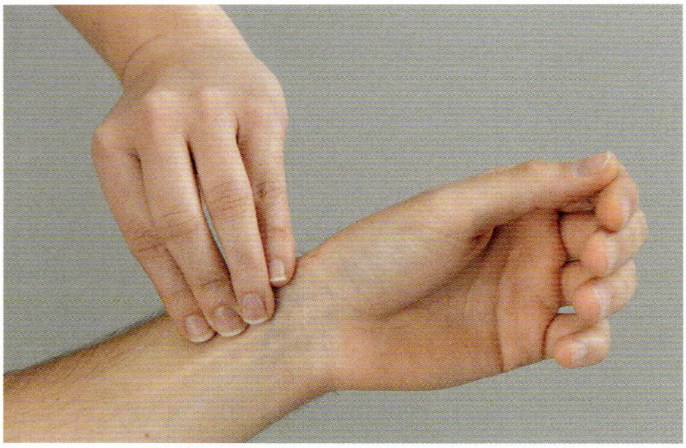

Figure 13.10 *Palpating a radial pulse.*

aspect of the forearm. It is lateral to the long flexor tendons of the forearm (Figure 13.10) (Allan, 2004).

Brachial Pulse

There are two locations for measuring this pulse. The first is in the mid-arm and can be found medially in the cleft between the biceps and triceps muscles (Figure 13.11). However, this is where a blood pressure cuff is usually placed, so in that

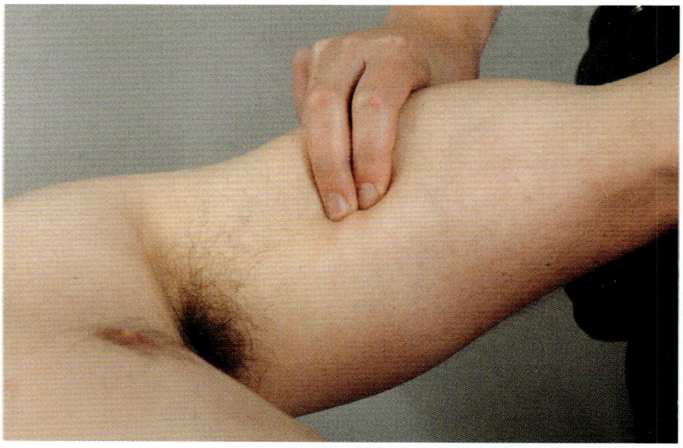

Figure 13.11 *Palpating a brachial pulse between the biceps and triceps muscles.*

instance you can also palpate the pulse in the crease of the elbow (antecubital fossa) (Figure 13.12). The pulse can be palpated just medial to the biceps tendon (Drake, 2005).

Carotid Pulse

The carotid artery can be palpated between the larynx and the sternocleidomastoid muscle. Gently press to feel the pulse (Figure 13.13) (Gregory, 2010b).

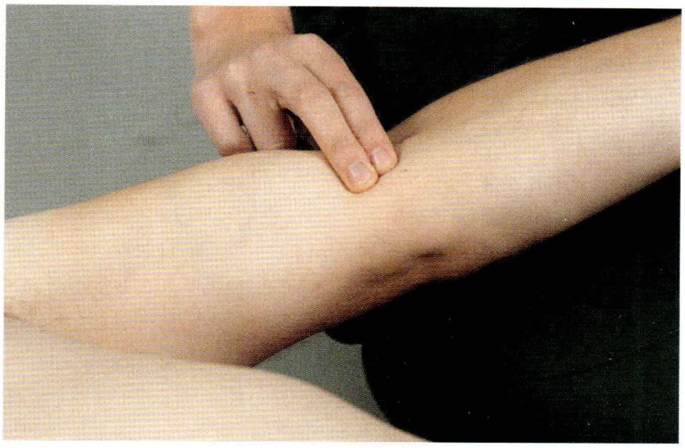

Figure 13.12 *Palpating a brachial pulse in the crease of the elbow.*

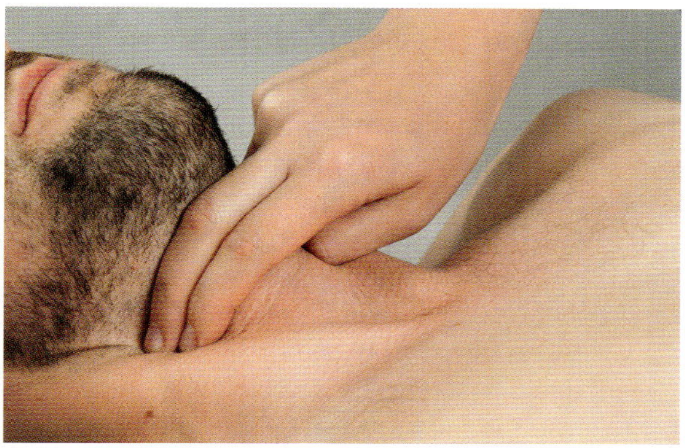

Figure 13.13 *Palpating a carotid pulse.*

Assessment

When you assess a patient's pulse, you are looking for four things:

- rate
- rhythm
- volume
- character.

Rate

The normal pulse rate for an adult is 60–100 beats/min (Allan, 2004). If the pulse rate is less than 60 beats/min this is termed bradycardia, and if greater than 100 beats/min, tachycardia (Talley, 2006; Douglas, 2005).

Causes of bradycardia include:

- sleep
- athletic training
- hypothyroidism
- medications such as beta-blockers
- hypothermia
- some types of arrhythmia (abnormal electrical activity within the heart).

Causes of tachycardia include:

- exercise
- pain
- excitement/anxiety
- hyperthyroidism
- fever
- some types of stimulant drugs such as caffeine and cocaine
- some arrhythmias.

Rhythm

In healthy patients, the rhythm should be regular. However, in certain arrhythmias this regularity can be interrupted. Try to identify whether the irregularity is regular, i.e. seems to occur in a pattern, or the beats are apparently completely random, i.e. irregularly irregular (Gregory, 2010b).

Volume and Character

The volume reflects the strength of the pulse. A high volume is typically noted during times when the cardiac output is high, such as during exercise, stress, heat and pregnancy. On the other hand, a low-volume pulse can be due to heart failure or peripheral vascular disease. A weak (also described as 'thready') pulse is most often seen in patients who are suffering from a decreased blood volume (hypovolaemia, or shock) (Douglas, 2005).

The character of the pulse is slightly different as you need to picture how the pulse changes during the cardiac cycle. This is tricky to master and will require practice.

Recording a Pulse

Procedure

Take the following steps to record a pulse (Gregory, 2010b):

1. Explain the procedure and obtain consent from the patient.
2. Place your index, middle and ring fingers along the artery and press gently. Avoid using the thumb as it has its own pulse. Don't push too hard, or you will occlude the artery. As a general rule, palpate the radial pulse first in

conscious patients, and the carotid pulse first in unconscious patients.
3. In pulses with a regular rhythm, count for 15 seconds and then multiply by 4. If the pulse is very fast or slow and/or irregular, then count for a full 60 seconds.
4. Record the pulse rate on the patient record.

Capillary Refill Time

Capillary refill time (CRT) is defined as the time taken for a distal capillary bed to regain its colour after pressure has been applied to cause blanching (Pickard, 2011). It was introduced during World War 2 to estimate the degree of shock in battlefield survivors. In 1981, an upper limit of 2 seconds was arbitrarily chosen as the acceptable upper limit; this has become the acceptable normal value and is published widely (King, 2014).

This presents a problem, because subsequent research has generally determined that it is not a good indicator of the degree of hypovolaemia in seriously ill and injured adult patients, and should not be used (Lewin, 2008).

It does have a place in the assessment of children, although it should not be taken in isolation, i.e. take into account the other aspects of patient assessment that you will undertake, such as pulse rate, respiratory rate, work of breathing, level of consciousness etc. (King, 2014).

As the usefulness of CRT is uncertain, you will need to follow local guidance about when to use CRT and in which age group.

Assessment

Be aware of the following external factors that can affect the accuracy of CRT measurement in children and neonates (King, 2014):

- **Temperature**: Children in cool environments will have a prolonged CRT, even when they are completely healthy. There is no evidence that CRT is affected by a child's body temperature, such as when they are feverish due to an illness.
- **Ambient light**: Assessing CRT in poor light leads to errors. Ensure you are somewhere well lit.
- **Site**: CRT is longer in neonates if the heel is used. One study demonstrated that fingertip and sternum CRTs are different in children (Crook, 2013). Current paediatric guidelines advocate only using the sternum to assess CRT in children (Skellett, 2016).
- **Pressure application**: It is not known how long pressure should be applied prior to assessing CRT, but current paediatric guidelines suggest pressing on the sternum for 5 seconds (Skellett, 2016).
- **Observer**: When different people (observers) measure CRT at the same time, on the same child, they end up with different results. As a rule of thumb, try to ensure that the same clinician assesses CRT each time.

Recording the Capillary Refill Time

Procedure

Follow these steps to obtain a capillary refill time (Gregory, 2010b; King, 2014):

1. Ensure the environment is warm and well lit.
2. Explain the procedure to the parent, and to the child if they are able to understand.
3. Apply pressure to the sternum for 5 seconds to compress blood from the tissues. Only apply enough pressure to cause blanching of the skin.
4. Release the pressure and count how long it takes for the colour of the skin to return to that of the surrounding tissues. This is the CRT.
5. Document your findings.
6. Consider this result in the light of other assessments of the child's cardiovascular status.

Blood Pressure

Blood pressure (BP) is the measurement of the pressure exerted by the blood on the walls of a blood vessel. It is highest in the aorta and large systemic arteries and lowest in the large veins (Tortora, 2008).

A BP that you record consists of two measurements (Gregory, 2010b):

- **Systolic blood pressure**: The BP during the systole phase of the cardiac cycle, when the ventricles contract and blood is forced out of the heart. This is the higher reading of blood pressure.

- **Diastolic blood pressure**: The BP during the diastole phase of the cardiac cycle, when the ventricles are relaxed. This is the lower reading of blood pressure.
- It is usually measured in millimetres of mercury (mmHg) and recorded as the systolic value over the diastolic, for example 120/80 mmHg.

Assessment

Blood Pressure (BP) Values

The normal range for adult BP is a systolic value of 120–139 mmHg and/or dia.stolic of 80–89 mmHg. Hypertension (high BP) is defined as a systolic value of 140 mmHg or higher and/or a diastolic of 90 mmHg or higher (Mancia, 2013). Hypotension is usually defined as a systolic blood pressure of less than 90 mmHg in adults (JRCALC, 2016).

Measurement of BP

Blood pressure can be measured directly, by inserting a sensor into a patient's artery, or indirectly using a cuff, which is applied to a patient's arm. The advantage of direct measurement is that it is accurate and continuous; it is typically used in hospital intensive care units. This method is not practicable outside of hospital and so non-invasive methods are used.

Non-Invasive Blood Pressure (NIBP) Measurement

There are two methods of NIBP measurement that you are likely to use in the pre-hospital setting (Gregory, 2010b):

- **Auscultatory**: This method uses a stethoscope and an aneroid sphygmomanometer, a device consisting of an inflatable cuff and an aneroid manometer to measure the pressure on a dial (Figure 13.14).
- **Automated**: This consists of an inflatable cuff with a sensor inside that detects the oscillations generated by turbulent blood flow and calculates systolic and diastolic values using an algorithm.

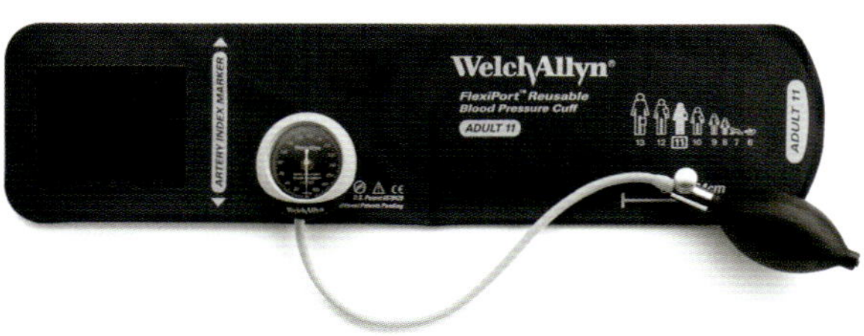

Figure 13.14 *An aneroid sphygmomanometer – image reproduced by the kind permission of Welch Allyn®.*

Korotkoff Sounds

When using the auscultatory method of measuring BP, you will place a stethoscope over the patient's brachial artery and listen for turbulent blood flow, known as the Korotkoff sounds, after a Russian surgeon, Nikolai Korotkoff, who first described them in 1905 (Talley, 2006).

The sounds are split into five phases (O'Brien, 2003):

1. The first appearance of faint, repetitive, clear tapping sounds that gradually increase in intensity for at least two consecutive beats is the systolic blood pressure. This corresponds to the restoration of blood flow, and is confirmed by the presence of a palpable pulse.
2. A brief period may follow during which the sounds soften and acquire a swishing quality. In some patients, sounds may disappear altogether for a short time.
3. The return of sharper sounds, which become crisper, to regain or even exceed the intensity of phase 1 sounds.
4. The distinct, abrupt muffling of sounds, which become soft and blowing in quality.
5. The point at which all sounds finally disappear completely is the diastolic pressure.

Note that in some groups of patients, the Phase 4 sounds may be heard until the BP measurement reaches 0 mmHg. In these cases, the onset of Phase 4 is taken to be the diastolic BP measurement (O'Brien, 2003).

Blood Pressure Measurement

Manual Blood Pressure Measurement Procedure

Take the following steps to manually record a blood pressure (Mancia, 2013; Kauffman, 2014; Gregory, 2010b; O'Brien, 2003):

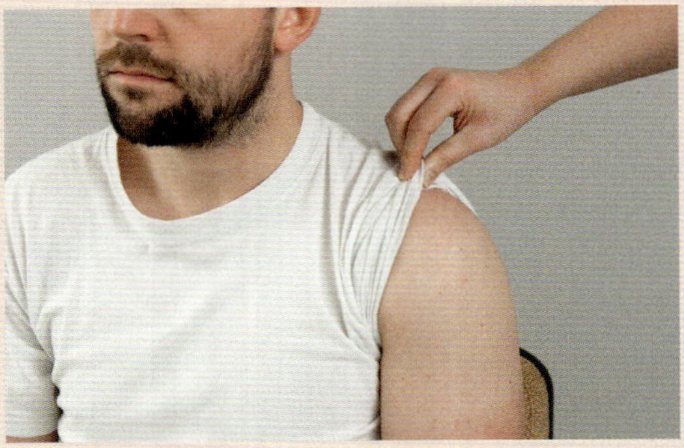

1. Ideally, allow the patient to sit for 3–5 minutes before measuring, and obtain consent.

   Ask about any medical conditions that might prevent a BP being recorded on a particular arm, e.g. mastectomy or arterio-venous shunts in dialysis patients.

   Ensure the arm is free of restrictive clothing and bare the arm. Do not apply a cuff over clothes.

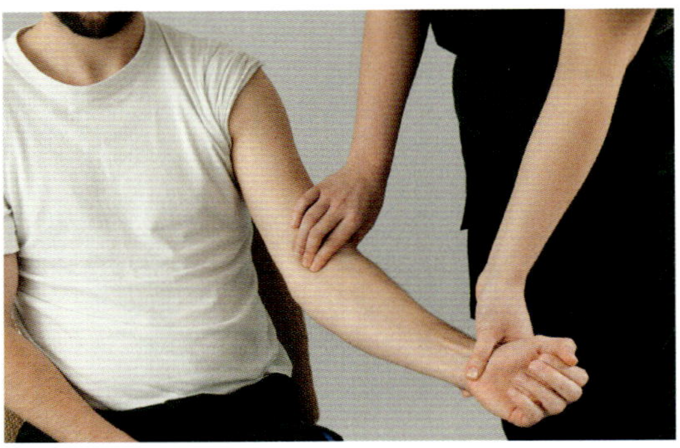

2. Palpate the brachial artery. This can be found by placing the pads of the index and middle fingers of one hand on the biceps tendon and then move medially and press deeply. If you have trouble locating the brachial pulse, ask the patient to extend their arm, which will bring the artery into a more superficial position. Once it is located, ask the patient to relax their arm so that their wrist rests on their thigh.

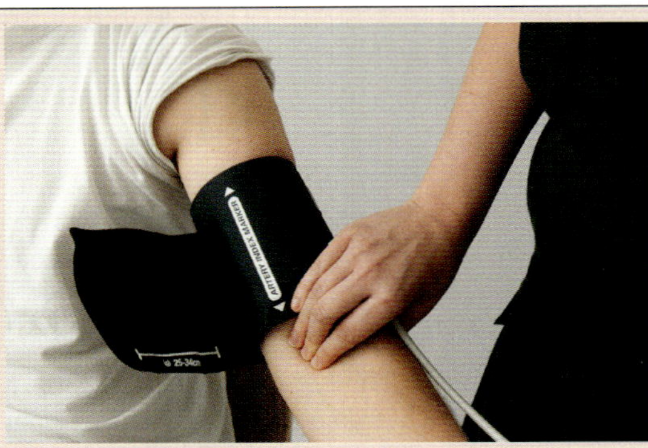

3. Ask the patient to remain still and not talk during the BP measurement.

   Select the appropriate cuff size. A standard bladder is 12–13 cm wide and is 35 cm long, but have smaller and larger sizes available.

   Ensure the cuff is at heart level and wrap snugly around the patient's upper arm and clear of the antecubital fossa, so that the cuff will not touch the stethoscope.

   Place the artery marker on the cuff over the patient's brachial artery.

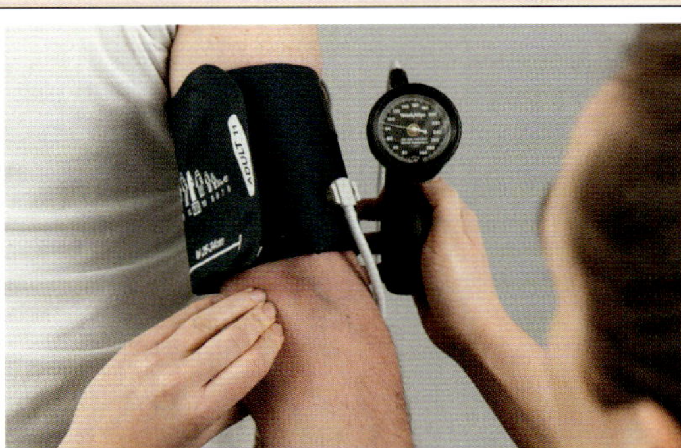

4. Palpate the brachial artery and inflate the cuff until the pulse disappears. Continue to inflate 30 mmHg above this point.

   Slowly deflate the cuff and note when the pulse returns. This gives an estimation of the systolic blood pressure.

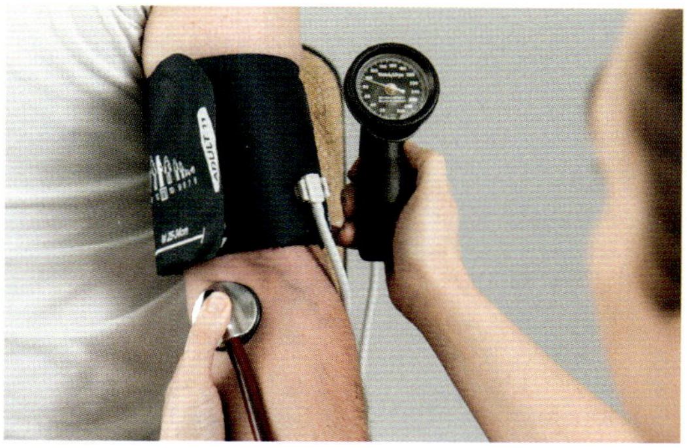

5. Wait 30 seconds and then place the diaphragm of the stethoscope over the brachial artery.

Rapidly inflate the cuff 30 mmHg above your estimation of the systolic blood pressure.

Deflate at a rate of 2–3 mmHg per pulse beat.

Note the pressure at which you first hear the Korotkoff sounds (systolic BP), the point at which they become muffled (Phase 4) and then disappear (Phase 5). The disappearance of sounds is usually taken to be the diastolic blood pressure.

Document the blood pressure, including which arm the measurement was taken from.

Automated Blood Pressure Measurement Procedure

Follow the manufacturer's instructions for the measurement of an automated blood pressure. The steps below apply to recording a BP using a LifePak 15 monitor/defibrillator (Physio-Control, 2009):

1. Press ON.
2. Select the appropriately sized cuff and apply it snugly to the arm.
3. Connect the tubing to the cuff and to the NIBP port on the monitor.
4. Change the initial inflation pressure, if necessary.
5. Position the arm in a relaxed and supported position at approximately the same level as the patient's heart. Inform the patient that the cuff will inflate and cause a 'big squeeze' around the arm and that the patient's fingers may tingle.
6. Press NIBP to start the measurement, and check that the patient's arm is not moving. When the measurement is complete, the blood pressure measurements are displayed.

Cardiovascular System Disorders

Learning Objectives

By the end of this section you will be able to:

- Describe the following conditions of the cardiovascular system and their management:
  - coronary artery disease
  - stable angina
  - acute coronary syndromes
  - heart failure.
- Explain the types, causes and stages of shock and their management.

Introduction

Many of the cardiovascular conditions you are going to learn about in this section are most commonly caused by the consequences of coronary artery disease (CAD), which worldwide is the most common cause of death, with around 7 million people dying from it each year (Steg, 2012).

Coronary Artery Disease

Coronary artery disease (CAD, sometimes called ischaemic heart disease) is almost always caused by atherosclerosis of the coronary arteries. This is a systemic, lipid (fat) driven immune/inflammatory disease of the medium and large arteries. Over time (usually decades), atherosclerosis causes the formation of plaques: collections of lipids and cholesterol that accumulate in the intimal layer of arteries, some of which attract macrophages (a type of white blood cell). The macrophages secrete protein-dissolving enzymes and engulf the lipids, leaving behind a lipid-rich 'necrotic core' (Falk, 2003).

The interface between the plaque and the lumen of the artery is known as the fibrous cap. If it becomes thickened it can cause narrowing of the artery lumen (stenosis), which if significant leads to cardiac ischaemia, particularly when myocardial oxygen demand rises, such as when the patient exercises. This can lead to stable or exertional angina. If the plaque ruptures, the artery can become occluded (blocked), leading to an acute coronary syndrome (Aaronson, 2004).

Stable Angina

Angina is a pain or discomfort usually felt across or in the centre of the chest as a tightness or indigestion-like ache. This can radiate to one or both arms, the neck, back or epigastrium (the portion of the abdomen between the diaphragm and umbilicus or belly button). It can be accompanied by belching, which may be wrongly assumed to be due to indigestion (Nolan, 2012).

To be classed as stable it should be (Montalescot, 2013):

- classic chest discomfort as described above
- provoked by exertion or emotional stress
- relieved by rest and/or nitrates (drugs that dilate the vessels) within minutes.

Stable angina is caused by significant stenosis (> 70%) of at least one coronary artery due to CAD. This causes narrowing of the artery, which at rest still allows sufficient oxygenated blood to the myocardium. However, during exercise or stress, coronary oxygen demand increases. This demand can be met by increasing blood flow through increasing the diameter of the arteries. However, this is not possible in stenosed vessels and the resulting imbalance of oxygen supply and demand leads to myocardial ischaemia (Aaronson, 2004).

Acute Coronary Syndrome

Acute coronary syndrome (ACS) represents a spectrum of three dangerous conditions, all of which constitute medical emergencies and result from a sudden decrease in coronary artery blood flow (Aaronson, 2004). These three conditions, in order of increasing severity, are:

- unstable angina (UA)
- non-ST-segment elevation myocardial infarction (NSTEMI)
- ST-segment elevation myocardial infarction (STEMI).

Since the treatment of UA and NSTEMI is similar, they are usually considered together. The ST-segment in NSTEMI and STEMI refers to the portion of an ECG complex that may change (STEMI) or not (NSTEMI) during a myocardial infarction (heart attack).

Pathophysiology

The steps that lead to an ACS are as follows (Aaronson, 2004):

1. Rupture of the fibrous cap leads to platelet aggregation (clumping together).
2. Intraplaque thrombus (blood clot) expands the plaque and can occlude the artery if large enough.
3. Intraluminal thrombus resulting in partial or complete occlusion of the artery.
4. Release of vasoconstricting substances associated with platelet aggregation, which makes the vessel constrict and narrow.
5. Endothelial damage promotes further vasoconstriction.

Assessment

The most common presentation of ACS is chest pain felt just under the sternum (sub-sternal) that may be described as heavy, squeezing, crushing or tight, that has lasted for more than 15 minutes and has not been relieved by glyceryl trinitrate (GTN). The pain radiates to the left arm in about 40% of patients, although it can also radiate to the right arm/shoulder or both left and right arms (Body, 2010). In addition, it can also radiate to the neck, jaw, upper back or epigastrium. The pain can be confused with indigestion and patients may even have tried antacid medication to relieve the discomfort. Pain is not typically altered by deep breathing or coughing. The patient may have other symptoms, such as (JRCALC, 2016):

- nausea and vomiting
- marked sweating (diaphoresis)
- pale, clammy skin
- shortness of breath
- a feeling of impending doom.

Note that up to 5% of patients do not have chest pain (Valensi, 2011). These are more likely to be women, and have diabetes or a history of heart failure (Canto, 2012).

Aspirin – Extended Skill

The indications and contra-indications listed below are taken from the UK Ambulance Services Clinical Practice Guidelines (JRCALC, 2016). However, you should be familiar with your own service guidelines, as restrictions on administration may exist. You must not administer any medication unless you are competent and authorised to do so.

Presentation

- 300 milligram (mg) aspirin (acetylsalicylic acid) in tablet form (dispersible).

Actions

- Has an anti-platelet action, which reduces clot formation.
- Analgesic, anti-pyretic and anti-inflammatory.

Indication

- Adults with clinical or ECG evidence suggestive of myocardial infarction or ischaemia.

Contra-Indications

- Known aspirin allergy or sensitivity.
- Children under 16 years (see additional information).
- Active gastrointestinal bleeding.
- Haemophilia or other known clotting disorders.
- Severe hepatic disease.

Cautions

- As the likely benefits of a single 300 mg aspirin tablet outweigh the potential risks, aspirin may be given to patients with:
    - asthma
    - pregnancy
    - kidney or liver failure
    - gastric or duodenal ulcer
    - current treatment with anti-coagulant.

Side Effects

- Gastric bleeding.
- Wheezing in some asthmatics.

Dosage and Administration

- Route: Oral – chewed or dissolved in water.
- 300 mg tablet, no repeat dose.
- In suspected myocardial infarction, a 300 mg aspirin tablet should be given regardless of any previous aspirin taken.

GTN – Extended Skill

The indications and contra-indications listed below are taken from the UK Ambulance Services Clinical Practice Guidelines (JRCALC, 2016). However, you should be familiar with your own service guidelines as restrictions on administration may exist. You must not administer any medication unless you are competent and authorised to do so.

Presentation

- Metered dose spray containing 400 micrograms glyceryl trinitrate per dose.
- Tablets containing glyceryl trinitrate 300, 500 and 600mcg for buccal administration (depends on local ordering).

Actions

- A potent vasodilator drug resulting in:
    - dilatation of coronary arteries/relief of coronary spasm
    - dilatation of systemic veins resulting in lower pre-load
    - reduced blood pressure.

Indication

- Cardiac chest pain due to angina or myocardial infarction.

Contra-Indications

- Hypotension (systolic blood pressure < 90 mmHg).
- Hypovolaemia.
- Head trauma.
- Cerebral haemorrhage.
- Sildenafil (Viagra) and other related drugs – glyceryl trinitrate must not be given to patients who have taken sildenafil or related drugs within the previous 24 hours. Profound hypotension may occur.
- Unconscious patients.

Side Effects

- Hypotension.
- Headache.

Dosage and Administration

- Route: Sublingual for spray and buccal for tablets.
- Sublingual spray: 1–2 sprays providing 400–800 micrograms of GTN.

- Buccal: 300, 500 and 600mcg tablet.
- Repeat every 5–10 minutes.
- No maximum dose, although side effects may limit repeat dosages.

Management

The management of ACS includes (JRCALC, 2016):

- correction of major ABC problems
- oxygen, if the patient has oxygen saturations of less than 94% on air
- administration of aspirin
- assisting the patient to take their own GTN
- being prepared to resuscitate the patient if they suffer a cardiac arrest.

Heart Failure

Heart failure is an abnormality of cardiac structure or function, leading to failure of the heart to deliver oxygen at a sufficient rate to meet cell and tissue metabolic needs, despite normal filling pressures (McMurray, 2012).

Patients who have been suffering from heart failure for some time are classed as having chronic heart failure. If their signs and symptoms have not changed in the past month, then it is considered to be stable. On the other hand, if there is an acute deterioration in these patients, they are considered to be suffering from acute decompensated heart failure (often just called acute heart failure, AHF) (Allen, 2007).

Although the most common cause of AHF is sudden worsening of chronic heart failure, about 20–30% of cases are a new-onset heart failure, with a small percentage due to malignant hypertensive crisis (blood pressure that is high enough to damage the body's organs) or cardiogenic shock. Up to 25% of cases are caused by an acute coronary syndrome, although these are normally considered separately from 'typical' AHF because of the differing presentation, pathophysiology and treatment (Howlett, 2011).

Assessment

Heart failure can be difficult to diagnose in the pre-hospital environment, since many of the symptoms are non-specific (Table 13.1), making it difficult to differentiate AHF from other conditions, such as pneumonia, chronic obstructive pulmonary disease (COPD) and pulmonary oedema (Williams, 2013). The more specific symptoms (such as orthopnoea, paroxysmal nocturnal dyspnoea and haemoptysis) are less common (Dobson, 2009).

Management

The management of acute heart failure includes (JRCALC, 2016):

- correction of major ABC problems
- oxygen, if the patient has oxygen saturations of less than 94% on air.

Table 13.1 History, signs and symptoms of heart failure

History	Signs	Symptoms
Patient age	Tachypnoea	Shortness of breath
Coronary artery disease	Crackles	Dyspnoea
Hypertension	Dullness to percussion	Orthopnoea
High cholesterol	Reduced SpO_2	Fatigue
Valvular disease (e.g. mitral regurgitation or aortic stenosis)	Haemoptysis	Paroxysmal nocturnal dyspnoea
Known heart failure or myocardial injury	Tachycardia	Reduced exercise tolerance
Loop diuretic use (e.g. furosemide)	Peripheral oedema	Ankle swelling
Arrhythmias	Enlarged liver	

Aortic Dissection

An aortic dissection occurs when the innermost layer of the aorta is breached, allowing blood to enter the medial layer of the vessel (Nienaber, 2012; Thrumurthy, 2012).

Aorta

The largest artery in the body is the aorta. Although a continuous vessel, it is often divided anatomically into the thoracic aorta, above the diaphragm, and the abdominal aorta, below. The thoracic portion of the aorta can be further subdivided into the ascending aorta, which arises from the left ventricle and heads upwards, backwards and to the left, arching over the pulmonary arteries (imaginatively called the arch of the aorta) and becoming the descending aorta, which continues through the thorax and abdomen before finally bifurcating into the common iliac arteries in the pelvis (Drake, 2005).

Pathophysiology

In order for aortic dissection to occur non-traumatically, the medial layer has to degenerate, either due to ageing or genetics.

Aortic dissection occurs when the intima (inner layer) is torn, typically at the sites of greatest wall stress, and is classified according to which part of the aorta is affected (Figure 13.15). In the ascending aorta, the point of greatest wall stress occurs close to the aortic valve on the right lateral wall of the aorta, and in the descending aorta near the ligamentum arteriosum (Ahmad, 2006).

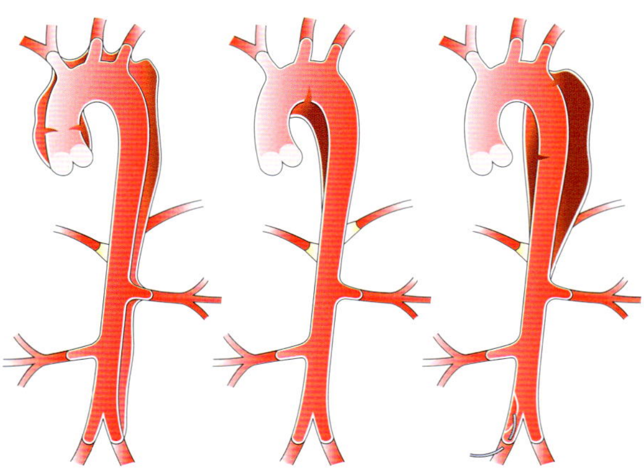

Figure 13.15 *DeBakey classification of aortic dissection. (Left) Type I: Originates in ascending aorta; expands to the aortic arch and often beyond into the descending aorta. (Middle) Type II: Originates and is confined to the ascending aorta. (Right) Type III: Originates and is confined to the descending aorta.*

Blood under high pressure is able to split (dissect) the media, forming a false channel, or lumen. Depending on the blood pressure and rate of acceleration of the blood flow, the dissection extends in the direction of blood flow (although can propagate in the opposite direction as well). The blood pressure in the new, false lumen can be high enough to compress and even obstruct the true lumen. Ultimately, the false lumen will either be occluded by thrombus, re-communicate with the true lumen or work its way into other potential spaces, such as the pericardium and pleural or peritoneal cavities (Patel, 2008; Ahmad, 2006). As the dissection extends, arteries branching off from the aorta can become affected, leading to cerebral, coronary, mesenteric, renal and limb ischaemia.

Assessment

Patients are more commonly men over 60 years of age (Ranasinghe, 2011). Pain is the most common presenting symptom of acute aortic dissection, which is typically of sudden onset and very severe (Nienaber, 2012). However, around 10% of patients will have no pain, particularly if they are diabetic (Thrumurthy, 2012). Although the textbook description of the pain is tearing or ripping, patients are more likely to describe their pain as sharp (Ramanath, 2009). Pain location varies depending on the type of dissection. Patients with type II dissections (involving the ascending aorta) are more likely to complain of anterior chest pain, whereas type III dissections (which do not involve the ascending aorta) are more commonly associated with back and abdominal pain. Pain can radiate into the neck (type II) or interscapular area (type III), and can change as the dissection progresses along the aorta (Thrumurthy, 2012).

Other signs and symptoms to look out for include neurological deficits (for example, loss of consciousness), symptomatic limb ischaemia, pulse deficits between limbs and a systolic blood pressure differential between arms of more than 20 mmHg (Ranasinghe, 2011).

Frustratingly, there are a number of differential diagnoses to consider, which not only mimic the signs and symptoms of aortic dissection, but can also be caused by a dissection (Thrumurthy, 2012):

- acute chest pain:
  - myocardial infarction
  - pulmonary embolism
  - spontaneous pneumothorax
- acute abdominal or back pain:
  - renal colic
  - perforated viscus
  - mesenteric ischaemia
- pulse deficit:
  - non-dissection-related embolic disease
- focal neurological deficit:
  - stroke
  - cauda equina syndrome.

Management

Without surgery, 50–91% of type A dissections (those involving the ascending aorta) will die within a week. Even with surgery, the mortality rate is 15–35% (Thrumurthy, 2012). Type B dissections (those not involving the ascending aorta), on the other hand, are usually managed medically, unless there is organ or limb malperfusion, and/or uncontrollable pain or hypertension.

Initial treatment common to both types includes strong analgesia (usually opiates, but if you are not working with a paramedic, Entonox is a reasonable alternative) and trying to calm and reassure your patient while getting them to hospital as quickly as possible (Pilbery, 2013).

Shock

Shock is a clinical state in which the delivery of oxygenated blood (and other nutrients such as glucose) to the body's tissues is not adequate to meet metabolic demand (Skellett, 2016).

The types of shock vary between textbooks, but five types are included here:

- hypovolaemic shock
- distributive shock
- cardiogenic shock
- obstructive shock
- dissociative shock.

Hypovolaemic Shock

This is an acute loss of circulating blood volume either from dehydration (loss of fluids and electrolytes) or from bleeding (haemorrhage) externally or internally. Shock due to blood loss (haemorrhagic shock) has been classified into four classes (stages) (NAEMT, 2014):

- **Class 1**: The body is able to cope with losses and there are no obvious clinical signs.
- **Class 2**: This is the compensated stage. Blood loss is more significant, but the body has mechanisms to maintain blood pressure despite the reduction in blood volume.
- **Class 3**: This is the decompensated stage. Despite the compensatory mechanisms, blood loss is now too severe to maintain blood pressure. These patients require blood and urgent surgical intervention to stop the bleeding.
- **Class 4**: The irreversible stage. Even if the circulation is restored, the patient is still likely to die.

Signs of Hypovolaemic Shock

The classic signs of hypovolaemic shock include (JRCALC, 2016):

- pallor
- cool peripheries
- anxiety and abnormal behaviour
- increased heart and respiratory rates.

Note that these may not appear until 1,000–1,500 ml of blood has been lost, and even later in some patient groups, such as pregnant women, patients on medication such as beta-blockers, and fit individuals.

Distributive Shock

This type of shock is caused by widespread dilation of the peripheral vascular system because of dilation of the arterioles and/or venules. This in effect creates a larger container for the same blood volume, leading to decreased tissue perfusion. In addition, in causes such as anaphylaxis and sepsis, the vessels become 'leaky', allowing fluid to escape into the tissues and so becoming removed from the general circulation (Pilbery, 2013).

Common causes of distributive shock include:

- anaphylaxis
- sepsis
- nervous system related cause, such as spinal cord injury.

Cardiogenic Shock

This is due to a primary cardiac problem when the heart is unable to circulate sufficient blood to meet the body's metabolic needs. This is most common following a myocardial infarction, but can also be caused by acute heart failure or arrhythmia (Pilbery, 2013).

Obstructive Shock

This is an uncommon cause of shock and is due to an obstruction of blood flow to/from the heart. It can be caused by a tension pneumothorax, cardiac tamponade or a massive pulmonary embolism (Evans, 2012).

Dissociative Shock

This occurs when the oxygen-carrying capacity of the blood is affected because of inadequate numbers of red blood cells available to carry sufficient oxygen (anaemia) or when competing molecules take up space on the red blood cells that would normally be used to carry oxygen, such as in cases of carbon monoxide poisoning (Skellett, 2016).

Management

Your management of shock will include the following actions (JRCALC, 2016; Zideman, 2015):

- Identify and control sources of external bleeding.
- Administer high levels of supplemental oxygen via a non-rebreathe mask.
- Place patients supine and, if there is no history of trauma, raise their legs. Note that this is only likely to provide transient improvement in vital signs (typically less than 7 minutes).

Chapter 14

Disability

Nervous System Anatomy and Physiology

Learning Objectives

By the end of this section you will be able to:

- State the functions of the nervous system.
- Describe the anatomy and physiology of the nervous system.

Introduction

The nervous system performs three main functions in order to carry out a complex range of tasks including controlling body movements, regulating heart rate, creating memories and producing speech (Tortora, 2008; Briar, 2003):

- **Sensory function (perception)**: Receptors located around the body detect internal stimuli, such as a change in blood pressure, and external stimuli, such as a bad odour, and transmit this via afferent nerves through the cranial and spinal nerves and into the brain and spinal cord.
- **Information transfer and processing**: Nerve cells (neurons) have special projections (axons) that allow the conduction of electrical impulses. These can be delivered to other neurons, and/or modified by or integrated with other impulses to create a complex web that can process sensory information received from afferent neurons.
- **Motor function**: This is the nervous system's response to the processing stage and is communicated via efferent nerves, which carry electrical impulses from the brain via cranial or spinal nerves. This enables the brain to control the body as well as control ventilation and circulation.

Anatomy and Physiology

The nervous system (Figure 14.1) consists of the brain and spinal cord (generally referred to as the central nervous system, CNS) and a network of peripheral nerves either originating from the brain (as 12 pairs of cranial nerves) or the spinal cord (as 31 pairs of spinal nerves). Together with small collections of neurons known as ganglia, these form the peripheral nervous system (PNS).

The PNS consists of two divisions. The first is the sensory, or afferent, division, which is composed of large numbers of sensory receptors in the skin. Their nerve impulses are conveyed by somatic sensory fibres, as well as internally around the body (impulses from which are transmitted by visceral sensory fibres), and an extensive network of neurons around the gastrointestinal tract, collectively known as the enteric plexus, which helps regulate digestion. The other division of the PNS is the motor, or efferent, division. This is split

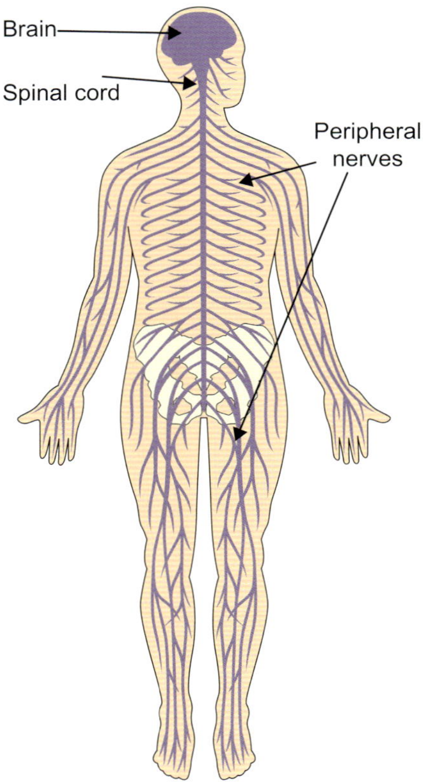

Figure 14.1 *The nervous system.*

into the somatic nervous system and the autonomic nervous system (Marieb, 2013; Tortora, 2008).

Brain

The portion of the central nervous system that is contained within the skull is known as the brain. The brain occupies 80% of the cranial vault, with the remaining 20% made up of cerebral blood (12%) and cerebrospinal fluid (8%). It has a wide range of functions as well as serving as the centre for intellect, emotions, behaviour and memory. The brain is generally divided into four major sections (Figure 14.2) (Tortora, 2008):

- brain stem
- cerebellum
- diencephalon
- cerebrum.

Brain Stem

The brain stem consists of the medulla oblongata, pons and midbrain. Their functions include:

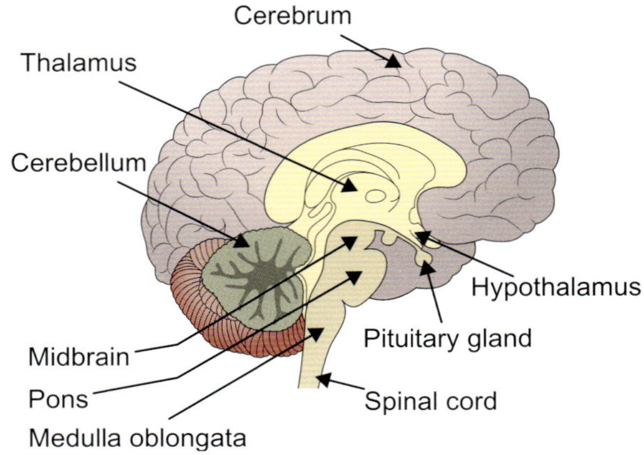

Figure 14.2 *The brain.*

- Medulla oblongata:
  - relays sensory and motor input between other parts of the brain and spinal cord
  - together with pons and midbrain, controls level of consciousness
  - contains centres to manage heart rate, blood pressure and breathing
  - contains origins of a number of cranial nerves.
- Pons:
  - relays nervous impulses from one side of the cerebellum to the other and between medulla and midbrain
  - contains origins of a number of cranial nerves
  - contains centres to regulate breathing.
- Midbrain:
  - relays motor output from the cerebral cortex and sensory input from the spinal cord to the thalamus
  - controls and co-ordinates movement
  - contains origins of two cranial nerves.

Cerebellum

This part of the brain is responsible for co-ordinating complex and skilled movements and regulates posture and balance.

Diencephalon

The diencephalaon consists of two of the brain's structures:

- Thalamus:
  - relays sensory input to the cerebral cortex
  - provides perception of touch, pressure, pain and temperature.

- Hypothalamus:
  - controls and integrates autonomic nervous system activity
  - regulates behavioural patterns and circadian rhythms
  - controls body temperature
  - regulates eating and drinking behaviour.

Cerebrum

The cerebrum allows you to read, write and speak. Various regions are responsible for a range of other functions:

- Sensory areas are involved in the perception of sensory information.
- Motor areas control muscular movements.
- Association areas are responsible for complex functions such as memory, personality and intelligence.

The cerebrum is split into two hemispheres and consists of an outer rim of grey matter and an internal region of white matter. The outer rim of grey matter contains the cerebral cortex which, although thin, contains billions of neurons. Each hemisphere can also be further divided into four lobes: frontal, parietal, occipital and temporal.

Meninges

In addition to the skull, the brain is protected by the meninges. There are three of them (Tortora, 2008):

- **Dura**: Tough outer layer consisting of connective tissue.
- **Arachnoid**: Middle layer; the sub-arachnoid space (between arachnoid and pia layers) is filled with cerebrospinal fluid.
- **Pia**: Delicate inner layer containing small blood vessels, which supply oxygen and nutrients to the brain.

Cerebrospinal Fluid

Cerebrospinal fluid (CSF) is a clear, colourless liquid, which protects the brain and spinal cord from physical and chemical injury. It also carries oxygen, glucose and other nutrients that are essential for normal brain function, as well as removing waste products (Tortora, 2008).

Spinal Cord

The vertebral column consists of 33 vertebrae: 7 cervical, 12 thoracic, 5 lumbar, 5 sacral and 4 coccygeal. Part of their function is to provide physical protection for the spinal cord, which the vertebrae encapsulate. Additional protection is provided by vertebral ligaments, meninges and the cerebrospinal fluid (CSF) (Tortora, 2008). Rather confusingly, there are 31 pairs of spinal nerves: 8 cervical, 12 thoracic, 5 lumbar, 5 sacral and 1 coccygeal (Figure 14.3).

The spinal cord is almost cylindrical in shape, although slightly squashed in the anterior–posterior dimension. Its average diameter is just 12 mm, and in adults it extends from the medulla oblongata to the superior border of the second lumbar vertebra (L2), i.e. it does not extend the full length of the vertebral column. Instead, it tapers to form a cone-like structure called the conus medullaris (Tortora, 2008). Nerves that originate distal to the conus medullaris form the cauda equina (meaning horse's tail). These nerves have a dorsal root containing afferent fibres which transmit sensation, and a ventral root containing efferent motor fibres (Gitelman, 2008).

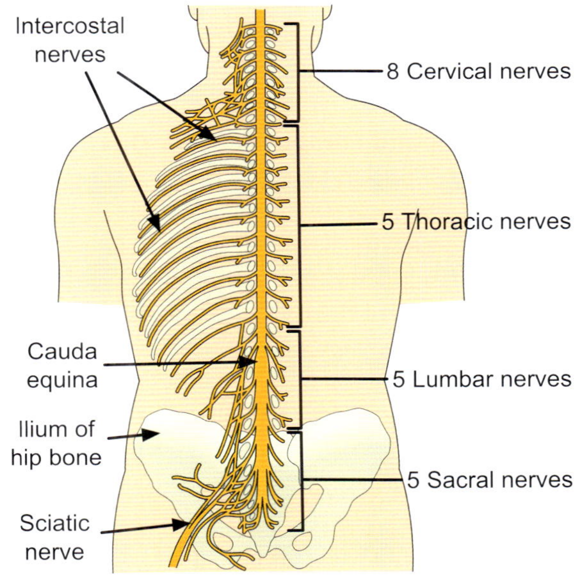

Figure 14.3 *Spinal nerves.*

Somatic Nervous System

The somatic nervous system is also sometimes known as the voluntary nervous system, since it allows the person to consciously control their skeletal muscles thanks to somatic nerve fibres, which conduct impulses from the central nervous system to skeletal muscles (Marieb, 2013). However, the somatic nervous system also includes an involuntary component: reflexes. These are primarily a protective mechanism, for instance removing your hand when you touch something hot (Tortora, 2008).

Autonomic Nervous System

The autonomic nervous system (ANS) is divided into three parts. These are the sympathetic, parasympathetic and enteric nervous systems. They are called autonomic because it was originally believed that they functioned completely independently from the CNS. However, it is now known that the hypothalamus and brain stem regulate ANS activity (Tortora, 2008). The enteric division is an extensive network of neurons that reside within the walls of the gastrointestinal (GI) tract, pancreas and gall bladder. It has a sensory nervous function enabling the monitoring of the mechanical state of the alimentary canal and the chemical status of the stomach and intestines. In addition, it can output motor signals to modify the motility and secretions of the gut, as well as controlling the diameter of local blood vessels (Briar, 2003).

Sympathetic and Parasympathetic Divisions

The sympathetic and parasympathetic divisions of the ANS are often thought of as being at either end of a see-saw. This is true in some organs such as the heart, but in reality this is rather a simplistic view. Some parts of the body receive inputs from only one division, whereas in others, the effects of the sympathetic and parasympathetic divisions are similar. However, their actions are carefully controlled and co-ordinated by the hypothalamus.

The sympathetic division is often referred to as the fight-or-flight division, as its actions prepare the body to respond to stress, facilitating sudden strenuous exercise and increased vigilance. In addition, it helps control blood pressure, thermoregulation, and gut and urogenital function.

The parasympathetic division is often referred to as the rest-and-digest division. Actions of the parasympathetic division include antagonising some effects of the sympathetic division, for example heart rate, gut motility and bronchiole diameter, and controlling many body functions in non-stress states, such as GI secretion to aid digestion, micturition and defaecation. Another important difference between the sympathetic and parasympathetic divisions is their structure. Parasympathetic neurons are clustered at either end of the spinal cord, whereas the sympathetic neurons originate from the thoracolumbar section.

Assessment of Disability

Learning Objectives

By the end of this section you will be able to:

- Describe how to undertake and record the following:
  - level of consciousness
  - pupillary response
  - face, arm, speech test.

Introduction

A complete assessment of the nervous system is involved and requires a number of tests, which is beyond the scope of the emergency medical responder. However, there are a couple of useful and simple tests that you can perform, which will uncover the presence of serious neurological problems in your patient and help determine the most appropriate management for them. You have already met one of them, AVPU, in Chapter 10: Patient Assessment.

Level of Consciousness

A rapid assessment of the patient's level of consciousness (LOC) can be undertaken using the acronym AVPU:

- **A**: alert. Patient's eyes are open and they interact with their surroundings and/or people on scene, including you
- **V**: responds to verbal stimulus. Patient opens their eyes or responds to you when you issue a verbal greeting or command

- **P**: responds to pain. Makes a verbal and/or motor response to a pain stimulus, such as opening their eyes, or moving their limbs
- **U**: unresponsive. No response to verbal commands or pain stimulus.

Painful stimuli

The aim of a pain stimulus is to assess the level of consciousness and depth of coma, but not to cause long-term pain or damage, which could be considered battery (Waterhouse, 2009)! The preferred pain stimulus is the trapezius pinch (Figure 14.4), (Middleton, 2012). Note that a patient with a spinal injury that affects the arms should not have a trapezius pinch applied.

Pupillary Response

Before switching on your pen torch to check the patient's pupils, have a look at the pupils' relative size to determine whether they are unequal. This is known as anisocoria and is a normal finding in around 20% of the population (Kaeser, 2010). Look for changes in shape (e.g. oval in acute angle-closure glaucoma, asymmetrical in a penetrating injury).

Pupillary Reactions

Test pupillary reaction by assessing direct response to light (James, 2011):

- Shine your pen torch directly on each eye in turn for 3 seconds. This should cause a prompt constriction of the pupil and the opposite pupil. Failure of either pupil to constrict could be a sign of serious disease and should be reported to the ambulance crew when they arrive.

Face, Arm, Speech Test

With the advent of clot-busting drugs (thrombolytics) for the management of acute stroke, the need for prompt recognition of stroke has never been greater. A simple tool that can be used to identify a patient suffering from a stroke is the Newcastle face, arm, speech test (FAST) (NAO, 2010).

The FAST consists of three components (Harbison, 2003):

- **Facial palsy**: Ask the patient to smile or show their teeth. Look for new lack of symmetry. This is positive if there is an unequal smile, grimace or obvious facial asymmetry.
- **Arm weakness**: Lift the patient's arms together to 90° (45° if they are lying on their back) with the palms uppermost (Figure 14.5). Ask them to close their eyes and hold that position for 5 seconds. Look for one arm drifting or falling rapidly.
- **Speech impairment**: During the course of a conversation (if the patient can speak), look for new speech disturbance. This may require asking someone who knows the patient. Specifically, look for slurred speech and word-finding difficulties. Ask the patient to identify common objects (such as keys, a cup, chair and pen). If the patient has a severe visual disturbance, place the object in the patient's hands and ask them to name it.

The presence of one or more of these signs constitutes a positive FAST (Figure 14.6).

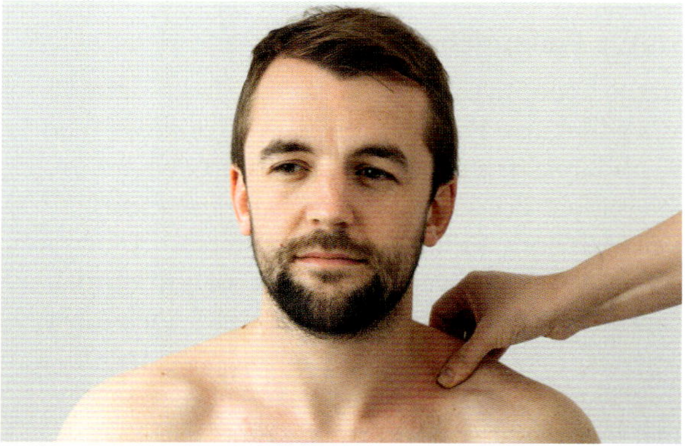

Figure 14.4 *Trapezius pinch.*

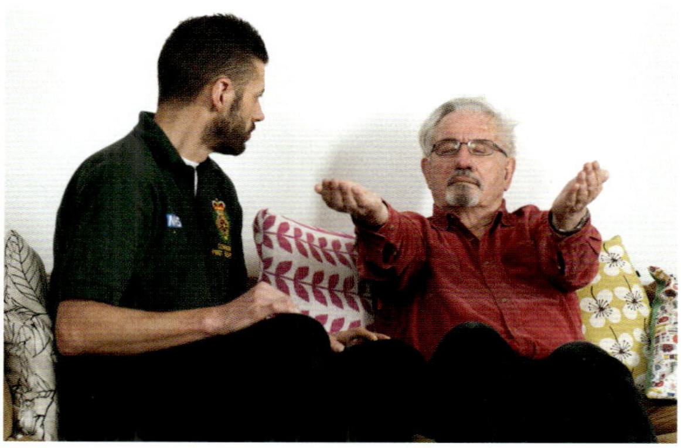

Figure 14.5 *A patient performing the FAST.*

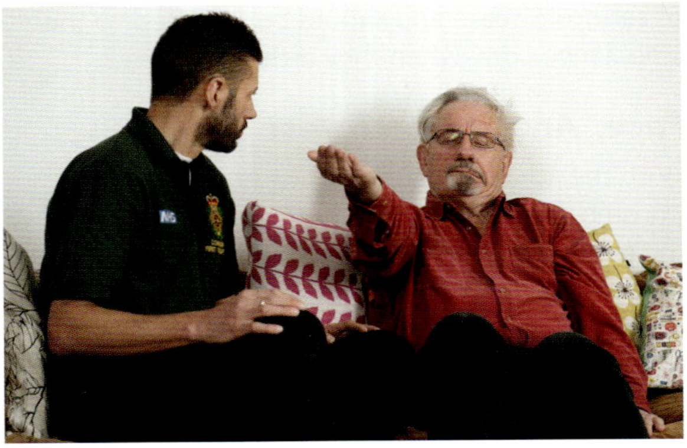

Figure 14.6 *A positive FAST, due to a facial palsy and arm weakness.*

Disorders of the Nervous System

Learning Objectives

By the end of this section you will be able to:

- Explain the pathophysiology relating to a range of neurological disorders.
- Describe the management of a range of neurological disorders.
- List several causes of coma.

Introduction

In this section, you will learn about a range of nervous system disorders. The nervous system is extremely complex and you will learn about only a few of the many disease processes. However, it is important to be able to recognise patients with epilepsy, stroke, meningococcal disease and patients who are unconscious. Timely and appropriate management can result in better outcome: in some cases, literally the difference between life and death, and/or life-altering disability.

Epilepsy

Epilepsy is not a single condition, but a term used to describe a tendency to have recurrent, unprovoked convulsions (also called seizures and fits). It is the commonest of the serious neurological conditions (Smithson, 2012).

Convulsions result from the synchronised and excessive activation of neurons in the cerebral cortex. How this presents clinically depends on where this activity starts and how far and fast it spreads through the brain (Briar, 2003). Convulsions are divided into two broad categories:

- **Partial (focal) convulsions**: As the name suggests, these originate from a specific area of the cortex, typically the temporal or frontal lobes. They are split into two subtypes (Smithson, 2012; Briar, 2003):
    - **Simple partial**: Patients remain conscious but may complain of 'butterflies' in their stomach, fear, illusions and hallucinations. These are usually brief.
    - **Complex partial**: Complex refers to an altered level of consciousness and is characterised by the patient chewing, lip-smacking and fiddling with their hands. These usually resolve within a few minutes.
- **Generalised convulsions**: These convulsions are also divided into two subtypes:
    - **Tonic-clonic**: These convulsions consist of two phases. In the tonic phase, the patient goes stiff (and may cry out), falls (if standing) and bites their tongue as the jaw clenches. This is followed by the clonic phase, characterised by regular jerking movements, which start in the upper limbs. These eventually slow and stop, which may herald the onset of incontinence. Patients typically experience a post-ictal period following a tonic-clonic convulsion, where they may be sleepy and confused. This usually resolves within 20 minutes.
    - **Absence convulsions**: These typically begin in childhood and adolescence and consist of 'day-dreaming', with a few seconds of staring into space, eyelid fluttering, swallowing and head flopping.

Status Epilepticus

Status epilepticus has traditionally been defined as a generalised convulsion lasting for more than 30 minutes, or a series of convulsions, where the patient does not become fully conscious between convulsions, lasting more than 30 minutes (ILAE, 1993). However, it has been suggested that shortened timescales should be used since most convulsions last less than 5 minutes and those that last more than 5 minutes generally require therapeutic intervention, because they will not stop on their own (Brophy, 2012).

In adults and children, common causes of status epilepticus are withdrawal from or sub-therapeutic doses of anti-epileptic drugs. In children, the most common cause is febrile illness, whereas in adults, stroke is the most common cause. Approximately 16–38% of children diagnosed with status epilepticus are known epileptics. In adults, this figure increases to 42–50% (Chin, 2004; Neligan and Shorvon, 2010).

Post-Ictal Phase

For patients who suffer a generalised tonic-clonic convulsion, they typically enter a post-convulsion (post-ictal) phase, which is characterised by a period of unresponsiveness and then a gradual return of consciousness. The patient is likely to be drowsy and disorientated, which can last 15 minutes to an hour (and in some cases, longer). Complaints of a headache are common (Kumar, 2012).

Management of Convulsions

As with all patients, start by ensuring they have a patent airway. This can be achieved by a combination of patient positioning (e.g. the recovery position) and airway adjuncts. An oropharyngeal airway can be difficult to insert when patients are convulsing and should not be forced into the patient's mouth (JRCALC, 2016).

Administer high-concentration oxygen (as close to 100% as possible) via a non-rebreathe mask (or bag-valve-mask) at a flow rate of 15 l/min. In adults, once a reliable pulse oximetry reading has been obtained, oxygen administration can be titrated to maintain saturations of 94–98%. Children should continue to receive high concentrations of oxygen irrespective of the pulse oximeter reading (JRCALC, 2016).

Stroke

Stroke is a syndrome consisting of rapidly developing (usually seconds or minutes) symptoms and/or signs of focal central nervous system (CNS) function. The symptoms last more than 24 hours or lead to death. A transient ischaemic attack is essentially the same thing as a stroke, with the exception of the duration of symptoms, which last less than 24 hours and are not caused by a haemorrhage (Ginsberg, 2004). Stroke is the third most common cause of death in England; around 110,000 strokes occur in England every year, a quarter of them in people under 65 years of age (NAO, 2005).

Anatomy and Physiology

The brain cannot store oxygen or glucose and so is dependent on a constant supply of blood, which is provided by two pairs of vessels – the vertebral and internal carotid arteries (Figure 14.7). These arteries are interconnected in the cranial cavity to produce an arterial circle (the circle of Willis), which provides an alternative pathway for blood flow should one of the vessels become occluded (Drake, 2005).

Risk Factors

Non-modifiable risk factors for stroke include age, sex, race and family or previous medical history of stroke, transient ischaemic attacks or myocardial infarction. The chance of having a stroke roughly doubles each decade after the age of 55 years,

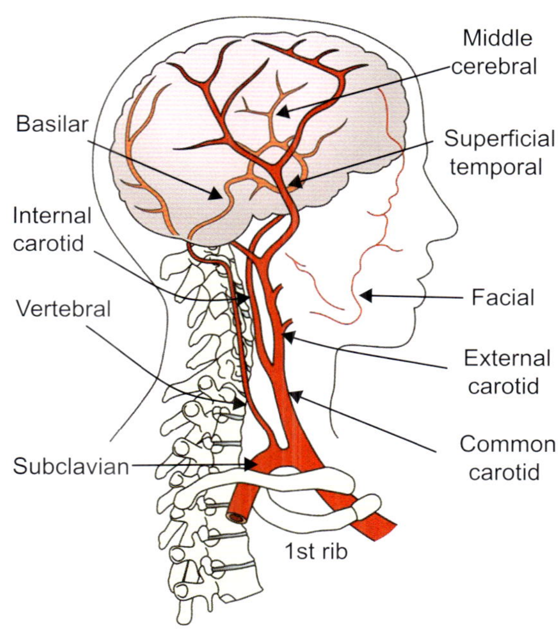

Figure 14.7 *Arteries supplying the brain. Note all arteries shown are right-sided except the basilar artery.*

and although it is more common in men, over half of all stroke deaths occur in women. People of South Asian, African or Afro-Caribbean origin are more likely to suffer from a stroke (O'Donnell, 2010). Modifiable risk factors include hypertension, smoking, atrial fibrillation, diabetes, diet, physical activity, alcohol consumption, blood cholesterol and obesity (Rodgers, 2004).

Types of Stroke

Strokes can be classified as either ischaemic or vascular in origin. Ischaemic strokes are the most common and are caused by atherosclerosis or an embolus from the heart, for example. They are responsible for around 80% of all new strokes (O'Donnell, 2010; EROS, 2009). Less common are strokes of vascular origin, caused by haemorrhage. Time is critical for the brain, and with each passing minute 1.9 million neurons, 14 billion synapses and 12 km (7.5 miles) of myelinated fibres are destroyed. This equates to the premature 'ageing' of the brain to the tune of 3.6 years for each hour without reperfusion treatment (Saver, 2006).

Assessment and Management of Stroke

- Assess ABCDE as for all patients.
- Determining the time of onset in stroke is very important for subsequent treatment. Find out when the patient was last free of stroke-like symptoms.
- Oxygen is not recommended unless the patient is hypoxic.
- Record a blood sugar if trained to do so; hypoglycaemia is a common stroke mimic.

Meningococcal Disease

Meningococcal disease is an umbrella term for a systemic bacterial infection caused by *Neisseria meningitidis* (meningococcus). It presents as meningitis (inflammation of the meninges), septicaemia or a combination of both (PHE, 2014).

Although uncommon, of those affected around 10% will die (increasing to 50% in patients with septicaemia without meningitis), and over 10% of those who survive will suffer long-term effects, such as convulsions. It is most common in children under 4 years of age, with a smaller peak in incidence in teenagers aged 15–19 years (PHE, 2017).

Pathophysiology

Meningococci inhabit the nasopharynx in around 10% of the population, although it is less common in infants (under 5%) and most common in 19-year-olds (over 23%). If the meningococci manage to penetrate the protective mucosa of the nasal passages and enter the bloodstream they rapidly multiply, doubling in number every 30 minutes.

In some people, meningococci cross the blood–brain barrier, where the bacteria are free to multiply inside the cerebrospinal fluid. This leads to inflammation and swelling in the meninges and brain tissue, raising intracranial pressure, which can result in nervous system damage and even death. Surprisingly, patients with meningococcal meningitis do better than those who go on to develop septicaemia. This is thought to be because the body's immune response has prevented the bacteria from causing an overwhelming sepsis (Ninis, 2010).

Signs and Symptoms

A major issue in the recognition of meningococcal disease is the non-specific nature of the signs and symptoms in the initial stages of the disease. These include (NICE, 2010b):

- fever
- nausea/vomiting
- lethargy
- irritable/unsettled
- ill appearance
- refusing food/drink
- headache
- muscle ache/joint pain
- respiratory signs and symptoms.

However, the diagnosis window is short. Many children will have non-specific signs and symptoms in the first 4–6 hours, but can be close to death after 24 hours (Thompson, 2006a).

Sepsis and Shock

The first specific clinical signs to appear are likely to be those of sepsis (covered in Chapter 16: Medical Emergencies) and shock and include leg pain, abnormal skin colour, cold hands and feet and, in older children, thirst. Parents of younger children may also report drowsiness and difficulty in breathing (described as rapid or laboured) (Thompson, 2006a). Don't forget to enquire about how much urine a child has been passing or if they have had a wet nappy recently. Oliguria (low output of urine) is an early sign of shock (Ninis, 2010).

Fever

Many children with septicaemia will become acutely ill with a fever. This can be complicated by a trivial viral illness that precedes this, but look for a sudden change in the history. Remember that not all children with meningococcal disease have fever, and you should not dismiss a fever responsive to anti-pyretics (such as paracetamol and ibuprofen) as of viral origin (Ninis, 2010). Rather counter-intuitively, infants can actually develop hypothermia in sepsis (Wells, 2001).

Rash

The classic sign is a petechial non-blanching rash (Figure 14.8). However, only 10% of children presenting with the rash will have meningococcal disease. The remainder will have a viral infection. On the other hand, febrile and ill children with a purpuric rash (a non-blanching rash of greater than 2 mm in diameter) are very likely to have meningococcal disease (Wells, 2001). Care needs to be taken with blanching rashes, such as a maculopapular rash, as up to 30% of children may initially present with this, although careful examination will generally yield some non-blanching elements (Figure 14.9) (Hart, 2006). On dark skin, you may have to check the soles of the feet, palms of the hand, abdomen or conjunctivae and palate. You must fully undress the child and be thorough in your search. Petechial rashes may not be widespread initially and can be easily missed.

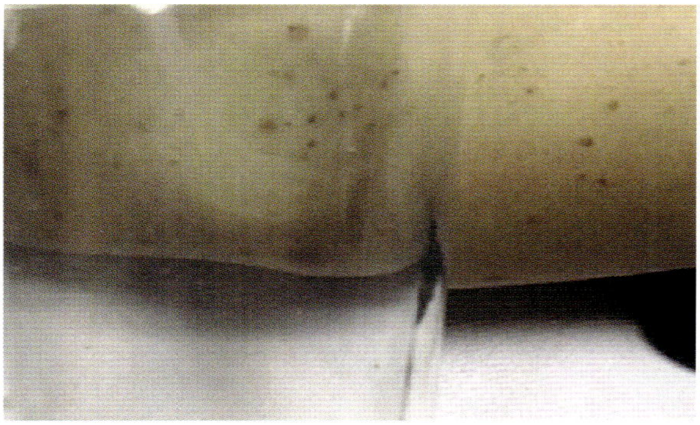

Figure 14.8 *Petechial non-blanching rash. Note how this does not blanch under the pressure of a glass.*
Courtesy of the Meningitis Research Foundation, www.meningitis.org.

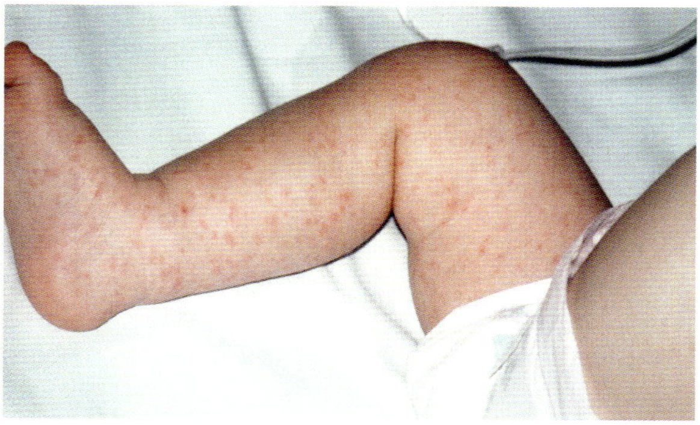

Figure 14.9 *Maculopapular rash with scanty petechiae.*
Courtesy of the Meningitis Research Foundation, www.meningitis.org.

Management

Patients with meningococcal disease need to be transported to hospital as soon as possible (JRCALC, 2016). While you wait for an ambulance you should:

- Ensure a patent airway.
- Administer high levels of oxygen to all patients via a non-rebreathe mask.
- Assist ventilations if necessary.

Paralysis

In medical terminology, paralysis is typically represented by the suffix *-plegia*. This is not to be confused with paresis, which is used to refer to muscle weakness, or incomplete loss of muscle function (Porth, 2003). Four common terms that you will hear used are (Macleod, 2005):

- **Monoplegia**: Paralysis in a single limb.
- **Hemiplegia**: Paralysis of both limbs on the same side of the body.
- **Quadriplegia** (also tetraplegia): Paralysis of all four limbs.
- **Paraplegia**: Paralysis of both the lower limbs.

Coma

Coma is the absence of consciousness (i.e. unconscious) and is often referred to as a loss of consciousness (LOC). This presents as a completely unaware patient, unresponsive to external stimuli, with only eye opening to pain and no eye tracking or fixation, and limb withdrawal to a noxious stimulus (usually pain) at best (often with reflex motor movements) (Wijdicks, 2010).

Full consciousness is an awake state in which one is aware of oneself and the environment, including the ability to perceive and interpret stimuli and to interact and communicate with others in the absence of motor deficits (Young GB, 2018).

Common causes of coma include:

- stroke – ischaemic and haemorrhagic
- cardiac arrest
- alcohol abuse
- substance abuse and overdose
- carbon monoxide poisoning
- sepsis
- bacterial meningitis
- syncope (faint)
- convulsions
- traumatic brain injury
- hyper-/hypoglycaemia.

Uncommon causes of coma include:

- subarachnoid haemorrhage
- brain abscess or tumour
- burns
- hypo-/hyperthermia.

It may not always be possible to determine the cause of coma and the management of the patient may just be supportive. However, for reversible causes, such as hypoglycaemia, convulsions and overdose, it is important to recognise these conditions as the patient can then receive the appropriate treatment out-of-hospital (JRCALC, 2016).

Chapter 15

Exposure/ Environment

Extremes of Temperature

Learning Objectives

By the end of this section you will be able to:

- State the normal temperature range for an adult.
- Explain the terms 'hypothermia' and 'heat-related illness'.
- Describe the appropriate management for a patient with signs of hypothermia and heat-related illness.

Introduction

Despite being exposed to a wide range of environmental temperatures, the human body maintains a stable temperature of around 37°C which is maintained in the range 35.8–38.2°C. Normal fluctuations of about 1°C occur over a 24-hour period, with highest temperatures recorded in the afternoon and early evening, and lowest temperatures in early morning (Marieb, 2013).

Thermoregulation is primarily the job of the hypothalamus, which receives sensory information from peripheral and central thermoreceptors. This is necessary because the different body regions have differing temperatures (Tortora, 2008):

- **Core**: Consisting of organs within the skull, thorax and abdomen.
- **Shell**: The skin.

By controlling the flow of blood to the shell, the hypothalamus can control the amount of heat generated and lost.

Heat-Promoting Mechanisms

When the external temperature falls, the heat-promoting centre is activated. This maintains core body temperature by (Marieb, 2013):

- constricting peripheral cutaneous blood vessels
- causing shivering – involuntary contractions of skeletal muscle, which generate heat
- increasing the body's metabolic rate.

In addition, there are a number of behavioural changes that can be promoted, such as:

- putting on warmer clothes
- drinking hot fluids
- increasing physical activity.

Heat-Loss Mechanisms

Most heat loss occurs via the skin by dilation of cutaneous blood vessels and/or enhanced sweating, allowing for heat loss to occur by (Marieb, 2013):

- **Radiation**: Infrared waves (thermal energy).
- **Conduction**: Direct contact with cooler objects (such as cold water).
- **Convection**: Since warm air expands and rises, warm air around the body is constantly replaced with cooler air, which absorbs the heat. This process can be enhanced by moving air more rapidly across the body surface, for example by the use of a fan.
- **Evaporation**: As water absorbs heat from the body, it becomes energetic enough to escape the body as a gas, called water vapour.

Assessment of Temperature

There are a range of different thermometers on the market and you may need to use a different type of thermometer depending on the age of the patient, as shown in Table 15.1 (JRCALC, 2016; NICE, 2013a). Common types include electronic thermometers (Figure 15.1) and tympanic thermometers (Figure 15.2).

Out-of-hospital, a peripheral temperature is gained to provide an estimation of what the temperature is in the core of the patient.

Table 15.1 Thermometers according to age

Age	Thermometer
Infants under 4 weeks of age	• Electronic thermometer in axilla
4 weeks to 5 years of age	• Paediatric infra-red tympanic thermometer
	• Electronic thermometer in axilla
	• Chemical dot thermometer in axilla
Over 5 years	• Infra-red tympanic thermometer
	• Electronic thermometer in axilla

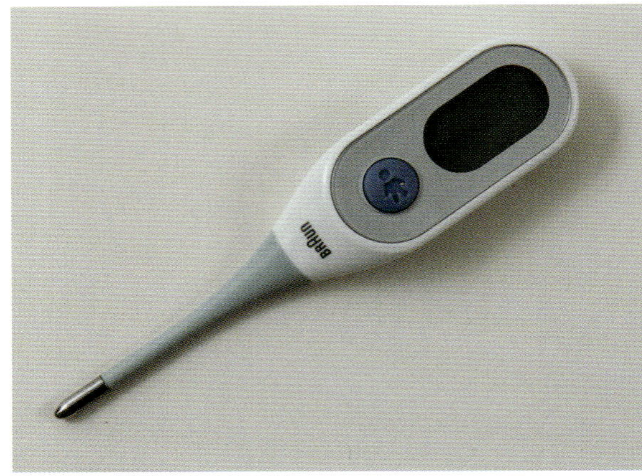

Figure 15.1 *Electronic thermometer.*

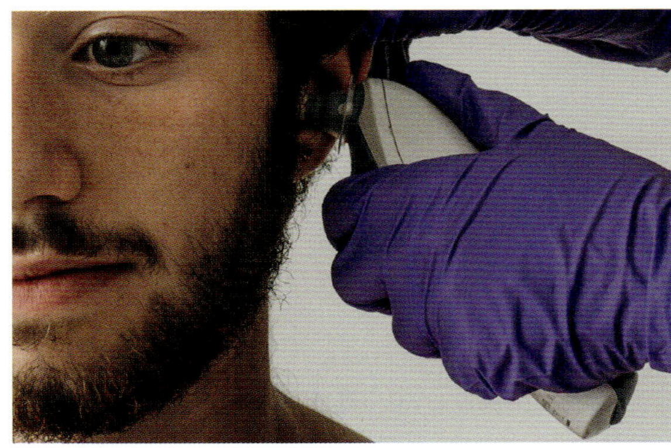

Figure 15.2 *Tympanic thermometer.*

Temperature readings are broadly accurate, but they can be impacted by factors including:

- build-up of ear wax
- lying on one side for a prolonged period
- wearing ear defenders or muffs prior to temperature being taken
- standing outside for a prolonged period
- water or snow in the ear.

When taking a series of temperature measurements, always use the same site and procedure to try and improve accuracy. For example, if you are using the tympanic thermometer and you take the first reading from the right ear, you should use the right ear for all further temperature assessments.

Procedure – Electronic Thermometer in Axilla

1. Turn on the thermometer, check it is clean and functional and apply a fresh cover to the probe.

Once you have turned it on, the thermometer will be able to perform any self-checks.

2. Place the tip of the thermometer high in the axilla, in the fold where the arm meets the chest. Get the infant to bring their arm down to the side so the thermometer is covered.
3. Leave in place until the thermometer has finished measuring. Usually there will be a visual or audible indication that this has happened.
4. Remove and read the temperature.

Procedure – Infra-Red Tympanic Thermometer

The below is a general description on how to use an infra-red tympanic thermometer. You may need to vary this procedure based on different models available.

1. Turn on the thermometer, check it is clean and functional and apply a fresh cover to the probe. Once you have turned it on, the thermometer will be able to perform any self-checks.
2. The thermometer works by taking an infra-red reading of temperature directly from the tympanic membrane. As the ear canals are not straight, you should first try to just straighten the canal slightly.
   a. For children under one, gently pull the pinna of the ear directly backwards.
   b. For children over one and adults, pull the ear gently upwards and backwards.
3. Place the probe into the ear. It should be placed straight down in the canal so the tip of the device is facing the tympanic membrane. At this point some devices will pre-warm the tip of the measuring probe to help ensure the results are accurate. They will emit a beep and the screen display will change when they are ready to use.
4. Push the button that measures temperature and hold the probe still until it has completed; this can take a few seconds.
5. Remove from the ear and read the temperature.

Hypothermia

Hypothermia is defined as a core body temperature of less than 35°C. It is classified into three categories, based on temperature (JRCALC, 2016):

- **Mild**: 32–35°C.
- **Moderate**: 28–32°C.
- **Severe**: Less than 28°C.

However, without a low-reading thermometer, it can be difficult to record accurate core body temperature. Therefore, it is important to suspect that hypothermia might be a factor in the following cases (JRCALC, 2016):

- older patients (over 80 years of age)
- children
- some medical conditions, for example, hypothyroidism and stroke
- intoxicated patients (alcohol and/or recreational drugs)
- drowning
- patients suffering from exhaustion
- injured and immobile patients
- decreased level of consciousness.

As patients succumb to hypothermia, they move through five stages (Durrer, 2003):

1. conscious and shivering
2. decreased level of consciousness and not shivering
3. unconscious
4. not breathing
5. death due to irreversible hypothermia.

Management

The mainstay of treatment is to prevent further heat loss (Figure 15.3). In the mildly hypothermic patient, this is likely to be enough, but severely hypothermic patients will require active rewarming, which realistically can only be performed in hospital (Nolan, 2012). Adopt the following principles when managing a patient with hypothermia (JRCALC, 2016):

- Administer oxygen if the patient is hypoxaemic.
- If using a foil blanket, ensure that you wrap the patient in a fabric blanket first and place the foil blanket over the top.
- Give the patient hot drinks/food if they are conscious, but NOT alcohol.
- Do not rub the patient's skin: as with alcohol, this leads to peripheral vasodilation, which worsens hypothermia.
- Avoid rough handling as it can cause arrhythmias and cardiac arrest.
- Patients with a decreased level of consciousness should not be encouraged to walk, but managed horizontally.

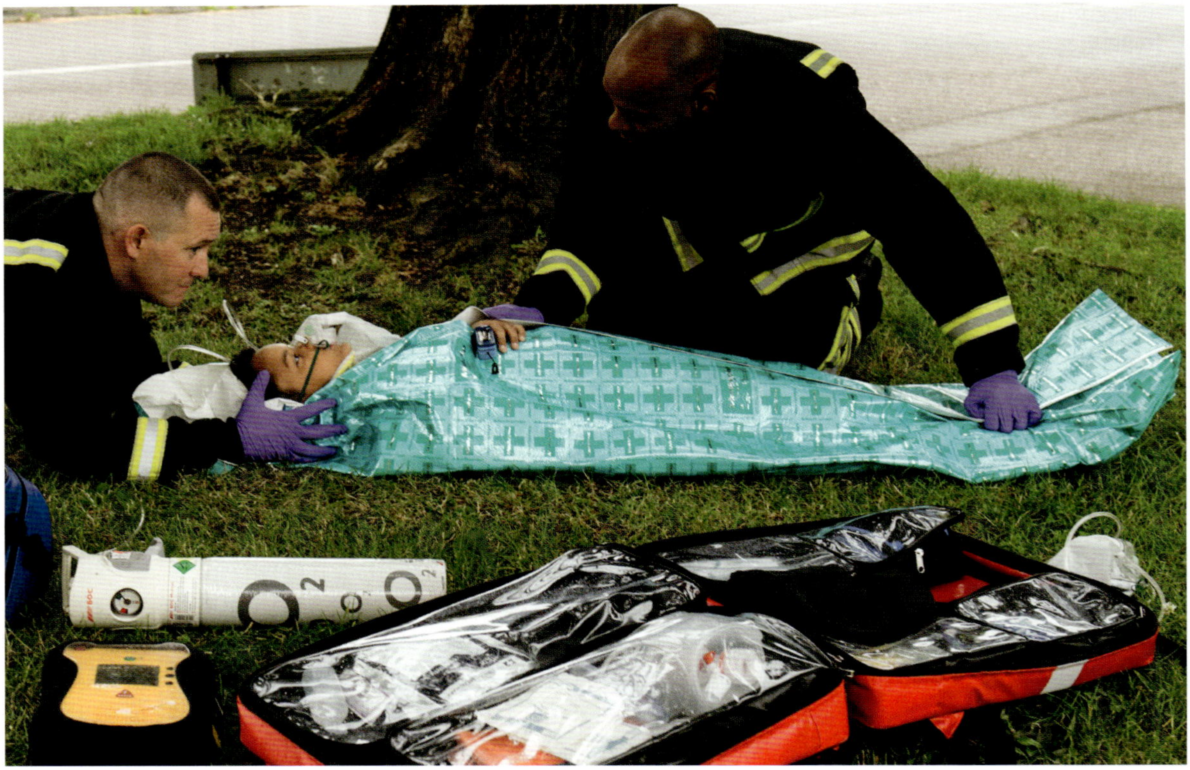

Figure 15.3 *Prevent further heat loss in hypothermic patients.*

Heat-Related Illness

Heat-related illnesses can occur as a result of external factors such as the sun, or internal factors such as drugs and exercise. It presents on a continuum, with heat stress the least serious heat-related illness, through to multi-organ dysfunction and even death at the other extreme (JRCALC, 2016):

- heat stress
- heat exhaustion
- heat stroke
- multi-organ dysfunction.

Heat Stress

This is a mild form of heat-related illness and is characterised by (Truhlar, 2015):

- normal temperature or mild temperature elevation
- heat oedema – swelling of feet and ankles
- heat syncope – vasodilation causes hypotension
- heat cramps – depletion of salts leads to muscle cramps.

Heat Exhaustion

This is a more severe form of heat-related illness, with symptoms mostly as a result of fluid loss and electrolyte imbalances (Truhlar, 2015):

- systemic reaction to prolonged heat exposure (hours to days)
- core body temperature over 37°C and less than 40°C
- headache, dizziness, nausea and vomiting, tachycardia, hypotension, sweating, muscle pain, weakness and cramps
- can progress quickly to heat stroke.

Heat Stroke

Heat stroke is a systemic inflammatory response to a core body temperature of 40°C or higher, and is associated with altered level of consciousness and organ dysfunction (Truhlar, 2015). It comes in two types: non-exertional heat stroke, which is caused by high external temperatures and/or high humidity; and exertional heat stroke, which is caused by excess heat production. Non-exertional heat stroke tends to occur in the elderly, very young and chronically ill, whereas exertional heat stroke is more typical in active groups such as athletes, manual workers and military recruits (JRCALC, 2016).

Clinical features include (Truhlar, 2015):

- core body temperature of 40°C or more
- hot dry skin (although sweating is present in around half of all cases)
- early signs and symptoms: extreme fatigue, headache, fainting, facial flushing, vomiting and diarrhoea
- arrhythmias and hypotension
- respiratory distress
- liver and kidney failure.

Management

Heat Stress and Exhaustion

The management of patients with heat-related illness broadly consists of cooling the patient and replacing lost fluid and electrolytes. For patients with signs and symptoms of heat stress consider the following (Lipman, 2013):

- Remove the patient from the heat source.
- Passively cool: Move the patient into the shade or an air-conditioned room. Loosen or remove tight-fitting clothing.
- Provide oral isotonic fluid replacement.
- Elevate oedematous extremities.

If the patient has developed heat exhaustion, similar management principles apply, except that depending on the patient's level of consciousness, fluid rehydration may have to be intravenous. In addition, cooling should be active, using conductive, evaporative and convective methods. Cold-water immersion is ideal for the ambulant, co-operative patient, but may not be practical otherwise. Alternatives include removing the patient's clothes and spraying or dousing the patient with water. Air movement can be augmented by fanning the patient (Lipman, 2013).

Heat Stroke

While supporting the patient's airway, breathing, circulation and disability, begin rapidly cooling the patient (Truhlar, 2015). Ice water immersion is useful, but not practical, so consider the same techniques as for heat exhaustion to cool the patient. Ice packs are useful if they cover the body, not just the neck, axillae and groin, but should not be applied directly to the skin (Lipman, 2013). Rehydration is safest intravenously as an altered level of consciousness increases the chance of aspiration (Soar, 2010).

Drowning

Learning Objective

By the end of this section you will be able to:

- Explain the pathophysiology and management of drowning.

Introduction

The definition of drowning has been complicated in the past and so in 2002 (at the World Congress on Drowning, held in Amsterdam) a single definition was agreed. As a result, drowning is now defined as a process resulting in primary respiratory impairment from submersion/immersion in a liquid (Idris, 2003). Whether the victim lives or dies after this process is irrelevant, they have still drowned. If they do not survive, then they have fatally drowned (Szpilman, 2012).

Pathophysiology

When a drowning victim is unable to keep water (the most common liquid in drowning incidents) from their mouth, it is spat out or swallowed. If still conscious, victims will then attempt to hold their breath, but this is likely to continue for less than a minute, depending on levels of panic and the temperature of the water. Once the inspiratory drive is too high to resist, the victim will take a breath and water will be aspirated into the airways (Szpilman, 2012). Laryngospasm may occur, but this is rapidly terminated by cerebral hypoxia, and active ventilation, with aspiration of water, will resume. It was once thought that laryngospasm might be responsible for suspected victims of drowning who were found not to have aspirated (so called dry-drowning). The theory was that the victim died due to hypoxic cardiac arrest because of laryngospasm or breath holding (Layon, 2009). However, autopsy studies have concluded that this is unlikely, as water does not passively seep into the lungs (Modell, 1999; Piette, 2006). To drown therefore requires active ventilation while the victim is submerged (i.e. under the water and still alive).

Whether due to laryngospasm or breath holding, with no gas exchange the victim becomes increasingly hypoxaemic, hypercarbic and acidotic. Unless they are rescued, the victim will succumb to hypoxaemia, leading to loss of consciousness and apnoea (Layon, 2009). The cardiac rhythm deteriorates, usually following a sequence of tachyarrhythmias, bradyarrhythmias, pulseless electrical activity (PEA) and asystole (Szpilman, 2012).

Immersion in cold water produces large and rapid reductions in skin temperature, which in turn leads to cold shock. This term refers to a collection of physiological responses, including an inspiratory gasp (which can result in drowning if the victim's airway is submerged), hyperventilation, hypocapnia, tachycardia, peripheral vasoconstriction and hypertension (Datta, 2006). Cold shock is thought to be caused by stimulation of cutaneous cold thermoreceptors, which results in an excessive sympathetic nervous system response. The magnitude of the cold shock response is reduced by the victim's clothing, their habituation to cold (regular winter swimming in just Speedos, for example) and orientation on immersion (Shattock, 2012).

If the victim's face is submerged in cold water, the diving response may be activated. This is caused by cooling of the cold thermoreceptors on the face, which are innervated by the trigeminal nerve. This results in a profound sinus bradycardia due to parasympathetic nervous system stimulation of the heart, an expiratory apnoea due to inhibition of central respiratory neurons, and sympathetic nervous system-mediated vasoconstriction of the trunk and limbs. A similar response is also possible by stimulation of vagal receptors in the pharynx and larynx (Angell-James, 1975).

It has been suggested that simultaneous stimulation of both sympathetic and parasympathetic pathways of the autonomic nervous system results in an 'autonomic conflict', leading to life-threatening arrhythmias that may result in death in susceptible individuals (Figure 15.4) (Shattock, 2012).

Although the tonicity of the water (for example sea water versus fresh water) was once thought to be important, the effect on the lungs is ultimately the same, although with a different osmotic gradient. The fragile alveolar-capillary membranes are disrupted, leading to increased permeability and movement of fluid, plasma and electrolytes (Orlowski, 1989). Clinically, this leads to significant amounts of blood-stained pulmonary oedema and decreasing gaseous exchange of oxygen and carbon dioxide. Following drowning, the presence of additional fluid in the lungs and the loss of surfactant lead to increasing areas of the lungs becoming regions of low, or no, ventilation and perfusion (pulmonary shunting), and there is widespread atelectasis and bronchospasm (Layon, 2009). Similarly, the haemodynamic and cardiovascular effects seen in drowning are not related to tonicity either, but primarily are a consequence of anoxia (Orlowski, 1989).

Management

The Fire and Rescue Service have specifically trained Swift water rescue technicians with specialised training and equipment to carry out water rescue (Figure 15.5).

Once the victim is out of the water and in a place of safety, place them supine (on their back), with head and torso at the same level, and check for breathing. If they are breathing but unconscious, provide high-flow oxygen via a non-rebreathe mask as per clinical guidelines and place them in the recovery position. They are at high risk of gastric regurgitation, so ensure that you have suction available (JRCALC, 2016).

Victims of prolonged immersion in water (typically 30 minutes or more, but less as water temperature decreases) may also suffer the added complication of circum-rescue collapse (Golden, 1997). This is due to the increased hydrostatic pressure from

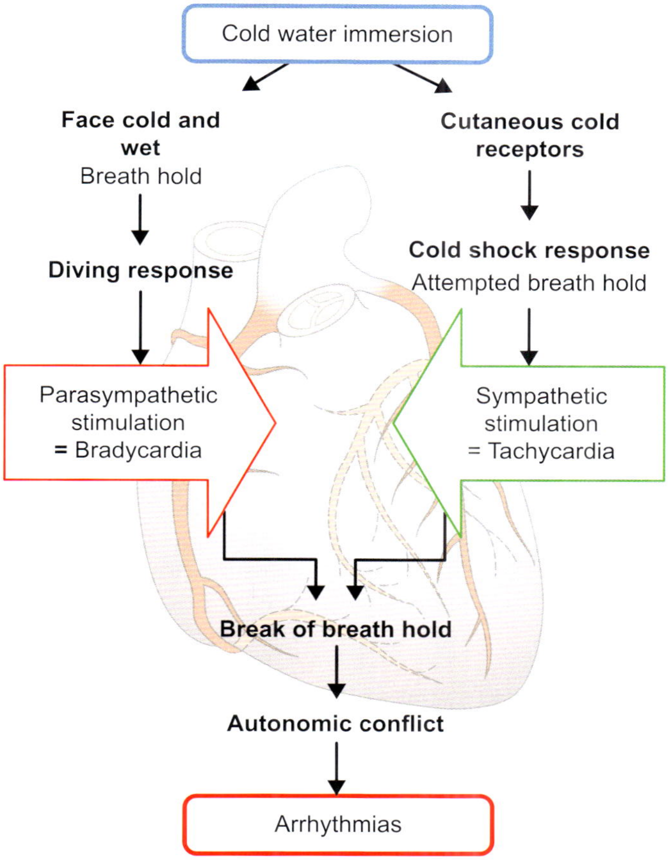

Figure 15.4 *Autonomic conflict.*

the water on the victim's legs and torso increasing venous return and cardiac output. Central baroreceptors mistake this for hypervolaemia resulting in increased diuresis. In addition, peripheral vasoconstriction will occur, as the water is cold relative to the body, which magnifies this response (Lord, 2005). Once the victim is removed from the water, the hydrostatic pressure is lost, exacerbating the hypovolaemia. This can also be compounded by hypothermia and physical effort (if the victim attempts to remove him- or herself from the water, for example). The sudden drop in venous return can reduce coronary perfusion enough to induce cardiac arrest. For this reason, it is advised to remove victims horizontally from the water if possible (Szpilman, 2012).

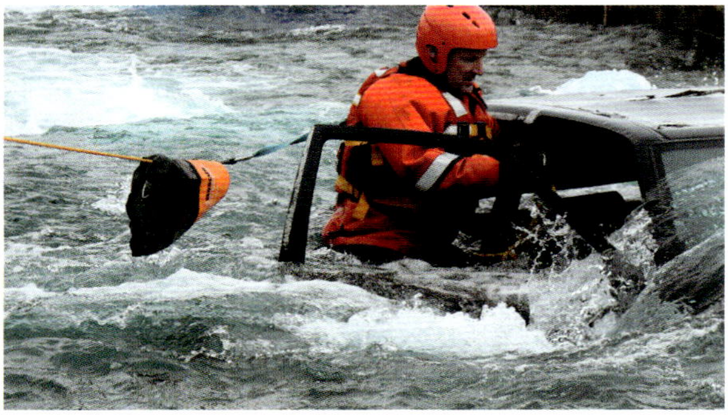

Figure 15.5 *Swift water rescue.*

Hypothermia is likely to occur and wet clothes should be cut off to minimise movement. Hypothermic patients are at risk of cardiac arrhythmias, including ventricular fibrillation, even with minor movement (Althaus, 1982). Get the patient covered with blankets and in a warm environment as soon as possible.

Cardiac Arrest Management

As before, once the patient is out of the water and in a safe location, place them supine (on their back), with head and torso at the same level, and check for breathing. If your patient is not breathing, or is breathing abnormally, administer five rescue breaths via a bag-valve-mask connected to high-flow oxygen. Note that this is different from the usual ABC approach that the current resuscitation guidelines advocate for adults, but reflects that correction of hypoxia is the most important aspect in the management of the drowned patient (see Chapter 18: Cardiac Arrest). It can be difficult to differentiate post-arrest gasping from initial respiratory efforts of the drowning patient, so if you are unsure, administer ventilations and start CPR. Pulse checks are unreliable, so if in doubt, commence chest compressions with ventilations at a ratio of 30:2. Compression-only CPR is not advocated (Truhlar, 2015).

Large amounts of foam can be generated by the mixing of moving air with water and surfactant from the lungs. If this occurs, do not waste time trying to suction it: continue to provide ventilations until an appropriate clinician can intubate the patient.

Note that the incidence of spinal injuries is very low (around 0.5%) and immobilising the spine delays effective resuscitation, so only immobilise the spine when there is a clear mechanism of injury that could cause spinal injury (such as diving into shallow water or water skiing) (Watson, 2001; Truhlar, 2015).

Resuscitation efforts should not be stopped unless it is clear that it would be futile to continue (see Chapter 18: Cardiac Arrest). There are no completely accurate prognostic indicators in drowning, although duration of submersion is correlated with risk of death or severe neurological impairment (Szpilman, 2012). In water above 6°C, survival after submersion for more than 30 minutes is unlikely. At 6°C or below, survival time can be extended up to 90 minutes, although this is more likely to apply to children and petite women immersed in ice-cold water (Tipton, 2011). As with hypothermia, the general rule is that your patient is not dead until they are warm and dead (Truhlar, 2015).

Chapter 16

Medical Emergencies

Anaphylaxis

Learning Objectives

By the end of this section you will be able to:

- Explain the term anaphylaxis and its common causes.
- Describe signs and symptoms with which a patient with anaphylaxis may present.
- State the management of anaphylaxis, including the administration of adrenaline using the patient's own auto-injector.

Introduction

Anaphylaxis is a serious allergic reaction that is rapid in onset and may cause death (Sampson, 2006). Its hallmark is rapidly developing, life-threatening airway/breathing/circulation (or any combination of the three) problem(s), and it is usually associated with skin and mucosal changes (Soar, 2008).

The exact incidence of anaphylaxis is unknown, as many episodes are not reported, but it is thought that around 1 in 1,333 of the population has an anaphylactic reaction at some point in their lives (Soar, 2008). Approximately 3,000 people a year are admitted to hospital in England with anaphylaxis, and it is estimated that there are 10–20 deaths per year in England and Wales (DoH, 2006b).

The most common causes (triggers) are food, medication and insect stings (Lee, 2011). In children, food is the most common cause of allergy, whereas in adults, it is medication (Capps, 2010). Death is unlikely more than 6 hours after exposure to a trigger, but cardiac arrest can occur in minutes, particularly if the trigger is medication that has been administered intravenously. Envenomation typically causes cardiac arrest within 15 minutes, and food takes a little longer on average, at around 30 minutes (Pumphrey, 2000).

Signs and Symptoms

Anaphylaxis is highly likely when any one of the following criteria is fulfilled (Sampson, 2006):

1. Acute onset of an illness (minutes to several hours) with involvement of the skin and/or mucosal tissue (e.g. generalised urticaria or flushing, and swollen lips/tongue/uvula, also known as angioedema) and at least one of the following:
   - respiratory compromise (e.g. difficulty breathing, wheeze, stridor)
   - reduced blood pressure or associated symptoms of end-organ dysfunction (e.g. collapse).
2. Two or more of the following that occur rapidly after exposure to a likely allergen for that patient (minutes to several hours):
   - involvement of the skin/mucosal tissue
   - respiratory compromise

  - o reduced blood pressure (BP) or associated symptoms
  - o persistent gastrointestinal symptoms (e.g. crampy abdominal pain, nausea, vomiting, diarrhoea).
3. Rapid onset of reduced BP after exposure to a known allergen for that patient (minutes to several hours):
  - o infants and children: low systolic BP
  - o adults: systolic BP of less than 90 mmHg.

Note: Up to 20% of anaphylaxis cases do not have skin and/or mucosal changes, particularly reactions that occur intraoperatively in adults and food/insect sting-induced reactions in children. Patients with severe anaphylaxis resulting in significant hypotension may not exhibit any cutaneous symptoms until their blood pressure is restored (Lee, 2011).

Management

Having conducted your standard ABCDE assessment and determined that your patient is likely to be suffering from anaphylaxis, you should identify the trigger and remove it if possible (e.g. remove bee stings). However, if this is not possible, then do not delay treatment. If you suspect food-induced anaphylaxis, encouraging the patient to vomit is **not** recommended (Soar, 2008).

Lie patient flat where possible with legs raised. Note that patients with A or B problems are likely to be more comfortable sitting up, but do not allow patients to sit or stand if they feel faint, as this can cause cardiac arrest.

If authorised to do so, give intramuscular (IM) adrenaline immediately to prevent cardiorespiratory arrest (JRCALC, 2016) via an auto-injector. Where possible, administer adrenaline into the anterolateral thigh as there is a greater margin of safety, it is quick to administer and the peak plasma concentration is higher when adrenaline is administered in the thigh compared to the arm (deltoid) (Simons, 2001). Doses of adrenaline can be repeated every 5 minutes depending on patient condition.

Administer high-flow oxygen at 10–15 l/min initially. If local guidelines allow, consider administering nebulised salbutamol (Figure 16.1) (Truhlar, 2015; JRCALC, 2016).

If you are working with a suitably qualified clinician (paramedic, nurse or doctor), they are likely to obtain IV access and administer fluid and second line treatments, such as antihistamines and steroids. In addition, you may be asked to set up a nebuliser to administer bronchodilators such as salbutamol and ipratropium (JRCALC, 2016).

Note: Adrenaline is also known as epinephrine, particularly in American texts.

Auto-Injectors

Patients who are known to have anaphylactic reactions may have been provided with their own adrenaline auto-injector. Common systems in the UK include Jext® and Epipen® and are typically available as 300 microgram adult and 150 microgram child doses.

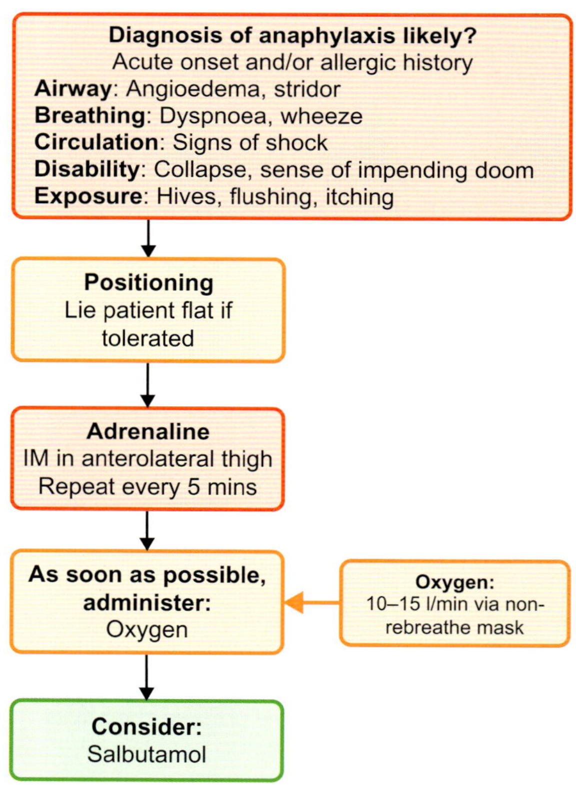

Figure 16.1 *Emergency management of anaphylaxis.*

Procedure for Jext® Auto-Injector

Take the following steps to administer adrenaline with a Jext® auto-injector (ALK-Abello, 2016):

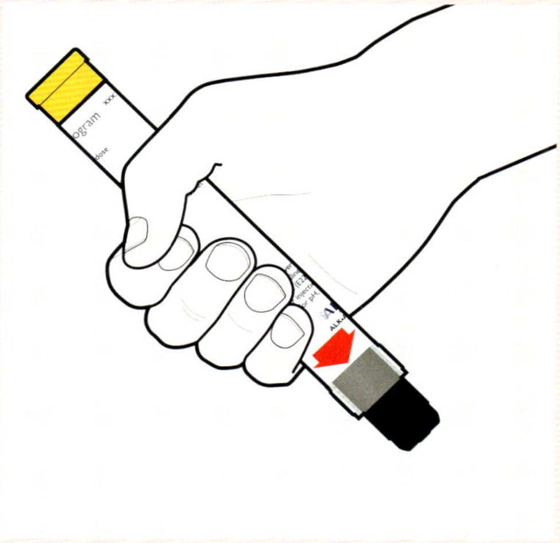

1. Grasp the Jext® injector in your dominant hand (the one you use to write with) with your thumb closest to the yellow cap.

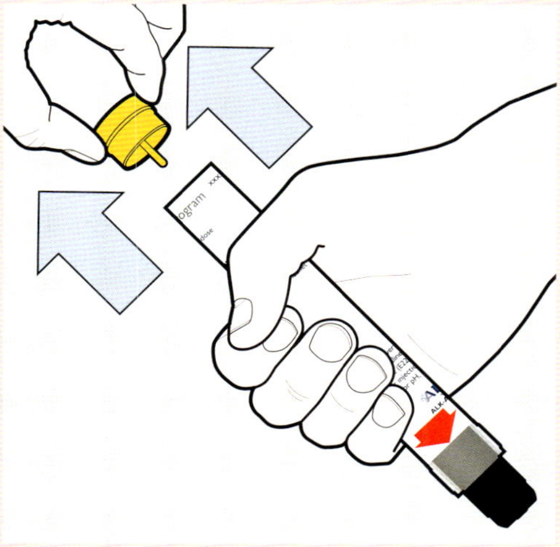

2. Pull off the yellow cap with your other hand.

Procedure – *cont*

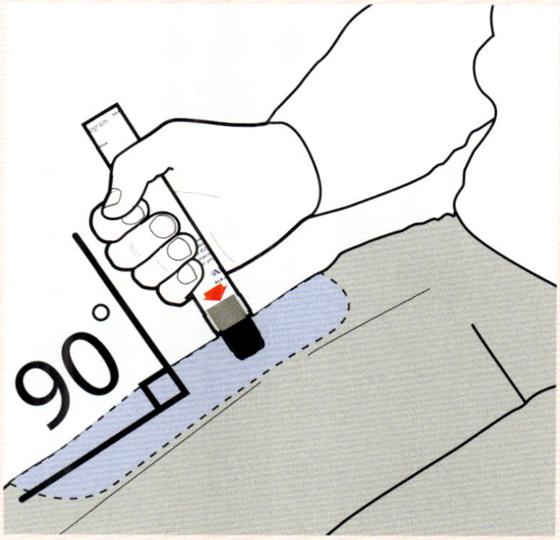

3. Place the black injector tip against your outer thigh, holding the injector at a right angle (approximately 90°) to the thigh.

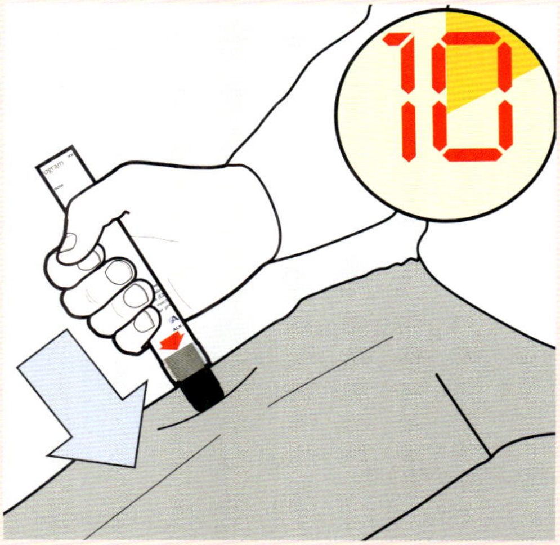

4. Push the black tip firmly into your outer thigh until you hear a 'click' confirming the injection has started, then keep it pushed in. Hold the injector firmly in place against the thigh for 10 seconds (a slow count to 10) then remove. The black tip will extend automatically and hide the needle.

Procedure – *cont*

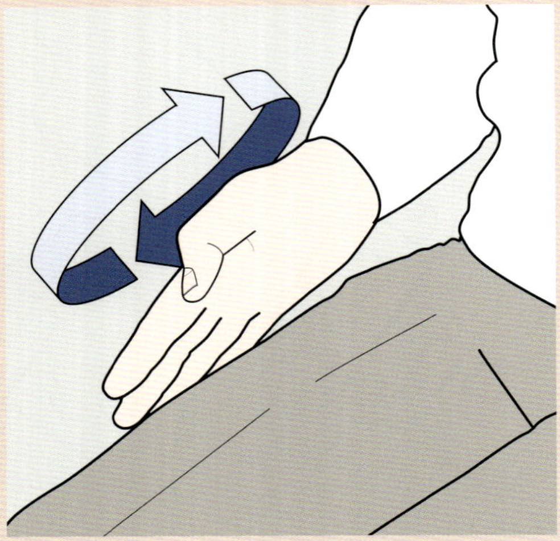

5. Massage the injection area for 10 seconds. Seek immediate medical help.

Sepsis

Learning Objectives

By the end of this section you will be able to:

- Explain what sepsis and red flag sepsis are and how they occur.
- State how you would recognise a patient with sepsis or red flag sepsis.
- Describe the out-of-hospital management of sepsis.

Introduction

Sepsis is a life-threatening condition that arises when the body's response to an infection injures its own tissues and organs. It leads to shock, multiple organ failure and death if not recognised early and treated promptly (Czura, 2011). Sepsis is estimated to cause 36,000–64,000 deaths a year and is responsible for more deaths than lung, bowel and breast cancer (Daniels, 2011a). Around 90% of patients with sepsis in the Emergency Department arrive by ambulance, most commonly presenting with a respiratory tract infection (Gray, 2013; Daniels, 2011b) and 35–40% of these patients will die in hospital (Daniels, 2011a; Vincent, 2006; Levy, 2010).

Recognition and Management

To simplify the identification of sepsis (particularly the more severe form, known as 'Red Flag Sepsis' (UKST, 2016a)), a screening tool has been developed for out-of-hospital use (Figure 16.2) (UKST, 2016b). The tool combines a specific assessment for sepsis and Red Flag Sepsis, with the NEWS score (RCP, 2015).

Sepsis Screening Tool

If the patient has a NEWS score of 3 or more (refer to Chapter 10: Patient Assessment for more information on how to calculate a NEWS score), a clinician believes a patient looks sick, or the patient presents with unexplained illness, they should be screened for sepsis (UKST, 2016a). The tool in Figure 16.2 (UKST, 2016b) is a useful way of screening for sepsis and 'Red Flag Sepsis'. Identifying sepsis early and, even more importantly, ambulance crews stating that they suspect the patient has sepsis reduces patients' time to receive antibiotics and the sepsis care bundle in the ED (Studnek, 2012; Band, 2011).

Sepsis Management

If you believe a patient may be suffering from sepsis then it is urgent that they receive a formal assessment, so you should immediately call for senior clinical support. It is likely that the patient will need to be conveyed to hospital, where blood tests can demonstrate the severity of the illness and, if required, patients can be given antibiotics.

As an emergency medical responder follow the ABCDE approach and administer high-flow oxygen (UKST, 2016b). Be prepared for the patient to deteriorate rapidly and consider that senior clinicians may choose to give other therapies, including intravenous fluids and antibiotics (NICE, 2017), with which they may need your assistance.

Endocrine System Disorders

Learning Objectives

By the end of this section you will be able to:

- Describe the relevant anatomy and physiology of the endocrine system.
- Describe the types and causes of diabetes.

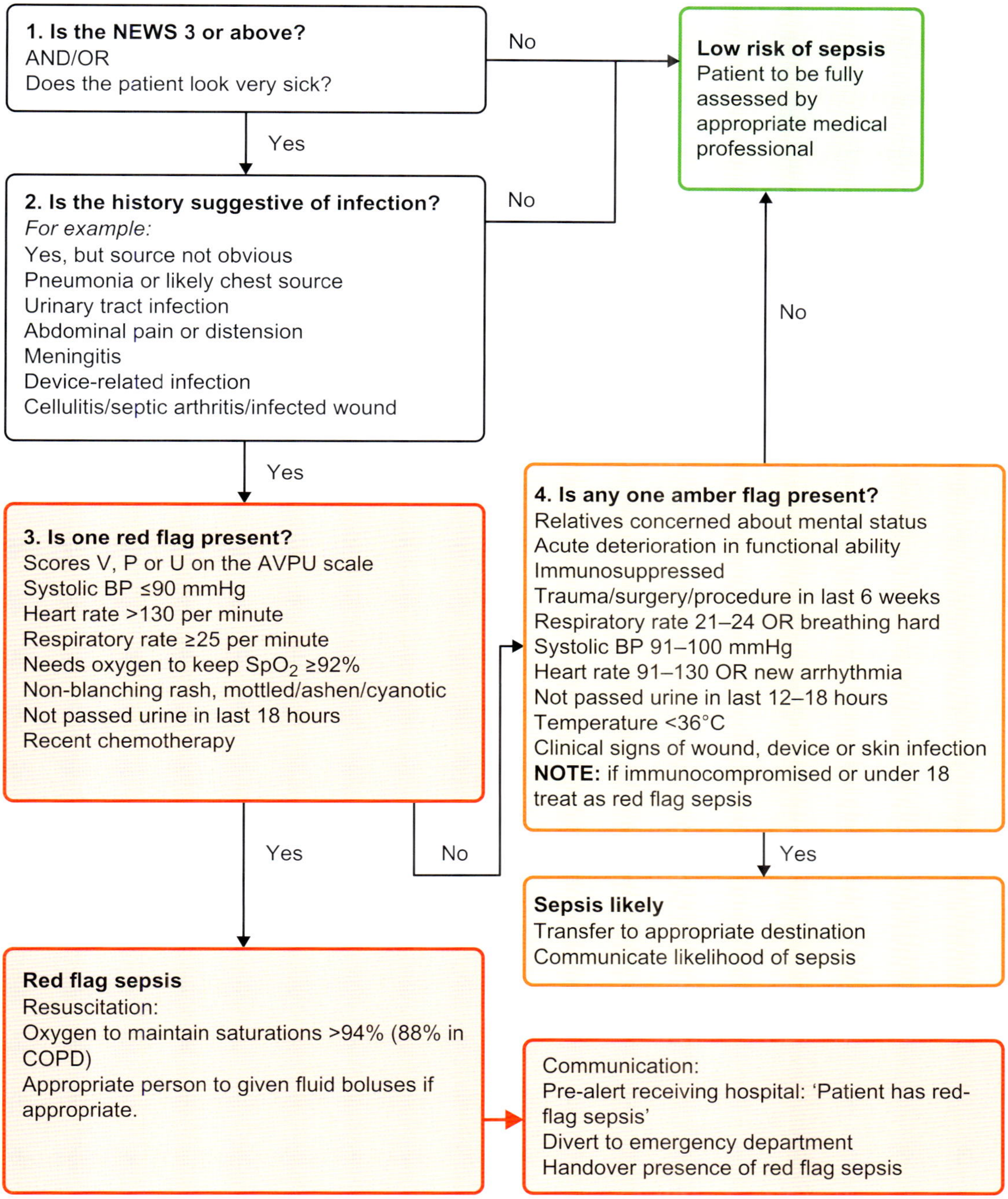

Figure 16.2 *Pre-hospital sepsis screening tool.*

- Describe two diabetic emergencies.
- Explain how to record a blood sugar measurement.

Introduction

The endocrine system consists of a collection of glands located throughout the body (Figure 16.3) that are responsible for the secretion of hormones – molecules that are released from endocrine glands and regulate the activity of cells in other parts of the body. The endocrine system works alongside the nervous system to help co-ordinate the function of all of the body's systems (Tortora, 2008).

The endocrine system consists of the pineal, pituitary, thyroid, parathyroid and adrenal glands. In addition, there are a number of organs and tissues that are not strictly endocrine glands, but do secrete hormones. These include the pancreas, ovaries, testes, liver and heart.

Anatomy and Physiology of the Pancreas

The pancreas is a mixed endocrine and exocrine gland, situated posterior to the stomach, and extends across the posterior abdominal wall from the duodenum on the right to the spleen on the left (Figure 16.4).

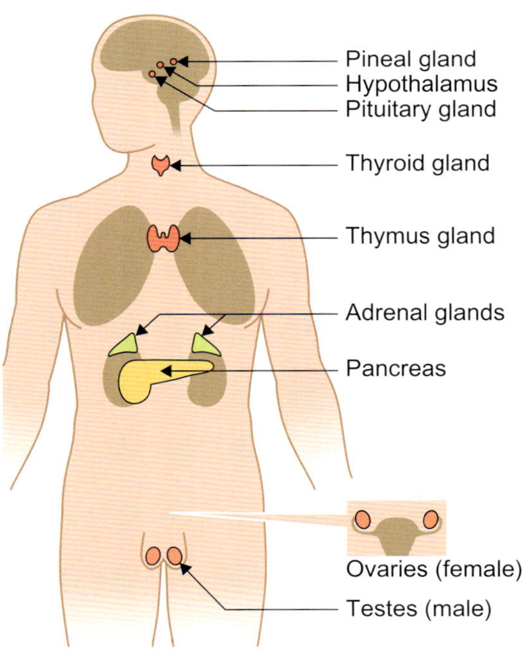

Figure 16.3 *The endocrine system.*

Around 99% of the cells in the pancreas are involved in the production of pancreatic enzymes. There are five main types of cells involved in the production of these enzymes, which have a range of functions, including regulation of blood glucose, however, the main two types of cell are alpha and beta cells (Table 16.1).

Blood Sugar Regulation

Falling blood glucose levels normally activate a series of processes to prevent, or quickly correct, hypoglycaemia (low blood sugar). This is crucial, given that the brain's demand for glucose is fairly constant and the intake of glucose from eating is intermittent. This is accomplished by the dynamic control of glucose by the liver and reduction of glucose consumption by non-neural tissue, such as muscle (Briscoe, 2006).

Hormonal control of blood glucose is largely dependent on the pancreas via the hormones insulin and glucagon. Insulin increases transport of glucose across cell membranes and is released by the pancreas beta cells. (Tortora, 2008). Glucagon targets the liver, promoting conversion of glycogen into glucose and the creation of glucose from lactic and amino acids. This results in increased glucose release by the liver into the blood. Glucagon release is inhibited by insulin and increased by falling blood glucose levels.

Defence against hypoglycaemia (also called glucose counter-regulation) can be broadly classified into physiological and behavioural responses (Briscoe, 2006). As blood glucose falls (although still within 'normal' limits), insulin secretion from the beta cells is reduced, leading to increased glucose production by the liver and virtual cessation of glucose use by tissue sensitive to insulin.

When blood glucose falls below approximately 4 mmol/l, glucagon release is increased from the alpha cells, further increasing glucose production and decreasing insulin release.

If blood glucose continues to fall, the adrenal glands release adrenaline causing a behavioural

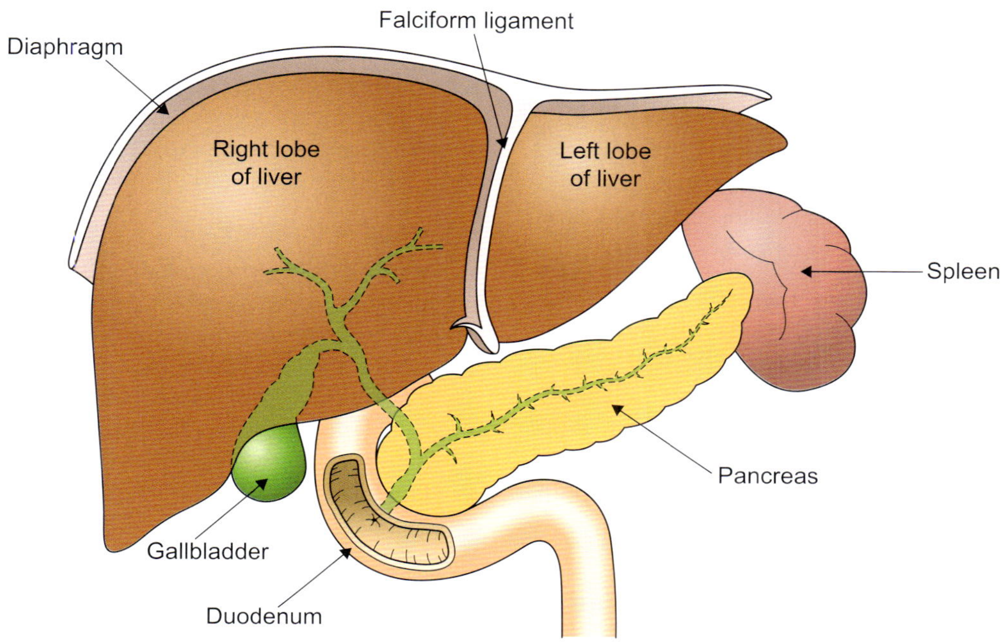

Figure 16.4 *The pancreas.*

response in the form of hunger, as well as other autonomic symptoms, such as palpitation and sweating (Graveling, 2009).

Diabetes

Diabetes mellitus is a common metabolic disorder typified by chronic high blood sugar (hyperglycaemia). It is a major cause of morbidity and premature death due to long-term complications, such as heart attack, stroke, kidney failure and blindness (Holt, 2010). There are around 3.6 million people in the United Kingdom known to have diabetes (Diabetes UK, 2016).

Diabetic Emergencies

Blood sugar is typically maintained within a narrow range of 3.0 to 5.6 mmol/l (JRCALC, 2016).

Table 16.1 Cells of the pancreatic islets

Cell	Hormone	Action
Alpha	Glucagon	Increases blood glucose.
Beta	Insulin	Reduces blood glucose.

When blood glucose becomes significantly outside of that range, diabetic emergencies can occur. There are two main types of diabetic emergency that you will encounter:

- hypoglycaemia
- severe hyperglycaemia.

Types and Causes of Diabetes

There are two types of diabetes (WHO, 1999):

- **Type 1**: Patients with type 1 diabetes are unable to produce any insulin, usually due to autoimmune disease, which destroys the insulin-producing beta cells in the pancreas (Holt, 2010). Insulin is a hormone that increases transport of glucose across cell membranes and is released by the beta cells. It targets the muscle, fat and liver cells to promote the creation of glucose (Tortora, 2008).
- **Type 2**: Patients with type 2 diabetes have a relative insulin deficiency due to varying degrees of insulin resistance. This is by far the most common type of diabetes, accounting for around 90% of all people with diabetes in the UK.

Another way to think about the two forms of diabetes is to imagine the membrane around the outside of cells in the body as locks and insulin as the key that unlocks them and allows glucose into the cells. In type 1 diabetes there isn't enough insulin (the key) to unlock cells, so glucose continues to be transported without making it into the cells and being converted into energy. The main priority of treatment is to replace the insulin, so patients often have injections or syringe pumps of insulin.

In type 2 diabetes diseases there is insulin, but the cell membranes have changed shape so the insulin (acting as the key) no longer fits in the lock and can't open the cell membranes. As type 2 diabetes progresses, the pancreas may also stop producing enough insulin. The priorities of treatment are to try and reduce this resistance to insulin and later to replace insulin if necessary.

Causes/Risk of Diabetes

Underlying causes of diabetes generally fall into four categories (Holt, 2010):

- **Genetic**: A family history of type 1 diabetes or other autoimmune disease is linked to a higher risk of developing type 1 diabetes in the family. Likewise, type 2 diabetes also has a familial component, although this connection is rather more complicated.
- **Obesity**: This increases the risk of developing type 2 diabetes, particularly in people with a body mass index over 25 kg/m^2 or a large waist circumference.
- **Age**: People are living longer and beta cell function declines with age, leading to a chance of developing diabetes in old age.
- **Ethnicity**: Some ethnic groups are at higher risk of developing diabetes, particularly those of South Asian and Afro-Caribbean origin.

Hypoglycaemia

Hypoglycaemia occurs when there is an imbalance between the amount of glucose available and the body's requirements for glucose or the amount of insulin available opening cell membranes. This can be brought about by a large variety of causes, including (NHS, 2017):

- taking too much diabetic medication, particularly insulin or oral anti-diabetic tablets including sulphonylureas
- skipping or delaying meals
- eating food that has fewer carbohydrates than usual
- unusually high levels of physical activity
- consuming excessive amounts of alcohol
- other illness causing increased stress on the body, i.e. pneumonia.

Signs and Symptoms

Although diabetic patients are generally encouraged to keep their blood sugar at 4.0 mmol/l or higher, some will experience symptoms of hypoglycaemia at blood sugar levels higher than this, making recognition important. Some signs and symptoms of hypoglycaemia include (Deary, 1993):

- sweating
- palpitations
- shaking
- hunger
- confusion
- drowsiness
- odd/aggressive behaviour
- speech problems
- headache
- nausea.

Management

If the patient is still conscious and able to take oral glucose, then administer 10–20 g of glucose. You can find 10 g of glucose in (BNF, 2014; JRCALC, 2016):

- 100 ml Coca-Cola
- 18 ml Ribena Blackcurrant (diluted to taste)
    - **NB**: should not be diet/sugar-free varieties
- 2 teaspoons of sugar
- 3 sugar lumps.

In addition, commercial preparations of glucose are available including Glucogel, Dextrogel and Hypo-Fit. Administration of oral glucose can be repeated after 10–15 minutes, if required.

If the patient is unable to take oral glucose due to impaired consciousness, is unco-operative or there is a risk of airway compromise, then either IM glucagon or IV glucose should be administered. This decision will be a judgement call by the senior clinician (if present) and will depend on whether IV access can be obtained.

Where it is not possible to administer oral or IV glucose, then glucagon can be administered

IM. This may not be effective in patients with inadequate stores of glycogen, such as those who are intoxicated, alcoholic or anorexic.

Diabetic patients who suffer an episode of severe hypoglycaemia will often fully recover and can be discharged at the scene safely by ambulance clinicians, as long as their blood sugar is above 5 mmol/l, they consume 20–40 g of carbohydrates and meet any local criteria for discharge at the scene. It is recommended that patients are referred to a diabetes specialist, as their treatment regimen may need to change (Walker, 2006; Roberts, 2003). It is also important that the senior clinician knows why the patient had a hypoglycaemic event, otherwise even if the patient has fully recovered, the hypoglycaemia could happen again.

However, patients should be encouraged to attend hospital in the following circumstances and as directed by local guidance (JRCALC, 2016; Roberts, 2003):

- elderly (although no specific age range is cited in the literature)
- not diagnosed as diabetic
- taking oral hypoglycaemic agents (mainly sulphonylureas such as glibenclamide or gliclazide (BNF, 2014; Ng, 2010))
- blood glucose < 5 mmol/l after treatment
- treated with glucagon
- co-morbidity (for example renal failure/dialysis, chest pain, arrhythmias, alcohol consumption, dyspnoea, seizures or focal neurological signs)
- signs of illness/infection.

Severe Hyperglycaemia

Severe hyperglycaemia (sometimes referred to as hyperglycaemic crisis) manifests as two conditions: diabetic ketoacidosis (DKA) and hyperosmolar hyperglycaemic state or syndrome (HHS, previously known as hyperosmolar non-ketotic coma, HONK) (Van Ness-Otunnu, 2013).

Signs and Symptoms

DKA and HHS typically present in different groups of patients and over differing time periods. DKA most commonly occurs in type 1 diabetes (although patients with advanced/severe type 2 diabetes are also at risk). HHS on the other hand is almost exclusively seen in type 2 diabetes and is more common in the elderly (Lupsa, 2014), although its incidence in teenagers and young adults is on the rise (Scott, 2015). DKA typically presents within hours to days of onset, whereas HHS can take far longer (Savage, 2011).

Typical signs and symptoms of severe hyperglycaemia are common to both DKA and HHS (except where highlighted in the list below) (Lupsa, 2014; Corwell, 2014):

- excessive urination (polyuria)
- excessive thirst (polydipsia)
- blurred vision
- fatigue
- weakness
- weight loss
- vomiting and abdominal pain (DKA) – probably due to delayed gastric emptying and ileus because of electrolyte abnormalities and/or acidosis
- fruity breath odour (DKA)
- Kussmaul breathing – deep, sighing respirations (DKA)
- focal neurological signs such as weakness of one side of the body (HHS)
- altered mental state, although this can range from confusion to coma
- signs of dehydration: dry mucous membranes, poor skin turgor, long furrows on tongue.

Management

Out-of-hospital management of a hyperglycaemic crisis is limited. Your focus should be on prompt recognition and transport of the patient to definitive care while managing ABCD (JRCALC, 2016; Skellett, 2016):

Airway

Ensure airway patency, with patient positioning, suction and adjuncts, as required, particularly in patients with a reduced level of consciousness.

Breathing

Adults need supplemental oxygen if the patient's SpO_2 is <94%. Children should receive high-flow oxygen titrated to a target range of 94–98%. Patients can expire CO_2 with spontaneous breathing far more effectively than with artificial ventilation, so avoid assisting/interfering unless the patient is in respiratory failure or arrest.

Circulation

Your senior clinician may commence rehydration en-route to hospital, since fluid deficits of patients with DKA are typically 100 ml/kg; in HHS, they can range from 100–220 ml/kg, i.e. up to 16.5 l in a 75 kg patient.

There are, however, risks of giving fluid too quickly, including fluid build-up on the brain, so fluids should only be given once a full assessment by a qualified clinician has been undertaken.

Disability

Assess level of consciousness and watch for the patient's general trend (e.g. decreasing AVPU score). In children, watch for signs of rising intracranial pressure (posturing in response to pain, reducing AVPU score, rising blood pressure with decreasing heart rate). Don't forget to record the patient's blood glucose, but be wary of results that do not fit the clinical picture, e.g. a low blood sugar reading in a patient with 'classic' signs of hyperglycaemia.

Blood Glucose Measurement

You will obtain blood glucose measurements as part of your clinical assessment, but as with all diagnostic tests, they are not perfect and are prone to error if the correct technique is not used. Common causes of error include (Lunt, 2010):

- Incorrect calibration chip used to read the test strips.
- Contamination of the test finger with glucose-rich foods or dilutional error due to inadequate hand drying or the patient licking their finger clean.
- Expired strips or strips stored in adverse environmental conditions, such as heat, humidity or extreme cold.
- Patient conditions, such as extremes of haematocrit (e.g. anaemia) and hypoxia. Shocked patients may have a reduced capillary blood glucose reading compared to a venous blood sample. Consider taking venous blood in these patients (particularly as you are likely to be cannulating them anyway).
- Aspirin, paracetamol and vitamin C can all raise blood glucose, although this may not be clinically significant.

Procedure

Take the following steps to record a blood sugar measurement with an Accu-Chek® Aviva blood glucose meter (other meters will have similar process but you should check manufacturer instructions):

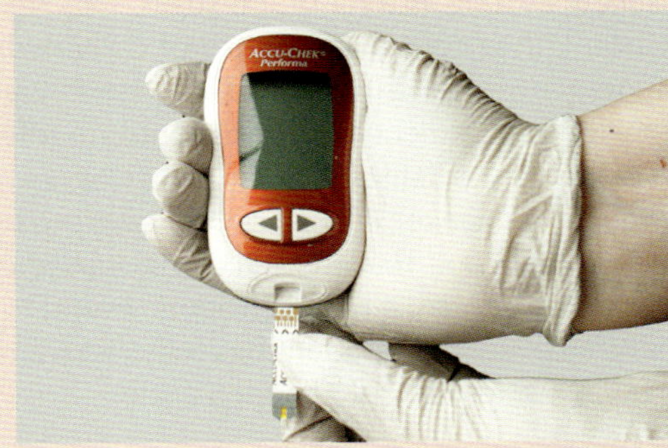

1. Wash and dry your hands or use alcohol gel and put on gloves. Select an appropriate site, which is typically the side of a finger in an adult or older child and the heel of the foot in a younger child or infant. Clean the area with water or a water-soaked gauze and dry thoroughly. Insert the test strip into the meter and check that the meter turns on automatically.

   Alcohol swabs do not remove traces of glucose as effectively as water, so hand-washing is preferable. Failing that, simple cleansing wipes are almost as effective.

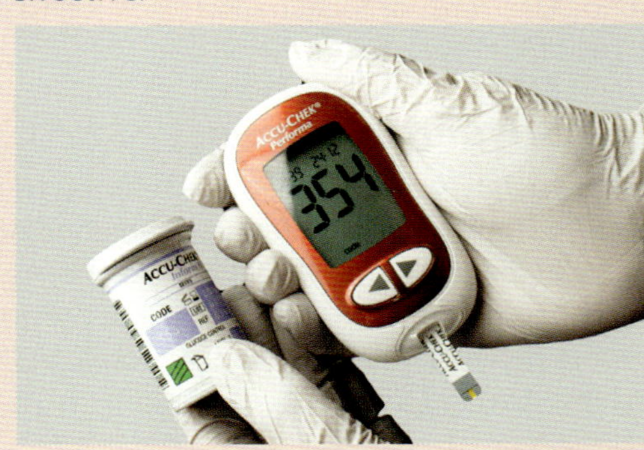

2. Ensure that the code number of the display matches the code number on the test strip container.

Procedure – *cont*

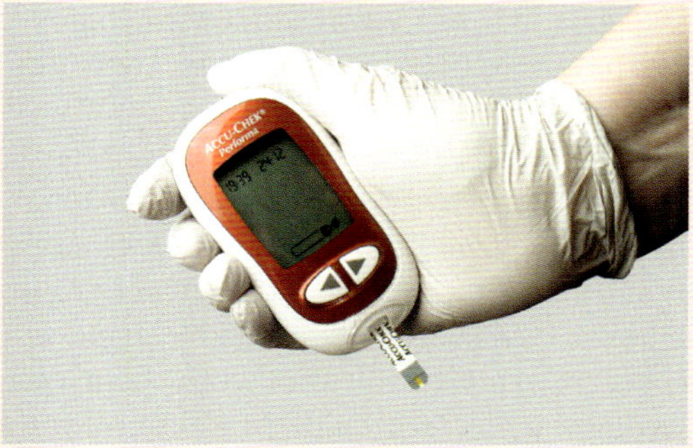

3. On the screen, an icon showing the test strip and a flashing blood drop will appear. Ask the patient to dangle their arm down at their side to encourage blood flow to their fingertips.

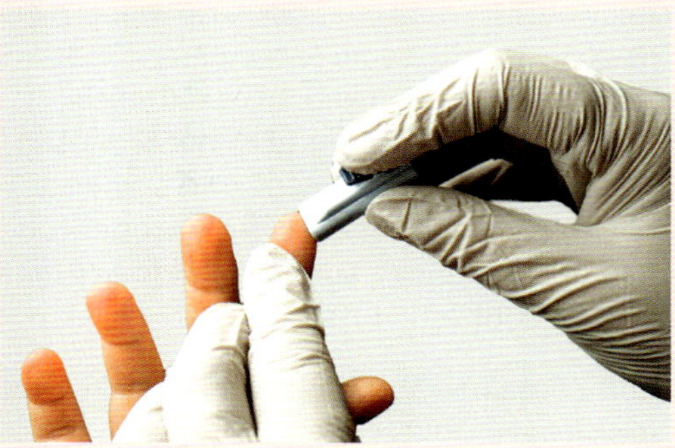

4. Prick the target area with a lancet, disposing of it in a sharps bin after use.

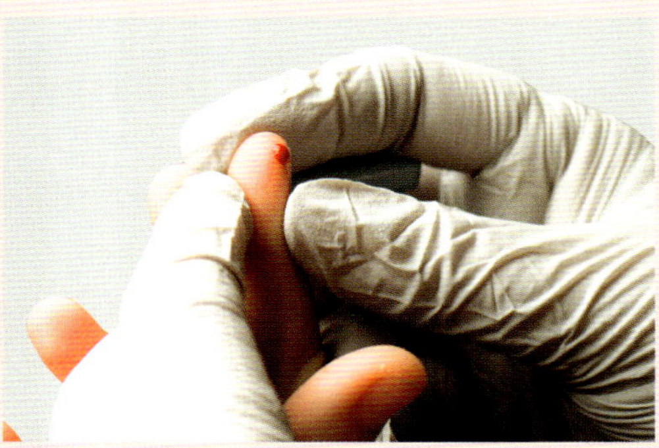

5. With the patient's hand facing downwards, gently squeeze their finger to assist the flow of blood.

Procedure – *cont*

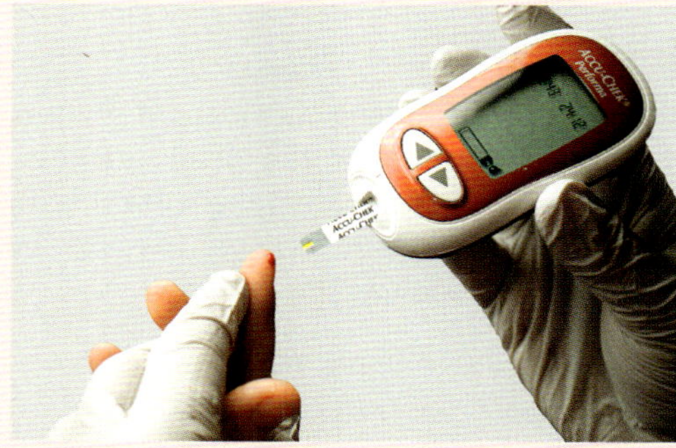

6. Touch the blood drop to the front edge of the yellow window of the test strip. When you have enough blood, you will see an egg timer icon flash.

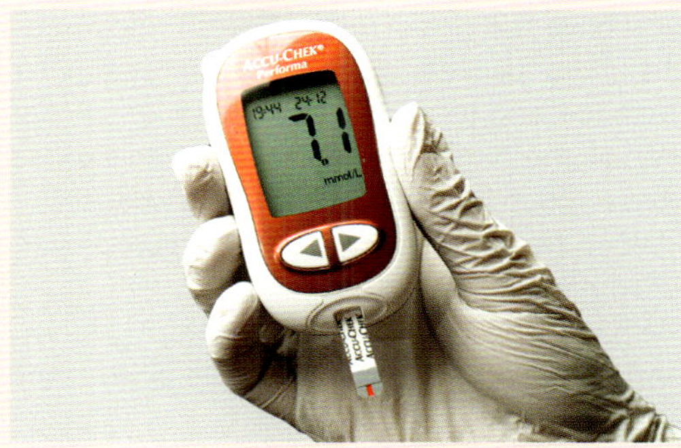

7. The blood sugar result will appear on the display. Note this value on the patient's clinical record.

Poisoning

Poisoning is the exposure by ingestion, inhalation, absorption or injection to a quantity of a substance or substances that may result in illness or death. Over 70% of emergency department (ED) admissions involving poisoning are deliberate, with paracetamol the most common drug involved (Baker, 2014).

Poisoning can take many forms, and can include:

- Prescribed medications
- Over-the-counter medications
- Herbal remedies and supplements

- Exposure to gases
- Contact with chemicals.

Management

In situations of poisoning consider carefully your own safety. It may be that the environment is unsafe (such as in an accidental chemical spill), so expert assistance may be required to make the area safe before approaching the patient.

You should follow the normal ABCDE approach to managing and supporting the patient whilst awaiting backup. You should not encourage the patient to ingest anything else and should not encourage vomiting as this can cause more injuries.

If you have the opportunity, you should keep hold of any packets or information relating to the substance, and record:

- What the patient has taken or been exposed to
- How much (number of tablets and dose)
- When (was it all at once, or staggered over a period of time)
- What with (i.e. water or milk etc.)
- Any first aid measures that have been taken.

Poisoning patients can deteriorate rapidly, so monitor closely and be prepared to resuscitate if necessary.

The Acute Abdomen

Learning Objectives

By the end of this section you will be able to:

- Describe the anatomy and physiology of the digestive system.
- List a number of causes of an 'acute abdomen' and describe their signs and symptoms.
- Explain the management of a patient with an 'acute abdomen'.

Introduction

The term 'acute abdomen' refers to abdominal conditions that are characterised by a rapid onset of severe symptoms, which require prompt admission to hospital and surgical intervention. Because of the number of organs and structures within the abdominal cavity, it can be difficult to make a diagnosis, but this does not matter out-of-hospital, as long as serious red flag symptoms have been recognised and acted on.

The Abdominal Cavity

The abdominal cavity extends from the diaphragm to the pelvic cavity, although it is continuous with this and some abdominal organs descend into the pelvic cavity. The arched dome shape of the diaphragm extends well above the costal margin, allowing the ribs to provide protection for the liver, spleen, upper poles of the kidneys and the adrenal (suprarenal) glands. The spine provides additional protection, although the anterior and lateral aspects of the abdomen are more exposed, since the abdominal muscles provide only modest protection. Organs are either suspended by double folds of the peritoneum (a membrane that lines the abdominal cavity) known as mesenteries, or bound to the posterior abdominal wall. In addition, some organs are located posterior to the peritoneum and are termed retroperitoneal, including the kidneys, adrenal glands and ureters (Tortora, 2008).

Organs contained within the abdominal cavity include (Drake, 2005):

- major elements of the digestive system (Figure 16.5)
- posterior end of oesophagus, stomach, small and large intestines, liver, pancreas and gallbladder
- components of the urinary system (kidneys and ureters)
- major neurovascular structures (e.g. abdominal aorta, inferior vena cava).

Locating Abdominal Organs

To make it easier to relate surface anatomy to the underlying organs, the abdomen is often divided into four regions (Figure 16.6).

The Digestive System

The digestive or gastrointestinal (GI) system performs six main functions (Tortora, 2008):

- ingestion
- secretion
- mixing and propulsion

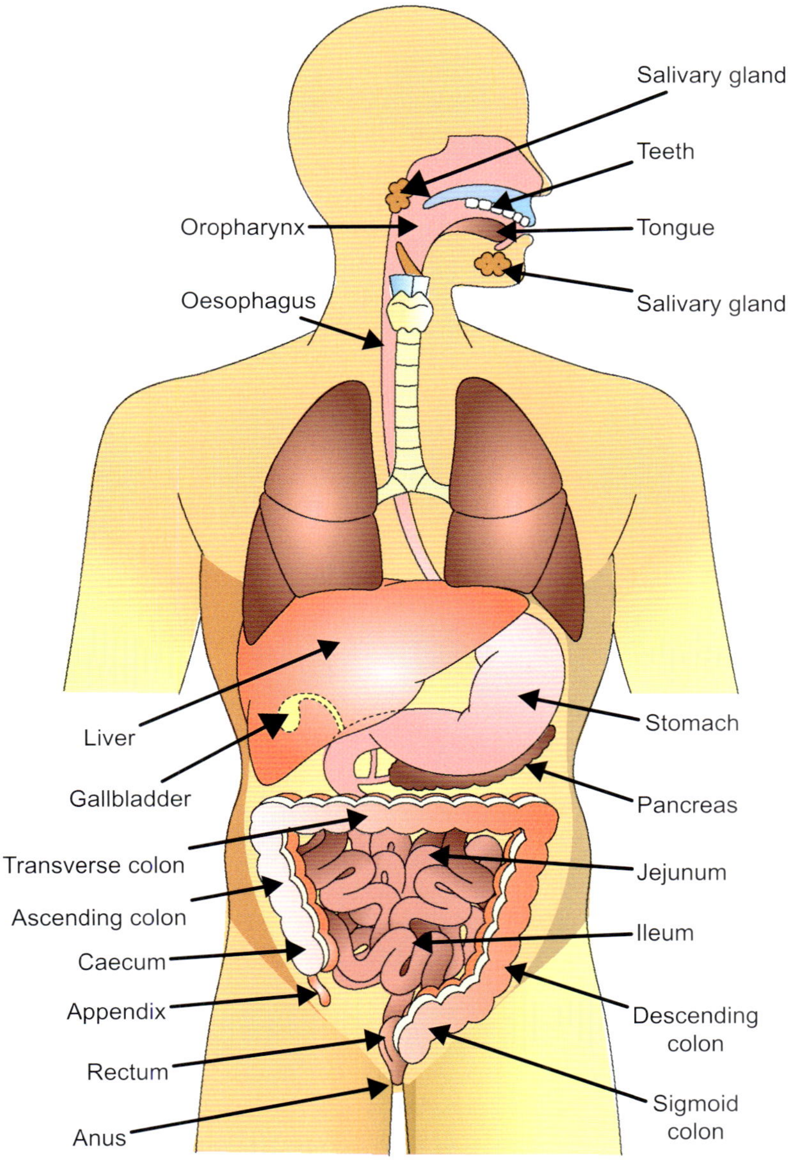

Figure 16.5 *Overview of the digestive system.*

- digestion
- absorption
- defaecation.

It consists of an alimentary canal (the GI tract) and associated accessory organs, forming a continuous tube that runs from mouth to anus. Starting at the oral cavity, the teeth pulverise, and saliva softens and partly digests the food that is in the mouth.

The tongue assists with mechanical manipulation of the food and flips what's left into the pharynx during swallowing.

Boluses of food move down the oesophagus due to regular peristaltic contractions, and enter the stomach, where the food is treated to mechanical and chemical digestion, resulting in the formation of a semi-fluid mass known as chyme. This enters

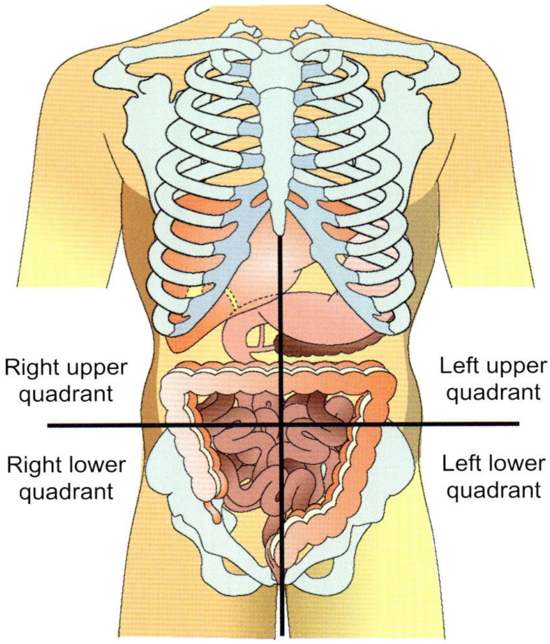

Figure 16.6 *Abdominal quadrants.*

the small intestine for further digestion, aided by bile from the gallbladder, which passes down the bile duct and into the duodenum and helps digest fat and neutralise stomach acid. In addition, digestive enzymes from the exocrine pancreas also enter the duodenum. Molecular sized nutrients are extracted from the small intestine and transferred by blood and lymph capillaries to the liver for processing.

Finally, the proximal half of the large intestine absorbs minerals and water, while the remaining portion acts as a storage unit for undigested and unabsorbed material, which continues to the rectum ready for discharge via the anus.

Abdominal Pain

Abdominal pain is a common presentation to emergency and urgent care services. As has already been discussed, diagnosing abdominal pain can be very challenging due not only to the sheer number of things that can go wrong with the abdomen, but also because of the arrangement of organs within, which makes it very difficult to pinpoint the exact issue.

It is likely that any patient with significant abdominal pain will need to be admitted to hospital for further examination, but in the initial phases, you should consider the following as part of your standard assessment (Kumar, 2012):

- the site, intensity, character, duration and frequency of the pain
- the aggravating and relieving factors
- associated symptoms, including non-gastrointestinal symptoms.

You should be particularly concerned when abdominal pain presents with altered vital signs (tachycardia, hypotension etc.) (Leath, 2017). Table 16.2 provides examples of conditions that cause abdominal pain (JRCALC, 2016).

Management of Abdominal Pain

The focus of management for abdominal pain patients is not to reach a definitive diagnosis, but to identify that the patient needs a more detailed assessment. Follow your normal initial assessment (see Chapter 10: Patient Assessment) and primary survey correcting any deficits as you progress.

While awaiting backup, you should pass an update back to the clinical hub. If you suspect any of the conditions listed above you should include this in your update.

You should avoid physical examination of the abdomen as this is a complex procedure that requires experience and training and if performed incorrectly can worsen some conditions.

Other treatment will include the following actions:

- Gather and frequently reassess vital signs – record these on your documentation.
- Place the patient in the position of most comfort.
- Administer adequate pain relief – consider if pain relief further than you are able to administer is required; if so, pass this information to the clinical hub as part of your update.
- Be prepared for the patient to deteriorate and to initiate resuscitation if necessary.

Table 16.2 Conditions that cause abdominal pain

Condition	Characteristics of pain	Associated symptoms
Leaking or ruptured abdominal aortic aneurysm (AAA) Consider AAA in patients >50 years who present with the symptoms listed. Most deaths occur in the elderly	Sudden severe abdominal pain or backache NB Given that <25% of all AAA patients present with classic signs and symptoms there is a risk of misdiagnosis	Collapse Hypotension with bilateral lower limb ischaemia History of smoking Hypertension and hypercholesterolaemia (high cholesterol)
Appendicitis Frequently misdiagnosed. Approximately one-third of women of childbearing age with appendicitis are considered as having pelvic inflammatory disease or UTI	A constant pain, increasing in intensity often starting in the periumbilical area Pain may settle in the right lower quadrant, but the location may vary in the early stages Older patients may present with generalised pain and distension	Nausea Vomiting Loss of appetite Constipation Increased temperature >37.5°C Diarrhoea
Acute cholecystitis Accounts for approximately 30% of patients attending the ED for acute abdominal pain	A sharp pain in the right upper quadrant of the abdomen May experience right shoulder-tip pain The pain is worse when breathing deeply	Nausea and vomiting Increased temperature >38°C History of fat intolerance
Intestinal obstruction A partial or complete obstruction of the small or large intestine	Abdominal pain that is cramping in nature	Abdominal distension Nausea and vomiting Absolute constipation (late stage)
Acute pancreatitis Inflammation of the pancreas	Constant pain in the upper left quadrant or middle of the abdomen The pain may radiate to the patient's back	Abdominal tenderness Hypotension Nausea and vomiting Dehydration Shock History of alcohol abuse or gallstones
Ectopic pregnancy Pregnancy is not implanted in the uterus. It affects around 1 in 80 pregnancies and accounts for 13% of all pregnancy-related deaths	Pain in the lower abdomen, pelvic area or back **NB** Patients may present atypically but pain is almost always present	Nausea Missed last menstrual period (though can occur before this) History of pelvic inflammatory disease Previous ectopic pregnancy If the pregnancy ruptures patients may report: • severe lower abdominal pain • shoulder-tip pain • feeling faint/collapse

Urinary System Disorders

Learning Objectives

By the end of this section you will be able to:

- Describe the anatomy and physiology of the urinary system.
- Explain the assessment and management of a patient with a urinary tract infection (UTI).

Introduction

The urinary system carries out a number of important functions, including (Tortora, 2008):

- regulation of blood volume and composition
- regulation of blood pressure
- glucose synthesis
- excretion of waste products in urine.

All of these functions are carried out by the kidneys. The other organs and tissues that make up the urinary system provide transport, storage and excretion of urine.

Anatomy and Physiology

The urinary system is made up of two kidneys, two ureters, a bladder and urethra (Figure 16.7).

Kidneys

The kidneys are red-brown kidney-bean-shaped organs that are located just above the waist and lie between the peritoneum and posterior wall of the abdomen. The right kidney is slightly lower than the left to accommodate the liver above. Due to the important functions of the kidney, they receive around 25% of resting cardiac output, about 1,200 ml per minute, via the renal arteries (Tortora, 2008). As with other blood vessels, these subdivide into smaller and smaller vessels, before reaching the glomerular capillaries in the nephrons (Figure 16.8).

As blood passes through the kidneys, water, vitamins, minerals and amino acids are reabsorbed back into the blood at different stages.

Ureters, Bladder and Urethra

The remaining fluid and solutes that leave the collecting duct of the kidney is urine. From here it drains into the ureters and moves into the bladder

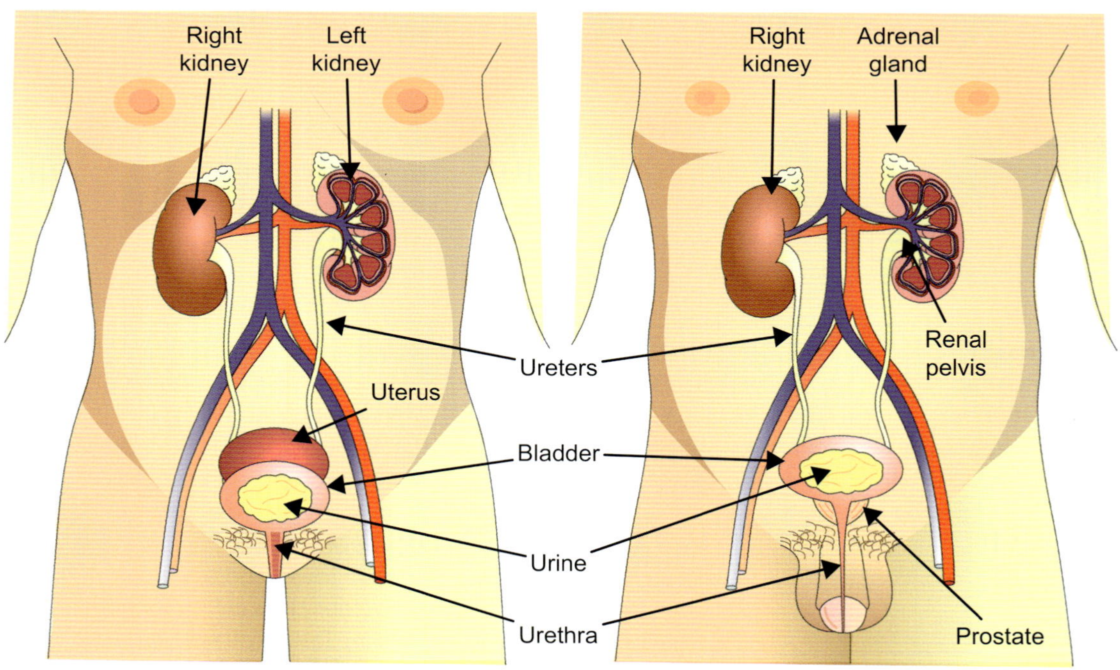

Figure 16.7 *The urinary system in females (left) and males (right).*

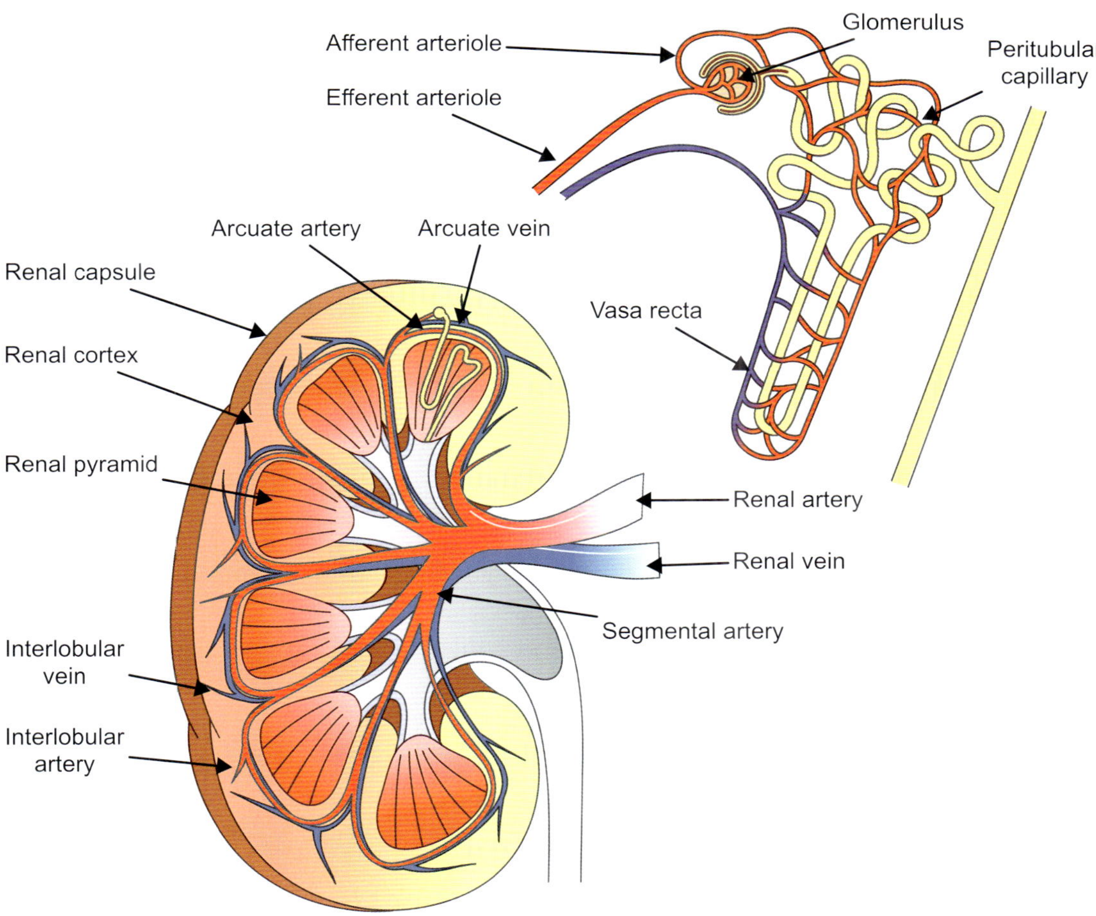

Figure 16.8 *Blood supply to the kidneys.*

by a combination of rhythmic contractions of its muscular walls (peristalsis), pressure and gravity.

The urinary bladder is sited in the pelvic cavity just posterior to the pubic symphysis. It is a hollow and expansible organ, which has a maximum capacity in the region of 700–800 ml. The last stage is the urethra, which allows urine to be excreted from the body.

Urinary Tract Infections

A urinary tract infection (UTI) occurs when there is microbial infiltration of the normally sterile urinary tract.

UTIs can affect the urethra (urethritis) and urinary bladder (cystitis), collectively termed lower UTIs, and/or ascend to the kidneys (pyelonephritis) where, unsurprisingly, it is termed an upper UTI.

UTIs are typically classed as mild or severe, which is defined by the number of symptoms the patient reports. Three or more symptoms are classed as severe, and this has implications for treatment. UTIs can also be classed as complicated or uncomplicated. In an otherwise healthy adult female, acute cystitis or pyelonephritis would be considered uncomplicated, and in 70–95% of cases are caused by *Escherichia coli* (*E. coli*). If the patient is male and/or has a structural or functional abnormality of the urinary tract, or suffers from kidney disease and certain other diseases, such as diabetes, then typically the UTI would be considered to be complicated.

Signs and Symptoms

The classic symptoms of a UTI include (Nickerson, 2007):

- **Dysuria**: Pain or a burning sensation when urinating.
- **Frequency**: Urinating more often.
- **Nocturia**: Having to get up in the night to urinate.
- **Urgency**: A reduction in the time between feeling the need to urinate and actually having to pass urine. If the patient cannot hold on until they reach a toilet, urge incontinence results.

Haematuria (blood in the urine) does sometimes occur (more common in upper UTIs) and the urine can also be offensive smelling, though offensive urine does not automatically mean a patient has a UTI as there can be many causes. Elderly patients may have minimal urinary symptoms, but consider this as a differential diagnosis if there is a history of new-onset confusion or incontinence.

Pyelonephritis

Upper UTIs classically present with loin to groin pain on the affected side, although some patients may just complain of back pain. The pain is often colicky and sharp in nature, with patients struggling to get comfortable and so are restless. Haematuria is more common, as are signs and symptoms of systemic illness, such as fever, rigors and profuse sweating (Nickerson, 2007).

Management

Conduct a full assessment including a NEWS score (refer to Chapter 10: Patient Assessment for more details) and pass your findings on to a senior clinician who will decide on the most appropriate course of action. A good history is important with all infections, so if you have the opportunity you should question about history relating to classic symptoms listed above as well as general medical history.

Remember to assess for sepsis (see the section on sepsis earlier in this chapter). UTI is a common cause of sepsis, especially in the elderly, so if you suspect it and are awaiting backup, you should contact the clinical hub to make them aware of your concerns.

In some circumstances patients with a UTI can be treated in the community (avoiding a hospital admission); this is a decision for a senior clinician once they have assessed the patient themselves.

Chapter 17
Trauma Emergencies

Introduction to Trauma

Learning Objectives

By the end of this section you will be able to:

- Define trauma and major trauma.
- Define mechanism of injury and outline the different types.
- Explain the kinetics associated with trauma.
- Define the mechanisms that can cause injury to the head, spine, chest, abdomen and pelvis.

Introduction

Trauma is the acute physiological and structural change (injury) that occurs in a patient's body when an external source of energy transfers to the body faster than the body's ability to sustain and dissipate it (Pilbery, 2013). The mechanism of injury (MOI) is defined as the physical forces that act on the body to cause damage (Pilbery, 2013). Since human tissue, organs and systems can only withstand a limited range of physical, environmental and physiological stress, when the energy delivery to the body exceeds these limits, injury occurs. This tolerance to external energy delivery is dependent on which type of tissue(s) have been targeted, the age and physical health of the patient, and the type, magnitude and duration of the energy that has been transferred (Greaves, 2008).

Types of Trauma

Trauma is generally divided into two types (NAEMT, 2014):

- **Blunt**: Injuries that do not cause penetration of the skin by an external object. Typical mechanisms of blunt trauma include road traffic collisions (RTC) involving vehicles, pedestrians, motorcyclists etc., fall from height, serious sports injuries and blast injuries (although this mechanism often also causes penetrating trauma). This is the most common type of trauma in the UK (NAO, 2010).
- **Penetrating**: Injuries caused by projectiles penetrating the skin. Examples include stab and gunshot wounds and blast injuries involving shrapnel and secondary projectiles.

Kinetics

Kinetics is the study of the relationship between motion and its forces.

In a road traffic collision there are three collisions. The first occurs when the vehicle a person is travelling in collides with another object. Newton's first law of motion states that a physical body will remain at steady speed and direction (i.e. velocity) or at rest until an external force acts upon it. In the case of a person driving their car, this force may be due to a collision with another vehicle or other object, such as a tree. During a head-on collision with a tree, for example, the vehicle stops abruptly, but the occupant inside will still be moving at the same velocity as they were prior to the collision until they come into contact with the vehicle (the second collision). The third collision occurs when the person's internal organs and tissues make contact with the body's hard surfaces, such as the skull or chest wall (NAEMT, 2014).

Newton's second law of motion states that the force an object exerts is equal to its mass multiplied by its acceleration, or in the case of a collision, mass multiplied by the deceleration. Thus, rapid decelerations, such as a car hitting an immovable object, or striking another vehicle travelling in the opposite direction at speed, for example, lead to large forces being exerted.

Newton's third law of motion states that for every force, there is an equal and opposite force, meaning that the force applied to the tree in our head-on collision example is exerted on the vehicle too, leading to damage to the vehicle and, potentially, the occupants (Pilbery, 2013).

Energy

Energy is a measure of an object's ability to do work, or transfer energy to another object. The law of conservation states that energy cannot be destroyed, only transformed.

Energy comes in at least five forms (Greaves, 2008):

- **Kinetic**: Related to motion, and the most common type of injury-causing energy.
- **Thermal**: Kinetic energy of molecular motion, measured as temperature. The cause of burns.
- **Electrical**: The flow of electrical charge. This type of energy mainly causes damage through conversion to thermal energy.
- **Chemical**: Energy created or consumed during the alteration of electrical charge in chemical reactions. Explosions are often due to chemical reactions.
- **Nuclear**: Energy released as a result of nuclear fission (the splitting of an atom into smaller parts, with associated energy release).

In trauma, it is usually kinetic energy that is of interest and this can be represented by the formula (NAEMT, 2014):

$$\text{kinetic energy} = \tfrac{1}{2}mv^2$$

where m is the mass of the object and v its velocity. From this, it is clear that it is the velocity of the object that makes the greatest difference to the amount of kinetic energy available to be transformed. Human tolerance to kinetic energy is influenced by the magnitude of the energy (the force applied) and the duration of the exposure, specifically the change in velocity. This is typically deceleration, for example a person's feet hitting the floor after a fall from height, or when a car strikes a large tree at speed. However, excessive acceleration can also cause injury, for example when a pilot is ejected from a jet aircraft (Greaves, 2008).

Energy Transfer

The energy exchanged during trauma is the same, whether it is blunt or penetrating. Cavitation, the formation of a cavity or hollow, occurs during trauma as tissues in the body move away from the point of impact and their usual position. If this energy is dispersed over a wide area, then penetration of the skin may not occur. Thanks to the elastic properties of tissues, body shape of the torso in particular often returns to its usual position, i.e. the cavitation is temporary. However, this may hide serious internal injury to organs and tissues that have had the kinetic energy of the impact transferred to them. Other denser tissues, such as bone, may remain deformed, giving clues to the presence of injury (Greaves, 2008).

In penetrating trauma, temporary cavitation also occurs, but there is also a permanent cavity that remains once the temporary cavity has collapsed due to the elasticity of the tissues. In low-energy penetrating trauma, such as a stab wound, temporary cavitation may be minimal, but with higher energies, such as those in a gunshot, the temporary cavity can become significant in terms of injury to surrounding tissues and by generating a sub-atmospheric pressure within, causing external debris and dirt to be 'sucked in' to the wound (Greaves, 2008).

The mechanical damage that remains after trauma does not necessarily correlate to the severity of injury either. For example, a screwdriver plunged through the chest that damages the heart may leave only a small external injury, but is likely to be more serious than a gunshot wound to the patient's knee (Figure 17.1).

Penetrating projectiles do not always follow a straight path and can ricochet off internal organs and bone as the projectile decelerates. Although entrance and exit wounds are sometimes visible, determining which is which is not clinically important. Note that the absence of an exit wound means that much of the projectile's kinetic energy has been transferred to the body (NAEMT, 2014).

Mechanisms That Cause Injury

There are many mechanisms that can result in a host of isolated and multiple injuries to the human body. Some of the more common mechanisms and the injuries they cause to the head, spine, thorax, abdomen and pelvis are covered in this section.

Head

If the head is travelling ahead of the body, such as during a headfirst fall, it is the first structure to receive the force of the impact and energy transference. The continued movement of the rest of the body results in compression, which can damage the scalp and skull. If the skull fractures, bony fractures can end up damaging the brain. The same damage can also be caused by the application of an external force, such as occurs as a result of a blow to the head during an assault (NAEMT, 2014).

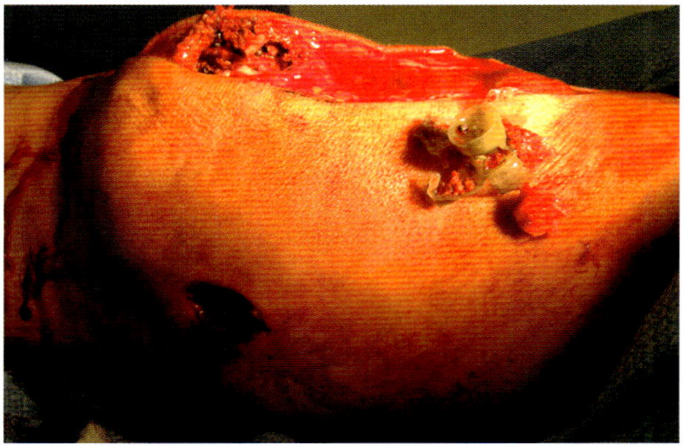

Figure 17.1 *A close-range gunshot wound to the right knee, with a shotgun. Note the smaller entrance wound towards the bottom of the picture and the much larger exit wound – by DiverDave (Own work) [CC-BY-SA-3.0 or GFDL], via Wikimedia Commons.*

The brain is soft and compressible and can move following the application of external forces. This can lead to shearing of brain tissue as well as rupture of the blood vessels surrounding the brain, leading to intracranial haemorrhage.

If a projectile penetrates the skull, the damage can be very severe as the kinetic energy is distributed within the confines of the skull. Small calibre bullets, for example, may not have enough energy to exit the skull, but instead contour around it, leading to extensive damage (NAEMT, 2014).

Spine

The main mechanisms that cause spinal injury can be divided into abnormal flexion, extension, rotation and compression. Extension or flexion with rotation are the main causes of injury to the cervical spine (Greaves, 2008; Pilbery, 2013; NAEMT, 2014).

Flexion

Hyperflexion injuries are typically caused by RTCs where lap-belts (rather than three-point belts) are used; direct blows to the occiput; and rapid deceleration in flexed positions, such as diving and contact sports like rugby. Hyperflexion on its own is uncommon in the cervical spine, since the chin abutting the chest limits flexion.

Flexion With Rotation

The design of the first two cervical vertebrae allows for significant rotation. Injuries due to this mechanism are considered unstable as there is little in the way of bony or soft-tissue support. Not surprisingly, this mechanism is much more likely to produce significant cervical injury and is often caused by lateral impact RTCs or direct trauma. Note that rotation rarely occurs in isolation.

Extension

These injuries are generally only found in cervical and lumbar regions and can be caused by hanging, striking the chin on a steering wheel during a collision or a rear impact collision where the headrest is improperly positioned (NAEMT, 2014).

Compression

Wedge fractures are the most common type of fracture of the lumbar and thoracic spines, but if a weight falls on the head or if the patient lands on their head after a fall, then the cervical vertebrae can be fractured and/or ligaments ruptured. Most fractures caused by compression are stable, but spinal cord injury can occur if the vertebral body is shattered and fragments of bone become embedded in the cord (Pilbery, 2013).

Thorax

Severe blunt thoracic trauma most commonly occurs as a result of RTCs (about 70–80%) where high speeds are involved, leading to rapid deceleration. This causes shearing forces that can rupture large blood vessels, tear the bronchial airways and damage the lungs, causing pneumothoraces, for example. Even with lower velocity mechanisms – such as direct blows to the chest – fractures of the rib cage and sternum as well as bruising to the underlying structures, including the heart and lungs, can occur (NAEMT, 2014).

In penetrating trauma, the most serious consequences arise as a result of rupture of the major blood vessels, which can lead to serious haemorrhage. Projectiles penetrating the chest wall can also cause open pneumothoraces (Greaves, 2008).

Abdomen

Abdominal injury is most commonly caused by blunt trauma, usually due to RTCs, and often as part of a multi-system pattern of injuries. If the abdomen comes into contact with the steering wheel during rapid deceleration, crush injuries can occur. Compression of the abdominal organs increases the intra-abdominal pressure, which in turn can rupture the hollow organs and/or the diaphragm. Penetrating trauma is less common, and in the UK is more likely to be a result of a stab wound than a gunshot. Fortunately, less than half of all stab wounds penetrate the peritoneum (the lining of the abdominal cavity) (Greaves, 2008).

Pelvis

As with any trauma patient, you should consider the MOI to provide an indication as to possible underlying injuries. Pelvic ring fractures usually require high forces, so it is no surprise that the most common cause is RTCs. Front-seat passengers in head-on collisions, and those on the side of impact in T-bone type collisions in cars, are most common. These are closely followed by motorcyclists, pedestrians and falls from heights (Gabbe, 2011; Papadopoulos, 2006). However, a significant sub-group are the elderly, who will typically fall from standing and may have osteoporosis (Garlapati, 2012).

Blast Injury

Blasts (or explosions) cause complex multi-system injury due to the significant transfer of kinetic, heat and other energies. Injuries are generally classified into the five types shown in Table 17.1 (NAEMT, 2014; JRCALC, 2016).

Table 17.1 Blast injury categories

Category	Cause	Possible Injuries
Primary	Injuries caused by patient contact with blast shock wave (Figure 17.2).	Gas-containing organs may be damaged, including lungs, gastrointestinal tract.
Secondary	Injuries due to flying fragments and debris striking the patient.	Entire body can be affected, leading to lacerations and fractures. Penetrating injuries.
Tertiary	Blast wave propels patient against objects. Crush injuries secondary to structural damage and building collapse.	Blunt and crush injuries.
Quaternary	Other explosion-related injuries and illnesses.	Burns.

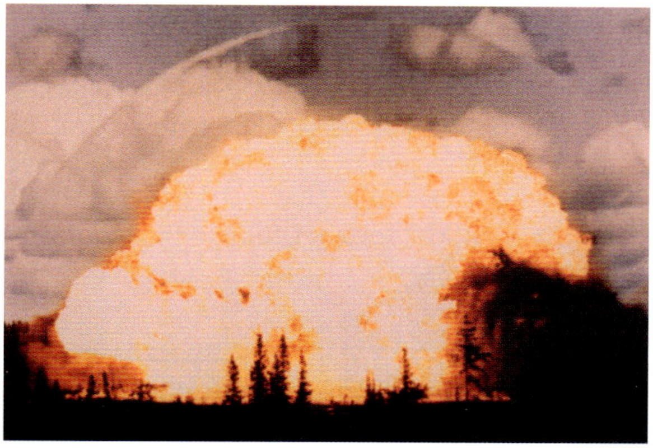

Figure 17.2 *An explosion, with visible blast wave.*

Suspension Trauma

The use of the word 'trauma' in suspension trauma is a bit of a misnomer, as there is often no physical injury. Instead, it is really a form of syncope that occurs when the body is held motionless in a vertical position for a period of time (5 to 30 minutes) (Lee, 2007c). This position causes venous pooling in the legs, which can result in a 20% reduction in circulating volume. The reduction in venous return leads to a reduced venous return to the heart, which reduces cardiac output and arterial blood pressure and leads to syncope (fainting). Ordinarily, a patient would collapse and assume a horizontal position, which would reverse this process. However, in suspension trauma, the victim is kept upright, typically due to being suspended in a harness from a rope, for example, and death can occur, although this appears to be uncommon (Thomassen, 2009).

Wounds and Bleeding

Learning Objectives

By the end of this section you will be able to:

- Describe the types of bleeding.
- Explain how to appropriately assess and manage bleeding.
- Explain how to detect concealed bleeding.
- Describe various types of wounds and how to manage them.
- Discuss the implications of foreign objects in wounds.
- Explain complications associated with bleeding and wounds.

Introduction

Wounds and bleeding are a common reason for an emergency call. Even in the emergency ambulance service, these calls will vary in their severity, from wounds and bleeding that require basic first aid only, through to life-threatening wounds and bleeding that require prompt and more advanced intervention in order to prevent death.

Bleeding

Bleeding is the loss of blood from a damaged blood vessel. You will often hear the term 'haemorrhage' used, which is bleeding, but in medical circles is usually reserved for severe bleeding. Bleeding is often classified by the type of vessel involved (i.e. artery, vein or capillary) or whether it is external or internal (SJA, SAA, BRC, 2014).

Assessment

Sources of Bleeding

Bleeding can be defined by whether it is visible on the outside of the body and/or which type of vessel is responsible (Gregory, 2010a; SJA, SAA, BRC, 2014):

- **Internal**: This bleeding is concealed within the body and can be hard to detect (Greaves, 2008). The thorax, abdomen, pelvis and long bones provide good hiding places for significant volumes of blood. The mechanism of injury and the presence of shock without signs of external haemorrhage can help with diagnosis. These patients need to be in hospital to stop the bleeding.
- **External**: This bleeding is visible and should be detected during your primary and/or secondary survey. This bleeding can usually be controlled.
- **Arterial**: Blood inside the arteries is under relatively high pressure and so bleeding can lead to significant blood loss. It is characterised by bright red (oxygenated) spurting, in time with the heart beat.
- **Venous**: Since veins carry blood back to the heart, they typically carry deoxygenated blood and so bleeding is a darker red. Since the pressure is lower, blood does not spurt but flows freely. However, blood loss can still be severe, particularly from veins in the neck and legs.

- **Capillary**: These are the smallest blood vessels in the body and carry a mixture of oxygenated and deoxygenated blood, so the colour of bleeding will vary. Blood loss tends to be small as blood oozes from wounds.

Estimating Blood Loss

Estimating blood loss accurately is very difficult (Frank, 2010; Bose, 2006; Tall, 2003; Moscati, 1999). Table 17.2 provides examples of what various volumes of blood loss look like (this was originally designed for estimating obstetric blood loss) (Bose, 2006). Fractures can cause significant blood loss, depending on the bone(s) affected and whether the fracture is open or closed (Table 17.3) (NAEMT, 2014). Remember to check for signs and symptoms of shock (this was covered in Chapter 13: Circulation).

Table 17.2 Visual guide to estimating blood loss

Blood Loss (ml)	
50	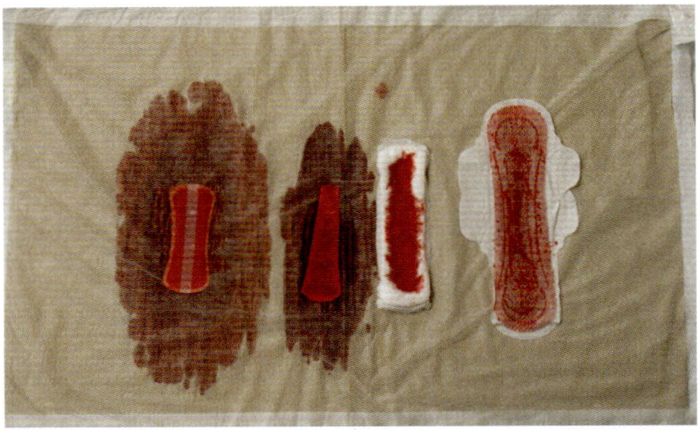
500	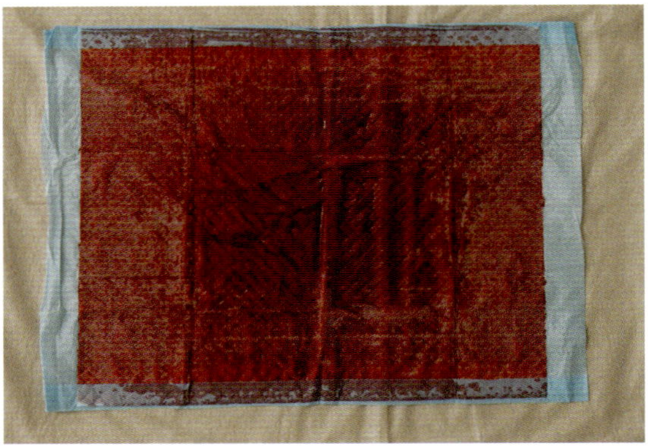

Table 17.3 Approximate internal blood loss due to fractures

Fracture	Blood Loss (ml)
Rib	125
Radius or ulna	250–500
Humerus	500–750
Tibia	500–1,000
Femur	1,000–2,000
Pelvis	1,000–5,000

Management

Once the scene assessment has been completed, you need to check for, and manage, any actual or potential catastrophic haemorrhage. Only once this has been completed can you return to the normal AcBC (i.e. airway with consideration of the cervical spine, breathing and circulation) approach.

During the assessment of circulation, any interventions to manage catastrophic haemorrhage must be reassessed to ensure that bleeding is being controlled appropriately. Don't forget the bleeding you cannot see. 'Blood on the floor plus four more' is a good way to remember the areas where significant blood loss can accumulate, i.e. the thorax, abdomen, pelvis and long bones (Greaves, 2010).

Most external haemorrhage can be controlled with simple first-aid measures, such as direct pressure and elevation of the bleeding extremity. In some cases, additional interventions are required, but these should be introduced in an incremental fashion, as shown in the haemostasis escalator (Figure 17.3) (Lee, 2007b; Moorhouse, 2007).

Catastrophic Haemorrhage Management

If you suspect the bleeding is likely to cause death in minutes (i.e. is a catastrophic haemorrhage), you are likely to ascend the haemostasis escalator rather faster than for non-catastrophic haemorrhage. If the haemorrhage involves a limb, then a tourniquet should be immediately applied. Should the first tourniquet not adequately control the bleeding, then a second tourniquet should be applied above the first. If bleeding continues, pack the wound with a haemostatic gauze and apply a fresh dressing. Apply firm direct pressure (JRCALC, 2016).

In other body areas, such as the head, neck and torso, it will not be possible to use a tourniquet. In this instance, you should apply a wound dressing to the site of bleeding and apply firm pressure directly over the wound. Elevation is unlikely to be appropriate with these types of bleeds. If direct pressure fails to stem the bleeding, then wound packing should be undertaken and may be supplemented with haemostatic agents. This is achieved by inserting a sufficient quantity of gauze into the wound to create mechanical pressure on the injured vessel and provide a structure for coagulation. Where haemostatic agents are used, they should be placed as close to the bleeding point as possible and then direct pressure should be applied for at least three minutes. Ideally, constant pressure should be applied with a suitable elastic bandage. If this fails to control bleeding, apply further dressings and more direct pressure.

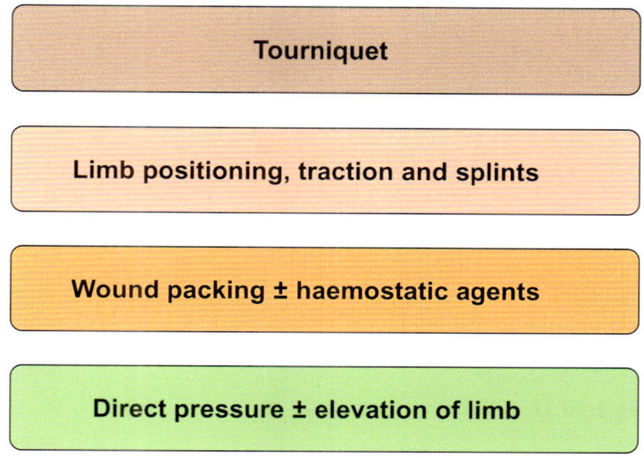

Figure 17.3 *The haemostasis escalator.*

Assess limb positioning and consider whether the use of splinting may help to reduce bleeding. Straightening angulated fractures and applying a pelvic binder may help to reduce blood loss (NICE, 2016).

Non-Catastrophic Haemorrhage

For other, non-catastrophic external haemorrhage, you can move up the haemorrhage escalator. Start by applying direct pressure, with or without a dressing and, if the injury is below the knee or elbow, consider elevating the affected limb above the level of the heart, if practicable. If this does not control the bleeding, consider applying a further dressing while continuing to apply firm direct pressure (JRCALC, 2016).

If bleeding continues, you should treat the haemorrhage as a potential catastrophic bleeding event. For limbs, this means applying a tourniquet and in the case of head, neck or torso wounds, packing with haemostatic dressing. As with catastrophic haemorrhage, consider whether splinting of a limb or applying a pelvic binder would help reduce blood loss.

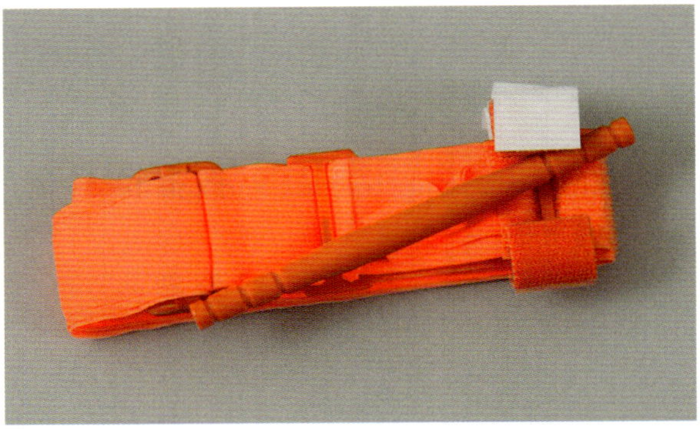

Figure 17.4 *A tourniquet.*

Tourniquets

Tourniquets can be a useful adjunct to stop haemorrhage as long as they are only used in the following situations (Lee, 2007b, Figure 17.4):

- Extreme life-threatening limb haemorrhage, or limb amputation/mangled limb with multiple bleeding points, to allow immediate management of airway and breathing problems. Following treatment of any airway or breathing problems, the need for a tourniquet can be reassessed in the circulatory assessment and may be converted to a simple method of haemorrhage control.
- Life-threatening limb haemorrhage not controlled by simple methods.
- Point of significant haemorrhage from limb is not peripherally accessible due to entrapment (and therefore it is not possible to initiate simple methods of haemorrhage control such as direct pressure).
- Major incident or multiple casualties with extremity haemorrhage and lack of resources to maintain simple methods of haemorrhage control.

However, incorrectly applied tourniquets can actually increase blood loss if venous, but not arterial, vessels are occluded. This is a risk for tourniquets sited below the knee and elbow joints, which may not be successful in controlling haemorrhage, as the arteries can run or slip between the tibia/fibula and radius/ulna and thus not be compressed by the tourniquet. Even correctly applied tourniquets, if used when not clinically indicated, can cause local tissue injury from direct contact with the tourniquet, and, when left in place for more than two hours, can lead to muscle and skin damage (Walters, 2005). In addition, tourniquets cause severe pain and patients must receive adequate analgesia.

Procedure – Tourniquet Application

The following steps are a suggested method for applying a tourniquet. (SWAST, 2013):

1. Identify the need for a tourniquet during the primary survey, assessing for catastrophic haemorrhage.
2. Apply the tourniquet above the injury, but as close as possible, leaving a gap of at least 5 cm between the injury and the tourniquet, except when injuries are close to the knee and elbow joints. In this case, apply the tourniquet above the joint.
3. Tighten the tourniquet until the bleeding stops.
4. Record the time of tourniquet application.
5. Reassess during the assessment of circulation. If bleeding continues, apply a second tourniquet proximal to the first and over a single bone (i.e. humerus or femur).
6. Frequently reassess and tighten tourniquet as required. Tourniquets are painful and some patients may even try to remove them. Provide analgesia and reassure.

Haemostatic Agents

Where direct pressure and wound packing are ineffective, and in areas such as the groin, neck and axilla, where tourniquet application is not possible, haemostatic agents can be used to control haemorrhage (Greaves, 2008; Cox, 2009; Rossaint, 2010). Haemostatic agents are usually impregnated into a dressing for ease of application. They work by either concentrating clotting factors or acting as a precursor to coagulation, or are mucoadhesive (Figure 17.5) (Granville-Chapman, 2011).

Procedure – Haemostatic Dressing Application

The following steps are a suggested method for applying a haemostatic dressing, but always follow manufacturers' guidelines if they differ to those given below (SWAST, 2016):

1. Locate the source of the bleeding and apply firm pressure with your fingers.
2. Remove any excess blood from the wound.
3. Pack gauze directly onto the bleeding point, ensuring the whole of the wound cavity is tightly packed. Use additional plain gauze

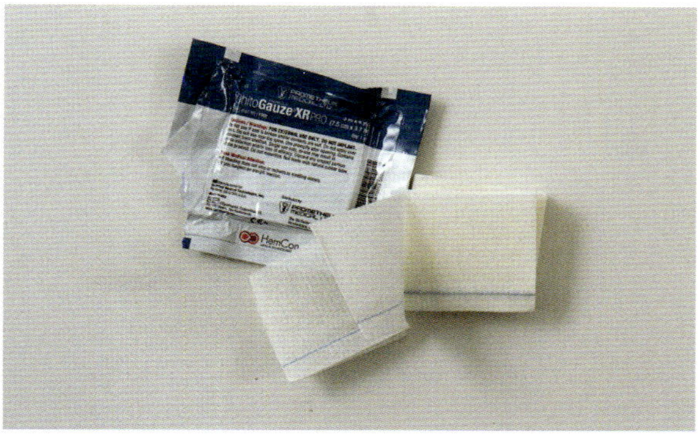

Figure 17.5 A haemostic dressing.

if necessary to achieve this. Do not blindly insert gauze into the thorax or abdomen if you cannot determine the source of the bleeding.

4. Apply firm pressure for 3 minutes, preferably with the help of a pressure dressing, applied circumferentially to the outer part of the gauze. This should help clot formation.
5. If bleeding continues, compress for a further 3 minutes.
6. Leave the gauze in place and if you have not already done so, apply a pressure dressing.

Wounds

A wound is an injury to living tissue, breaking its continuity. There are seven basic categories (Dougherty, 2011; Gregory, 2010b):

- **Contusion (bruises)**: Caused by bleeding from damaged blood vessels under the skin. They cause a bluish/purple discolouration beneath the skin and are typically caused by blunt trauma.
- **Abrasion (grazes)**: Injuries caused by friction shearing the skin away. These usually involve the superficial layers of the skin, but can go much deeper. They can be very painful and are often dirty, with embedded grit and mud.
- **Laceration (tear)**: Tearing or splitting of the skin due to blunt trauma. These cause a ragged wound, which can extend through the skin surface to the underlying structures.
- **Incision (cut)**: A break in the continuity of the skin by a sharp implement, such as broken glass or a knife. These are usually clean wounds (unless the implement is dirty) with neat edges.
- **Puncture (stab)**: A penetrating wound caused by an object that is pointed and narrow, such as a nail or knife. Although these wounds are typically small, they can be deep, causing serious damage to vessels and other body structures below the skin.
- **Burn**: An injury caused by energy transfer to the body's tissues, causing necrosis and an associated inflammatory reaction (covered in the burns section later in this chapter).
- **Gunshot**: A complicated wound caused by a projectile moving at speed. The wound consists of an entry point, with varying amounts of tissue destruction and cavitation underneath the skin, and, if there is sufficient energy left, an exit wound.

There are a range of external and internal factors that can lead to wound formation (Thompson, 2008):

- **External**: Mechanical (friction), chemical, electrical, temperature extremes, radiation and microorganisms.
- **Internal**: Circulatory system failure, endocrine (e.g. diabetes), neuropathy, haematological, malignancy (cancer).

Management

Wound management will be determined by the size and nature of the wound and the presence of complicating factors. The main initial problems are bleeding, pain and the risk of infection (Purcell, 2010). Always enquire about tetanus immunisation in any patient who has a wound with a higher risk of infection, such as a dirty wound, or a wound caused by a bite (human or animal) or involving a puncture by a dirty object (SJA, SAA, BRC, 2014). In addition, consider whether there has been damage to other structures, such as blood vessels, nerves, tendons and ligaments, which can have life-changing consequences if not managed appropriately. For example, consider a pianist who damages her hand causing damage to ligaments. Although the external wound may be minor, without prompt management of the ligamentous injury, her fingers may not function properly in the future.

If the wound is small and bleeding is easily controlled, clean the wound:

- Use a wet gauze to clean the edges of open wounds, wiping away from the wound to avoid contaminating it further. Continue until all visible dirt and blood has been removed.
- Irrigate wounds with tap water as rubbing or scrubbing can cause tissue damage and swabs or cotton wool can leave fibres in the wound.

Once cleaning is complete, cover with a sterile, non-adherent dressing. If the wound is suitable for treatment at home, or at a minor injuries unit, the clinician may advise that a wet dressing be applied over the wound, although this is typically reserved for wounds where treatment will commence promptly (for example within 30–90 minutes) (Pilbery, 2013).

If there is a foreign object in the wound, it should not be removed but left in place, and a sterile, non-adherent dressing applied. Focus your efforts on controlling bleeding and preventing further contamination.

Assessment and Management of the Trauma Patient

Learning Objectives

By the end of this section you will be able to:

- Explain the assessment and management of patients with a range of traumatic injuries.
- Describe the complications associated with a range of traumatic injuries.

Introduction

The approach to the trauma patient is similar to that of all patients, with an initial scene assessment, followed by a primary survey. However, there are some aspects of this process that are specific to trauma and they are going to be covered in this section. In addition, there are a range of complications that can arise as a result of traumatic injury to specific regions and a number of these are going to be covered in this section, specifically injuries to the head, spine, thorax, abdomen and pelvis.

Scene Assessment

The SCENE mnemonic can be used to ensure that you cover all aspects of an initial trauma scene assessment (JRCALC, 2016):

- **S: Safety**. A dynamic risk assessment should highlight current as well as potential dangers. If you are not equipped in terms of kit and expertise to deal with the scene, withdraw and request specialist help. Remember to continually reassess safety as the situation can change quickly. Make sure you are wearing appropriate personal protective equipment (PPE).
- **C: Cause**, including mechanism of injury (MOI). Finding out what happened is important in order to appreciate likely injuries and energy transfer. However, ensure that the scene matches the story you are being told, as you may have come across a crime scene or case of abuse.
- **E: Environment**. Consider whether there are any environmental factors that need to be taken into account. These may complicate your extrication by affecting access to and from the scene and/or increase the risk of harm to the patient, due to increased risk of hypothermia, for example.
- **N: Number of patients**. Determine the number of patients early on in your assessment to help you determine whether you can manage the scene on your own. It may also help to identify patients who have either wandered off from scene or who have been ejected from a vehicle, for example, and are currently hidden from view.
- **E: Extra resources needed**. Depending on the number of patients, the severity of their injuries and the nature of the incident, you may need additional help from other emergency services, such as the police to keep a scene safe, or additional ambulances, including the air ambulance, for patient transport.

Primary Survey

The aim of the primary survey is to identify threats to life promptly and intervene as soon as they are found. The steps of the primary survey should be undertaken sequentially, unless there are enough personnel to allow for simultaneous assessment and treatment (Greaves, 2008).

Procedure

Take the following steps to undertake a primary survey in the trauma patient:

1. **General impression**: As you approach the patient, perform a global assessment. Are they sitting up and watching you approach, with well-perfused skin, or are they lying unresponsive, pale and clammy with an expanding pool of blood leaking from a wound?
2. **Catastrophic haemorrhage**: This is bleeding that is likely to cause death within minutes, so cannot wait until airway and breathing have been addressed. Typically, bleeding can be controlled with direct pressure and elevation

of the bleeding site, but may require the use of a tourniquet (see the section on wounds and bleeding in this chapter).

3. **Airway with cervical spine consideration**: If a patient has suffered significant blunt trauma or the MOI suggests that the cervical spine may have been damaged, provide prompt manual in-line stabilisation. Assess the airway by looking for obvious obstruction, listening for noisy airflow (snoring or gurgling) and feeling for air movement.
4. Manage the airway using appropriate airway manoeuvres, such as:
   - jaw thrust–chin lift
   - suction
   - naso- and oropharyngeal airways.
5. **Breathing**: Administer high-flow oxygen to patients to obtain a target saturation of 94–98%, even if they have COPD.
6. Examine the neck for:
   - **T**: tracheal deviation
   - **W**: wounds and swellings
   - **E**: emphysema (surgical/subcutaneous)
   - **L**: laryngeal crepitus
   - **V**: veins (distended jugular veins).
7. If you have enough personnel, a cervical collar can be applied, if appropriate.
8. Look for obvious chest injuries, wounds, bruising or flail segments. Assess the rate, depth and quality of respiration:
   - Ventilate with a BVM if respirations are absent or less than 10 breaths/min.
   - If respirations are greater than 30 breaths/min, it may also be clinically appropriate to ventilate the patient.
   - If respirations are 10–30 breaths/min, monitor closely.
9. Feel for equality of chest movement and note any instability.
10. Manage breathing problems as you find them. This may include (depending on local guidance):
    - applying non-occlusive dressings to sucking chest wounds
    - positioning to support a patient with a flail segment (not possible if the patient has a suspected spinal injury).
11. **Circulation**: If a catastrophic haemorrhage was encountered at the start of the primary survey, reassess this now.
12. Assess both central and distal pulses (carotid and radial, typically), noting rate, rhythm and volume. Note the skin colour, temperature and the presence of clamminess. If additional personnel are available, the blood pressure can also be measured.
13. Assess for signs of blood loss, remembering the phrase 'blood on the floor plus four more':
    - **Externally**: Don't forget to consider bleeding into clothing, splints and dressings.
    - **Chest**: Completed during assessment of breathing.
    - **Abdomen**: Look for bruising or external marks and feel for rigidity and to elicit tenderness.
    - **Pelvis**: This should not be manipulated or 'sprung' to assess for instability. The MOI is sufficient to immobilise the pelvis.
    - **Long bones**: Assess long bones, particularly the femurs, but do not be distracted by fractures at this stage.
14. Manage bleeding appropriately. Ideally splint pelvic fractures prior to moving the patient. Limb fractures can wait until you are en-route if the patient is critically injured.
15. A clinician on scene may wish to gain intravenous access now if fluids and/or tranexamic acid are required.
16. To minimise clot disruption, patient movement should be kept to a minimum.
17. **Disability**: Assess level of consciousness with AVPU, and pupil size, equality and reaction to light. Don't forget to check the blood glucose if authorised.
18. **Exposure/environment**: Take care to prevent hypothermia, as this can dramatically increase mortality (up to 3 times higher if core body temperature drops below 35°C (Ireland, 2011)). It may be more appropriate to remove patients to a heated ambulance before completing this step.

Head Injuries

Common causes of traumatic brain injury (TBI) include road traffic collisions, direct blows to the head, falls from heights and sports-related injuries. The worst outcomes are associated with (Moppett, 2007):

- penetrating injuries
- non-accidental injury in children aged under 5 years
- pedestrians and pedal cyclists
- ejection from a vehicle.

Recognition

Suggestive signs and symptoms of TBI include (Pante, 2010):

- lacerations, contusions or haematomas to the scalp
- boggy areas when palpating the scalp
- visible fractures or deformity of the skull
- Battle's sign or 'panda eyes' (not apparent for several hours)
- cerebrospinal fluid and/or blood leaking from the nose or ears
- Cushing's triad: rising blood pressure, reducing heart rate and irregular respirations
- dizziness
- nausea and vomiting
- abnormal pupils and/or pupil reaction
- visual disturbances (double or blurred vision, seeing 'stars')
- severe headache
- altered level of consciousness
- perseveration (repeatedly asking the same questions)
- amnesia
- paraesthesia/paralysis of the extremities
- convulsions
- posturing
- abnormal respirations.

Management

The mainstay of management for patients with TBI is preventing hypoxia, treating hypotension and transporting patients quickly to definitive care. There is a link between head injury and injury of the cervical spine, so an assumption of spinal injury should be made, unless an ambulance clinician is on scene and, having examined the patient, is confident that a cervical spine injury is not present (NICE, 2014).

Airway compromise is common after severe TBI and needs to be managed with gentle suction. Provide 100% oxygen via a non-rebreathe mask and aim for oxygen saturations of 94–98% (JRCALC, 2016). Continuous monitoring of oxygen saturations is important. Assess adequacy of ventilation and provide assistance if required.

A single drop of systolic blood pressure to less than 90 mmHg doubles the patient's risk of death (Moppett, 2007). Make sure you share any blood pressures that you have recorded with the ambulance clinicians on scene.

Maxillofacial Injuries

Maxillofacial injury (i.e. involving the maxilla and/or face but referred to as just facial injury in this chapter) is common, with an estimated 500,000 facial injuries occurring each year in the UK, 180,000 of them serious (requiring specialist treatment or hospital admission). The commonest causes include falls (39%), assault (31%) and road traffic collisions (RTCs, 3%) (Jalo, 2009). There are regional variations: for example, a Scottish study found nearly 62% of facial injuries were caused by alleged assault (Hutchison, 2012). Alcohol is a common factor, particularly in assaults, where over 50% of patients had consumed alcohol in the preceding 4 hours (Hutchison, 1998).

Facial Structures and Injuries

Orbit

A blow to the eye can cause the orbit to 'blow out' and fracture. The most common location for this to occur is the inferior portion (floor). This injury may not necessarily lead to any external tenderness, but signs and symptoms of a blowout fracture include (Purcell, 2010; NAEMT, 2014):

- enophthalmos: the eyeball retracts into its socket
- double vision (diplopia) and/or loss of upward vision
- pupils at a different horizontal level to each other
- loss of sensation above eyebrow and over cheek.

Zygoma

Fractures of the zygoma, typically caused by assault and RTCs, lead to a depression of the cheek. They are commonly associated with orbital fractures, ocular injury and epistaxis (Purcell, 2010). Paraesthesia may be present as in orbit injury (Greaves, 2008).

Maxilla

The maxilla is most commonly fractured by RTCs, but other blunt injury causes include assault and sport injuries. Maxilla fractures are often associated with injuries to other middle facial structures.

Since the base of the skull is sloping, the bones forming the middle third of the face have a tendency to slide backwards and downwards, obstructing the airway and causing an anterior open bite, which splints the front teeth open (Greaves, 2008).

Mandible

The mandible and its associated structures form the lower third of the face. The necks of the mandibular condyles are a point of weakness and are often fractured following blunt trauma to the chin. The combination of bilateral condylar and midline (symphyseal) mandibular fractures is sometimes referred to as a guardsman's fracture.

Teeth

Teeth are frequently avulsed (knocked out) as a result of facial trauma, and can be inhaled if the patient is unconscious. In addition, avulsed teeth can displace into the soft tissues, including the lips. A fracture to the crown of a tooth is extremely painful and may prove to be the patient's main complaint.

Soft Tissue

The facial tissues have an abundant blood supply, which can lead to dramatic-looking wounds and bleeding. However, it is uncommon for these to result in hypovolaemia (except in children) and other causes should be assumed to be responsible, particularly in the initial stages of your assessment. Large lacerations on the face often gape due to muscle pull and those in the middle third of the face can swell rapidly, masking underlying fractures. If swelling involves the eyelids, this can prevent examination of the globe of the eye, potentially hiding damage to the patient's vision (Pilbery, 2013; NAEMT, 2014).

Management: General

The management of facial injuries follows the same principles as for any trauma patient, but the airway is likely to occupy a significant portion of your time. Follow the standard CABCDE approach, although note that catastrophic haemorrhage in isolated facial trauma is unlikely unless major arteries of the neck are involved.

Generally, patients with facial injuries are best managed sitting up and leaning forward, to allow for drainage of blood and debris from the mouth and reduce venous return. Cervical spine injury needs to be considered, but arguably, any conscious patient who asks to sit up should be allowed to do so on the basis of the following (Perry, 2008):

- A talking patient has intact airway reflexes and will be able to protect their airway if sitting forward.
- To be able to sit up, the patient requires sufficient muscle tone that will provide spinal stability.
- Persistent/repeated requests to sit up are an indication of either impending airway compromise or the desire to vomit, requests that can be misinterpreted as the patient being 'difficult' due to alcohol or brain injury.
- Spinal immobilisation is only appropriate for co-operative or unconscious patients. Agitated patients or those who actively resist your attempts to immobilise them should be left to adopt a position they choose. Forcible restraint against active movement increases forces applied to a potentially unstable spine.
- As always, follow local guidance and procedure.

Management: Airway

Unconscious Patients

Clear any debris from the mouth (e.g. broken teeth) using forceps or a careful finger sweep and suction. Although cervical spine injury needs to be considered, the lack of a patent airway will kill the patient first, and if neck movement is required then this is acceptable, although it is reasonable to try and keep this to a minimum (Kovacs, 2011). Even a jaw thrust results in some cervical spine movement, albeit less than a head tilt–chin lift manoeuvre (Prasarn, 2014). However, these can be difficult to perform in patients who have a face covered in blood.

If the maxilla has moved posteriorly, reduce it by holding the upper jaw and pulling forward firmly. If the mandible has become displaced due to bilateral condylar fractures, then this too should be reduced as the tongue is likely to end up resting on the posterior wall of the oropharynx, increasing the risk of airway occlusion. This can be achieved by pulling forward on the mandible and, if necessary, taking hold of the tongue with some gauze, although this position will have to be maintained (Greaves, 2008).

Oropharyngeal airways (OPAs) are not always helpful in facial injuries as they can easily dislodge, particularly with the alterations in airway anatomy that occur with facial fractures. In addition, they are not suitable for responsive patients. Nasopharyngeal airways (NPAs) are generally better tolerated, but should be used with caution in patients with fractures to the middle third of the face, as these are associated with fractures to the base of the skull. The use of a bag-valve-mask can also be challenging with fractures of the mid-face as the application of the mask to the face can displace the fractures and further occlude the airway. However, in serious facial injuries the real enemy is bleeding, and neither an OPA nor an NPA will prevent aspiration, and both can block with clots and other debris.

Conscious Patients

In awake supine patients, facial bleeding may not be obvious if the patient is able to swallow the blood. This is problematic as it increases the risk of the patient vomiting. Conversely, patients with mandibular fractures may actually have trouble swallowing efficiently, leading to difficulty in keeping the airway clear. Be wary of patients on anti-coagulants ('blood-thinning' medication), as significant airway-threatening swelling can occur, even in the absence of fractures. Retropharyngeal swelling is important to note as it is also a marker for cervical spine injury (Perry, 2008).

Watch for repeated requests/attempts to sit up. This may be a sign that your patient is going to vomit.

Management: Breathing

This should be managed as for other traumatic injuries, although facial injuries sustained as a result of a road traffic collision are often accompanied by chest and abdominal injuries, including diaphragmatic rupture.

Management: Circulation

With the exception of significant middle third fractures, bleeding from facial injuries is unlikely to lead to hypovolaemic shock, so look for an alternative cause. Mid-face fractures can be tricky, as this portion of the face has an extensive collateral supply from the internal and external carotid arteries. Reducing maxilla fractures may assist in staunching haemorrhage, which can be otherwise difficult to control. Asking the patient to bite on gauze may help, but nasal bleeding needs to be controlled with anterior and posterior nasal packing, if available.

Management: Disability

Many patients with facial injuries are going to be under the influence of alcohol, but don't assume that the abnormal neurology they display is due to this (and don't forget the blood sugar measurement either). If in doubt, treat agitation as a sign of hypoxia, unresponsiveness as a sign of hypercarbia, and cyanosis as hypoxaemia secondary to inadequate oxygenation (Ceallaigh, 2006).

Pupil signs can be misleading if the patient has cranio-orbital trauma, as mydriasis (pupil dilation) can occur even in the absence of raised intracranial pressure. Soft tissue swelling of the eyelids can prevent the eye being seen at all. In this case, holding a pen torch against the swollen eyelid can at least assist in the detection of blindness.

Speech is often poor and/or slurred, secondary to either alcohol, facial fractures, tongue swelling and/or dental malocclusion, so don't rush in deciding that your patient is FAST positive.

Specific Management: Eye Injuries

Eye injuries can be categorised into four types (Purcell, 2010):

- chemical burns
- corneal abrasions
- blunt trauma
- foreign bodies.

Chemicals splashed into the eye should generally be considered to be an emergency, as they can lead to severe corneal injury and blindness (Purcell, 2010). Ensure that you do not get contaminated by wearing the appropriate PPE, and then irrigate the eye with copious amounts of water, ensuring that you do not contaminate the unaffected eye. Don't waste time identifying the chemical at the expense of starting irrigation. In some work settings, specific antidotes may be available and can be used in place of water (Zideman, 2015).

A corneal abrasion is a superficial injury to the surface of the cornea. It can be caused by a foreign body, leaves or branches, fingernails and contact lenses, for example. This is not normally a serious injury, but is often very painful. Patients will require an ophthalmic assessment, but this may be able to be performed by a local minor injuries unit or advanced practitioners from the ambulance service. Similar injuries can be caused by flash burns. These are a form of radiation burn caused by sun lamps or a welder's flash, for example. However, the onset of pain and other symptoms can take several hours to develop (Purcell, 2010).

Blunt trauma to the eye is typically caused by mechanisms such as a blow from a fist or a small ball (for example a squash ball). It's important to assess visual acuity, and is typically undertaken with a Snellen chart – a chart containing letters of reducing size. This can be approximated, by asking the patient to read text from a book or newspaper, for example. Even if their vision appears unaffected, they still require a thorough eye examination.

Foreign bodies such as grit or a loose eyelash can safely be rinsed out of the eye. If the object is in the upper eyelid, instruct the patient to grasp the eyelashes of their upper eyelid and gently pull it over the lower lid (SJA, SAA, BRC, 2014). Any foreign bodies that are embedded in the cornea or are intraocular should not be removed, and the patient should be taken to hospital.

Specific Management: Nosebleed

A nosebleed, or epistaxis, is a common occurrence with multiple causes, including (Pope, 2005):

- direct trauma to the nose
- nose picking
- infection
- bleeding disorders, such as haemophilia
- anti-coagulant and anti-platelet drugs, such as warfarin and aspirin.

The source of bleeding in children and young adults is usually from the anterior portion of the nasal septum (called Little's area), whereas bleeding in older adults can occur anteriorly and posteriorly, which is more difficult to access (Purcell, 2010).

Assessment

Obtain a good history. This will provide clues as to whether this is a one-off occurrence due to aggressive nose picking, for example, or due to the patient having high blood pressure and poorly controlled anti-coagulant drug therapy.

Management

Take the following steps to control a nose bleed (Purcell, 2010):

1. Instruct the patient to sit down and lean forward to reduce the likelihood of blood entering the oropharynx and being swallowed.
2. Ask the patient to squeeze the soft part of their nose for 10 minutes. They must not release the pressure before this time.
3. Advise patients to breathe through their mouth and gently spit blood out of their mouth, rather than swallow it, as this can lead to vomiting.
4. Once 10 minutes are up, instruct the patient to release the pressure and see if the bleeding has stopped. If bleeding continues, reapply pressure for a further 10 minutes and reassess. If bleeding continues, reapply pressure for a further 10 minutes.
5. If bleeding continues for more than 30 minutes, appears to be from a posterior bleeding point, or the patient is on anti-coagulant medication, transport the patient to hospital unless you have access to advanced practitioners who can pack the nose.

Spinal Injuries

Spinal injuries, or more specifically spinal cord injuries (SCI), are rare, with around 1,000 new cases per year (Harrison, 2007). In adult major trauma, approximately 10% of patients will sustain a spinal fracture/dislocation, but less than 2% will sustain an SCI. The most common cause is a fall (46%), although, significantly, a third of these are falls of less than 2 m in height. Falls are closely followed in frequency by road traffic collisions (RTCs, 40%), whereas the other causes, such as sports injuries (under 3%), stabbings (1%) and shootings (0.6%), are much rarer. SCIs most commonly occur at the cervical level (45%), followed by thoracic (29%), lumbar (24%) and multi-level injuries (2%) (Hasler, 2011).

Risk factors for SCI include (Hasler, 2011):

- male sex
- under 45 years of age
- reduced Glasgow Coma Scale score
- accompanying chest injury
- dangerous mechanism (falls greater than 2 m, sports injury, RTC, shooting).

Recognition

The signs and symptoms also depend on the completeness of the SCI. The classic picture in complete SCI is vasodilation, flaccidity of muscles and loss of sensation below the injury, as well as loss of temperature regulation mechanisms such as vasodilation and sweating. This can lead to a poikilothermic state, where the body adopts the temperature of the surrounding environment (whether hot or cold). Depending on how high the SCI injury is, the blood pressure can dramatically fall – for example to 80 mmHg systolic in high cervical injuries – but there is no compensatory tachycardia, since the sympathetic signals are blocked. In fact, parasympathetic division dominance leads to bradycardia, further reducing cardiac output. In an incomplete SCI, there is a mixed picture of paralysis and paraesthesia, but not profound hypotension or bradycardia, making the absence of these signs unreliable in excluding SCI in unconscious patients (Harrison, 2007).

Management

All patients who are suspected of having a spinal injury should be immobilised as soon as possible. Remember that the whole spine must be immobilised. The techniques and equipment involved in order to perform this safely are described in the skeletal immobilisation section of this chapter (JRCALC, 2016).

Patients with isolated penetrating trauma to the head or limbs do not require immobilisation, but if, in torso or neck trauma, it is possible that the projectile could have passed near or through the spinal cord and there are signs of spinal cord injury, then immobilisation is appropriate.

In blunt trauma, there are guidelines that allow clinicians to discontinue immobilisation, so you may on occasion be asked to stop immobilising a patient once a thorough assessment has been completed (JRCALC, 2016).

Thoracic Injuries

Figures 17.6-17.8

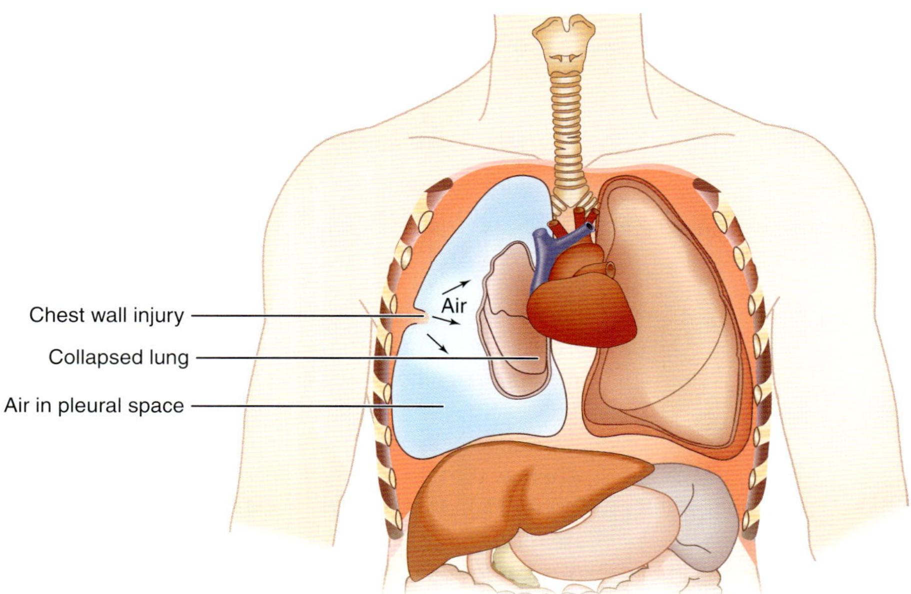

Figure 17.6 *An open pneumothorax. A penetrating chest injury has resulted in an opening between the outside and inside of the chest wall.*

Thoracic trauma accounts for 25–50% of all trauma and is a contributing factor to around half the deaths through injury. Major causes are road traffic collisions, industrial accidents and domestic and sporting injuries (Greaves, 2008). The most common problem associated with severe thoracic injury is hypoxia (JRCALC, 2016).

Pneumothorax

The lungs are surrounded by a pleural membrane. The outer layer (parietal pleura) lines the chest wall, and the inner layer (visceral pleura) covers the lungs. Between them is the pleural space, which is lubricated to ensure that the surfaces glide

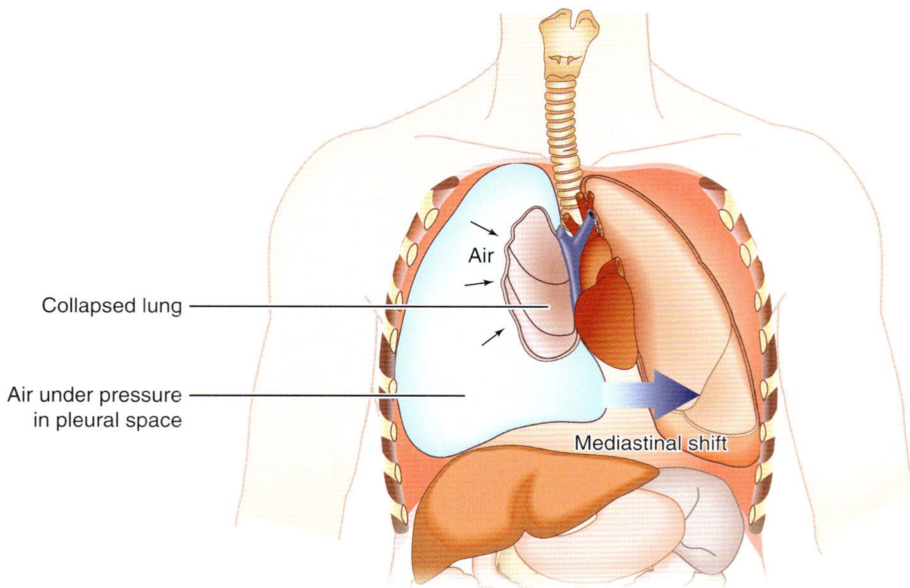

Figure 17.7 *A tension pneumothorax.*

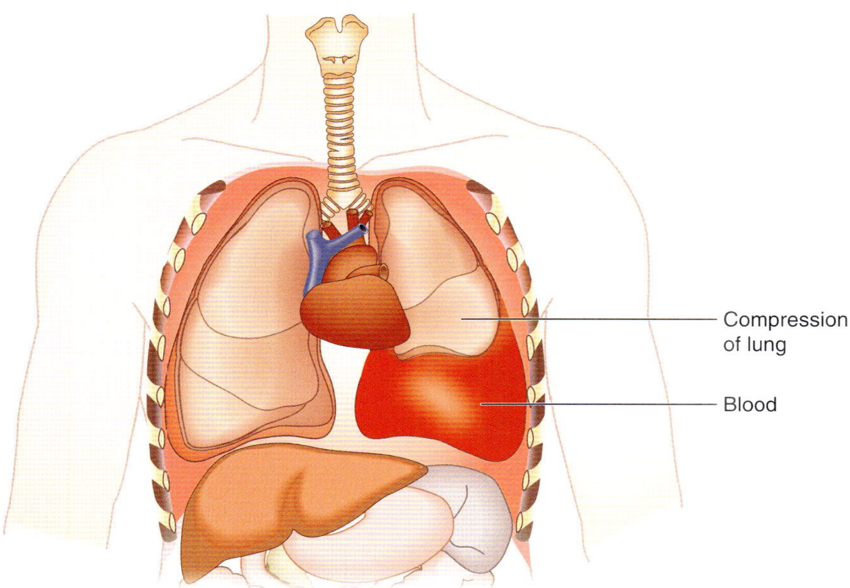

Figure 17.8 *A haemothorax.*

smoothly over one another, as well as creating a surface tension that results in the surfaces 'sticking together.'

Pneumothorax, or air in the pleural space, is generally classified as being spontaneous, if there is no obvious causal factor, or traumatic, if there is an external cause (Noppen, 2010). If air within the alveoli can escape into the pleural space, or there is an external breach of the thoracic cavity allowing atmospheric air to enter the pleural space, the normal physiology of ventilation is disrupted and the lung collapses.

Traumatic pneumothoraces are caused by penetrating trauma (such as stab and gunshot wounds or impalements), blunt trauma that leads to rib fractures and increased intrathoracic pressure, and bronchial rupture and barotrauma, where changes in pressure of the air delivered to the lungs leads to expansion (Figure 17.6). This phenomenon has been reported in air crew and SCUBA divers (Sharma, 2008).

Assessment

Arguably, the most important type of pneumothorax to recognise is one under tension (Figure 17.7). However, the clinical course of a tension pneumothorax is not the same for all patients, with the progression of clinical deterioration for an awake, spontaneously breathing patient likely to be considerably longer than for those who are being ventilated with positive-pressure ventilation (Leigh-Smith, 2005).

Signs and symptoms of a tension pneumothorax in awake patients include:

- pleuritic chest pain (sharp pain, worse on breathing in and out)
- air hunger
- respiratory distress
- tachypnoea (rapid breathing rate)
- tachycardia (rapid heart rate)
- falling oxygen saturations (SpO_2)
- agitation
- on the same side as the injury:
    - hyper-expansion
    - hypo-mobility
    - decreased breath sounds
- pre-terminal (near death):
    - decreasing respiratory rate
    - hypotension
    - decreasing level of consciousness.

Management

Patients with a simple pneumothorax with no signs of cardiovascular compromise, suggesting tension, can be managed conservatively out-of-hospital, but should be closely monitored en-route to hospital (Lee, 2007a). All patients with a pneumothorax should receive oxygen at the appropriate target range (usually 94–98%, except for patients at risk of carbon dioxide retention, who should be managed at either 88–92% or their usual range (JRCALC, 2016)). If there is an open pneumothorax, apply a commercial chest seal, if you have one. Alternatively, leave the wound open or apply a non-occlusive dressing (Zideman, 2015).

Haemothorax

Haemothorax, or blood in the thoracic cavity, usually occurs as a result of penetrating trauma (Figure 17.8). Life-threatening haemorrhage can occur in cases of severe lacerations of the lung, large vessels in the mediastinum and the heart. Each hemithorax (literally, half of the chest) can easily accommodate half of the patient's circulating blood volume before the physical signs are obvious (Greaves, 2008).

However, this amount of bleeding will lead to the signs and symptoms of shock, and since blood occupies space usually reserved for the lung, lung collapse occurs, leading to absent or decreased lung sounds and reduced chest wall expansion on the injured side (Greaves, 2008).

There are few treatment options available outside of hospital; usually, expedient transport to the nearest major trauma centre is indicated.

Flail Chest

Blunt chest trauma can lead to multiple rib and sternal fractures. In the event that two or more ribs are broken in two or more places, the chest wall will lose the rigid structure that usually supports the chest. A flail segment will start to move paradoxically, that is, it will move inwards during inspiration and outwards on expiration. If this area is large enough, it results in compromised ventilation. However, it is usually bruising of the underlying lung that leads to hypoxia and there can also be significant blood loss, with each rib fracture causing around 100 ml of blood loss (Greaves, 2008).

The flail segment is not always obvious, as muscular spasm can support the segment until the muscles are exhausted. Do not attempt to splint the flail segment, as this is likely to further impair ventilation (NAEMT, 2014).

Abdominal Injuries

The abdominal cavity extends from the diaphragm to the pelvic bones and from the vertebral column to the muscles of the abdomen and flanks (Figure 17.9). Organs are classed as peritoneal if they are covered by a lining called the peritoneum. These include the spleen, liver, stomach, gallbladder, the tail of the pancreas, parts of the large intestine and most of the small intestine, and the female reproductive organs (NAEMT, 2014). The retroperitoneal space is the area behind the peritoneum. This area contains the kidneys, ureters, pancreas (except the tail), parts of the small and large intestine and the aorta and inferior vena cava (JRCALC, 2016).

In blunt trauma, the spleen, liver and structures that are firmly fixed, such as the retroperitoneal organs, are most commonly injured due to shearing forces associated with rapid deceleration. Penetrating trauma can also cause serious damage and severe bleeding. Depending on the angle at which the penetrating object enters, thoracic injury is also possible, particularly in upper abdominal stab injuries (NAEMT, 2014).

Patients suffering from abdominal trauma may not exhibit many symptoms initially, although you should suspect internal injury in any shocked patient with a suggestive mechanism of injury. Look at the abdomen for signs of injury, such as bruising, abrasions and seat belt marks. Gently feel the abdomen for signs of tenderness, but don't be reassured by a normal examination (JRCALC, 2016).

There is no specific management of blunt abdominal trauma, but in penetrating trauma, if the injury has caused the bowel to protrude out of the abdomen, you should not push it back in. Instead, cover it with a dressing soaked in warm saline (NAEMT, 2014).

If the penetrating object is still in place in the patient's abdomen, do not attempt to remove it. Instead, secure it appropriately, although if it is pulsating, allow some movement of the object, but not its removal (JRCALC, 2016).

Pelvic Injuries

Fractures of the pelvic ring are uncommon, with around for 20–37 per 100,000 people suffering a fracture, about 2–8% of all skeletal injuries (Garlapati, 2012; McCormack, 2010). However, pelvic fractures are found in up to 20% of injuries involving a significant mechanism of injury resulting in multiple injuries. The major cause in the younger population is road traffic collisions (RTCs), with around 44–64% of pelvic ring fractures due to the patient being involved in an RTC. Vehicle speed and compartmental intrusion are important factors (Adams, 2002). The overall mortality rate is around 12%, although it can be as high as 50% for open pelvic fractures (Lee, 2007c).

All pelvic fractures cause some bleeding, although the source can vary. Bleeding from cancellous bone that has been fractured is common, but bleeding can also occur from lacerations to retroperitoneal veins and the internal iliac arteries. Arterial bleeding accounts for up to 25% of haemodynamically unstable pelvic ring fractures (McCormack, 2010), but most bleeding is, in fact, low-pressure bleeding (i.e. not arterial) and usually responds well to appropriate stabilisation (such as with a pelvic binder or external fixator) and tamponade (Abrassart, 2013).

Associated Abdominal Injuries

As well as the potential vascular damage that pelvic ring fractures can cause, the soft tissues are also vulnerable, and injuries to the anorectum, vagina, urethra and nerves can occur. The most common is bladder injury, typically caused by compression or tearing of the bladder wall. Urethral and anorectal

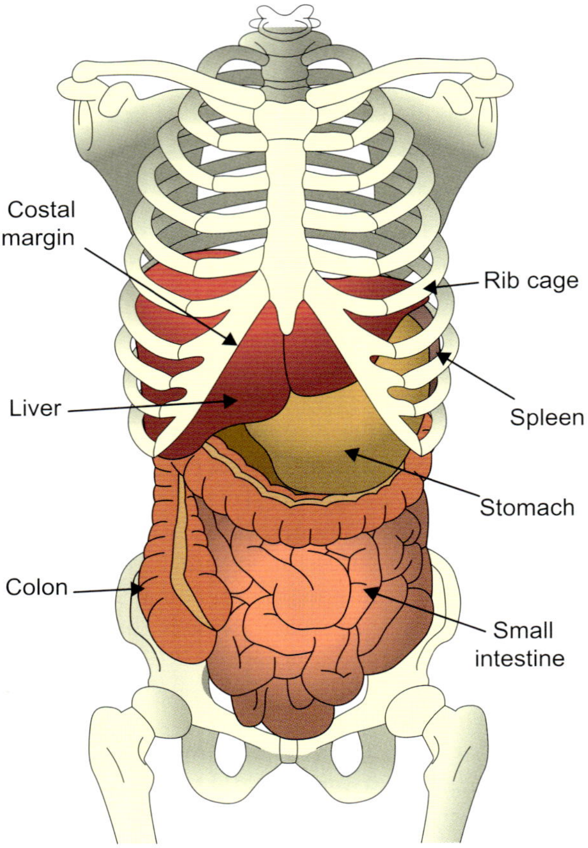

Figure 17.9 *The abdominal cavity.*

injuries are more common with straddle injuries, for example when a motorcyclist straddles the fuel tank during an RTC, resulting in the separation of the two pelvic bones and severe tearing of the pelvic floor (Luke, 2010).

Pelvic Binders

If you decide to apply a pelvic binder, make sure it is positioned correctly. Generally, the binder should be placed over the greater trochanters, but it is commonly placed too high (Bonner, 2011), such as over the iliac crests, which can actually compound pelvic fractures. Pelvic binders should be placed directly against the patient's skin. As with cervical collars, pelvic binders are not risk-free, so consider whether their application is appropriate. Follow local guidance for application of pelvic binders.

Fractures and Dislocations

A fracture is a break (or breaks) in a bone. There are a number of types (Figure 17.10) (Pilbery, 2013):

- **Transverse**: A single horizontal break through the bone, splitting it into two parts.
- **Comminuted**: A fracture that results in the bone being split into more than two parts.
- **Oblique**: The bone is broken diagonally along its shaft.
- **Spiral**: Caused by a twisting force.
- **Open**: Sometimes called a compound fracture. A fracture with a wound at the site of the injury caused by bone pushing through the skin.
- **Closed**: Sometimes called simple fracture. A fracture where no puncturing of the skin has occurred.
- **Greenstick**: An incomplete fracture where only one side of the periosteum fractures. This fracture is common in children because their bones are soft and porous.

A dislocation is an abnormal separation of joint surfaces. They can occur in isolation, or be associated with a fracture (or fractures). Since joints are kept in place by soft tissues such as ligaments, these will have been injured for a dislocation to have occurred. Prompt reduction of the dislocation to its original anatomical position is required, following analgesia and/or a local anaesthetic. A competent clinician is required for this procedure.

The management of fractures and dislocations follows the standard primary and secondary survey for the trauma patient, but specifically consider:

- splinting the affected limb
- providing analgesia: these injuries can be very painful
- covering open fractures with a sterile dressing.

Sprains and Strains

Sprains are ligamental injuries, that involve a partial or complete (depending on severity) tear of the ligament, whereas strains are tears in muscles. Their management is essentially the same, and consists of (Polzer, 2011):

- **P**: Protect the limb from further injury.
- **R**: Rest the injured limb.

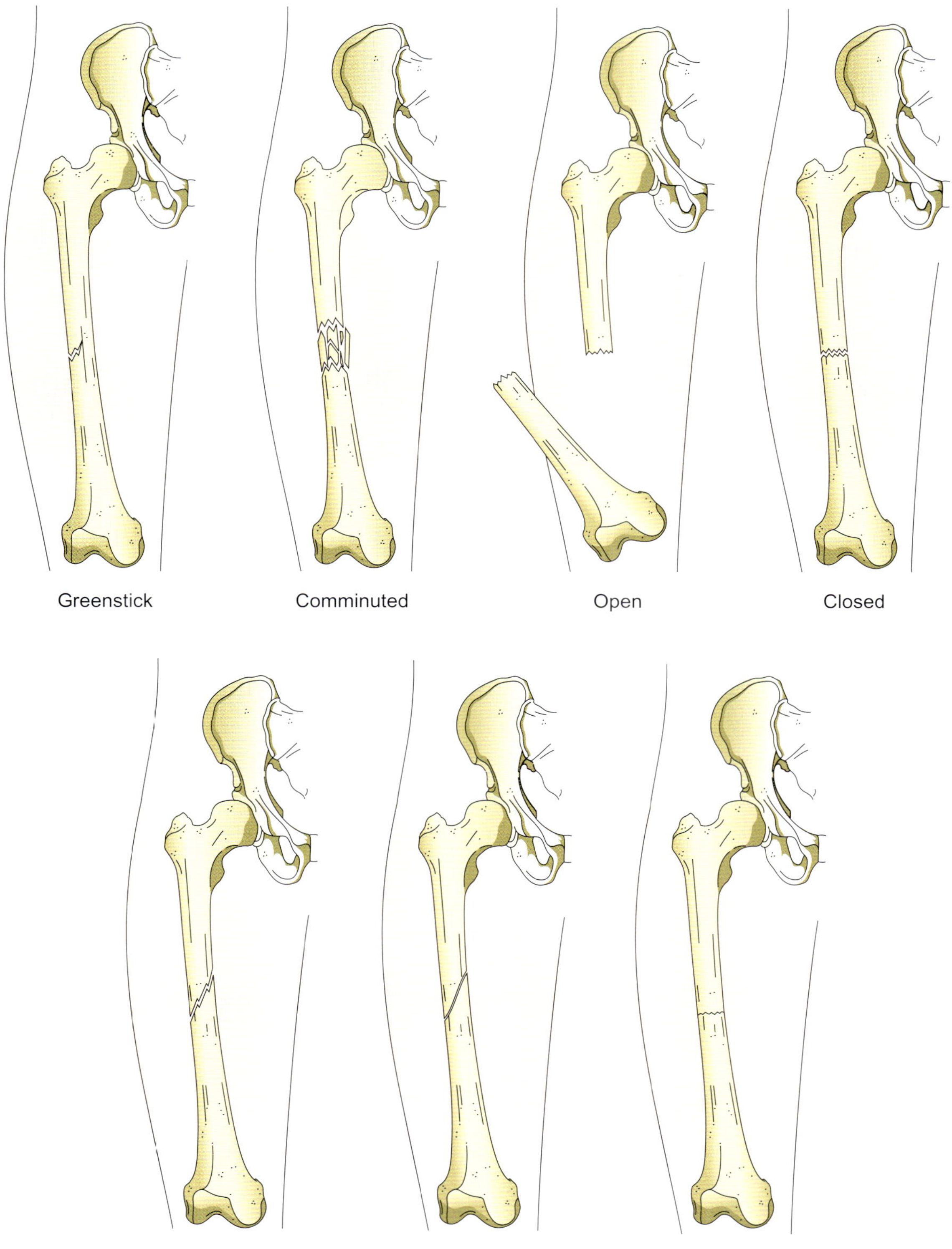

Figure 17.10 *Types of fractures.*

- **I**: Ice wrapped in a damp towel should be applied to the injury for 15–20 minutes.
- **C**: Compress with a simple elastic bandage or elasticated tubular bandage, which should be snug, but not tight.
- **E**: Elevate the limb above the level of the heart.

Skeletal Immobilisation

Learning Objective

By the end of this section you will be able to:

- Describe how to perform a range of skeletal immobilisation techniques.

Introduction

Skeletal immobilisation is an important skill to learn and has the following benefits when performed correctly (NAEMT, 2014; Greaves, 2008):

- reduces pain
- reduces risk of further damage to soft tissues, nerves and blood vessels
- helps to control bleeding
- reduces risk of fat embolism.

In this section you will learn how to perform the following techniques and/or use the equipment listed:

- first-aid techniques:
    - triangular bandages
- spinal immobilisation:
    - manual methods
    - cervical collar application
    - crash helmet removal
    - spinal board
    - orthopaedic (scoop) stretcher
- using splints:
    - box splint
    - pelvic splint
    - traction splint.

First-Aid Techniques

Effective splinting does not always require expensive equipment, which may or may not be available. Sometimes, it is preferable to use basic first-aid methods, such as triangular bandaging for the management of upper limb injuries.

Triangular Bandages

Triangular bandages have three main uses and can be:

- folded as a broad- or narrow-fold bandage to immobilise and support a limb or to secure a splint or bulky dressing
- opened to form a sling
- folded into a pad and used as a dressing.

You are most likely to use a sling to hold an injured limb close to the body and take some of the weight off that limb to prevent pain (Gregory, 2010b).

Spinal Immobilisation

Spinal immobilisation should be considered for any trauma patient with (EEAST, 2014):

- a mechanism of injury consistent with spinal injury (mechanism may be minimal in the elderly or those with fragility conditions, e.g. osteoporosis)

Procedure – Arm Sling

Take the following steps to apply an arm sling (SJA, SAA, BRC, 2014; Gregory, 2010b):

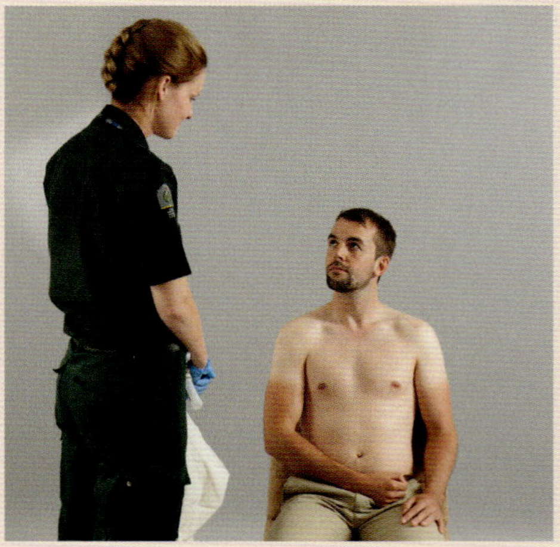

1. Explain the procedure to the patient and obtain informed consent. Provide analgesia as required to enable the sling to be applied. Prepare the triangular bandage.

Procedure – *cont*

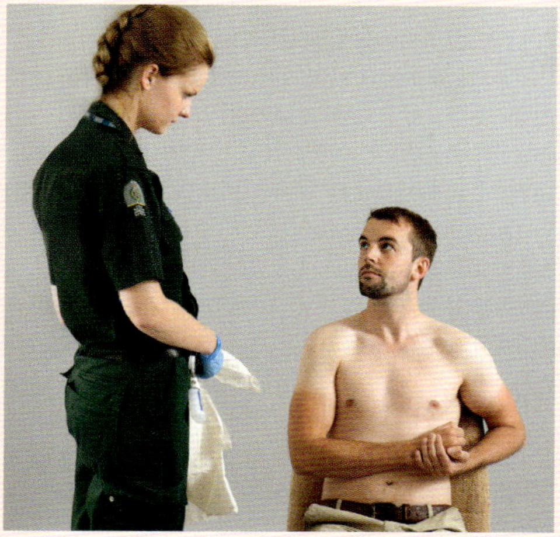

2. Ask the patient to support their injured arm with the uninjured arm and flex the elbow to 90° if possible.

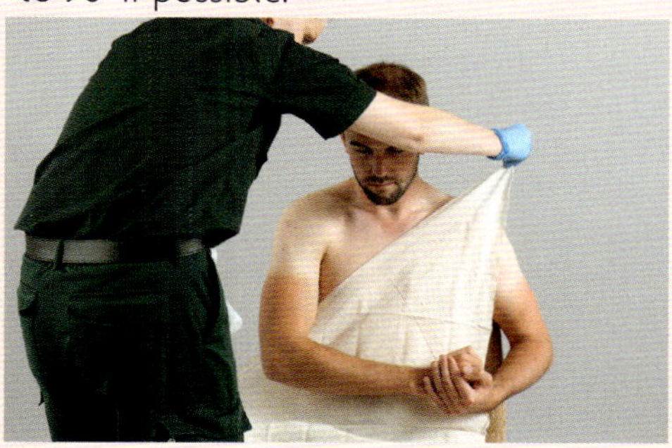

3. Slide the triangular bandage under the patient's arms so that the point is under the injured arm and the base (the long edge) is on the side of the uninjured arm.

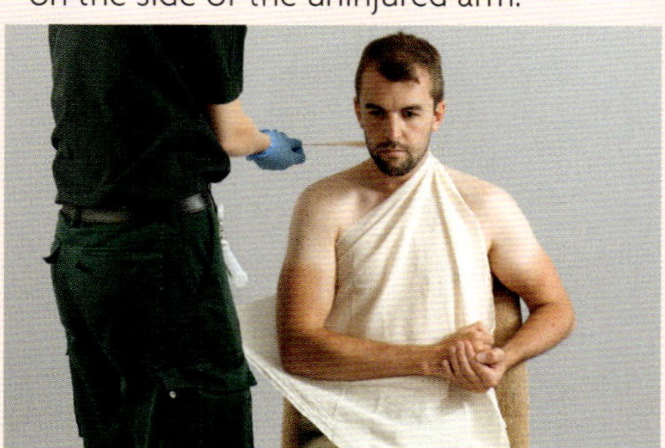

4. Slide the upper end of the triangular bandage around the neck towards the shoulder on the injured side.

Procedure – *cont*

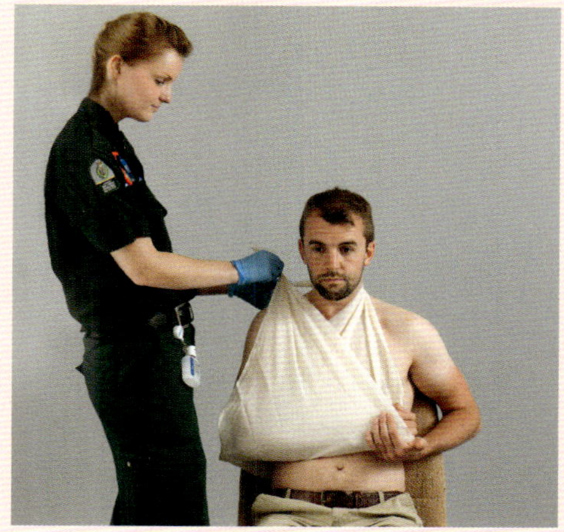

5. Fold the lower end of the bandage up over the forearm and bring it to meet the other end of the bandage at the shoulder.

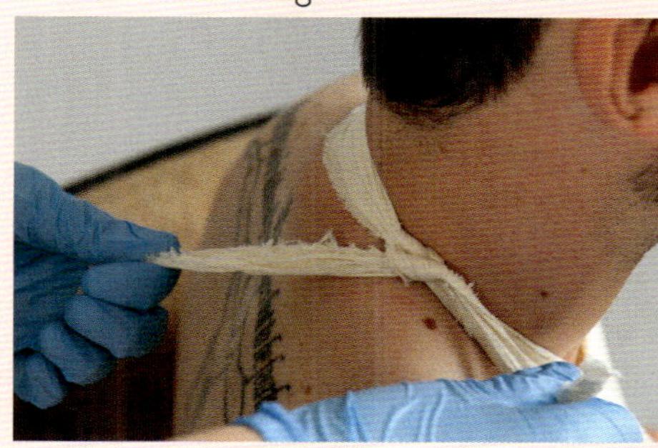

6. Tie the ends together using a reef knot. Consider applying a pad under the knot, if required.

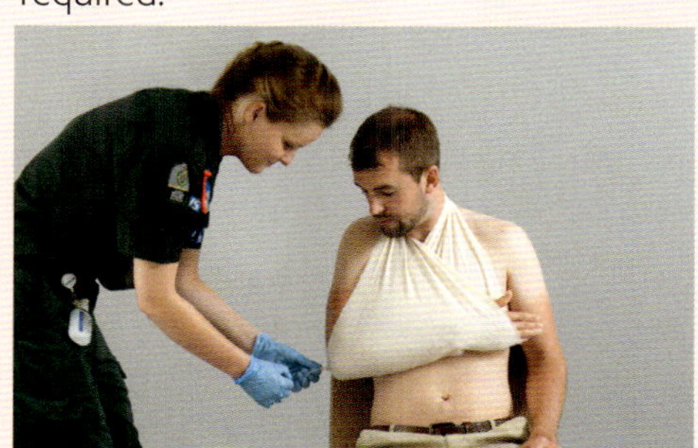

7. Holding the point of the bandage beyond the elbow, twist the point of the bandage until it fits the elbow snugly, then tuck it

(*continued*)

Procedure – *cont*

into the bandage. An alternative is to use tape or a safety pin.

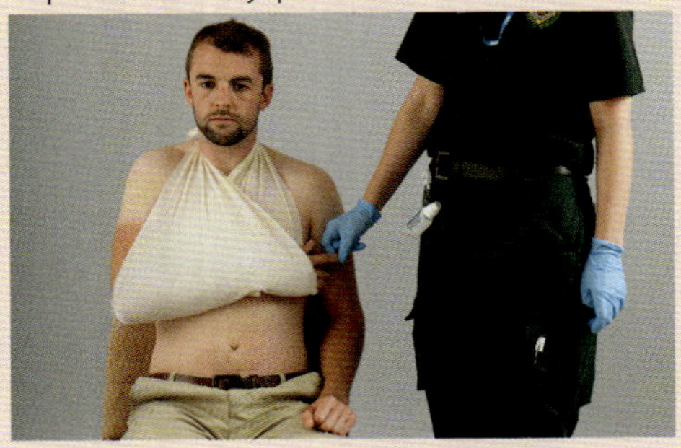

8. Re-check and record motor/sensory/circulation (MSC) function.

- Scores less than A on the AVPU scale
- complaints of neck or back pain
- signs or symptoms of spinal cord injury
- drug/alcohol intoxication.

Manual In-Line Stabilisation

Manual in-line stabilisation (MILS) with adequate back support is one of two acceptable methods of immobilisation. The other requires the use of several items of equipment (JRCALC, 2016). Therefore, MILS will almost always be the first form of spinal immobilisation to be applied to a patient with a suspected spinal injury.

Procedure

Take the following steps to apply manual in-line stabilisation (NAEMT, 2014; Pilbery, 2013):

1. Use appropriate PPE as required. Advise the patient not to move their head, explain that you are about to hold their head, and gain their consent if possible.
2. If the patient is supine (lying on their back) either kneel or lie on the ground behind the patient's head. If seated, move behind the patient. Hold the head firmly with both hands. Support the lower jaw with your fingers and support the head with your palms. Try to rest your lower arms on a surface (such as the ground or the back of a seat), as maintaining MILS can be tiring.
3. If the patient's head is not facing forwards and the patient is conscious, ask them to slowly move their head into a neutral, in-line position (eyes looking straight ahead and nose in line with umbilicus). If the patient is unconscious, gently move the head into a neutral position. If there is any pain or resistance to this manoeuvre, stop immediately.
4. Do not let go until instructed to do so by a clinician.

Cervical Collars

The most important thing to know about cervical (semi-rigid) collars is that they do not fully immobilise the cervical spine (NAEMT, 2014; James, 2004). Until head blocks and a back support are in place, manual in-line stabilisation must be used.

Orthopaedic (Scoop) Stretcher

Orthopaedic stretchers (Figure 17.11) are the preferred tool to immobilise and transport patients who require spinal immobilisation (JRCALC, 2016). This results in

Procedure in the SITTING Position – Ambu® Perfit Adjustable Collar for Extrication (ACE)

Take the following steps to apply a cervical collar when the patient is in a sitting position (Ambu, 2011):

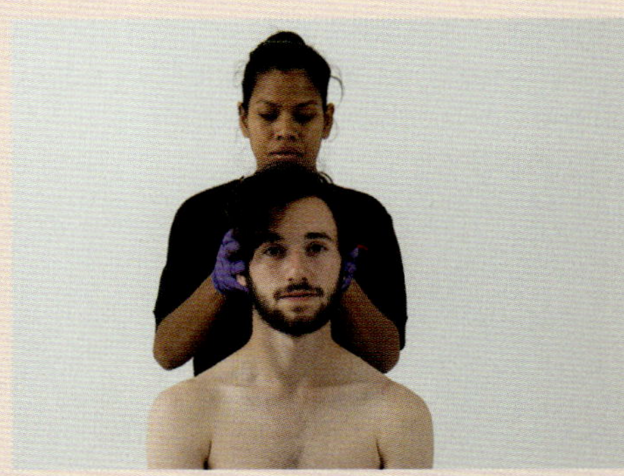

1. Use appropriate PPE as required. Inform the patient and obtain consent, if possible. One crew member should maintain manual in-line stabilisation while the other prepares the collar.

Procedure – *cont*

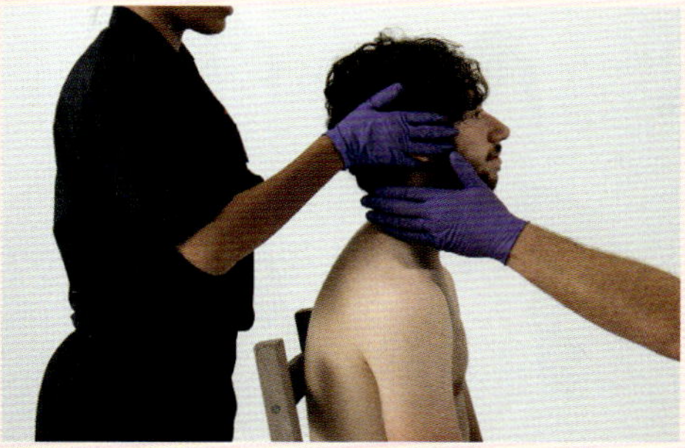

2. Ensuring the head is in a neutral position, size the collar by measuring the distance with your fingers between an imaginary line drawn horizontally and immediately below the patient's chin, and another immediately on top of the patient's shoulder.

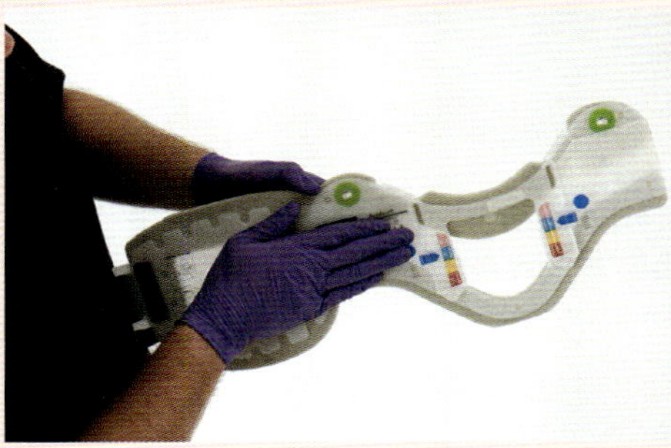

3. Compare this distance with the distance from the collar sizing line to the lower aspect of the plastic collar (NOT the foam).

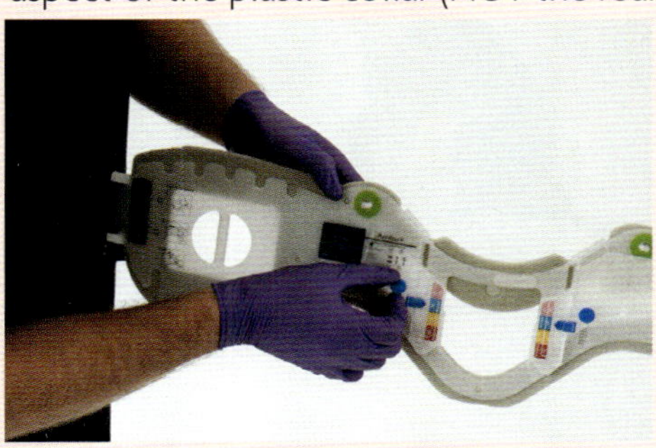

4. The Ambu® Perfit ACE collar is preset to neckless size 3. If a larger size collar is needed, disengage the safety locks by pulling UP on the buttons.

Procedure – *cont*

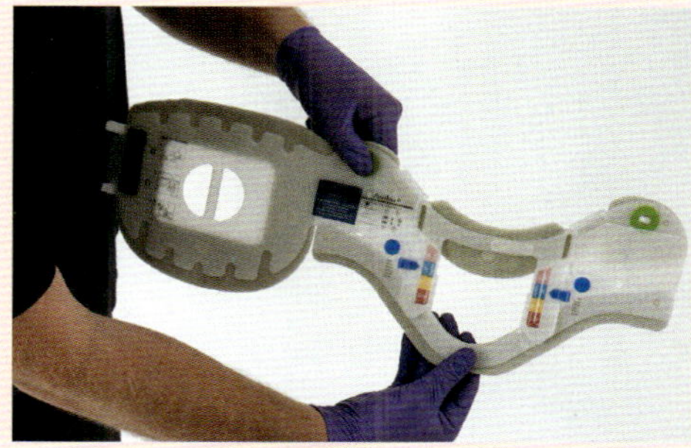

5. Adjust the collar to the correct size. There are 16 ratchet settings: simply pull the collar apart until the distance between the sizing line and the plastic collar body is the same as your finger measurement in Step 2.

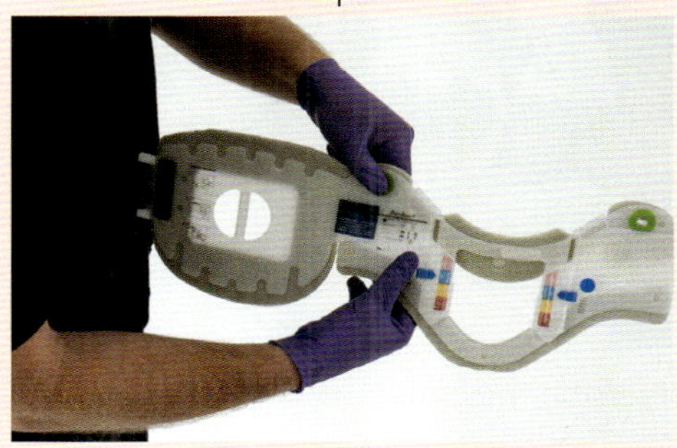

6. Engage the safety locks by pushing DOWN on the safety buttons.

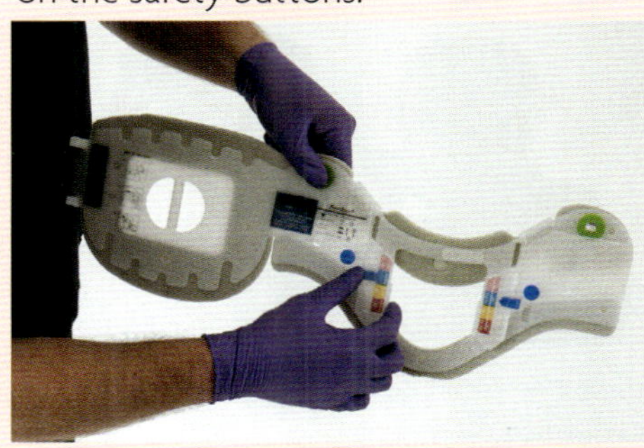

7. If the collar requires resizing, disengage the safety locks and pull OUT on the ratchet latches. Once resized, push the arrows IN and the safety locks DOWN.

(continued)

Procedure – *cont*

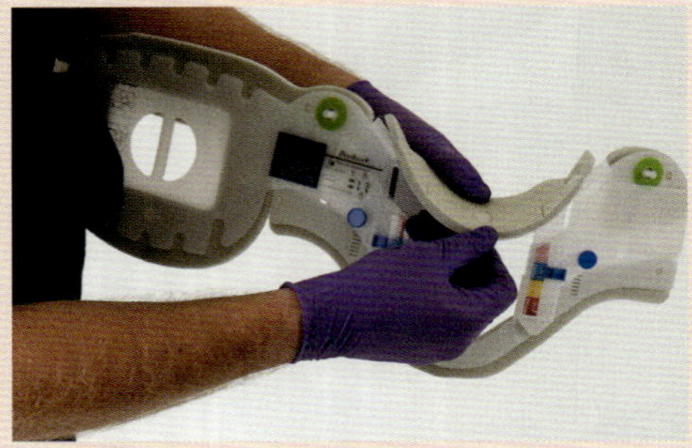

8. Assemble the collar by holding it near the tracheal opening and flip over the chin piece from the back of the collar to the front.

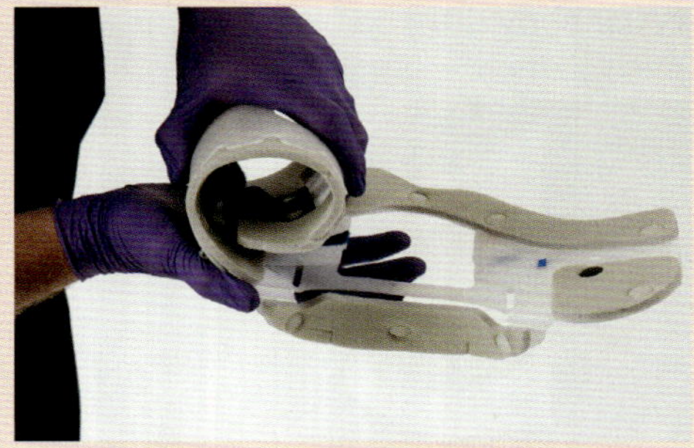

9. Preform the collar.

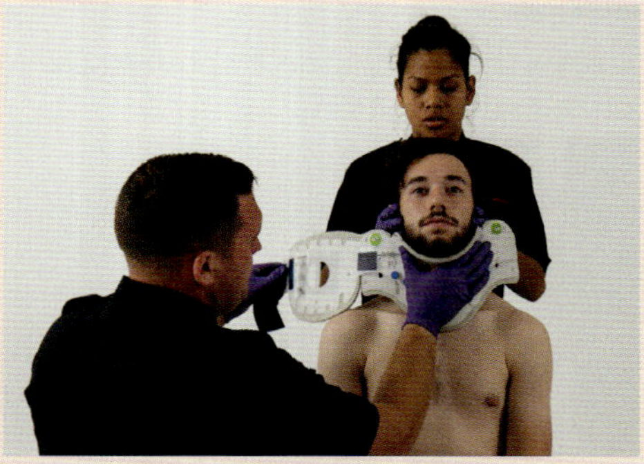

10. Slide the front of the collar along the patient's chest and position the chin piece so that the chin is supported. The collar body should rest on top of the patient's shoulder and against the sternum without gaps. The patient should remain in neutral alignment.

Procedure – *cont*

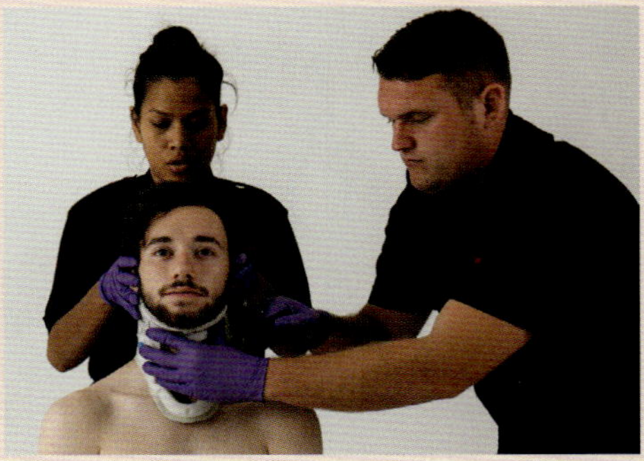

11. While holding the front of the collar in place, wrap the back of the collar around the back of the patient's head and neck and secure to the front of the collar with the Velcro tab. Maintain MILS.

Procedure in the SUPINE Position – Ambu® Perfit Adjustable Collar for Extrication (ACE)

Take the following steps to apply a cervical collar when the patient is in a supine position (Ambu, 2011):

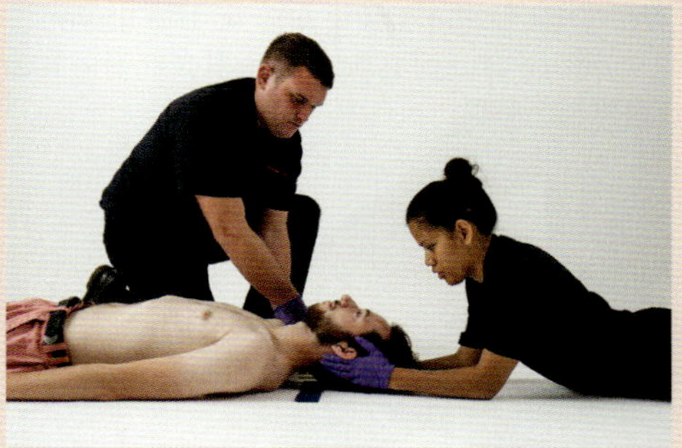

1. Follow steps 1 to 9 above. Slide the back portion of the collar directly behind the patient's neck until the Velcro can be seen on the opposite side of the patient's neck.

Procedure – *cont*

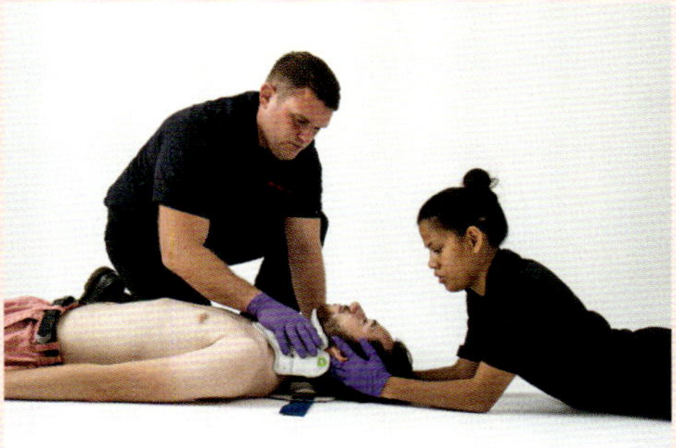

2. Position the chin piece under the chin.

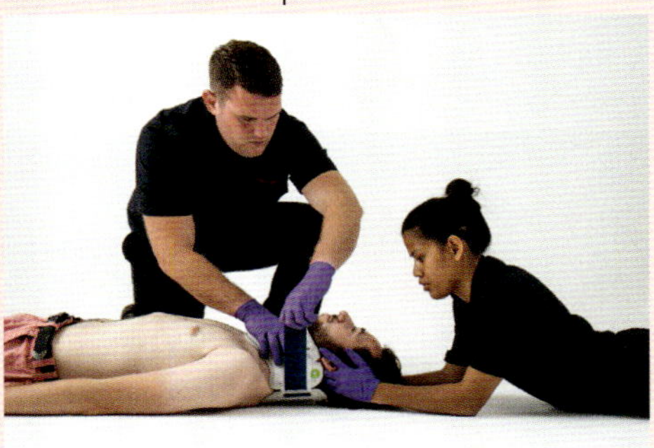

3. While maintaining proper positioning of the front of the collar with one hand, attach the Velcro with your other hand, to form a snug fit. Maintain MILS.

less movement of the spine while placing the patient onto the device, compared to the spinal board, and is also more comfortable (Krell, 2006).

Crash Helmet Removal

Patients who are wearing crash helmets need to have them removed in order to assess and manage their

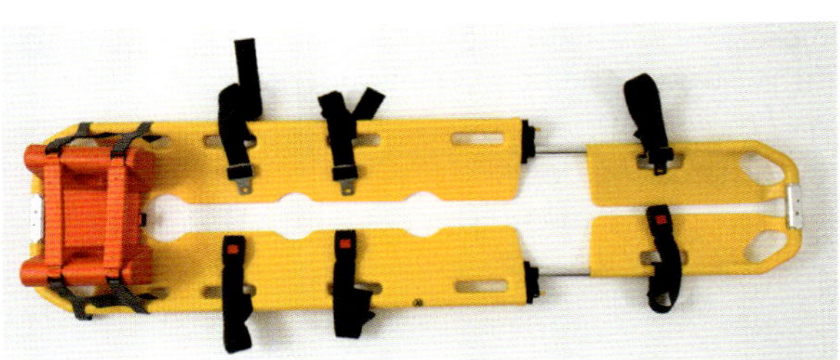

Figure 17.11 *Orthopaedic stretcher.*

Procedure

Take the following steps to apply the orthopaedic stretcher (Pilbery, 2013; Ferno, 2006):

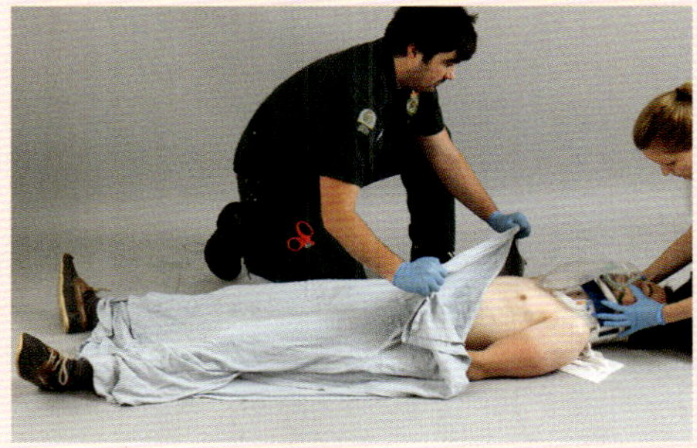

1. Explain the procedure and obtain the patient's informed consent, if possible. In major trauma, you should remove the patient's clothes ('skin to scoop') and maintain in-line stabilisation (MILS). Assess distal motor, sensation and circulatory (MSC) function in each extremity. Apply a cervical collar.

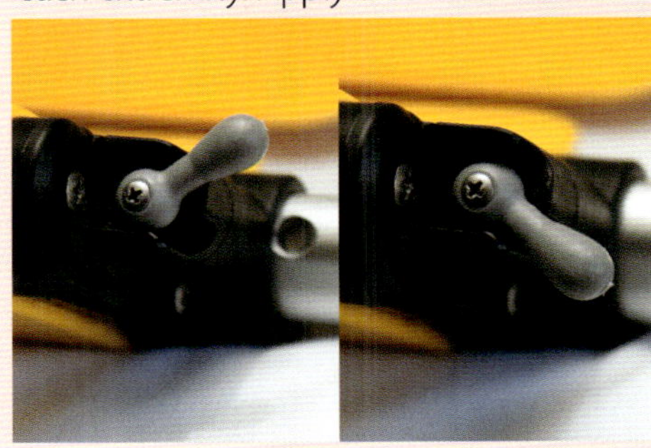

2. Adjust the length of the stretcher before uncoupling the halves. This ensures equal adjustment to both halves:
   - Move the lock-pin lever on each side of the frame to the unlocked position.
   - Pull the foot section outward to the desired length, stopping near one of the locking positions located at the holes along the foot-section frame.
   - Return both lock-pin levers to the locked position.
   - Push or pull the foot section a little until it locks into place.
   - Make sure both sides are securely locked.

(continued)

Procedure – *cont*

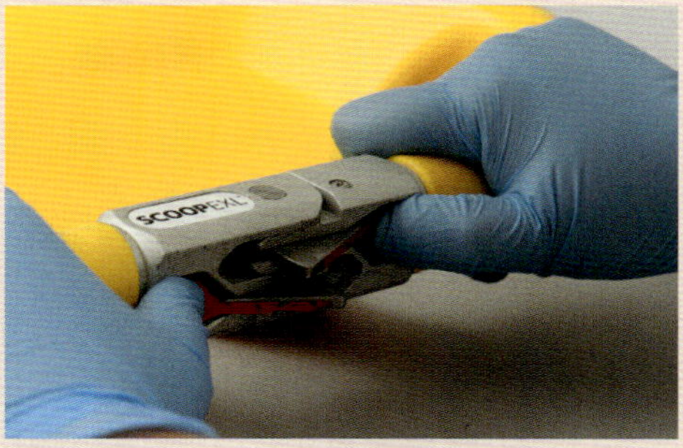

3. To separate the stretcher halves, unlock the Twin Safety Lock® coupling by pressing both levers of the Twin Safety Lock® and pull the coupling halves away from each other. Place one half on either side of the patient.

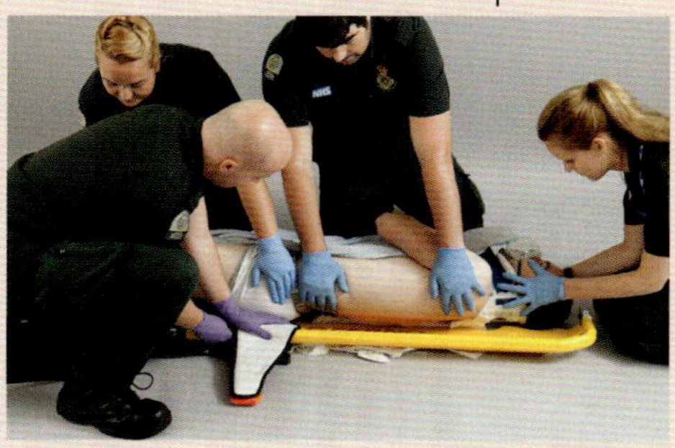

4. Gently insert each side of the orthopaedic stretcher under the patient. This may require a 10° tilt. If applying a pelvic binder to the patient, do this at the same time (NOTE: the tilt has been exaggerated in the photo and is in excess of 10°).

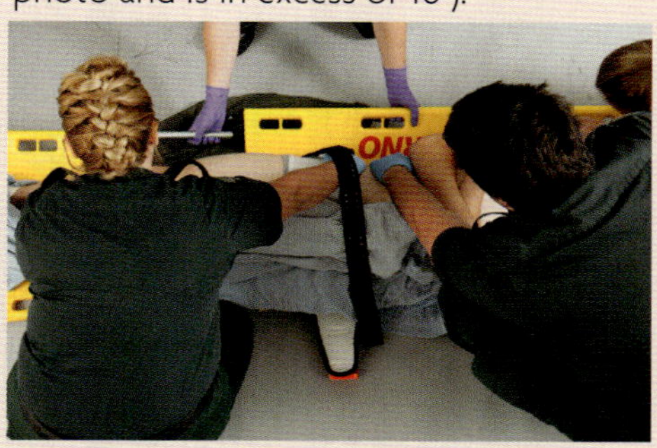

5. Return the patient to the supine position and repeat Step 4 with the other half of the orthopaedic stretcher.

Procedure – *cont*

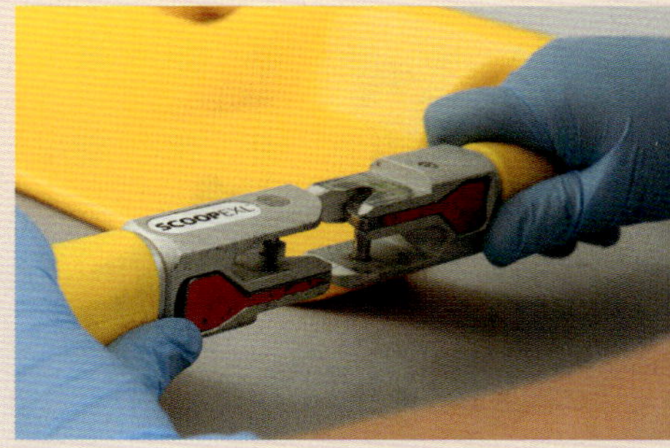

6. To rejoin the stretcher halves, align the right and left halves of the head and foot couplings and push them together until the Twin Safety Locks® engage.

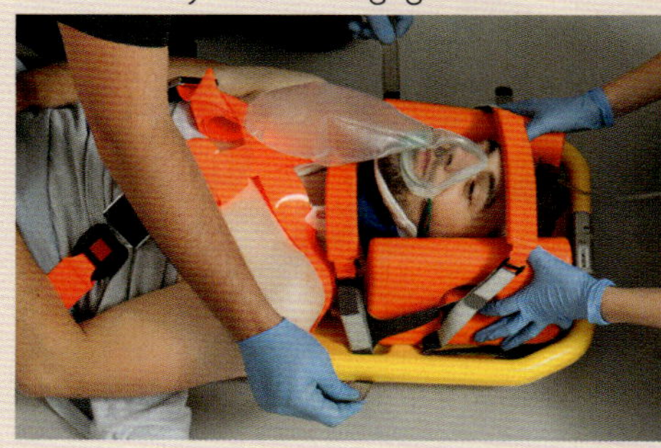

7. Insert appropriate head padding. Secure the patient to the stretcher by applying straps in the following order: chest, pelvis, thighs, ankles (tie the straps in a figure-of-eight), head blocks and straps. Reassess MSC function.
   If the patient is more than 20 weeks pregnant, tilt the stretcher 15–30° to the left, or manually displace the uterus to the left.

airway and ventilation. In addition, hidden bleeding at the back of the head can be identified and the head moved into a position of neutral alignment. Note that some degree of spinal motion will occur, even in optimal circumstances (NAEMT, 2014).

Procedure

Note: Unless immediate airway intervention is required, a single rescuer should not attempt helmet removal (Pilbery, 2013).

Take the following steps to remove a crash helmet:

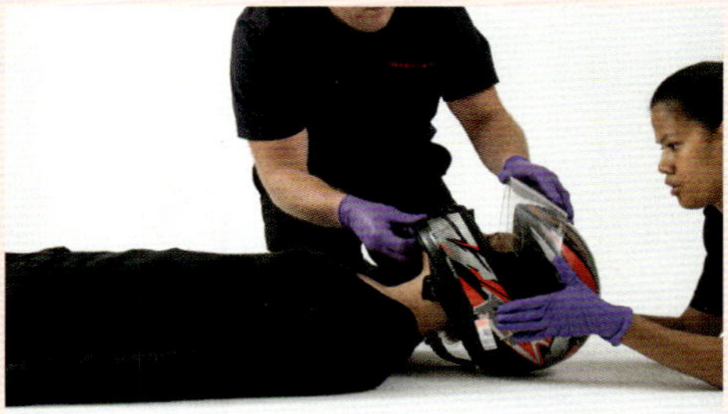

1. Explain the procedure and obtain the patient's informed consent, if possible. Rescuer One should position themselves above the patient's head. Their palms should be pressed on the sides of the helmet and fingertips curled underneath. The helmet, head and neck should be maintained in as near to an in-line neutral position as possible. Rescuer Two should remove the face shield, glasses (if worn) and chin strap.

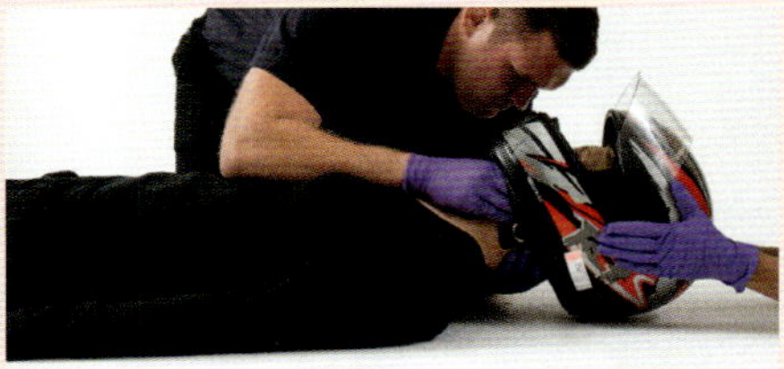

2. Rescuer Two should move their thumb and first two fingers up to support the mandible. Their other hand should be placed behind the head at the back of the helmet.

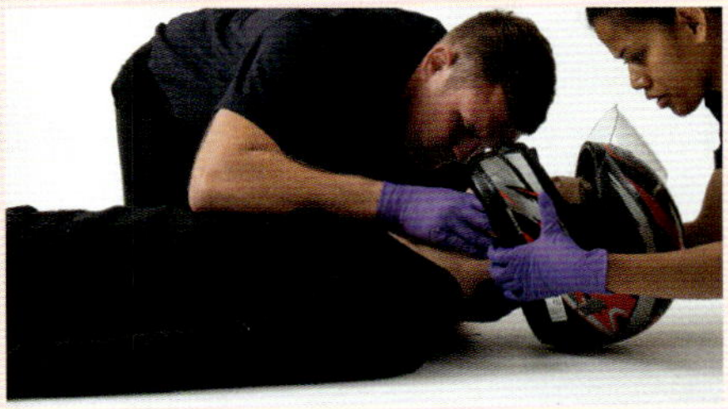

3. Rescuer One pulls the side of the helmet slightly apart and gently tilts the helmet up and down while applying traction to remove the helmet. This should be slow and deliberate. Take care as the helmet clears the patient's nose.

Procedure – *cont*

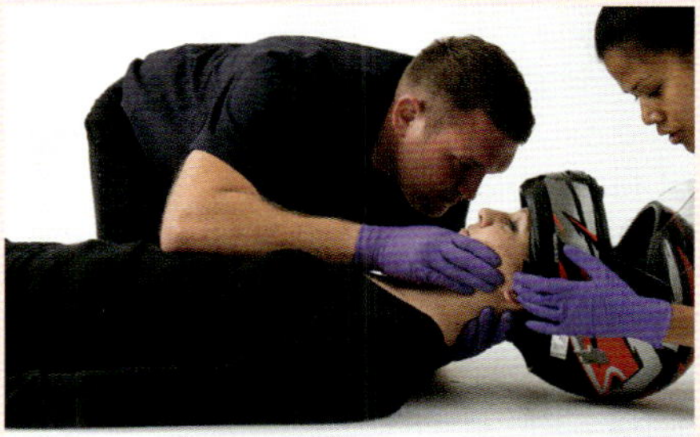

4. Once the helmet has reached the halfway point, Rescuer One should stop moving the helmet, while Rescuer Two repositions their hands from the back of the helmet to the occiput. Take care, the head is heavy.

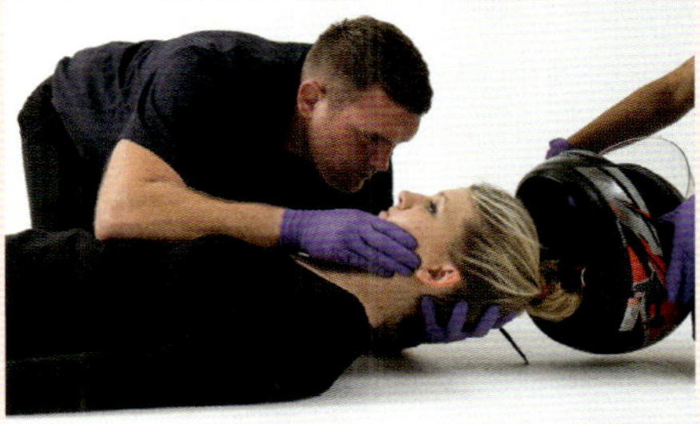

5. Once Rescuer Two has repositioned their hands and has control of the patient's head, Rescuer One should continue to remove the helmet.

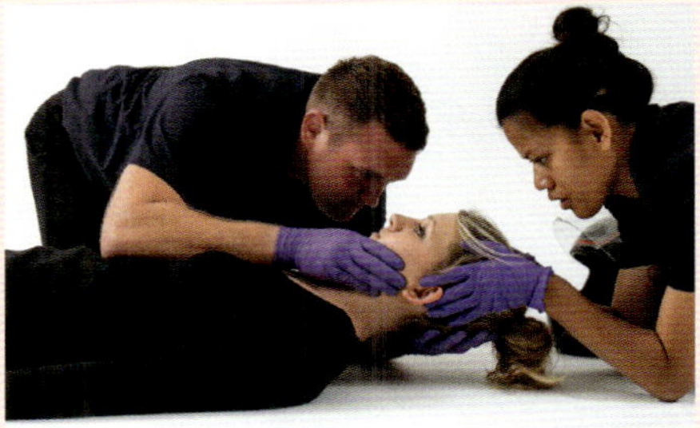

6. Once the helmet has been removed, Rescuer One takes back control of the head and gently moves it into an in-line neutral position.

Splints

Splinting forms an important part of fracture management, particularly in the lower limbs. The benefits of splintage include reducing (Greaves, 2008):

- pain
- blood loss
- pressure on skin
- pressure on adjacent neurovascular structures
- risk of fat embolism
- risk of further damage.

Basic principles of immobilisation should consist of assessment and reassessment of the neurovascular status before and after any manipulation or handling of the fracture, and immobilisation of the joints above and below the fracture.

Note: It is not possible to show the application of every type of splinting device in this text. Instead, a selection of commonly used devices is explained. This is not a substitute for hands-on training with your service's splints.

Box Splints

Box splints are simple devices that are most commonly used for lower leg fractures (Figure 17.12). They are only suitable for the immobilisation of straight limbs as they will not conform to the shape of deformed limbs (Gregory, 2010b).

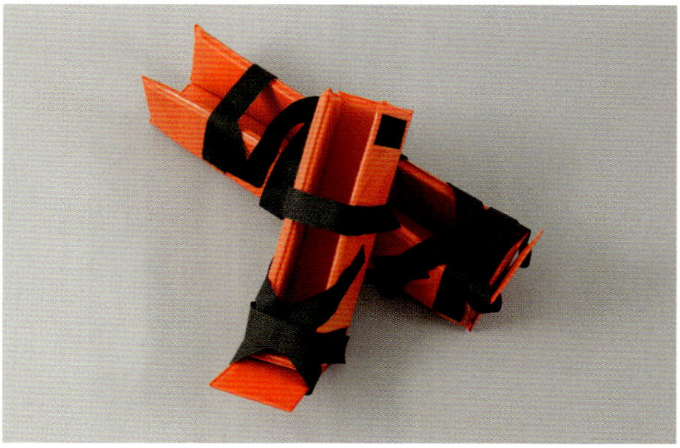

Figure 17.12 *A box splint.*

Procedure

Take the following steps to apply a box splint (EEAST, 2014; Gregory, 2010b):

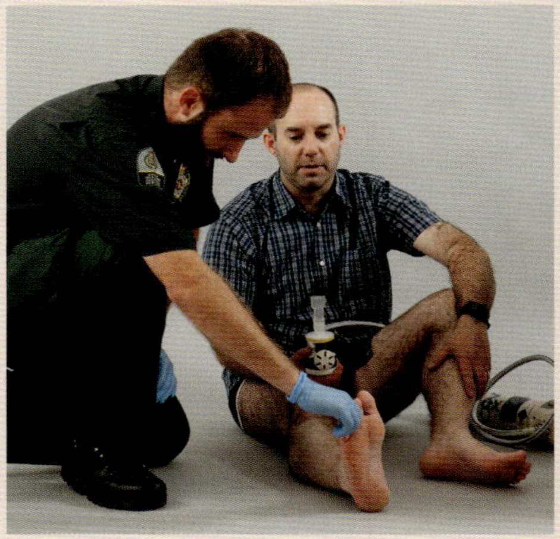

1. Gain the patient's informed consent. Provide analgesia if required prior to the procedure. Ensure the splint is clean and undamaged. Check motor/sensory/circulation (MSC) function.

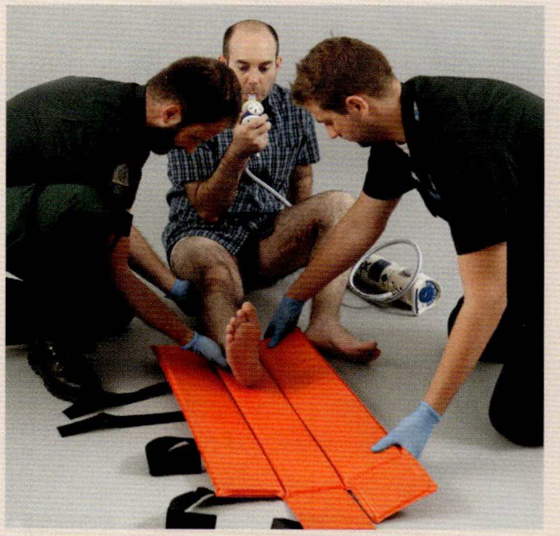

2. Expose the injured limb and remove footwear where possible. Support the limb manually and raise it carefully while the splint is passed under it.

Procedure – *cont*

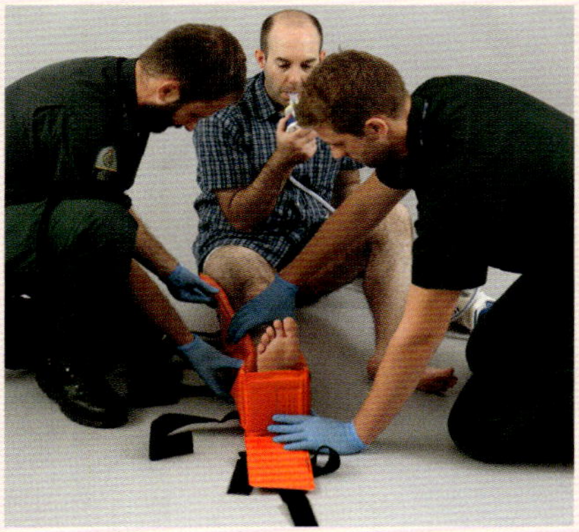

3. Fold the two sides of the splint around the limb to form a box to support the limb.

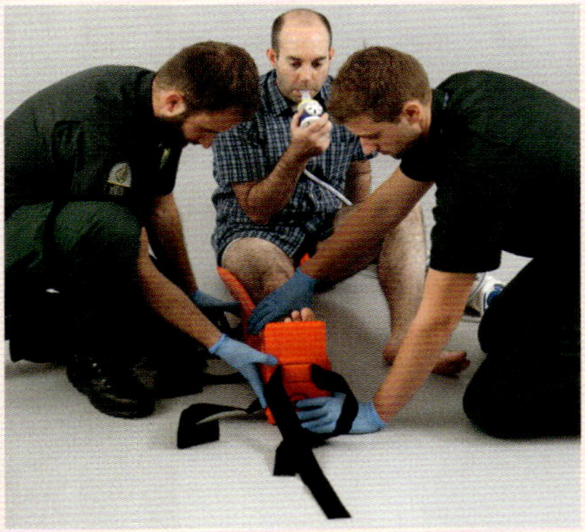

4. Ensure the foot piece is placed against the sole of the foot at 90° or in a position comfortable for the patient.

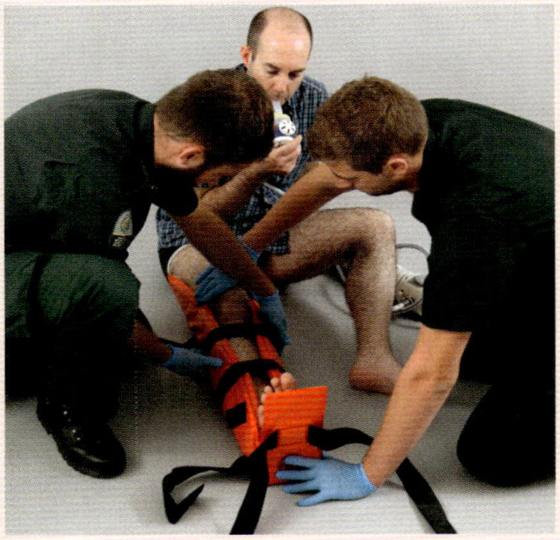

5. The Velcro straps should be carefully placed over the limb, avoiding the area of

Procedure – *cont*

injury. The foot strap should be passed over the top of the foot.

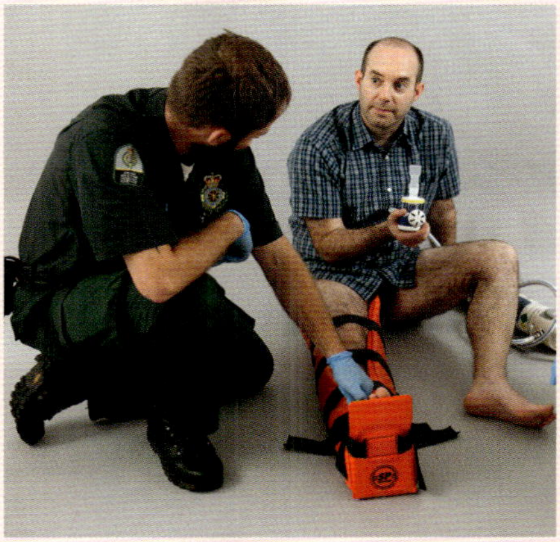

6. Re-check MSC function of the limb after application of the box splint.

Pelvic Splints

Commercial pelvic splints (commonly called pelvic binders) have been shown to reduce stable, 'open book' and rotational and vertically unstable fractures adequately (Figure 17.13), with no significant displacement of fractures, irrespective of device (Knops, 2011). Concerns have been expressed with their use in lateral compression fractures, but there is no good evidence that their use is detrimental to the patient with these fractures (Toth, 2012). That said, there is no conclusive evidence that the use of

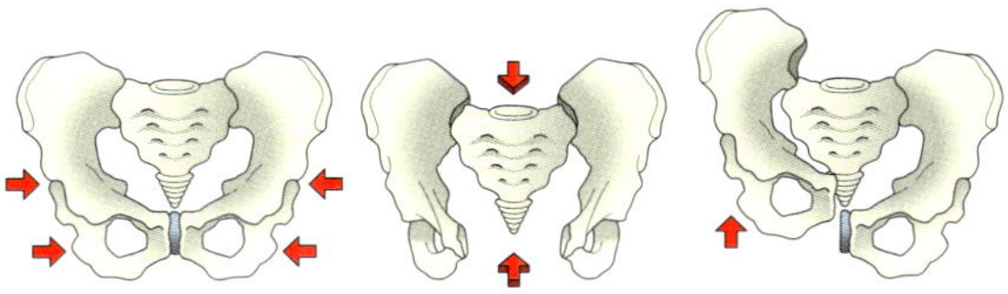

Figure 17.13 *Types of pelvic fracture. The red arrows indicate the direction of the force.*

pelvic binders reduces morbidity or mortality from serious trauma either (Stewart, 2013).

In the absence of a commercial device, sheets (and binding the legs together at the knee and ankles) (Simpson, 2002) or an inverted Kendrick Extrication Device® (KED) can be used, although these make access to the pelvis and abdomen difficult (McCormack, 2010).

Procedure – SAM Pelvic Sling II

Take the following steps to apply the SAM Pelvic Sling™ II (EEAST, 2014):

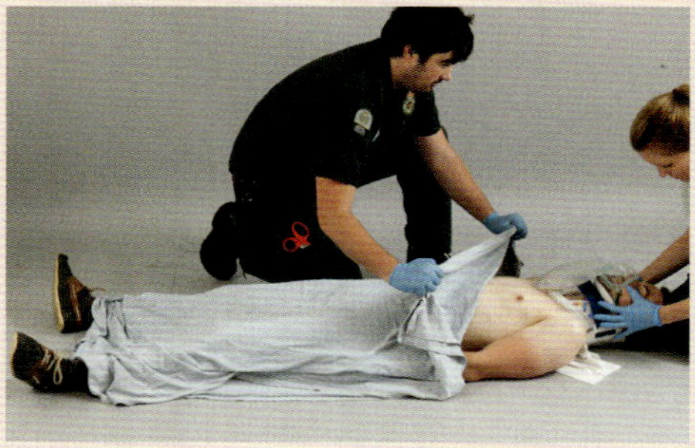

1. Use appropriate PPE as required. Inform the patient and obtain consent, if possible. Prepare the SAM splint. Fully expose the patient as the splint needs to be placed directly on the patient's skin. Cover the patient to preserve their dignity and prevent heat loss.

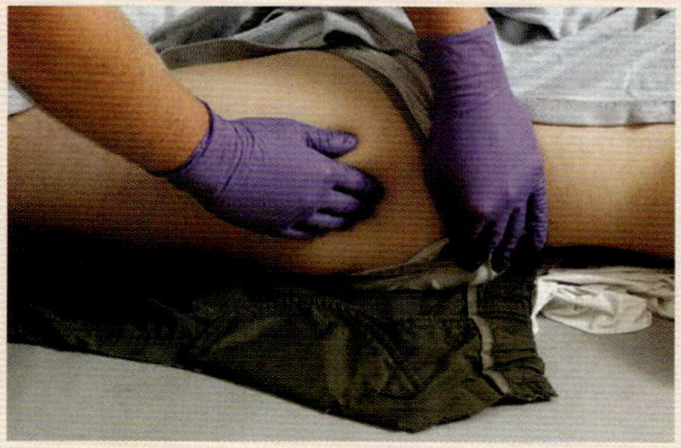

2. Identify the level of the greater trochanters.

Procedure – *cont*

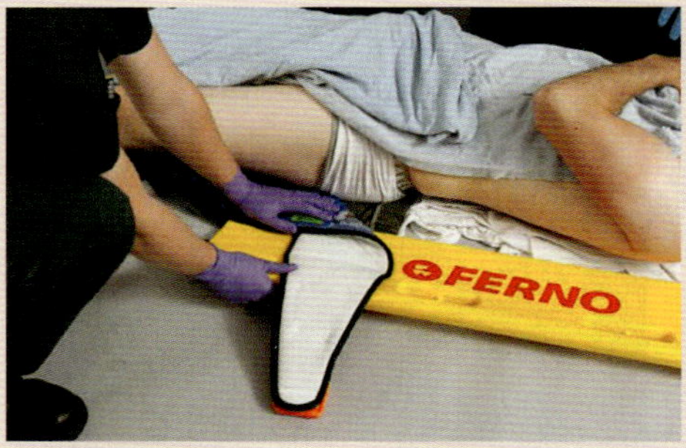

3. Place the buckle side of the device level with the greater trochanter and facing away from the direction of the first roll. Fold the tail end of the splint 90° so that the tail strap points down towards the patient's feet, forming an L-shape. Slide one half of the orthopaedic stretcher under the splint, so both can be inserted under the patient during the log roll.

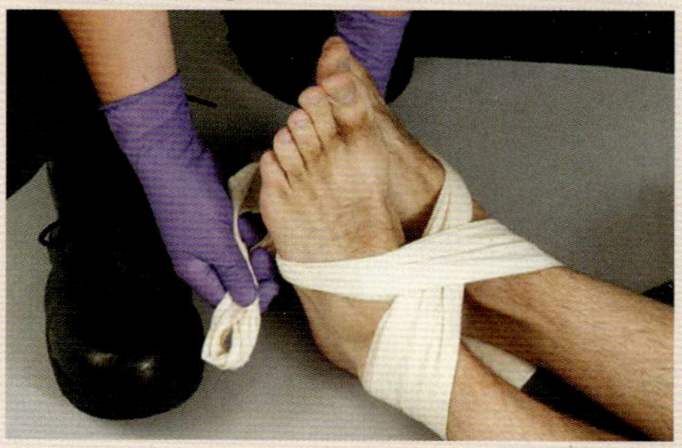

4. As long as there are no lower limb fractures, tie the patient's feet together prior to securing the splint.

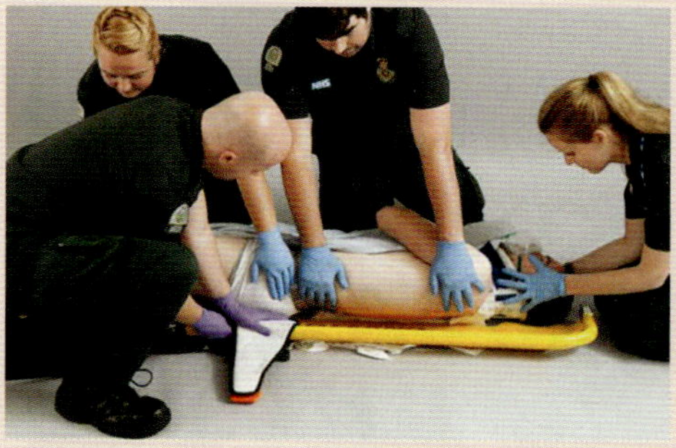

5. Log roll the patient 10°, place the SAM splint on the orthopaedic stretcher and insert

Procedure – *cont*

both items under the patient (NOTE that the degree of tilt has been exaggerated in this photo).

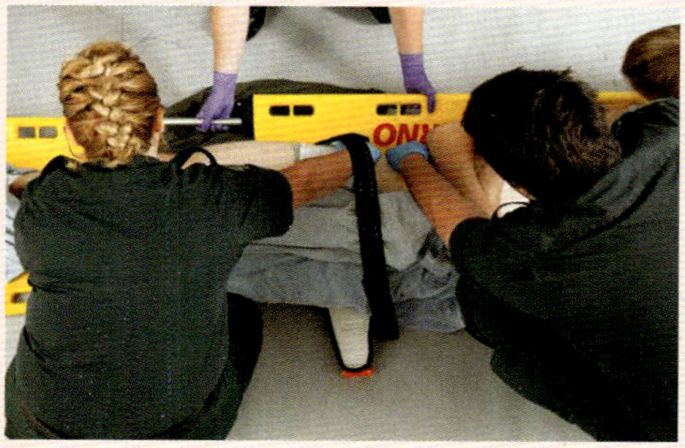

6. Roll the patient onto their back and then roll 10° in the other direction. Pull the tail of the SAM splint through and ensure it is at the correct level. Insert the remaining half of the orthopaedic stretcher and connect both together.

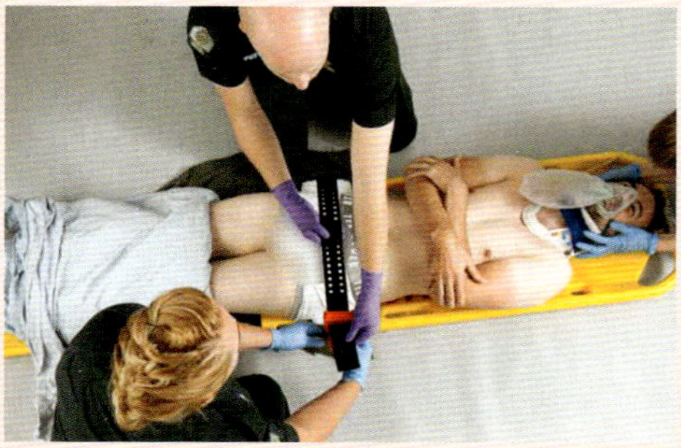

7. Log roll the patient onto their back. Place the black strap through the buckle and pull completely through.

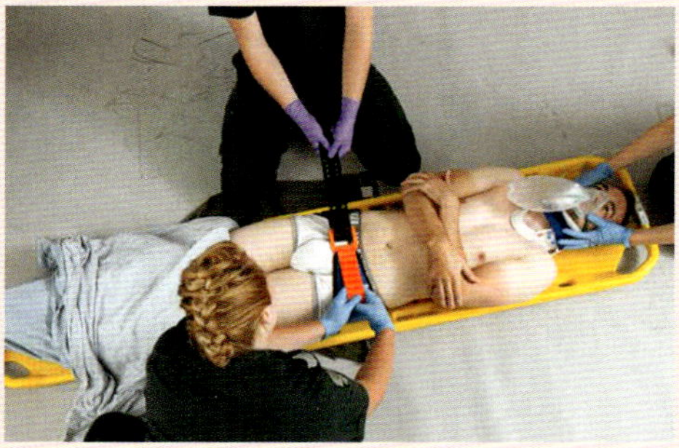

8. Hold the orange strap and pull the black strap in the opposite direction until you

Procedure – *cont*

hear and feel the buckle click. Maintain tension and immediately press the black strap onto the surface of the SAM splint to secure. You may hear a second click as the sling secures.

9. Re-cover the patient to maintain dignity and minimise heat loss.

Traction Splints

Traction splints apply longitudinal force to long bones (normally the femur). Correctly splinting the femur using this method helps to reduce (JRCALC, 2016):

- pain
- haemorrhage and damage to blood vessels and nerves
- movement of bone fragments and the risk of a closed fracture becoming an open fracture
- the risk of a fat embolus
- muscle spasm.

Indication:

- suspected fracture of the femoral shaft.

Contra-indications (NAEMT, 2014):

- suspected pelvic fractures (except the Kendrick Traction Device™)
- suspected femoral neck fracture
- avulsion or amputation of ankle and foot
- fractures close to, or below, the knee
- dislocated knee (not just patella).

Procedure – Kendrick Traction Device™ (KTD)

Take the following steps to apply the KTD (EEAST, 2014):

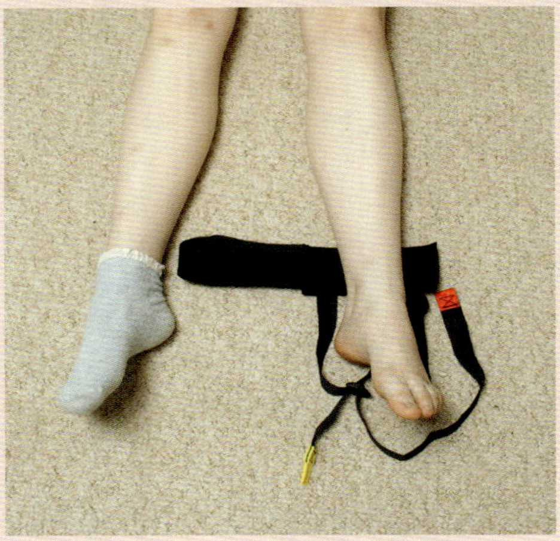

1. Use appropriate PPE as required. Inform the patient and obtain consent, if possible. Remove the patient's shoes and clothing to expose the injured leg. Check motor, sensation and circulation (MSC) function below the injury. Prepare the KTD.

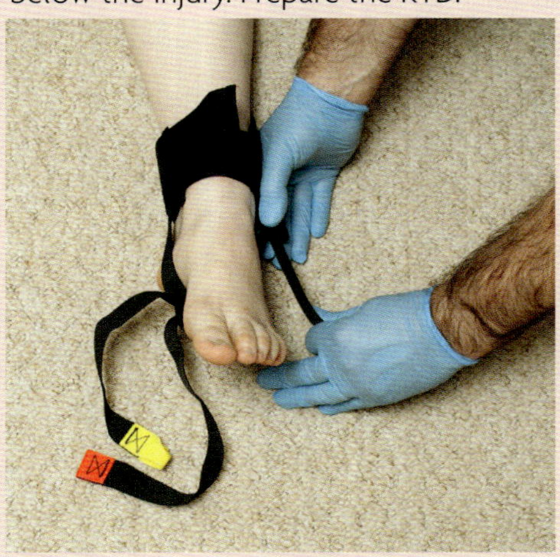

2. Apply the ankle hitch around the injured leg, just above the anklebone, and tighten the stirrup by pulling the GREEN tabbed strip until snug under the heel.

Procedure – *cont*

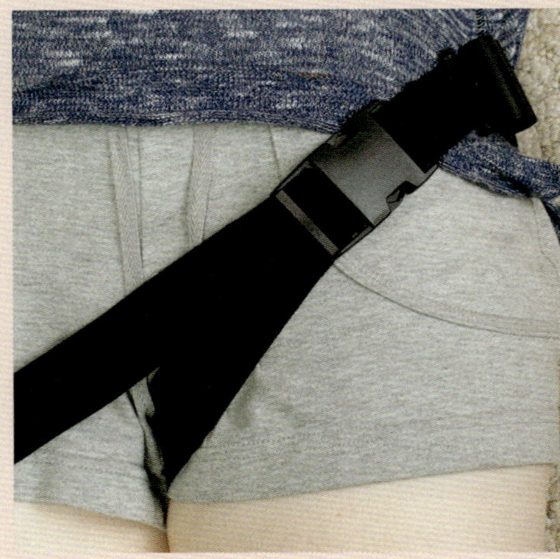

3. Apply the upper thigh strap by sliding the male buckle under the knee, 'see-saw' the strap upwards until it rests in the crotch area and click the ends together. Tighten the strap until the traction pole receptacle is positioned at the level of the pelvic crease. Make sure male genitals are clear of the strap.

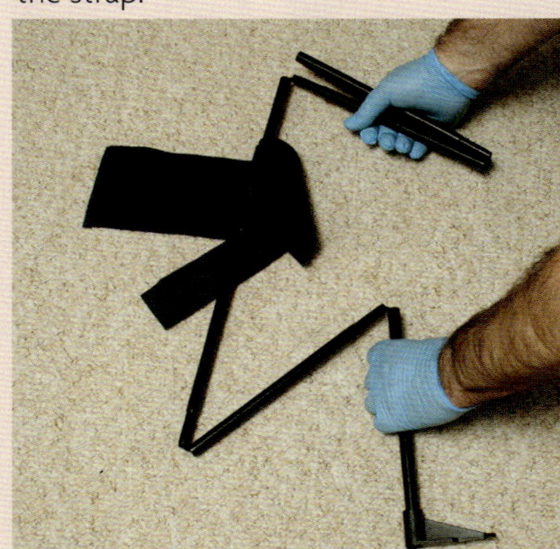

4. Snap out the traction pole, ensuring each joint is securely seated.

Procedure – *cont*

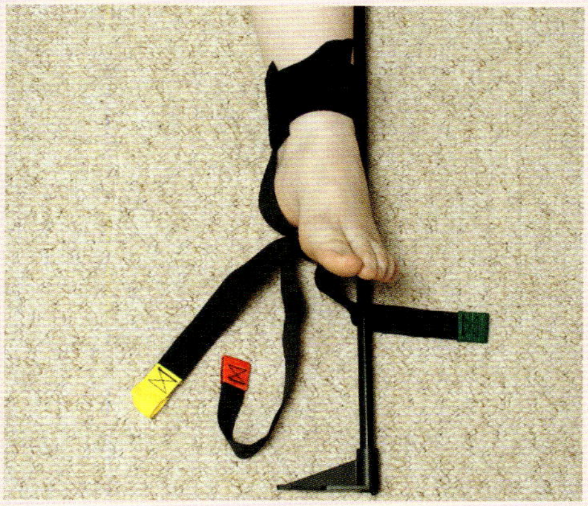

5. Place the traction pole alongside the leg so that one section extends below the foot.

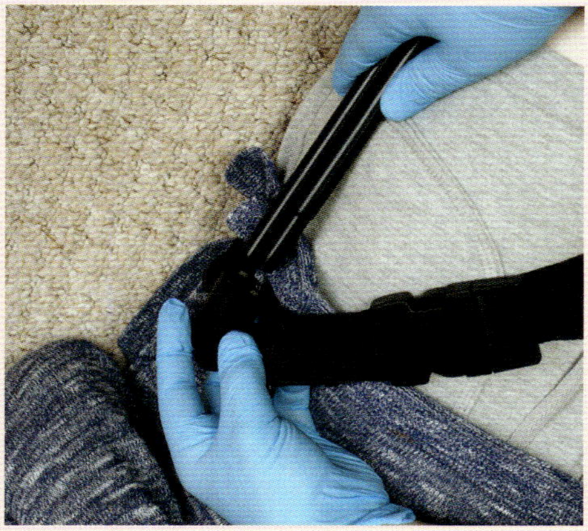

6. Adjust the length of the pole and place the ends into the traction pole receptacle.

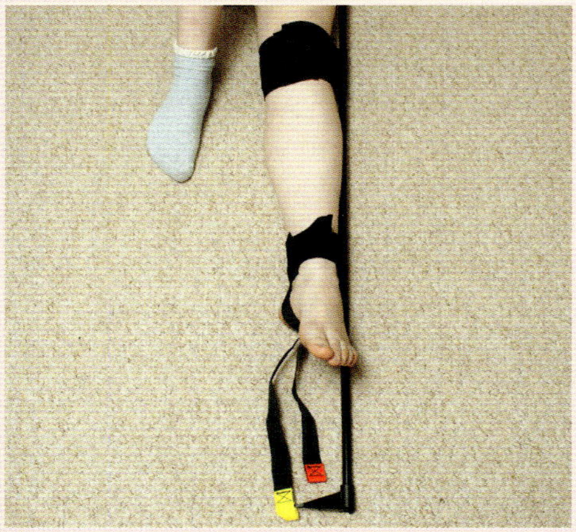

7. Secure the elastic strap around the knee.

Procedure – *cont*

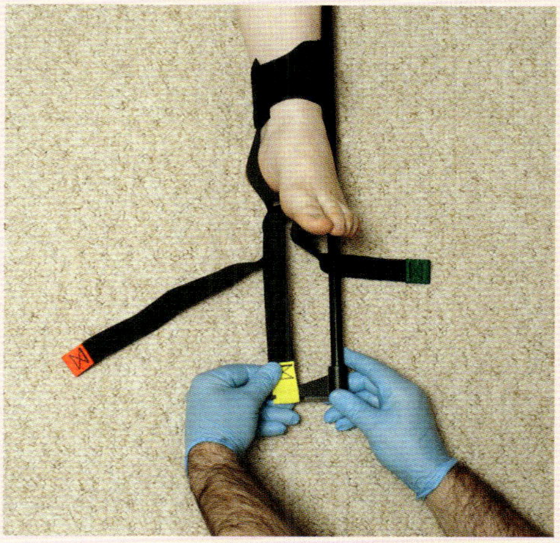

8. Place the YELLOW tab over the dart end.

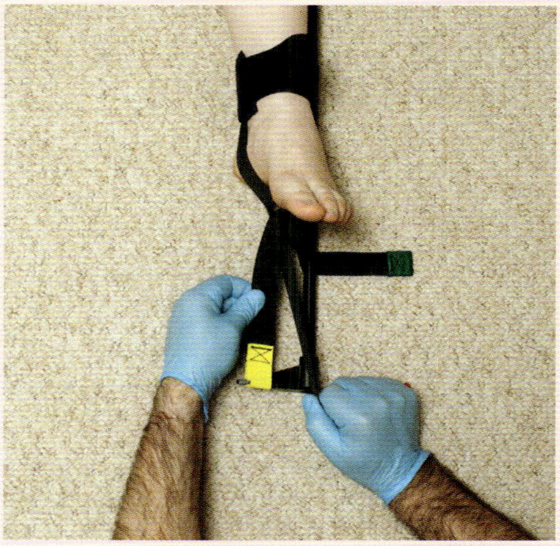

9. Apply traction by pulling on the RED tab. As a guide, apply around 10% of body weight (up to 7 kg) tension. Use patient comfort as the main objective. Traction can be applied smoothly by grasping the strap either side of the buckle and simultaneously feeding and pulling with equal pressure.

Procedure – *cont*

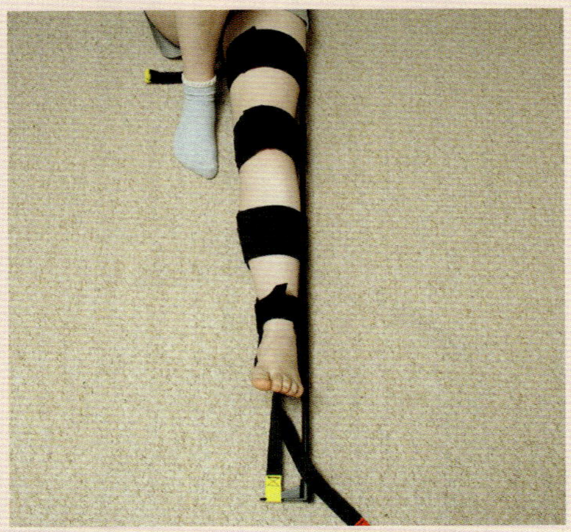

10. Finish packaging by applying upper and lower straps. Re-check and record MSC function.

Burns

Learning Objectives

By the end of this section you will be able to:

- Explain what is meant by the term 'burn'.
- Describe the types of burn and their causes.
- Explain the safety considerations when dealing with burns.
- State the rules associated with estimating the size of burns.
- Explain time-critical factors that affect the management of burns.
- Explain the complications associated with burns.
- Explain the treatment of burns.
- Explain why burns patients are transported to definitive care.

Introduction

A burn is an injury caused by energy transfer to the body's tissues, causing necrosis and an associated inflammatory reaction (Greaves, 2008).

It is estimated that there are 250,000 burn injuries a year in the United Kingdom, resulting in 175,000 visits to an emergency department (NBCRC, 2001). In England and Wales, serious burn injury (defined as requiring at least a 72-hour stay in hospital) is responsible for 5.4% of all serious trauma (Kalson, 2012).

Burn injury most commonly occurs in the home (over 30%) with the kitchen being the most frequent location. The most common sources of injury are (NBCG, 2008):

- cup of tea in children
- petrol ignition in adults
- bathing, kettle spills and central heating radiators in elderly people.

Burns are commonly split into a number of types (JRCALC, 2016):

- chemical
- cold
- electrical
- friction
- radiation
- thermal.

Assessment of Burns

History

It is important to identify the mechanism, including the cause of the burn, how it came into contact with the patient, and any first aid undertaken. Note when the injury occurred, how long the patient was exposed to the source and the duration of any cooling. Don't forget to be alert for signs of non-accidental injury.

Assessment

Pre-hospital estimation of total body surface area (TBSA) of burn injury is poor, with the 'rule of nines' (Figure 17.14) leading to an underestimating of burns less than 20% and an overestimating of burns over 40%; also, it is not suitable for children under 14 years of age (Hettiaratchy, 2004; JRCALC, 2016). Note, if using the 'rule of nines', it is important not to include areas of simple erythema (skin that is reddened, but not blistered).

The whole hand (palm and fingers) represents about 0.82% TBSA in adults and 0.77% in children, making accurate calculations tricky. However, the palm alone is 0.5% TBSA (Muehlberger, 2010) and is suitable for estimating burns less than 15% or greater than

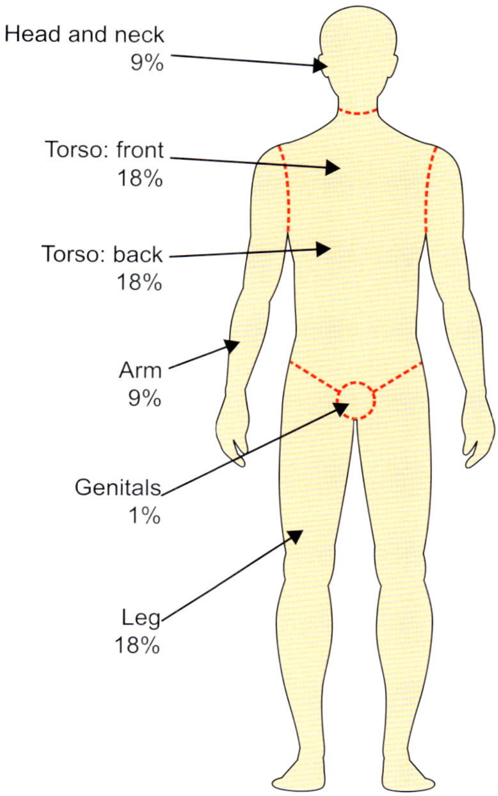

Figure 17.14 *The 'rule of nines'.*

85% TBSA. Note that these methods will generally underestimate %TBSA in obese patients (Berry, 2001).

Lund and Browder charts are more accurate, but these are cumbersome to complete out-of-hospital. An alternative that has been advocated is serial halving (Allison, 2004). This involves determining whether greater than or less than 50%, 25% and finally 12.5% of the TBSA is burnt. This approximation is sufficient to determine whether the patient requires referral to a burns unit (if direct access is an option) and the need for intravenous fluids. As before, erythema (reddening) should not be included when calculating TBSA of burn injury (Enoch, 2009).

Classification

Although important for subsequent burns management, the depth of a burn does not affect pre-hospital treatment, but may provide some indication as to the cause (Table 17.4) (NZGG, 2007).

Burns Requiring Transport to Hospital

The National Network for Burn Care (NNBC) has set out a suggested minimum threshold for patients who may require specialised burn care services.

Table 17.4 Burns classification

Classification	Other Names	Example Causes	Appearance	Sensation
Epidermal	Superficial, 1st degree	Ultraviolet light, scalds	Dry and red, blanches with pressure, no blisters	May be painful
Superficial dermal	Superficial, partial thickness, 2nd degree	Scald (spill or splash)	Pale pink, fine blisters, blanches with pressure	Very painful
Mid-dermal	Superficial, partial thickness, 2nd degree	Scald (spill), flame	Dark pink with large blisters, delayed capillary refill	May be painful
Deep dermal	Deep partial thickness, 2nd degree	Scald (spill), flame	Blotchy red, may blister, no capillary refill	No sensation
Full thickness	3rd degree	Scald (immersion), flame, steam, high-voltage electricity	White, waxy or charred. No blisters or capillary refill Children: dark lobster red with mottling	No sensation

These patients will usually require transport to hospital, but check with your own ambulance service's local arrangements (NNBC, 2012):

- all burns ≥ 2% TBSA in children or ≥ 3% in adults
- all full thickness burns
- all circumferential burns
- any burn not healed in 2 weeks
- any burn with suspicion of non-accidental injury
- all burns to hands, feet, face, perineum or genitalia
- any chemical, electrical* or friction burn
- any cold injury
- any unwell/febrile child with a burn.

*May not apply to low (domestic) voltage injury.

Thermal Burns

The most common type of thermal burns (sometimes referred to as thermal injuries) are flame, scald and contact. Flame burns are more common in adults and are often associated with smoke inhalation and other traumatic injuries. These are more likely to result in deep dermal or full-thickness burns.

Scalds are the most common cause of burns in children, usually due to spillages of hot drinks or immersion in hot bath water. They generally cause epidermal or superficial dermal burn injury (Hettiaratchy, 2004).

Direct contact burns are caused by brief contact with a very hot object, or (more commonly) prolonged contact with a cooler object. Typical patient groups include epileptics and those who misuse alcohol or drugs.

Irreversible damage to the epidermis can be caused by exposure to 44°C heat for 6 hours, or 65°C for 1 second (Moritz, 1947). Burns injuries are characterised by a local response and, if the total body surface area (TBSA) burnt is greater than 20%, a systemic response (Greaves, 2008).

Acute Smoke Inhalation Injury

Smoke inhalation is a killer. Between 80% and 90% of fire-related fatalities are attributed to smoke inhalation, and it has a greater contribution to overall mortality and morbidity of burn injuries than either %TBSA or age (Kimmel, 1999). Naso-oropharyngeal and mucosal burns are common (Toon, 2010), but thermal injury below the vocal cords is rare, since heat is effectively exchanged in upper airway passages (Prien, 1988). When air, steam and/or smoke are at sufficiently high temperatures to cause thermal injury to the lower airways, rapid oedema of the glottis develops, resulting in fatal airway obstruction.

Systemic toxins are the products of incomplete combustion and include carbon monoxide (CO) and hydrogen cyanide. CO is an odourless, colourless gas that binds to haemoglobin with 250 times the affinity of oxygen. This results in a decrease in the oxygen-carrying capacity of the blood. Cyanide adversely affects internal respiration by preventing aerobic production of adenosine triphosphate (ATP), the energy source for cells (Toon, 2010).

Friction Burns

Although friction burns are strictly speaking a thermal burn, they are the result of heat production caused by friction between the skin and another object. This can result in not just a burn, but abrasions too (see the section in this chapter on wounds and bleeding) (Gregory, 2010b).

Management

Safety first! The patient needs to be removed from the source of the burn if it is safe to do so, but don't get burnt yourself. Clothing should be removed unless it is sticking to the patient, as should jewellery, which may become constrictive as tissues swell.

Follow the CABCDE approach for burns as you would any traumatic injury. However, inhalation injury is a particular concern and occurs in around 22% of all burns, 60% if facial burns are present (Toon, 2010).

Signs of inhalation injury include (Singer, 2010):

- full-thickness or deep dermal burns to face, neck or upper torso
- singed nasal hair
- soot in sputum or oropharynx
- dyspnoea, hoarseness, cough or stridor
- cyanosis
- altered level of consciousness.

Administer high-flow oxygen via a non-rebreathe mask. CO poisoning may make pulse oximetry readings unreliable (JRCALC, 2016).

Cooling

Thermal burns should be cooled for 20 minutes (Bartlett, 2008), preferably with running water (between 8°C and 15°C) (NZGG, 2007). There is little evidence that ice causes damage to underlying tissues, but it runs the risk of making the patient hypothermic so is not recommended (Cuttle, 2008, 2009). Cooling should commence immediately after the burn has occurred, but there is limited evidence to suggest that cooling up to an hour after the burn has occurred is still beneficial (Cuttle, 2010). If running water is not available or practicable, then gel-based body blankets can be used without causing hypothermia (NZGG, 2007; Singer, 2006; Martineau, 2006).

Covering/Dressing

Patients with burns lose heat from non-epithelialised areas of skin (i.e. skin missing its outermost layer) due to evaporation. With the thermoregulatory function of the skin disrupted, patients are at risk of hypothermia, even on a warm day (AAOS, 2011). Hypothermia is part of the lethal triad in trauma, and for each 1°C reduction in body temperature the mortality rate increases significantly (Lonnecker, 2001), although there is no evidence currently to suggest that pre-hospital cooling causes hypothermia (Lonnecker, 2001; Singer, 2010). Once cooling has been completed, cover the burn with a clean sheet or cling film, but take care not to apply it circumferentially as it can become constrictive as oedema develops (NZGG, 2007).

Time-Critical Features

If a burns patient has any of the following signs, they are considered to be time-critical and will require blue light transport to an appropriate facility (JRCALC, 2016):

- any major ABCD problems
- airway burns
- history of hot air or gas inhalation
- respiratory distress
- evidence of circumferential (completely circling the neck, torso or limb) burns
- significant facial burns
- burns more than 15% TBSA in adults or 10% TBSA in children
- presence of other major injuries.

Chemical Burns

Chemical burns generally result from exposure to acids, alkalis and other corrosive materials. Alkali burns are generally more serious, as they penetrate more deeply than other chemicals (ATLS, 2008). Their severity depends on the concentration of the chemical, the duration of exposure and the speed in applying first-aid measures (Greaves, 2008).

Management

Safety first! It is important that you do not become exposed to the chemical. If in doubt, do not approach the scene but wait for the Hazardous Area Response Team (HART) or the fire and rescue service to attend.

Speed is of the essence when treating chemical burns, so flush the exposed area with copious quantities of water as soon as possible. However, brush off any chemical powder from the patient first. In industrial settings, decontamination showers may be available, but at home, the shower or a hosepipe is an alternative. While flushing, contaminated clothing should be removed, although do not pass anything over the patient's head; cut it off instead (Pilbery, 2013).

Chemical burns should be irrigated for at least 15 minutes, and ideally for up to an hour (although alkali burns may require much longer periods of irrigation), but watch out for hypothermia (NZGG, 2007).

Radiation Burns

Radiation burns are most commonly caused by ultraviolet radiation from the sun or sunlamps (sunburn). However, in rare cases, it can be caused by exposure to radioactive materials (Gregory, 2010b).

Approximately 80% of skin cancer is preventable, and avoiding sunburn is key (Simon, 2010):

- Take care not to burn.
- Cover up with loose cool clothing, a hat and sun glasses.
- Seek shade during the hottest part of the day.

- Apply high-factor sunscreen (at least sun protection factor 15) to sun-exposed body parts.
- Take extra care to protect children in the sun.

Management

Safety first! If the burns are due to exposure to radioactivity, do not approach but wait for specialist response teams.

Sunburn

Basic first-aid measures are usually sufficient (SJA, SAA, BRC, 2014):

- Cover the patient's skin with light clothing or a towel. Move them out of the sun, preferably indoors.
- Encourage them to drink frequent sips of cold water while cooling the affected area with cold water. If the area of sunburn is large, it may be more practical for the patient to soak the area in a cold bath for 10 minutes.
- If burns are mild, calamine or an after-sun lotion may help. Patients should be advised to stay inside or in the shade.

Most sunburn will manifest as reddening of the skin (erythema), but blistering is evidence of a partial thickness burn and transport to hospital should be considered if it meets the criteria for review by specialised burns care services (NNBC, 2012).

Electrical Injuries

Electrical injuries are thankfully uncommon, but they cause significant damage and even death when they occur. The majority of electrical injuries in adults occur in the workplace and involve high voltages, whereas in children most injuries occur in the home with domestic voltage. Electrocution from lightning strikes is very rare, leading to around 1,000 deaths each year worldwide (Nolan, 2010).

Electrical burns arise when a source of electrical power makes contact with the patient's body. They are frequently more serious than they appear, since rapid heat loss from the surface of the skin may leave it relatively undamaged, whereas the underlying tissues may have sustained serious injury, particularly between the entry and exit points (don't forget to look for both) (ATLS, 2008).

Management

Safety first! Do not approach the patient until you are certain that the source of electricity has been cut off.

When dealing with electrical injuries, the thermal burns sustained may not be your highest priority. The patient may be in cardiac arrest, have airway or facial burns and be traumatically injured (fractures, serious internal injuries) that will need addressing first. Associated thermal burns can be managed as previously described.

The Problem With Burns

Without appropriate intervention and management, patients with serious burns can die due to (Sheridan, 2012):

- burn shock owing to excessive fluid loss in the first 24 hours
- respiratory failure in the subsequent 3–5 days
- burn wound sepsis in the following few weeks.

Thankfully, because of prompt transfer by ambulance staff to burn centres and the subsequent specialised management that patients receive, this is less common. However, it does underline the importance of transporting patients to definitive care.

There are four general phases of burn care, with the ambulance service only playing a small part in the initial management stage (Sheridan, 2012):

- initial evaluation and resuscitation (0–72 hours)
- initial surgery and temporary closure of wounds created by removal of full-thickness burns (days 1–7)
- definitive wound closure (weeks 1–6)
- rehabilitation and reconstruction (up to 2 years).

Chapter 18

Cardiac Arrest

Adult Basic Life Support

Learning Objectives

By the end of this section you will be able to:

- Explain the benefits of the chain of survival to basic life support.
- Explain common types and causes of cardiac arrest in adults.
- Explain the procedure for providing basic life support to adults.

Introduction

Cardiac arrest is the ultimate medical emergency, but you will have the ability to undertake the two most effective treatments for this: cardiopulmonary resuscitation (more commonly called basic life support in healthcare circles) and defibrillation. However, the role of the Fire and Rescue Service is just one link in a chain that maximises the patient's chance, not only of a return of spontaneous circulation (ROSC), but also of surviving to hospital discharge neurologically intact (i.e. with normal or near-normal brain function) (Perkins, 2015). That chain is known as the chain of survival (Nolan, 2006).

Chain of Survival

The chain of survival encompasses four key principles that are required if a resuscitation is to be successful in adults (Figure 18.1) (Perkins, 2015):

- early recognition and call for help
- early bystander cardiopulmonary resuscitation (CPR)
- early defibrillation
- post-resuscitation care.

Early Recognition and Call for Help

This relies on patients and the public calling for help early and can be influenced by the ambulance service with public education and training sessions. Recognition of cardiac chest pain is particularly important as around 21–33% of patients with acute myocardial ischaemia will suffer a cardiac arrest in the first hour following onset (Müller, 2006).

Early CPR

Performing CPR immediately following cardiac arrest can double or triple the chance of the patient surviving (Perkins, 2015). When someone calls 999 they will be given advice on how to perform chest compressions only, as this has been shown to produce higher survival rates in adults

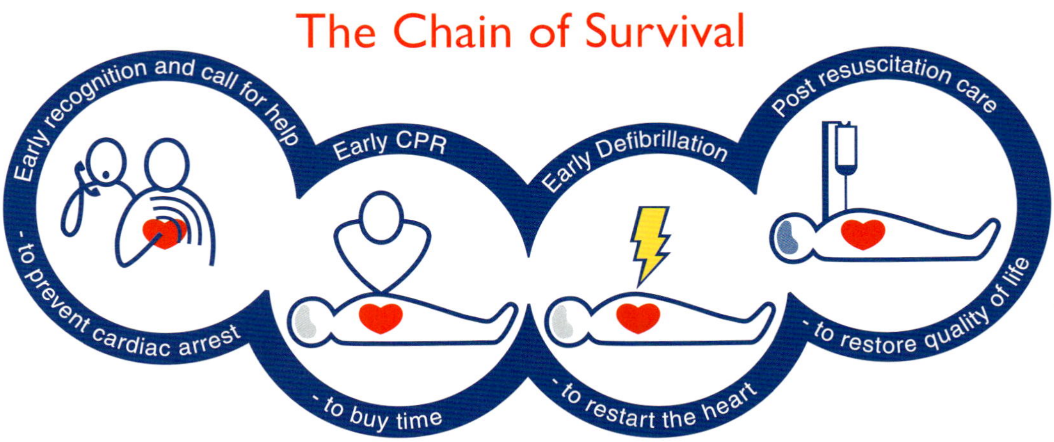

Figure 18.1 *The chain of survival – Image reproduced by the kind permission of Laerdal Medical.*

than conventional CPR (chest compression and mouth-to-mouth ventilation) (Hüpfl, 2010).

Early Defibrillation

Providing good quality CPR and defibrillating in the first 3–5 minutes of a cardiac arrest can produce a survival rate of 50–75%, but, conversely, the chance of surviving to hospital discharge falls by 10–12% for every minute of delay (Perkins, 2015).

Post-Resuscitation Care

Restarting your patient's heart and palpating a pulse (ROSC) is a great feeling, but the patient is not out of the woods yet. The true measure of success is returning the patient to their pre-cardiac-arrest state, with brain function intact so that they can leave hospital. Providing post-resuscitation care on scene, en-route and in hospital is crucial if this is to happen (Nolan, 2012).

Children

In stark contrast to adults, children usually suffer a cardiac arrest secondary to hypoxia. The outcomes from these secondary cardiac arrests are very poor and the emphasis with children is to intervene before their heart arrests (Skellett, 2016).

Adult BLS

Basic life support (BLS) refers to maintenance of airway patency, and supporting breathing and circulation, with artificial ventilation and chest compressions as required (JRCALC, 2016).

The procedure described is for a single rescuer, but tasks are usually shared when there is more than one rescuer on scene, such as when you are working as a crew.

Procedure

Take the following steps to perform adult BLS (Perkins, 2015; JRCALC, 2016):

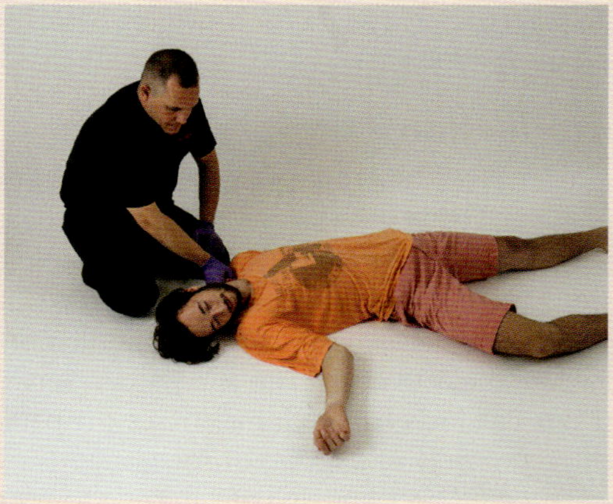

1. Ensure the scene is safe for you, your colleague, the patient and other bystanders. Check the patient to see if they are responsive by gently shaking their shoulders and asking if they are all right.
   If the patient responds, obtain a history and undertake a further patient assessment.

Procedure – *cont*

If the patient does not respond, inform your colleague so they can assist. Turn the patient onto their back, if required.

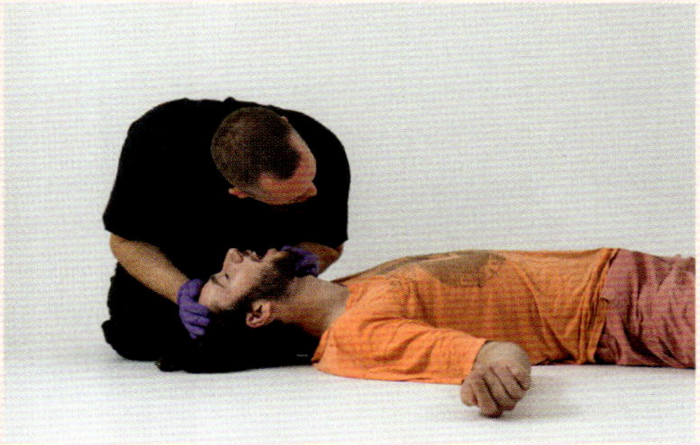

2. Open the patient's airway and look, listen and feel for breathing for no more than 10 seconds. Note that agonal breathing (occasional gasps) is common immediately following cardiac arrest and should not be confused with normal breathing or taken as a sign of life. If the patient is breathing, place them in the recovery position.

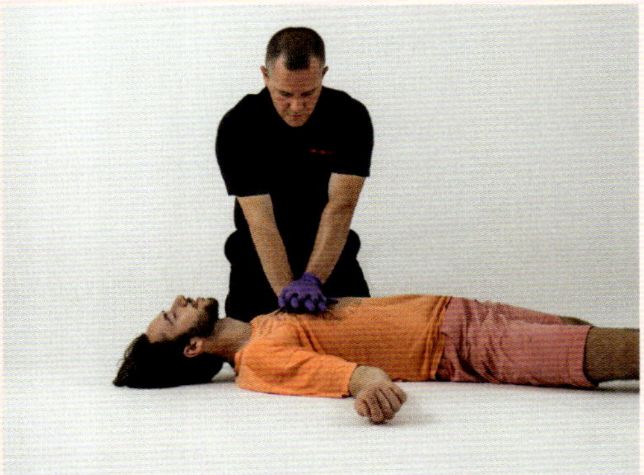

3. If the patient is not breathing or there are no signs of life (not moving, no normal breathing or coughing), start chest compressions:
   - Kneel beside the patient.
   - Place the heel of one hand in the centre of the chest (lower half of the sternum).
   - Place the heel of your other hand on top of the first.
   - Interlock your fingers and ensure that pressure is **not** applied over the patient's ribs.

Procedure – *cont*

   - Keeping your arms straight and with you positioned directly over the patient's chest, apply downward pressure to compress the chest to a depth of 5 cm but not more than 6 cm.
   - After each compression release the pressure on the chest, but maintain contact with the patient's skin.
   - Repeat at a rate of 100–120 compressions/min.

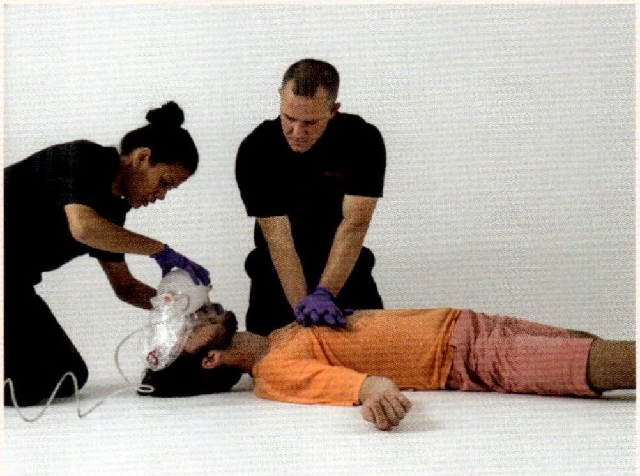

4. Continue with chest compressions and ventilations at a ratio of 30:2. You should alternate chest compressions with your colleague every two minutes, but keep the changeover time to a minimum.

Paediatric Basic Life Support

Learning Objectives

By the end of this section you will be able to:

- Explain how the causes of cardiac arrest in children are usually different from adults.
- Explain the procedure for providing basic life support to paediatric patients.

Introduction

Unlike adults, who experience a primary cardiac arrest typically due to a cardiac arrhythmia, infants and children usually suffer a secondary cardiac arrest (Maconochie, 2015). This is not the sudden event experienced by adults, but a progressive worsening of the patient's condition until they cannot continue to compensate. Outcome from secondary cardiac arrest is poor.

Paediatric basic life support (BLS) is different from that of adults, and there are also some differences between infants (paediatric patients under 1 year of age) and children (between 1 year of age and puberty), and so they are presented separately here.

Infant BLS

Procedure

Take the following steps to perform basic life support on an infant (Maconochie, 2015; JRCALC, 2016):

1. Ensure the scene is safe for you, your colleague, the patient and other bystanders. Check for responsiveness by placing a hand on the infant's forehead to stabilise it and tug their hair while calling their name. If they do not have hair, consider flicking the soles of their feet. Never shake an infant.
2. If the patient responds, assess their ABCDE, call for assistance and reassess regularly. If they do not respond, summon additional assistance.
3. Open the infant's airway by placing one hand on their forehead and gently tilt it back until it is in a neutral position (Figure 18.2). Perform a chin lift by placing the fingertips of your other hand on the bony part of the lower jaw and lift upwards. Don't compress the soft tissues under the jaw as this will occlude the airway. Placing a towel under the infant's shoulders and upper body can help keep their head in a neutral position.
4. If a head tilt–chin lift does not effectively open the airway, you can use a jaw thrust:
   - Position yourself behind the infant.
   - Place two fingers under both angles of the jaw.
   - Rest your thumbs on the infant's cheeks.
   - Lift the jaw upwards.
5. Look, listen and feel for normal breathing by placing your face close to the infant's face:
   - Look for chest and abdominal movements.
   - Listen for airflow at the mouth and nose.
   - Feel for airflow at the mouth and nose.
6. If the infant is breathing normally, turn them onto their side and monitor their breathing.
7. If the infant is not breathing or there are no signs of life (not moving, no normal breathing or coughing), check for, and carefully remove, any airway obstruction and provide five rescue breaths:
   - Ensure the head is in a neutral position and apply a chin lift.
   - Either place a bag-valve-mask over the infant's mouth and nose (Figure 18.3), or take a breath and place your mouth over the mouth and nose of the infant.
   - Ventilate the chest steadily for 1 second, just enough to make the chest rise.
   - Maintain head tilt–chin lift and watch the chest fall.
   - Repeat this sequence five times.
8. If the infant's chest is not rising and falling in a similar fashion to normal breathing, open the infant's mouth and check for any visible

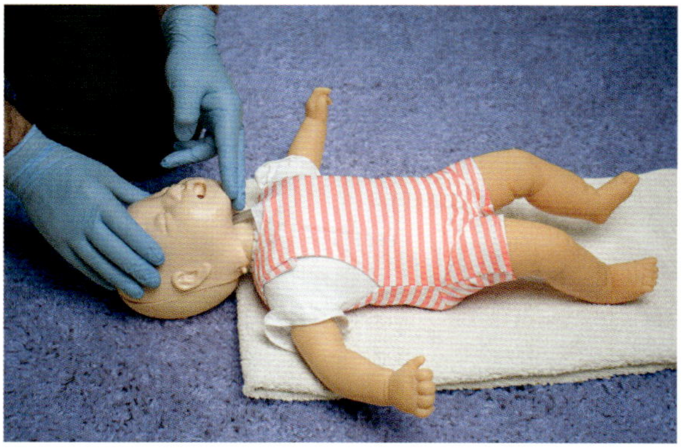

Figure 18.2 *Neutral alignment.*

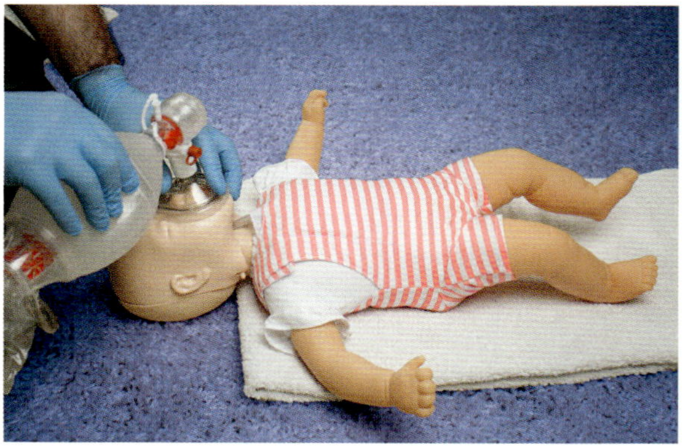

Figure 18.3 *Ventilating with a bag-valve-mask.*

obstruction. Do not blindly sweep in the infant's mouth. Reposition the head to ensure it is in the neutral position, using a jaw thrust if the head tilt–chin lift manoeuvre is not effective. Make no more than five attempts to achieve effective ventilation before moving on to chest compressions.

9. Check for signs of life (movement, coughing or normal breathing). If you are confident in checking for a pulse, feel for a brachial pulse in the medial aspect of the infant's arm. Unless you are sure you can feel a pulse, assume it is absent and start chest compressions. If there are signs of circulation, reassess airway and breathing and manage appropriately.
10. If there are no signs of life and/or no pulse or a pulse rate of less than 60 beats/min, start chest compressions:
    - If you are on your own, use the tips of two fingers (Figure 18.4), otherwise adopt the encircling technique by placing both thumbs side by side on the lower sternum and spreading the remaining fingers around to the infant's back (Figure 18.5).
    - Avoid compressing the abdomen, by placing your fingers one finger's width above the xiphisternum.
    - Compress the sternum at least one-third of the depth of the chest (or by 4 cm) and then fully release the pressure while maintaining contact with the sternum.
    - Repeat the compressions at a rate of 100–120/min for 15 compressions and then give 2 ventilations.

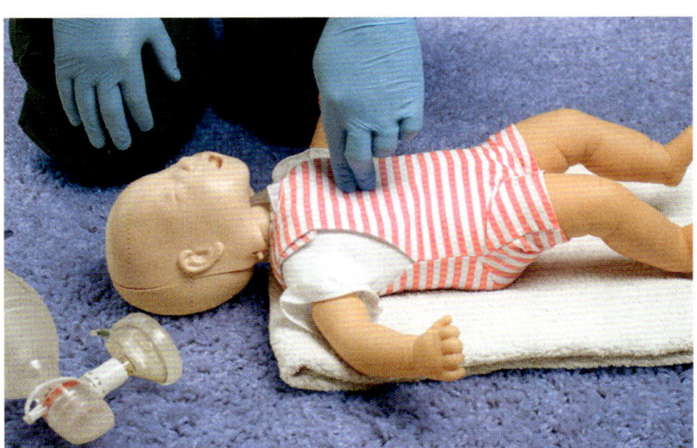

Figure 18.4 *Chest compressions using the two-finger technique.*

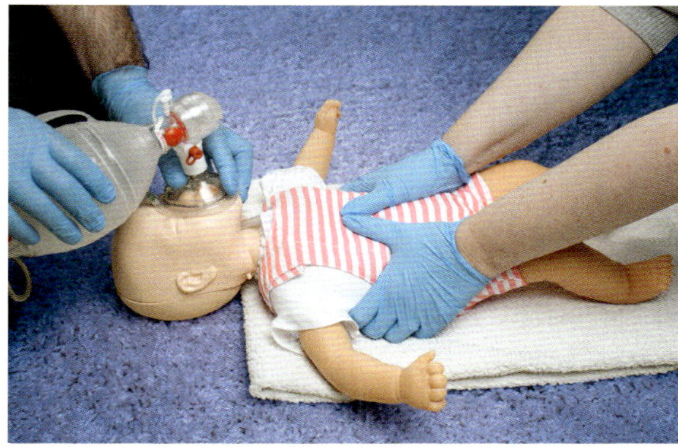

Figure 18.5 *Chest compressions using the encircling technique.*

    - Continue compressions and ventilations at a ratio of 15:2 unless you are on your own, in which case a ratio of 30:2 may be easier.
    - If you are on your own, continue until the infant shows signs of life or you become exhausted. Alternatively, if you have a colleague present, alternate chest compressions with your colleague every two minutes, but keep the changeover time to a minimum.

Child BLS

Procedure

Take the following steps to perform basic life support on a child (Maconochie, 2015; JRCALC, 2016):

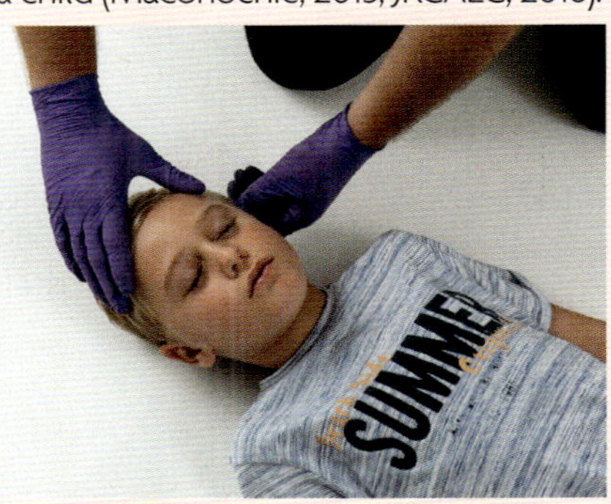

1. Ensure the scene is safe for you, your colleague, the patient and other bystanders. Check for responsiveness by placing a hand on the child's forehead to stabilise it and tug their hair while calling their name or telling them to wake up. Never shake a child.

Procedure – *cont*

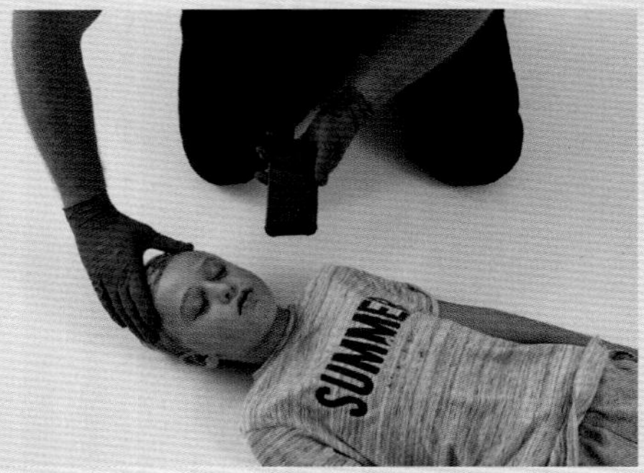

2. If the patient responds, assess the child's ABCDE, call for assistance and reassess regularly. If they do not respond, summon additional assistance.

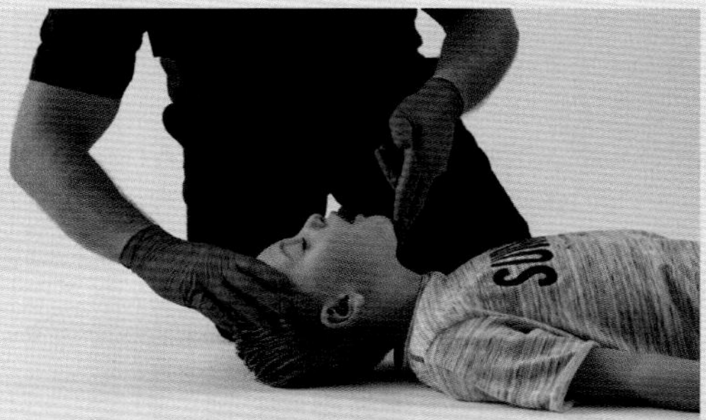

3a. Open the child's airway by placing one hand on their forehead and gently tilt it back until it is in a 'sniffing' position. Perform a chin lift by placing the fingertips of your other hand on the bony part of the lower jaw and lift upwards. Don't compress the soft tissues under the jaw as this will occlude the airway. Do not use a head tilt–chin lift technique in children who you suspect have a cervical spine injury: use a jaw thrust instead.

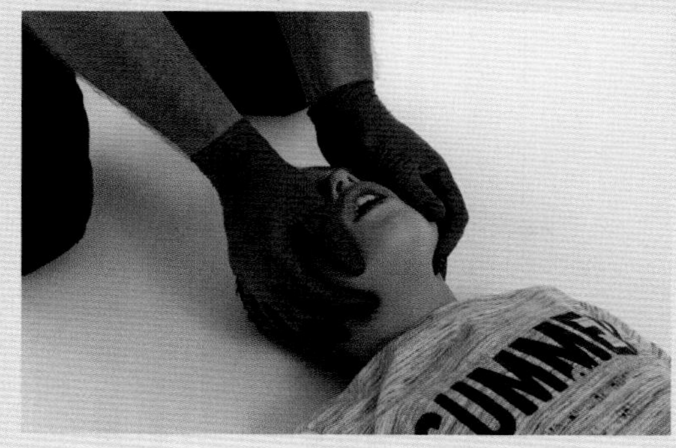

Procedure – *cont*

3b. If a head tilt–chin lift is not effectively opening the airway, or you suspect a cervical spine injury, use a jaw thrust to open the airway.

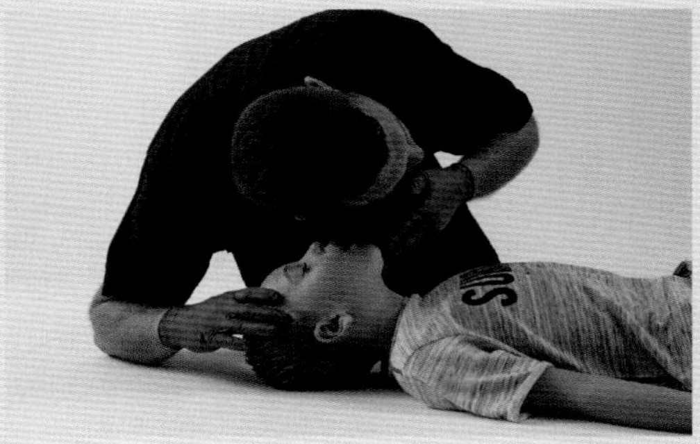

4. Look, listen and feel for normal breathing for no more than 10 seconds, by placing your face close to the child's face:
   - Look for chest and abdominal movements.
   - Listen for airflow at the mouth and nose.
   - Feel for airflow at the mouth and nose.

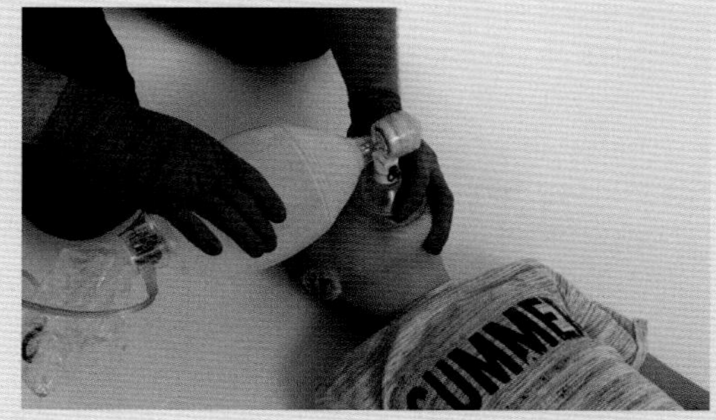

5. If the child is not breathing or there are no signs of life (not moving, no normal breathing or coughing), check for, and carefully remove, any airway obstruction that is visible and provide five rescue breaths:
   - Apply a head tilt–chin lift.
   - Either place a bag-valve-mask over the child's mouth and nose, or take a breath and place your mouth over the mouth of the child and pinch their nose to prevent air from escaping.
   - Ventilate the chest steadily for 1 second, just enough to make the chest rise.
   - Maintain head tilt–chin lift and watch the chest fall.
   - Repeat this sequence five times.

Procedure – *cont*

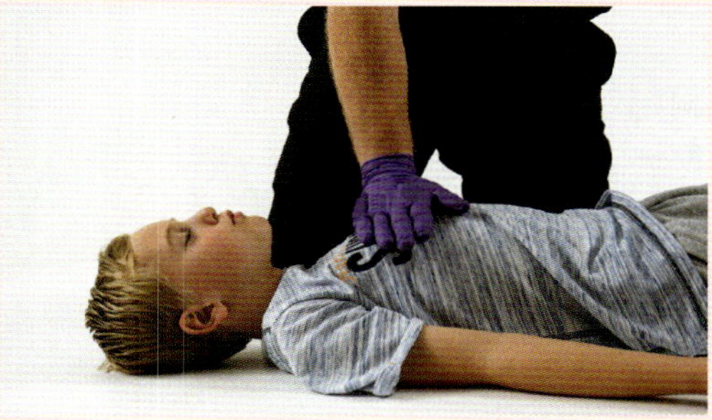

6. Check for signs of life (movement, coughing or normal breathing). If you are confident in checking for a pulse, feel for a carotid pulse at the neck. Unless you are sure you can feel a pulse, assume it is absent and start chest compressions. If there are signs of circulation, reassess airway and breathing and manage appropriately.

If there are no signs of life and/or no pulse or a pulse rate of less than 60 beats/min, start chest compressions:

- Position yourself at the side of the child.
- Avoid compressing the abdomen, by locating the xiphisternum and placing the heel of one hand one finger's width above this point.
- Lock your elbows and position your body so that your shoulders are directly over the child's chest.
- Compress the sternum at least one-third of the depth of the chest (or by 5 cm) and then fully release the pressure while maintaining contact with the sternum. If this is difficult, use the two-handed technique as you would for adults.
- Repeat the compressions at a rate of 100–120/min for 15 compressions and then give 2 ventilations.
- Continue compressions and ventilations at a ratio of 15:2 unless you are on your own, in which case a ratio of 30:2 may be easier.
- If you are on your own, continue until the child shows signs of life or you become exhausted. Alternatively, if you have a colleague present, alternate chest compressions with your colleague every two minutes, but keep the changeover time to a minimum.

Defibrillation

Learning Objectives

By the end of this section you will be able to:

- Describe the types of cardiopulmonary arrest.
- Recognise when it is appropriate to use a defibrillator.
- Explain the safety considerations when using a defibrillator.

Introduction

Heart rhythms associated with cardiac arrest are divided into shockable and non-shockable rhythms, depending on whether they should receive an electric current across the myocardium (heart muscle) to depolarise a sufficient amount of the heart muscle simultaneously and allow the normal heart pacemaker (the sino-atrial node) to resume control of the electrical conduction system. Delivering electricity to the heart in this way is known as defibrillation (Nolan, 2012).

In patients who have a shockable rhythm, the sooner they receive defibrillation, the greater the chance it will be successful and the patient will survive. However, it is equally important to ensure that defibrillation minimises the interruption of cardiopulmonary resuscitation (CPR). For each 5-second delay in CPR prior to delivering a shock, the chance of the shock being successful is halved (Nolan, 2012).

Shockable Rhythms

There are two shockable rhythms: ventricular fibrillation and ventricular tachycardia. Ventricular fibrillation (VF) is a rapid and disorganised ventricular rhythm and is never associated with a palpable pulse (Figure 18.6). Your automated external defibrillator (AED) will always advise a shock with this rhythm.

Ventricular tachycardia (VT) usually originates from the ventricles, is monomorphic (has one shape), and has a regular rhythm at a rate of 100–300/min (Figure 18.7) (Nolan, 2016; Garcia, 2004). Most AEDs will shock VT as long as it meets certain criteria (such as a heart rate >150 bpm for example).

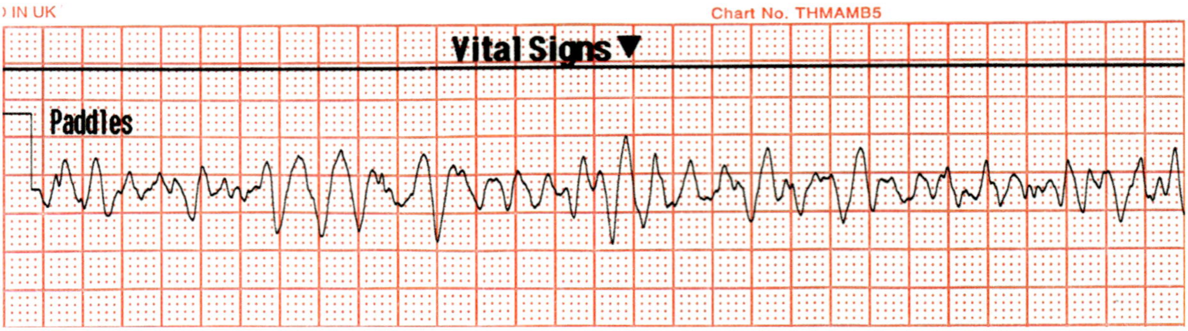

Figure 18.6 *Ventricular fibrillation.*

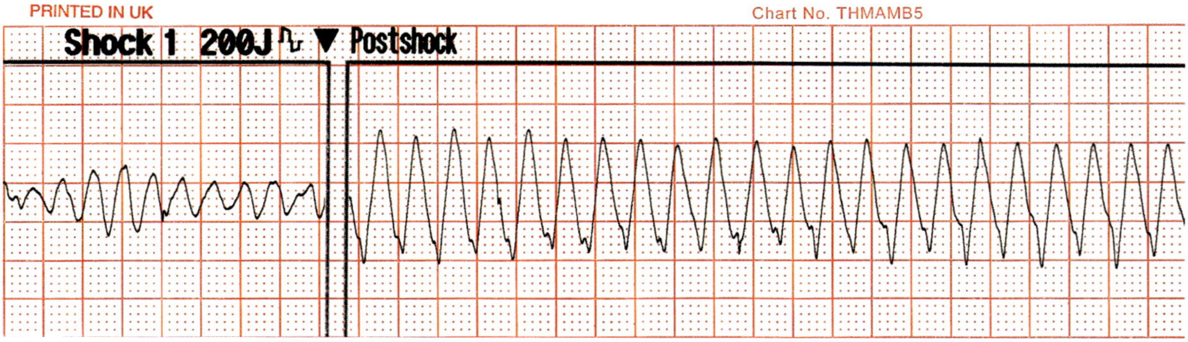

Figure 18.7 *Ventricular tachycardia following a 200 J shock. The patient was in VF prior to the shock.*

Non-Shockable Rhythms

As with shockable rhythms, there are two non-shockable rhythms: asystole and pulseless electrical activity. As the name implies, these are patients who will not benefit from defibrillation.

Asystole

Asystole is the term given to the absence of electrical activity from the heart. On an ECG, you will see a flat (isoelectric) or almost flat line (Figure 18.8) (Garcia, 2004). A variant of asystole is an agonal rhythm, which is characterised by a slow

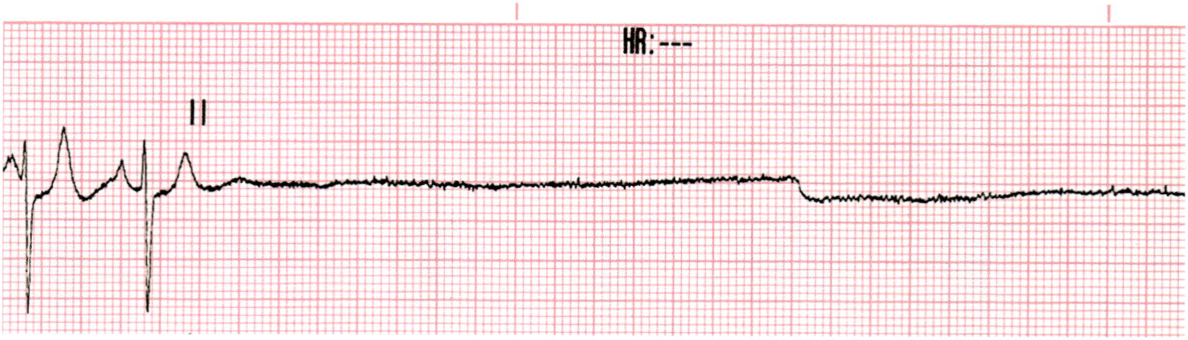

Figure 18.8 *Asystole. Note the two complexes on the left-hand side of the ECG before the start of asystole. The baseline is not always completely straight in asystole.*

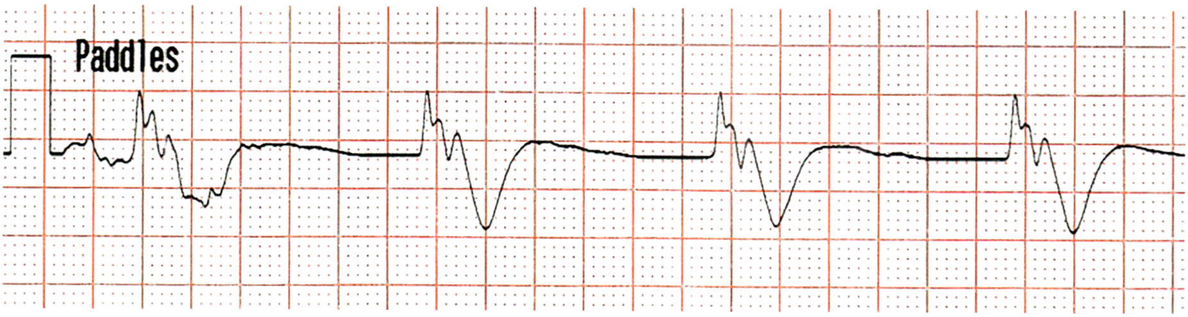

Figure 18.9 *An example of an ECG showing PEA.*

(a rate of <10/min), broad, sinusoidal complex, which interrupts the otherwise isoelectric line on the ECG (SWAST, 2014c).

Pulseless Electrical Activity (PEA)

PEA is organised electrical activity in the absence of a palpable pulse (Figure 18.9). Typically, patients in PEA will have some mechanical myocardial activity, but it is not sufficiently strong to produce adequate cardiac output to lead to a detectable pulse or blood pressure (Nolan, 2016).

Defibrillators

There are many brands and types of defibrillator on the market and it is important that you are familiar with the equipment you have available to you. Broadly, they fall into two types: automated external defibrillators (AEDs) and manual defibrillators. You will be issued with an AED.

Automated External Defibrillators (AEDs)

These 'shock boxes' are devices that provide voice and visual prompts to guide the public and healthcare professionals to defibrillate safely. AEDs are now widely available in public places such as shopping centres, sports centres, airports and railway stations (BHF, 2017). Despite their name, some AEDs can be manually overridden by healthcare providers capable of rhythm interpretation, but they are capable of recognising shockable and non-shockable rhythms (Nolan, 2016).

Difficult Environment and Defibrillation

You will frequently encounter challenging environments, which make resuscitation difficult. In terms of defibrillation, some of these can increase the risk of injury due to inadvertent electrocution. However, prompt defibrillation is life-saving and so it is important that you make a dynamic risk assessment and do not delay a shock unnecessarily.

Specific defibrillation scenarios include (Deakin, 2015):

- **Wet surfaces**: This is safe as long as you are not in contact with the patient and the patient's skin (if wet) is dried to ensure good contact is made by the self-adhesive pads to the patient's chest.
- **Metal surfaces such as gantries and mezzanine floors**: As before, this is safe as long as you are not in contact with the patient. Metal surfaces actually conduct any current that leaks from the pads through the metal and away from the crew and bystanders.

Safety

The only person who should receive a shock when a defibrillator is used is the patient. This can be achieved as long as members of the resuscitation team communicate well, so that everyone is well clear of the patient at the time of defibrillation.

Other ways of maximising safety include (Nolan, 2016; EEAST, 2014; Kerber, 2012):

- Use self-adhesive pads.
- Do not defibrillate patients while they are in water or near an explosive or combustible environment.

- Ensure that the rescuers do not hold intravenous infusion equipment or the ambulance trolley during defibrillation.
- Wear gloves.
- Shave the patient's chest, if required, to obtain a good skin-to-electrode contact.
- Avoid placing the pads over jewellery, piercings, medication patches, wounds and tumours.
- Ensure that the pads are well away from pacemaker sites (8 cm in adults and 12 cm in children).
- Remove oxygen from the patient unless the ventilation bag is directly connected to an endotracheal tube or supraglottic airway device. It should be at least 1 metre away from the patient's chest (Deakin, 2015).

Adult Defibrillation

Pad Placement

The standard placement for defibrillator pads is one just below the right clavicle, to the right of the sternum, and the other in the left mid-axillary line, or female breast. This should ensure that it is clear of breast tissue (Soar, 2015). There are often illustrations on the pads to indicate correct placement.

AED Procedure

Take the following steps to defibrillate using an AED (Perkins, 2015):

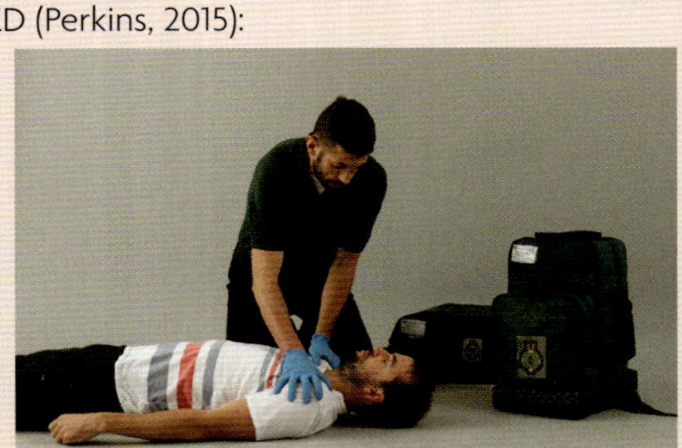

1. Check for danger and ensure that you, your colleagues, the patient and bystanders are safe. Assess the patient's responsiveness.

Procedure – *cont*

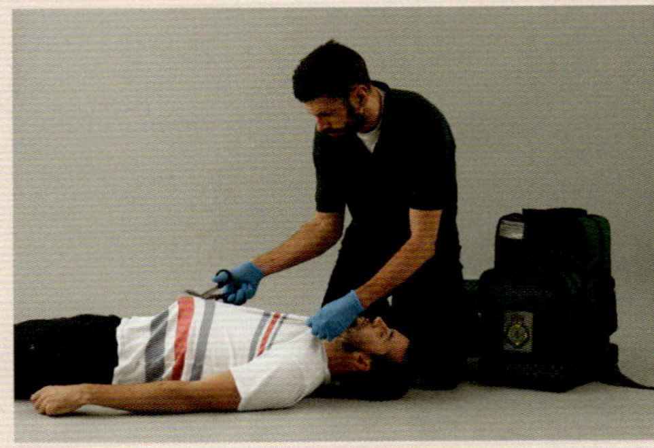

2. If the patient is unresponsive and not breathing normally and there is another person who can provide chest compressions, instruct them to commence CPR at a ratio of 30 compressions to 2 ventilations (30:2).

Bare the patient's chest and ensure that the pad sites are free from jewellery, piercings, medication patches, pacemakers, wounds and tumours. Shave the chest if required.

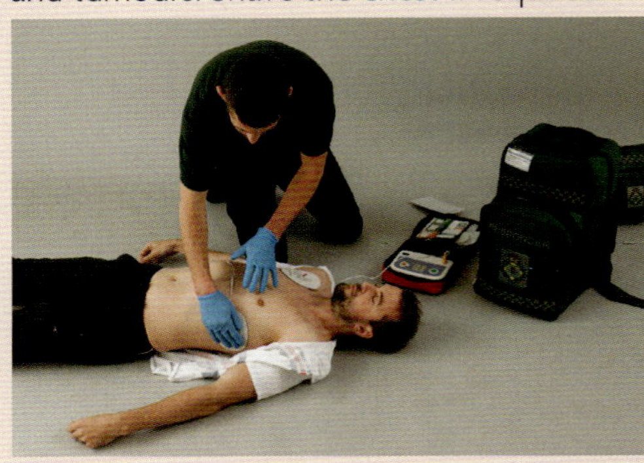

3. Switch on the AED and attach the pads to the patient, ensuring they make a good contact.

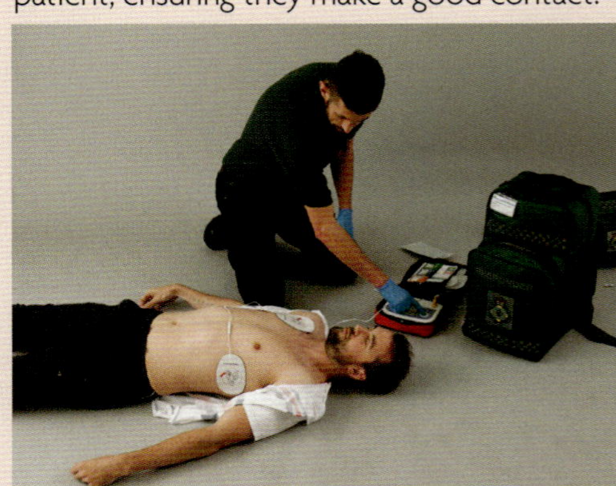

Procedure – *cont*

4. Follow visual/voice prompts, ensuring that no-one touches the patient while the AED is analysing the rhythm.

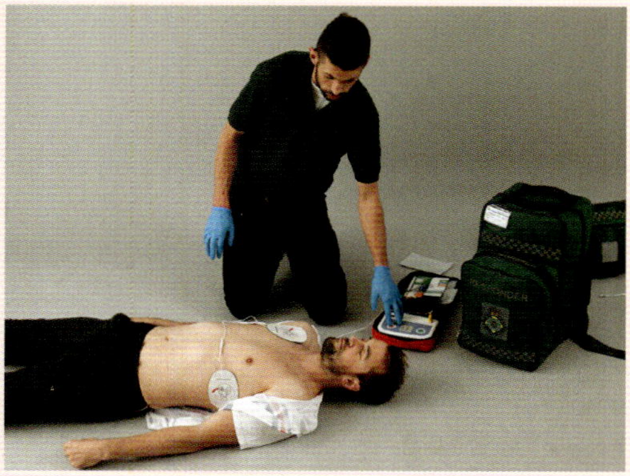

5. Shock?
   - If a shock is advised, make sure everyone is clear of the patient and push the shock button. Follow visual/voice prompts.
   - If a shock is not advised, restart CPR at a ratio of 30:2.

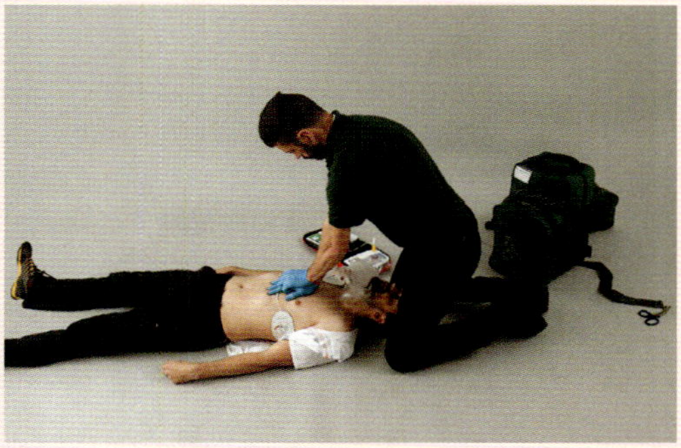

6. Continue until senior help arrives and takes over, the patient shows signs of life or you become exhausted.

Paediatric Defibrillation

Pad Placement

The standard placement for defibrillator pads is one just below the right clavicle, to the right of the sternum, and the other in the left mid-axillary line. Adult defibrillator pads can be used on children who are >25 kg (about 8 years of age), but they must not touch each other. Use paediatric pads for children under 25 kg (under 8 years of age), if available, but adult pads can be used in smaller children if there is no alternative (Maconochie, 2015).

If a sufficient gap between the defibrillator pads is not possible due to patient size, place the pads in the anterior–posterior position, with one pad over the left precordium and the other on the back, just under the left scapula (shoulder blade).

Procedure

Take the following steps to defibrillate a child with an AED (Maconochie, 2015):

1. Check for danger and ensure that you, your colleagues, the patient and bystanders are safe.
2. Start basic life support (BLS). For solo responders, opening the airway and providing effective ventilation takes priority over attaching an AED.
3. Bare the patient's chest and ensure that the pad sites are free from jewellery, piercings, medication patches, pacemakers, wounds and tumours.
4. Switch on the AED and attach the pads to the patient, ensuring they make a good contact. Use paediatric pads on patients under 25 kg if available.
5. Follow visual/voice prompts, ensuring that no-one touches the patient while the AED is analysing the rhythm.
6. Shock?
   - If a shock is advised, make sure everyone is clear of the patient and push the shock button. Follow visual/voice prompts.
   - If a shock is not advised, restart CPR at a ratio of 15:2 (30:2 if you are on your own).
7. Where possible, alternate chest compressions every 2 minutes with another person on scene to avoid fatigue. Continue until senior help arrives and takes over, the patient shows signs of life or you become exhausted.

Cardiac Arrest in Special Circumstances

Learning Objectives

By the end of this section you will be able to:

- Explain the considerations for a pregnant patient in cardiac arrest.
- Explain the considerations for a hypothermic patient in cardiac arrest.
- Explain the management of a patient who has suffered a traumatic cardiac arrest.

Introduction

In this chapter, you have been introduced to the principles and techniques of resuscitation of a patient in cardiac arrest. However, in some circumstances, the techniques need to be modified and/or alternative techniques used. Note that cardiac arrest associated with drowning is covered in the drowning section within Chapter 15: Exposure/Environment.

Cardiac Arrest in Pregnancy

The general procedure for resuscitating a pregnant patient is the same as for any other patient. However, for patients who are more than 20 weeks pregnant, there is a risk that their growing uterus can press down on the inferior vena cava and aorta, restricting venous return and leading to a reduction in cardiac output and uterine perfusion (Nolan, 2012).

To prevent this from occurring, the pregnant patient must not lie supine. In the conscious patient, the left lateral position is often used, but this is not practicable in a cardiac arrest when chest compressions need to be provided. Instead, the uterus should be manually displaced to the left (ALSG, 2010). This is achieved, by positioning a rescuer, or other person at scene, on the patient's right, level with the pregnant uterus. They then need to place both hands on the patient's uterus and push to the patient's left (JRCALC, 2017, Figure 18.10).

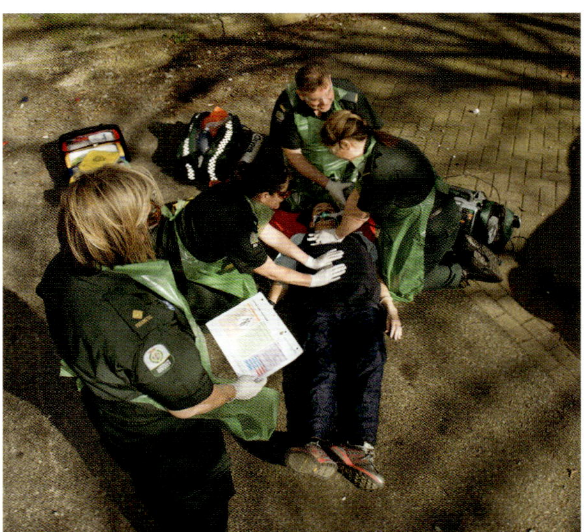

Figure 18.10 *Manually displacing the uterus.*

The hand position for patients in advanced pregnancy (over 28 weeks) may need to be 2–3 cm higher on the sternum. In addition, you may not be able to place the defibrillator pads in their usual position, due to enlarged breasts. In these cases, use alternative pad placement, such as the anterior–posterior position (Deakin, 2015).

During the latter stages of pregnancy, the patient is more likely to regurgitate their stomach contents and aspirate them into the lungs, particularly with over-enthusiastic bag-valve-mask ventilation. Consider using a supraglottic airway device early on in the resuscitation and keep suction close by. Intubation is ideal, if you have a clinician capable, but anatomical changes in pregnancy can make this difficult (ALSG, 2010).

Remember, the focus of resuscitation in pregnancy is on saving the mother, not the fetus, although sometimes it is possible to save both. High quality CPR will ensure the highest chance of a good outcome.

Cardiac Arrest in Hypothermic Patients

In cases of moderate and severe hypothermia, signs of life can be difficult to identify. Unless there is a clear indication that the cardiac arrest has been caused by a lethal injury or fatal illness, patients should be resuscitated based on the principle that 'no one is dead until warm and dead' (Truhlar, 2015).

Traumatic Cardiac Arrest

Surviving a traumatic out-of-hospital cardiac arrest is uncommon. However, survival rates of 6–7% have been reported, so it is important to manage these patients effectively. The key to success is to identify and treat the reversible causes of the cardiac arrest (Deakin, 2015).

Traumatic cardiac arrest may develop as a result of (JRCALC, 2016):

- hypoxia due to airway obstruction or breathing problems (e.g. facial injuries or pneumothorax)
- hypoperfusion due to hypovolaemia (internal or external haemorrhage) or injury to the heart, such as cardiac tamponade.

Management

All trauma patients in cardiac arrest should be resuscitated unless there is a clear indication that attempts would be futile (e.g. injuries incompatible with life). Patients who have suffered blunt trauma are likely to be resuscitated on scene, but those with penetrating injury must be rapidly transferred to an emergency department (JRCALC, 2016).

Follow the principles of standard trauma patient management (JRCALC, 2016):

- **C**: Control catastrophic haemorrhage.
- **A**: Ensure the airway is open and clear.
- **B**: Search for and manage sucking chest wounds. A tension pneumothorax will need to be decompressed by a suitably qualified clinician. Use high-flow oxygen during the resuscitation attempt.
- **C**: Hypovolaemia needs to be addressed with fluid (preferably blood). Clinicians on scene are likely to request repeated boluses of 0.9% saline and administer tranexamic acid.

Post-Resuscitation Care

Learning Objectives

By the end of this section you will be able to:

- State clinical signs that indicate an ROSC.
- Explain the management of the post-resuscitation patient.

Introduction

A return of spontaneous circulation (ROSC) in a patient you have resuscitated is a great feeling, but it is just the first step on the path to complete recovery from a cardiac arrest. A complex pathophysiological process occurs as a result of whole body ischaemia during a cardiac arrest and subsequent reperfusion when ROSC is achieved. This is known as post-cardiac arrest syndrome (Deakin, 2015).

During the resuscitation attempt, if the patient shows signs of life, including purposeful movement, normal breathing or coughing, and preferably confirmed by the presence of a central pulse, chest compressions may be discontinued.

Management

The following steps should be taken once ROSC is achieved (EEAST, 2014; SWAST, 2014c; Deakin, 2015):

- Reassess the patient's airway and breathing:
  - Provide ventilation, if required, at a rate of 10–12 breaths/min.
  - Oxygen therapy should be titrated to maintain an SpO_2 of 94–98%, except in trauma, where high-flow oxygen should continue to be administered.
- Reassess the patient's circulation:
  - Perform frequent pulse and blood pressure checks if trained to do so.
- Check blood glucose, if trained to do so.
- Aim for a core temperature no higher than 36.0°C. Do this by passively cooling the patient, i.e. don't cover the patient in blankets.
- Record all observations on the patient's care record.

Cardiac Arrest Decisions

Learning Objective

By the end of this section you will be able to:

- Explain when a resuscitation attempt may be stopped or not commenced.

When to Start and Stop Resuscitation

Whenever there is a chance that a patient may survive from a cardiac arrest, resuscitation should be attempted unless a patient has stated, via an 'advance decision to refuse treatment' (ADRT), that this should not occur, or there is a valid 'do not attempt cardiopulmonary resuscitation' (DNACPR) order (JRCALC, 2016). These documents vary from region to region, so ensure you are familiar with the type used in your area.

However, there are certain patients who have an injury or presenting condition that is unequivocally associated with death, irrespective of age (JRCALC, 2016; SWAST, 2014c). You should not attempt resuscitation in the following cases:

- **Massive cranial and cerebral destruction**
- **Hemicorporectomy** (complete amputation of the body below the waist) or similar massive injury
- **Decomposition/putrefaction** – tissue damage suggesting that the patient has been dead for hours, days or even longer

- **Incineration** – full thickness burns and charring covering more than 95% of the total body surface area (TBSA)
- **Hypostasis** – the pooling of blood in the dependent part of the body (i.e. below the level of the heart) after death
- **Rigor mortis** – stiffness of the body and limbs following death
- **Fetal maceration.**

End of Life Decisions

Advance Care Planning

In terminal conditions, death can often be anticipated, which provides patients with the opportunity to consider their wishes and preferences about future care, particularly as they are likely to be unable to do so when close to death. Unfortunately, only 5% of people put these wishes and preferences in writing by means of an advance care plan (ACP, sometimes also called a preferred priorities for care document) (NatCen, 2013). The contents of an ACP are not legally binding, but any best-interests decision about patients must take into account the patient's wishes and preferences (Watson, 2009).

Advance Decisions to Refuse Treatment (ADRT)

ADRTs (also known as living wills) are documents that outline specific aspects of care that the patient does not wish to receive. This is then typically referred to when the patient is unable to make these wishes clear. Examples of the interventions that a patient may refuse include being ventilated, being tube fed, receiving antibiotics and being admitted to hospital unless they are suffering from a complaint with a treatable cause.

Unlike the ACP, this is a legal document and, as long as the phrase 'even if life is at risk' is present, and the document is signed, dated and witnessed, the contents must be respected by all responders. Note that treatment can only be declined and not requested, and the ADRT only comes into effect once the patient loses mental capacity (Henry, 2008).

Do Not Attempt Cardiopulmonary Resuscitation (DNACPR) Decisions

DNACPR decisions are made by a senior clinician, usually with involvement from the patient's clinical team. This will normally be a consultant, GP or suitably experienced nurse (BMA, 2007). There are four broad situations when a DNACPR decision will be made (Dimond, 2011):

- A mentally competent patient refuses resuscitative treatment.
- A valid advanced directive clearly states that the patient does not want CPR.
- CPR is unlikely to be successful.
- Successful CPR is possible, but the length and quality of life following resuscitation is not in the patient's best interests.

Ideally, this is written and agreed ahead of time and documentary evidence of the decision will be presented to you before you commence resuscitation. Follow local procedures for how to approach a patient who has a DNACPR. Ultimately, if you are unsure about the validity of previously made decisions, then commencing resuscitation is defendable (JRCALC, 2016).

Chapter 19

Children and Infants

Why Paediatric Patients are Different

Learning Objective

By the end of this section you will be able to:

- Explain how paediatric patients are anatomically, physiologically and developmentally different from adults.

Introduction

Paediatrics is a speciality of medicine that looks after people from birth to age 18 years. Children are generally divided into five main groups (Lissauer, 2007):

- **Infants**: From birth to 12 months of age. In the first 4 weeks after birth, infants may also be called neonates.
- **Toddler**: Approximately 1–2 years of age.
- **Pre-school**: This is a young child aged 2–5 years.
- **School-age**: Generally 5–12 years (or the onset of puberty).
- **Teenager**: Also called adolescents. Generally from the onset of puberty to 18 years, when, in the UK, they become an adult. Some guidance (such as for resuscitation or the administration of some drugs) treats this group the same as adults.

Note that for the purposes of resuscitation, an infant is a patient under 12 months of age and a child is a patient who is 1 year to the onset of puberty (around 12 years) (Skellett, 2016).

Anatomy and Physiology

As children get older, their bodies change anatomically and physiologically. This is important to remember when undertaking your assessment as you may need to modify your plan for their management.

Airway

Most of the changes in the infant and child airway have been covered in Chapter 11: Airway. However, some extra points to consider are provided here.

Face and Mouth

Infants' faces are small. This makes sizing of a face mask for resuscitation important if a good seal is to be achieved. It is important that pressure on the eyes is avoided as this can result in damage and a reflex bradycardia. The floor of the mouth is also easy to compress, so care must be taken not to apply pressure to the soft tissues under the mandible during airway opening and positive-pressure ventilations (Figure 19.1) (Skellett, 2016).

Nose and Pharynx

In the first 6 months, infants breathe through their nose, meaning that any nasal obstruction can result in increased work of breathing and respiratory compromise (AAP, 2013).

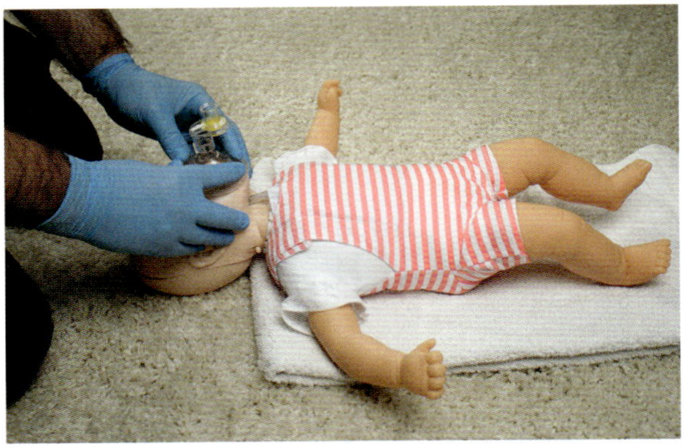

Figure 19.1 *Infant positive-pressure ventilation.*

Breathing

Infants and small children have relatively small resting lung volumes, which means they have less oxygen capacity in reserve than adults and have a higher oxygen consumption. In cases of respiratory compromise, therefore, the blood oxygen levels in these infants and small children will rapidly decline, making the prompt administration of supplemental oxygen crucial (Skellett, 2016).

The ribs of infants are cartilaginous and so are very pliable. In addition, they have weak intercostal muscles, which means that the diaphragm is their main muscle of respiration. If the diaphragm is impeded in any way, such as by gastric distension, for example, their ventilation may become ineffective (AAP, 2013).

As children get older, their intercostal muscles become more developed, contributing more to mechanical ventilation. Their ribs ossify, hardening and acting as an anchor for the developing intercostal muscles, making them less likely to collapse during periods of respiratory distress. As a result, intercostal recession in any child over the age of 5 years should be seen as an ominous sign of severe respiratory distress (Skellett, 2016).

Infants have a relatively high metabolic rate, oxygen consumption and carbon dioxide production, requiring a higher respiratory rate than older children. This can be further increased by pain, fever and anxiety, resulting in changing 'normal' respiratory rates for infants and children (Table 19.1) (Skellett, 2016).

Table 19.1 Respiratory rate ranges in infants and children

Age (years)	Respiratory rate (breaths/min)
<1	30–40
1–2	26–34
2–5	24–30
5–12	20–24
>12	12–20

Circulation

The circulating blood volume in an infant is about 80 ml/kg, which means that in a newborn baby weighing 3 kg, their blood volume is only 240 ml, making small blood losses significant.

Another important point to note is that oxygen delivery to the tissues is dependent on the arterial blood oxygen content multiplied by the cardiac output. In respiratory failure, a reduction in arterial blood oxygen can be compensated by increasing cardiac output. However, in circulatory failure, it is not possible to increase arterial blood oxygen content, so tissue oxygen delivery falls immediately (Fuchs, 2012).

The stroke volume at birth is small, only 1.5 ml/kg, so increasing cardiac output is mainly achieved by increasing heart rate. Thus heart rates in infants and small children are higher than in older children (Table 19.2). In addition, systemic vascular resistance increases as children get older, a change reflected by increased 'normal' blood pressures (Table 19.3) (Skellett, 2016).

Table 19.2 Paediatric heart rate ranges

Age	Awake (beats/min)	Deep sleep (beats/min)
0–3 months	85–205	80–140
3 months to 2 years	100–180	75–160
2–10 years	60–140	60–90
>10 years	60–100	50–90

Table 19.3 Paediatric blood pressure ranges

Age	Systolic blood pressure (mmHg)
0–1 month	> 60
1–12 months	80
1–10 years	90 + (2 x age in years)
> 10 years	120

Cognitive Development

Children are also challenging because their brain develops as they age. This means that during your assessment of a child, you will expect different levels of interaction and abilities in a 1-year-old compared with a 12-year-old child (Lissauer, 2007; AAP, 2013; Fuchs, 2012).

Infants

Under 2 Months

Infants in this age group will spend most of their time feeding and sleeping. They are unable to tell the difference between their parents/carers and others, so do not display stranger anxiety. They will exhibit primitive reflexes, such as grasping objects placed in the palm of their hand, or turning their head towards a gentle stimulation of the side of their mouth (rooting).

2–6 Months

Infants become more active during this period, making assessment a little easier. They begin to make eye contact, will smile and follow the light of your pen torch or a toy with their eyes. They will also turn their head in response to a loud noise or the voice of their parent/carer. Their motor skills develop and they will start to roll over and reach for objects. They will vocalise with coos and laughs when spoken to.

6–12 Months

Infants are much more socially interactive at this age. They may be able to say single words such as 'mama' or 'dada', but will also develop stranger anxiety in the latter stages (typically after 9 months), so keep the infant with their parent/carer if possible. They will be able to feed themselves, sit unsupported, reach for objects and pass them between hands.

Toddlers

There is a rapid change in growth and cognitive development at this age. By 18 months, children will have a vocabulary of around 6–10 words, and will know the name of, and be able to point to, several parts of their body. They should be able to walk steadily and feed themselves with a spoon.

As they reach 2 years of age, children may be able to combine several words together to make a simple phrase. They will start to engage in symbolic play, feeding their teddy for example. Stranger anxiety may be extreme and they are typically illogical thinkers, learning by trial and error, but have no sense of danger. They are self-centred and will be able to label objects as 'mine'. Toilet training may lead to children being dry during the day.

Pre-School

These children are creative and illogical thinkers, often confusing fantasy and reality. They are likely to have misconceptions about illness, injury and bodily functions. In addition, they may fear the dark, being left alone and the presence of monsters under the bed. They have good language skills and can participate in parallel play, taking it in turns with others, but their attention span is short.

School-Age

Children at this age understand cause and effect and are capable of abstract thought. They can tell you about the progress of their current illness or injury but their ability to understand the seriousness of the situation is limited. They can be involved with their care if explanations are kept simple and clear. Peer-group support becomes important at this age, but they will still have separation anxiety from their parents/carers when ill, and fear pain and loss of control.

Teenagers

Teenagers (adolescents) are sometimes compared to toddlers: highly mobile but lacking common sense! However, they are able to rationalise and express themselves and their feelings in words. This is also a period of experimentation and risk-taking.

Children at this age will typically transition from relying on their parents/carers for psychological support and development to their friends and peers. This typically leads to feelings of anxiety if they are 'different' from their peers. In addition, they may struggle with anxiety of independence, body image, sexuality and peer pressure.

Initial Assessment and Management of the Paediatric Patient

Learning Objectives

By the end of this section you will be able to:

- Conduct an initial assessment of the paediatric patient, including the assessment of pain in the child.
- Identify problems with a paediatric patient's airway, breathing, circulation and neurological status.
- Describe the principles that underpin the support of a seriously ill paediatric patient.
- Demonstrate the procedures to support a clinician to manage a seriously ill paediatric patient.
- Describe the assessment and management of the paediatric patient with a febrile illness.

Introduction

The assessment of the paediatric patient is much the same as for adults, and you will follow the standard procedure you learnt about in Chapter 10. As before, the primary survey is a chance to identify and correct life-threatening problems. In infants and children, prompt recognition and intervention when there are signs of respiratory and/or circulatory failure can prevent most paediatric cardiorespiratory arrests (Skellett, 2016).

Developmental Approach to the Paediatric Patient

A child's cognitive development changes as they age, which requires modification to your method of assessment. In this section, you will be provided with some suggestions about how to assess the paediatric patient. Don't forget that you will also need to manage and reassure an often anxious and distressed parent/carer.

Infants

Conduct your assessment by taking account of the following principles (AAP, 2013):

- Keep the environment comfortable, in terms of temperature and security for the infant. Familiar toys and blankets can help.
- Use the name of the patient while conducting your assessment.
- Where possible, assess an infant in the arms of a parent/carer.
- Approach the infant slowly and calmly. Loud voices and fast movements may scare them.
- Do not stand over an infant, but sit or kneel at their eye level.
- Look, listen and feel, in that order, to minimise infant distress.
- Warm your hands and tools such as stethoscopes.
- Be flexible in your assessment. If the infant is calm, count the respiratory rate and listen to the chest first. This is not possible to do accurately when the infant is crying.
- Observe the interaction between parent/carer and the infant. Consider if child abuse is a possibility.
- Toys can be used to distract the infant.
- Older infants may display stranger anxiety, so if you need to expose the infant, ask the parent/carer to do this. Don't let the infant get cold, though.
- Save painful procedures (such as blood sugar measurement) until last.

Toddlers

Conduct your assessment taking account of the following principles (AAP, 2013):

- Use the name of the patient while conducting your assessment.
- Approach slowly and don't touch them until they are familiar with you.
- Communicate using a firm, but friendly, tone of voice.
- Do not stand over a toddler, but sit or kneel at their eye level.
- Where possible, place the toddler on the lap of a parent/carer.
- Use play and distraction to help you conduct your assessment.

- If you need to use equipment, such as a stethoscope, let them hold it and become familiar and comfortable with it.
- Communicate directly with the toddler. Admire their clothes or ask about pets. Remember they are self-centred at this age.
- Provide limited choices. For example, 'Do you want me to listen to your belly or chest first?'.
- Avoid questions that can be answered with a 'No'.
- Examine a toddler from toe to head.
- Involve the parent/carer. For example, place the pulse oximeter probe on their finger first, and ask them to remove the toddler's clothes or hold an oxygen mask near the toddler.
- Do not expect toddlers to sit still and co-operate. Be patient and opportunistic.

Pre-School

Conduct your assessment taking account of the following principles (AAP, 2013):

- Use the name of the patient while conducting your assessment.
- Use simple terms to explain what you are going to do.
- Choose your words carefully. Use age-appropriate language and avoid scaring the child.
- Teddy or dolls can be helpful to explain what you are going to do.
- Set limits on behaviour, if required. For example, 'You can cry or scream, but not kick or bite'. Praise good behaviour.
- Use games and toys to provide distraction. Ambulance bandages can be useful for this.
- Focus on one thing at a time and minimise the time between explaining a procedure, especially a painful one, and carrying it out.

School-Age

Conduct your assessment taking account of the following principles (AAP, 2013):

- Use the name of the patient while conducting your assessment.
- Privacy becomes important in this age group. Make sure the environment is appropriate, and if you need to expose the child to examine them, cover them up afterwards.
- Speak directly to the child first, then include the parent/carer. Ask older children if they would like their parent/carer present.
- Involve the child in their care if they want this. Feeling out of control can distress children in this age group. However, do not negotiate unless the child really does have a choice.
- Anticipate the fears that the child has and address them straight away. Assure them that becoming ill or injured is not a punishment.
- Explain in simple terms what is wrong and what is going to be done.
- Explain procedures just prior to undertaking them. Don't lie to the child, for example telling them a procedure won't hurt, when it will.
- Praise the child for being co-operative, but do not chastise them if they are not.
- Physical assessments in this age group can usually be conducted head to toe.

Teenagers

Conduct your assessment taking account of the following principles (AAP, 2013):

- Use the name of the patient while conducting your assessment.
- Speak directly to the teenager and ask them first for information. If they do not know the answer, for example the name of their GP, check with them if it is okay to ask their parent/carer.
- Respect their modesty and privacy. Be confidential unless you have a duty to report or pass on their disclosures.
- Be honest and non-judgemental. Provide accurate information and allay fears, particularly concerns over body image or being 'different' because of their current illness or injury.
- Do not mistake the size of the teenager as a measure of their maturity.
- Avoid becoming frustrated or angry if the teenager does not want to communicate or is unco-operative.
- Enlist the help of their friends to assist when the teenager is being unco-operative, although keep in mind the teenager's right to confidentiality.

Recognising the Sick Infant and Child

Unlike adults, infants and children generally have a cardiac arrest secondary to respiratory and/or circulatory failure. Outcome from cardiac arrest in infants and children is significantly worse than in adults, and intervening early on can prevent this from occurring.

Respiratory Failure

Respiratory failure can be either compensated or decompensated. Compensated respiratory failure (sometimes known as respiratory distress) is characterised by increased work of breathing to overcome a respiratory problem, e.g. bronchiolitis. Respiratory failure is termed decompensated when the respiratory system can no longer maintain appropriate blood levels of oxygen (O_2) and carbon dioxide (CO_2). Since blood gases are not available out-of-hospital, a rough equivalent is a pulse oximetry (SpO_2) reading of less than 90% when breathing room air (Skellett, 2016).

Occasionally, respiratory failure can be present in the absence of increased work of breathing, for example due to a decreased level of consciousness or a morphine overdose.

Cardiac Failure

As with respiratory failure, cardiac failure can also be compensated or decompensated. In compensated failure, vital organ (heart and brain) perfusion is maintained and blood pressure remains within normal limits. This is mostly achieved by peripheral vasoconstriction. Once there is insufficient circulation to deliver O_2 to the tissues (i.e. in shock), the infant or child will become hypotensive and their level of consciousness will reduce.

Pain in Children

Pain is 'an unpleasant, subjective, sensory and emotional experience, associated with actual or potential tissue damage or described in terms of such damage' (IASP, 2017). Using a pain score to quantify a patient's level of pain is important, as their pain tends to be underestimated by healthcare professionals otherwise, leading to the provision of inadequate analgesia (Jennings, 2009). The situation is even worse for children, who have pain scores recorded, and analgesia administered, much less often than adults (Hennes, 2006).

Wong and Baker Faces Pain Rating Scale

The Wong and Baker faces pain rating scale is probably the most common method of pain assessment in children over the age of 3. It consists of 6 faces with a happy face at one end, through to a crying and distressed looking face at the other. To use the scale, point to each face using the words to describe the pain intensity. Ask the child to choose the face that best describes their own pain and record the appropriate number (JRCALC, 2016).

Primary Survey

The primary survey in the infant and child is the same as for adults, except for the general impression component, which should include use of the paediatric assessment triangle (PAT). The PAT is advantageous in children because it can be undertaken without touching the child and be performed 'across the room' to avoid increasing a child's anxiety by getting too close initially (AAP, 2013).

General Impression

It is important to gain a general impression of the health of an infant or child from 'across the room', before your presence has an adverse effect on their level of anxiety or distress. To help you achieve this, use the paediatric assessment triangle (PAT) (Dieckmann, 2010). As the name suggests, it consists of three key components:

- appearance
- work of breathing
- circulation to skin.

Appearance

The child's general appearance is probably the most significant aspect of the PAT as it provides information about the perfusion of the brain. The parts of this component can be remembered using the mnemonic TICLS (AAP, 2013):

- **T**one: Is the infant/child moving spontaneously or are they floppy and listless?
- **I**nteractiveness: Does the infant/child respond to people, objects and sounds or are they uninterested in their surroundings?
- **C**onsolability: Can the infant/child be consoled by their parent/carer?

- **L**ook/Gaze: Does the infant/child look at you or do they have a 'glass-eyed' stare into the distance?
- **S**peech/Cry: Is their speech or cry strong or weak, muffled or hoarse?

Work of Breathing

In children, it is their work of breathing that provides a better indication as to the adequacy of oxygenation and ventilation, rather than the more traditional respiratory rate and/or auscultation in adults (AAP, 2013). Look for signs of increased work of breathing, as well as listening for abnormal airway sounds:

- **Abnormal airway sounds**: These include snoring, muffled or hoarse speech, stridor, grunting and wheezing.
- **Abnormal positioning**: Children who can sit up may adopt a 'sniffing the morning air' position, tripod position and/or refuse to lie down.
- **Recession**: Recession of the chest muscles provides an indication of increased work of breathing, as does head bobbing in infants. Beware the child over 5 years who has signs of recession, as this is a sign of serious respiratory compromise (Skellett, 2016).
- **Flaring**: Look for nasal flaring, an exaggerated opening of the nostrils during laboured inspiration.

Circulation to Skin

When cardiac output is not sufficient to meet the body's metabolic demands, the circulation to non-essential organs, such as the skin, reduces. This can manifest in children as (AAP, 2013):

- **Pallor**: White or pale skin indicating a reflex shunting of blood away from the skin. This may be the only sign of compensated shock.
- **Cyanosis**: This is blue discolouration of the skin caused by inadequate oxygenation. Note that blue hands and feet in newborns and infants under the age of 2 months (acrocyanosis) is a normal finding.
- **Mottling**: This is caused by abnormal blood vessel tone in the capillary beds of the skin. There are patchy areas of pallor and cyanosis. This can be normal when the child is exposed to a cold environment.

Airway

Obstruction of the airway is common in seriously ill children, causing hypoxia, which can lead to unconsciousness and cardiorespiratory arrest (such as in cases of choking) (Skellett, 2016). It is important to remember that chest movement does not imply a clear airway: you need to listen and feel for air movement.

Look for apparent difficulty in breathing or increased work of breathing. In conscious children, they may be in visible distress. Listen for additional noises, such as stridor, a high-pitched (usually) inspiratory sound (Skellett, 2016).

Management

Children who are conscious should be allowed to adopt a position of comfort, ideally one that they themselves adopt to maximise the efficiency of their airway, and supplemental high-flow oxygen via a non-rebreathe mask should be administered.

For unconscious children, their head needs positioning appropriately to open the airway and prevent the tongue from falling backwards and occluding the airway. This can be achieved in children using a head tilt–chin lift, or jaw thrust manoeuvre. Remember that in infants, their head should be placed in the neutral position, with padding under the shoulders to account for their proportionally larger head (Figure 19.2). Care must be taken not to compress the soft tissues under a child's jaw as this can also occlude the airway (Skellett, 2016).

Oropharyngeal airways (OPAs) can be used in children as for adults. For small children and

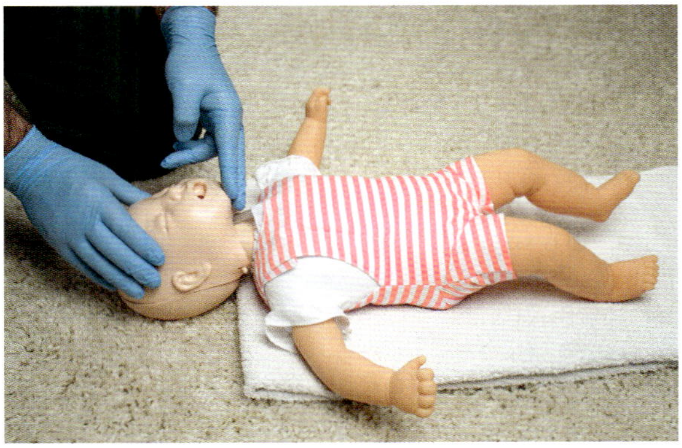

Figure 19.2 *An infant with the airway in neutral alignment.*

infants, it is generally recommended that the OPA is introduced the 'right way round' and not rotated 180°. This is likely to require a tongue depressor (Gregory, 2010b).

Breathing

Assessment

The most effective way of determining whether the airway is obstructed is to look, listen and feel (Biarent, 2010):

- **Look** for chest (and abdominal) movements.
- **Listen** at the child's mouth and nose for breath (plus added) sounds.
- **Feel** for air movement on your cheek.

Note that the chest may move in children, even with an obstruction, making it important to listen and feel.

As part of gaining a general impression, you will already have considered the patient's work of breathing, which includes (AAP, 2013):

- abnormal airway sounds
- abnormal positioning
- recession
- flaring.

Other signs of increased work of breathing include elevated respiratory rates and accessory muscle use.

Abnormal Airway Sounds

Stridor is a high-pitched inspiratory sound that indicates an upper airway obstruction. This may be an object, or swelling due to infection. In severe cases, it can also occur on expiration. A wheeze, on the other hand, is usually an expiratory sound and is a sign of lower airway obstruction. You may be able to hear it with just your ears, but often it will only be heard on auscultation (AAP, 2013).

Grunting is usually heard in neonates and small infants, although it can occur in small children. It occurs when the infant exhales against a partially closed glottis. This generates a small amount of end-expiratory pressure, keeping the small airways from collapsing at the end of expiration. It is an indication of severe respiratory compromise (Skellett, 2016).

Abnormal Positioning

Children in respiratory distress typically adopt a position that maximises their respiratory efficiency. In upper airway obstruction, this will be a 'sniffing the morning air' position. In lower respiratory problems they may adopt a 'tripod' position, sitting forward with their arms outstretched and resting on their knees (Skellett, 2016).

Recession

Recession can be sternal, subcostal and/or intercostal. Note that significant recession can be seen in infants and young children, even in mild respiratory distress, due to their compliant chest wall (Figure 19.3). However, as previously mentioned, it is a serious sign in children over 5 years of age (AAP, 2013).

Flaring

Nostril flaring in infants and young children is a sign of increased respiratory effort.

Respiratory Rate

An increased respiratory rate (tachypnoea) is often the first sign of respiratory problems, although it can be difficult to assess in the crying infant/child (Table 19.1) (Skellett, 2016).

Accessory Muscle Use

Additional muscles are often recruited when the work of breathing increases. One group is the

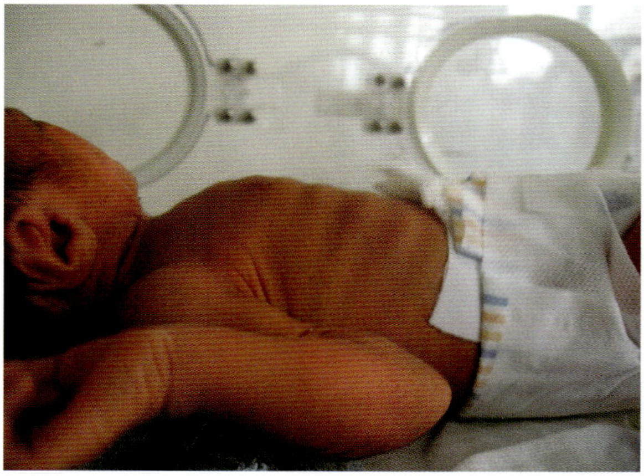

Figure 19.3 *A newborn with intercostal recession – by Bobjgalindo (Own work) [CC-BY-SA-3.0-2.5-2.0-1.0], via Wikimedia Commons.*

sternocleidomastoid muscles in the neck. These cause 'head bobbing' in infants, who will nod their head up and down with each breath. However, this is not an efficient method of breathing (Skellett, 2016).

Pulse Oximetry

This can be unreliable when a child has poor peripheral circulation, but if obtainable, a reading of less than 90% on air, or 95% on high-flow oxygen, is a sign of decompensated respiratory failure and urgent intervention is required (Biarent, 2010). Use a dedicated paediatric probe where possible.

Management

All seriously ill children should receive high-flow oxygen via a non-rebreathe mask, unless their ventilation is insufficient. In this case, assistance should be provided with bag-valve-mask ventilation. For children who are conscious, placing a mask over the child may be distressing. In this case, attempt administration using the least-threatening method, for example by asking the parent/carer to hold an oxygen mask close to the patient's mouth and nose (JRCALC, 2016).

Watch for signs of decompensation, which include:

- changes to respiratory rate – increasing or sudden decrease
- reducing level of consciousness/interaction with you and parents/guardians
- exhaustion.

Unconscious children and infants whose airway is clear, and who are breathing normally, should be turned on their side into the recovery position (Maconochie, 2015). While the adult recovery position can be used in children, modification is required for infants. Adopt the following principles when placing an infant in the recovery position:

- Place the child in as near true lateral position as possible, with their mouth suitably positioned to assist in the free drainage of fluid.
- The position needs to be stable. This may require a small pillow or a rolled-up blanket to be placed along the infant's back to maintain the position, to prevent the infant from rolling on to their back or front.
- Avoid any pressure on the infant's chest that might impair breathing.
- Whatever the position, it should be possible to turn the infant from their side on to their back (and vice versa) easily and safely.

Circulation

Assessment

When assessing circulation, look for signs of blood and other fluid losses, which are causing shock. Children can compensate very well, maintaining their blood pressure until they have significant fluid losses. However, you can spot the child in compensated circulatory failure by examining the following (Skellett, 2016):

- heart rate
- pulse volume
- capillary refill time.

Heart Rate

Tachycardia is common in children and has several causes including pain, anxiety and fever. It is also often the first sign of circulatory failure. Bradycardia, defined in an infant as a heart rate less than 80 beats/min and in a child, a heart rate less than 60 beats/min, is a serious sign (Skellett, 2016). A heart rate of less than 60 beats/min in infants and children is normally an indication to start chest compressions.

Pulse Volume

When a child develops shock, peripheral pulses will become weak and thready. If central pulses (such as a carotid pulse) become weak and thready, the child is in cardiorespiratory failure and arrest is imminent (Skellett, 2016), so always ensure you compare central and peripheral pulses.

As children become peripherally vasoconstricted in response to shock, their extremities will become cool. Sometimes there is a clear demarcation line between cool skin and warm skin, that will either move towards the torso if shock progresses, or move distally if perfusion and circulation improve (JRCALC, 2016).

Capillary Refill Time

Capillary refill time (CRT) can be a useful indicator of circulatory status, as was covered in Chapter 13: Circulation.

Skin

Skin perfusion can provide valuable clues as to the infant's or child's circulatory status. Note the temperature of the skin, particularly the level of warm/cold demarcation lines on the limbs. This occurs due to peripheral vasoconstriction and reduced perfusion to the limbs. Over time, if the patient condition does not improve, the demarcation line will move up the limb towards the torso. Monitor this level frequently to see whether things are improving or heading to circulatory failure. The colour of the skin should also be assessed if it wasn't covered in the PAT.

End-Organ Perfusion

Although you will conduct a formal assessment of level of consciousness (LOC, reviewed in Chapter 14: Disability), consider if there are any signs of poor cerebral perfusion. Early signs of compromise include a loss of interaction with the infant's or child's surroundings and irritability and agitation. Late signs include a loss of consciousness and loss of tone (e.g. a 'floppy' baby).

The kidneys are an essential organ and one clue that they are not being adequately perfused is a reduction in urine output. A simple way of assessing this is to ask about the number of wet nappies or the number of times the child has passed urine.

Management

The principal method of maintaining circulation is to ensure that airway and breathing are adequately addressed and any life-threatening conditions, such as tension pneumothorax, are identified and treated. However, for seriously fluid-depleted children, intravenous access will be required so that fluid replacement can commence (JRCALC, 2016).

As with breathing, watch for signs of decompensation:

- changes in heart rate: increasing or sudden fall
- increasing peripheral vasoconstriction:
  - CRT increasing
  - warm/cold demarcation line moving up the limb towards the body
  - loss/reduction of peripheral pulses
- reduced level of consciousness
- hypotension (late sign).

Disability

Assessment

Often, you will already have an idea about the patient's level of consciousness (LOC) from the general impression. Use the AVPU mnemonic to quickly gauge the child's LOC:

- **A**: alert
- **V**: responds to voice
- **P**: responds to pain
- **U**: unresponsive.

Pupils should be checked for dilation, equality and reactivity. Seriously ill children are typically hypotonic and floppy, but in cases of serious brain dysfunction, children may become abnormally stiff and rigid (Skellett, 2016).

Management

Ensure that airway, breathing and circulation are managed adequately. Don't forget to check blood glucose if you are authorised, and during the history determine whether there is a risk of poisoning or meningococcal septicaemia (JRCALC, 2016).

Exposure/Environment

In order to complete the primary survey it may be necessary to remove some of the child's clothing, but be mindful that children lose heat rapidly, particularly infants. Use this time to thoroughly examine infants and children who are ill for rashes (Pilbery, 2013). Keep in mind the possibility of a non-accidental injury, and check for bruises and other signs of injury (see Chapter 5: Safeguarding for further details).

Febrile Illness in the Paediatric Patient

Fever is defined by the National Institute for Health and Care Excellence (NICE) as an elevation of body temperature above normal daily variation (NICE, 2013a). There is no actual temperature value specified in the guidelines for fever, although temperatures of 38°C and above in infants under three months are classed as high risk. For older infants, temperatures of 39°C and above are classed as an intermediate risk. It is the most common medical complaint in childhood and is suggestive of an underlying infection (JRCALC, 2016).

Table 19.4 NICE 'traffic light system' for establishing risk of serious illness

	Green low risk	Amber intermediate risk	Red high risk
Colour (of skin, lips or tongue)	Normal colour.	Pallor reported by parent/carer.	Pale/mottled/ashen/ cyanosed.
Activity	Responds normally to social cues. Content/smiles. Stays awake or awakens quickly. Strong normal cry/ not crying.	Not responding normally to social cues. No smile. Wakes only with prolonged stimulation. Decreased activity.	No response to social cues. Appears ill to a healthcare professional. Does not wake or, if roused, does not stay awake. Weak, high-pitched or continuous cry.
Respiratory		Nasal flaring. Tachypnoea: RR >50 breaths/ min, age 6–12 months. RR >40 breaths/ min in children. Oxygen saturations 95% or less in air. Crackles on chest auscultation.	Grunting. Tachypnoea: RR >60 breaths/ min. Moderate or severe recession.
Circulation and hydration	Normal skin and eyes. Moist mucous membranes.	Tachycardia: >160 beats/min, age <12 months. >150 beats/min, age 1–2 years. >140 beats/min, age 2–5 years. CRT 3 seconds or more. Dry mucous membranes. Poor feeding in infants. Reduced urine output.	Reduced skin turgor.
Other	No amber or red signs or symptoms.	Age 3–6 months, temperature 39°C or higher. Fever for 5 days or more. Rigors. Swelling of a limb or joint.	Under 3 months of age, temperature 38°C or higher. Non-blanching rash. Bulging fontanelle. Neck stiffness. Status epilepticus. Focal neurological signs. Focal convulsions.

Key: RR — respiratory rate; CRT — capillary refill time

Assessment

As with all children, you should conduct an initial ABCDE assessment and correct any immediate life-threatening findings. Once this has been undertaken, obtain a history, ensuring that you cover the following (JRCALC, 2016):

- duration of illness
- associated symptoms
- urinary symptoms
- abdominal pain
- headache, photophobia, neck stiffness
- painful joints, sore throat, ear pain
- adequacy of fluid intake
- existing medical problems
- current medication
- other illness in the family/school/nursery
- recent foreign travel.

NICE have produced a helpful table utilising a 'traffic light' system' to highlight signs and symptoms most associated with level of risk (Table 19.4). Children with fever and any of the signs and symptoms in the red column should be considered to be high risk. Similarly, children with fever and signs and symptoms only in the yellow column, are classed as intermediate-risk and for signs and symptoms in the green column only, low-risk (NICE, 2013a).

Management

All paediatric patients who meet any one of the red, high-risk criteria should receive high-flow oxygen. In addition, paediatric patients who have any of the adverse respiratory and/or circulatory signs of the amber, intermediate-risk criteria may also benefit from the administration of high-flow oxygen. Follow local guidance on oxygen administration. Sometimes, rapid changes in body temperature can cause children to have a convulsion. Management is the same as for convulsions from other causes (see Chapter 14: Disability).

Anti-Pyretics

Giving a patient anti-pyretics, such as ibuprofen or paracetamol, for fever is not necessary if the child is otherwise asymptomatic. However, they are useful for treating other symptoms associated with infection, such as aches, pains and generally feeling unwell, and may also reassure concerned parents, who in turn can relay their anxiety to the child (Bont, 2014; Williams, 2014). There is no evidence that anti-pyretic drugs prevent febrile convulsions occurring, or are beneficial in preventing further episodes when a child has suffered from a convulsion (Oluwabusi, 2012). Follow local guidance with regards to the administration of anti-pyretics.

Chapter 20

Mental Health

Mental Health Legislation and Codes of Practice

Learning Objectives

By the end of this section you will be able to:

- Define mental health and mental disorder.
- Explain a number of important roles specified by the Mental Health Act.
- Explain the guiding principles that are used when applying the Mental Health Act.
- Outline how a person is detained under the Mental Health Act.

Introduction

As an emergency medical responder you will be exposed to individuals who suffer from mental ill health. It is important to understand what mental health is, how to recognise it and how to safeguard those individuals who need support.

Mental health is defined by the World Health Organization as 'a state of well-being in which every individual realizes his or her own potential, can cope with the normal stresses of life, can work productively and fruitfully, and is able to make a contribution to her or his community' (WHO, 2014).

However, around 1 in 4 people will suffer from mental ill health at some point in their lifetime, such as anxiety, depression, phobias and obsessive compulsive disorder (OCD), for example, and these conditions are collectively referred to as mental disorders. Most of these conditions are managed between the patient and their general practitioners (GPs) (HSCIC, 2009), without the need for specialist mental health treatment.

The Mental Health Act 1983 (as amended 2007, MHA)

If a person has a mental disorder (defined as any disorder or disability of the mind (UK, 2007)) and is required to be detained against their wishes, specific sections of the MHA will be used to admit patients without their agreement. You will commonly hear these patients being referred to as being 'sectioned' or 'detained' under the MHA. This is in contrast to patients who agree to attend a psychiatric ward, whose admission may be referred to as 'informal' or 'voluntary' (UK, 1983).

Roles Defined by the MHA

Approved Mental Health Professional (AMHP)

An AMHP is usually a social worker (although since the amendment to the MHA in 2007, appropriately trained nurses, occupational therapists and psychologists can also become an AMHP (UK, 2007)) who has been approved by the local social services authority to carry out a number of activities specified in the MHA (DoH, 2008).

Their role includes the following (Dimond, 2011):

- informing the nearest relative about the admission of the patient and their right to discharge
- consulting the nearest relative about admission for treatment or guardianship and discontinuing the application (in the case of detention under Section 3 of the MHA) if the relative objects
- applying for admission or guardianship if they are satisfied that the application is necessary
- interviewing patients to determine that detention in hospital is the most appropriate way to care for the patient
- reporting on the patient's social circumstances.

Section 12 Doctor

This is a senior doctor (typically a middle-grade or higher psychiatrist, that has specialist experience in the diagnosis or treatment of mental disorder) who is an approved clinician, i.e. has been approved by the Secretary of State (England) or Welsh minister (Wales) (Mind, 2012).

Nearest Relative

This is an important role according to the MHA. The nearest relative is defined as the highest in the following hierarchy (UK, 1983):

- relative who usually resides with or cares for the patient
- husband, wife or civil partner
- son or daughter
- father or mother
- brother or sister
- grandparent
- grandchild
- uncle or aunt
- nephew or niece.

They have a range of powers including (Dimond, 2011):

- applying for admission of the patient for assessment, treatment and guardianship (although this is unlikely: this is virtually always undertaken by an AMHP)
- objecting to an AMHP's proposed application for treatment under Section 3
- discharging the patient having given 72 hours' notice in writing to hospital managers
- applying to a mental health review tribunal.

Guiding Principles

When deciding on a course of action to take using the MHA, AMHPs must take into account the five overarching principles. They are (DoH, 2015):

- **Least restrictive option and maximising independence**: This may include home treatment, staying at a crisis house, staying with a relative or friend, for example, or offering the patient the chance to attend hospital informally.
- **Empowerment and involvement**: Patients should be involved in decisions about their care. In addition, the views of family members, carers and others, if appropriate, should be taking into consideration.
- **Respect and dignity**: Patients, their families and carers should be treated with respect and dignity and listened to by professionals.
- **Purpose and effectiveness**: Care and treatment need to conform to current best practice guidelines and have clear therapeutic aims.
- **Efficiency and equity**: Provision of services should be of a high quality and be given the same priority as physical ill health.

MHA Sections

Section 2

This section provides the power to admit a patient to hospital and detain them for up to 28 days for the purposes of assessment on the grounds that they are suffering from a mental disorder severe enough to warrant the admission, and that detention is appropriate for maintenance of the health and safety of the patient and others. The applicant needs to be an AMHP or the nearest relative and requires the agreement of two doctors, one of whom must be approved under Section 12 of the MHA (UK, 1983).

Section 3

This section provides the power to admit a patient to hospital and detain them for a period of 6 months initially (although it can be renewed) for the purposes of treatment, on the grounds that they are suffering from a mental disorder severe enough to receive treatment in hospital, that detention is appropriate for maintenance of the health and safety of the patient and others, and that an appropriate treatment is available. As before, the applicant needs to be an AMHP or nearest relative and requires the agreement of two doctors, one of whom must be approved under Section 12 of the MHA.

Section 4

This section is rarely used as it is viewed as an incomplete Section 2 or 3 by mental health professionals. It allows for the emergency admission of a patient for the purposes of assessment, requires the applicant to be an AMHP or nearest relative, but only requires one Section 12-approved doctor to recommend detention.

Section 135

If a patient believed to have a mental disorder is being ill-treated, neglected or not kept under proper control, or is unable to care for themselves and living alone, an AMHP can obtain a warrant from a magistrate to enter any property where the patient is believed to be located, and, if necessary, remove them to a place of safety. This requires a police officer to execute the warrant and gain access to a property, with force if necessary, but they must be accompanied by a doctor and AMHP (Mind, 2012).

Section 136

If a police officer encounters a person in a public place who appears to be suffering from a mental disorder and in immediate need of care or control, they can remove that person to a place of safety (UK, 1983). This should be a hospital or other health-based location where mental health services are provided. However, other locations, such as residential care homes, may be appropriate. Police stations should not be used as a place of safety other than in exceptional circumstances and must never be used if the patient is a child. Remember, patients detained by the police under Section 136 are not being detained for criminal acts; they are patients and should receive the same standard of care and compassion as all other patients.

Transporting Patients

Generally, it falls to the ambulance service to transport patients, as use of police personnel and vehicles has been highlighted as bad practice, and their use should be reserved for physically violent patients (DoH, 2014).

Mental Disorders

Learning Objectives

By the end of this section you will be able to:

- Describe a range of mental disorders.
- Explain the aims and components that make up mental health first aid.
- State some general principles to consider when assisting a patient with a mental disorder.

Introduction

Traditionally, mental disorders were divided into neuroses – illnesses that are severe forms of 'normal' experiences, such as anxiety and depression – and psychoses – illnesses that result in misperception of thoughts that arise from the patient's own mind/imagination as reality, and include delusions and hallucinations, such as schizophrenia (Kumar, 2012).

Although the terms are still used, definitions provided by the International Classification of Diseases version 10 (ICD-10) organise disorders according to common themes. Disorders covered in this chapter include (Cooper, 2012):

- organic disorders
- schizophrenia and delusional disorders
- mood (affective) disorders
- neurotic, stress-related and somatoform disorders
- personality disorders.

Organic Disorders

Organic disorders occur as a result of physical brain disease, such as occurs in dementia (see Chapter 21: Older People), or from disturbed central nervous system (CNS) function, for example a fever-induced delirium (Kumar, 2012).

Delirium

Delirium is a common form of psychosis, and is characterised by incoherent thoughts and speech, impaired memory and episodes of hallucinations and delusions. Common causes of delirium include systemic infection, metabolic disturbances, endocrine diseases and intracranial causes, such as trauma, haemorrhage or epilepsy, for example. In addition, toxic doses of the patient's usual medication, as well as drug and/or alcohol withdrawal can cause delirium.

Schizophrenia and Delusional Disorders

The most common type of schizophrenia is the paranoid subtype, which includes delusions and auditory hallucinations. Delusions typically consist of the following characteristics (Cooper, 2012):

- **persecutory**: someone or some group is out to harm the patient
- **delusions of reference**: the patient is mentioned on the TV news or in a newspaper.

Disorders of thought can occur including:

- **derailment**: seemingly random connections between verbal statements in conversation
- **neologisms**: the patient uses made-up words, or uses words in a special way
- **word salad**: jumbled nonsense
- **concrete thinking**: inability to deal with abstract ideas.

Mood (Affective) Disorders

Mood can be thought of as a temporary state of mind or feeling. Patients with mood disorders sit somewhere on a continuum from severe depression to severe mania, with 'normal' mood in the middle. Mood disorders can be bipolar or unipolar (Kumar, 2012).

Bipolar Affective Disorder

This disorder (formerly called manic depression) is characterised by recurring episodes of altered mood and activity, typically swinging between depression and mania.

The classic features of a manic episode are an elevated mood (although the patient can become irritable too) and the presence of the following associated features (Cooper, 2012):

- exaggerated optimism and inflated self-esteem
- decreased social inhibition, e.g. sexual over-activity, reckless spending, dangerous driving
- rapid thinking and speech (flight of ideas)
- lack of insight into disorder.

Depression

Everyone experiences a low mood from time to time, but this is not depression. Depressive illness occurs when symptoms become severe enough to affect a person's ability to carry out daily activities or go to work, for example, and lasts for more than 2 weeks.

Patients often describe symptoms in physical terms and complaints of fatigue and headache are common. Other descriptions used by patients include describing the world as looking grey, and of being without anything pleasurable or interesting to do or look forward to. Anxiety attacks are common, and phobic and/or obsessive disorders can also result (Kumar, 2012). In more severe forms, suicide can become a persistent and intrusive thought.

Neurotic, Stress-Related and Somatoform Disorders

Disorders in this category range from phobic and general anxiety disorder, panic disorder, obsessive compulsive disorder and post-traumatic stress disorder to somatoform disorders (whereby the patient complains of physical symptoms that are medically unexplained) such as hypochondriasis.

Panic Disorder

This mental disorder is characterised by episodes of severe panic (anxiety) attacks, which can occur without an obvious trigger. These can be very frightening for patients, who experience fear and feelings of impending doom and have signs of sympathetic nervous stimulation (fight or flight), such as palpitations, sweating, chest pain and nausea. They may feel they're 'losing control' or dying (Cooper, 2012).

Personality Disorders

Personality disordered (PD) patients make frequent contact with emergency services (police and ambulance), GPs and emergency departments. They can be a chaotic and challenging patient as they have a tendency to experience many pseudo-psychiatric symptoms, and so are often referred to as 'borderline', which implies a condition that is fleeting in nature but not chronic. They are usually worse when there is some form of social/relationship stressor as a backdrop (Cooper, 2012).

The nature of the personality disorder is about frantically avoiding perceived isolation and abandonment, which typically manifest as becoming engaged in risky behaviour in order to prompt rescue. This can elicit 'knight in shining armour' behaviour in emergency services personnel, and is in stark contrast to mental health staff, who are likely to be more consistent and stick to the patient's care plan, becoming unpopular in the process. A common strategy adopted by patients with PD is to 'divide and rule' (known as splitting) to help them take control of a seemingly intolerable situation. Watch for comments relating to a comparison between how caring and understanding you are versus how bad mental health or hospital staff are.

Suicide and Deliberate Self-Harm (DSH)

In England, there are around 4,500 suicides each year, 77% of whom are male. Only 30% of those had contact with mental health services in the year prior to suicide (DoH, 2014). People who regularly self-harm will continue to be at risk of future self-harm, but not typically suicide. Although DSH is regarded as taboo and unfathomable by many people, including clinicians, it may help you to think of DSH as a method of coping with incredibly difficult feelings rather than as a serious wish to die (RCP, 2010). People who regularly overdose and/or engage in risky behaviour – designed to elicit a response – are more at risk via misadventure of accidental death, and it is not uncommon for a coroner to give a narrative verdict in such cases. Predicting who will commit suicide is very difficult, and scales, such as the SAD PERSONS scale, do not accurately predict the risk of death by suicide (Warden, 2014; Bolton, 2012).

IPAP Suicide Risk Assessment

Although suicide risk assessment tools are generally not recommended to be used by non-mental health professionals, it is helpful to have some guidance relating to the factors that suggest your patient is at risk. Current UK Ambulance Services Clinical Practice Guidelines recommend using 'IPAP' (JRCALC, 2016):

- **Intent**: Any thoughts of killing self?
- **Plans**: Does the patient have a plan about how they would kill themselves?
- **Actions**: Has the patient ever attempted suicide before?
- **Protection**: Does the patient have any support, such as family and friends? Are there any restraints that would stop the patient taking their own life, such as family, pets, work, religion?

Although there is no scoring system associated with IPAP, it is important to recognise that each element that is present increases the patient's risk.

Assessment of Patients with Mental Health Problems

Patients with mental health problems can still have physical illnesses, so ensure that you conduct a primary survey on all patients to identify any life-threats. Once these have been excluded, you are going to need to slow down – making and implementing a plan for a patient with a mental disorder can take time and will require seeking advice from senior clinicians and mental health experts.

As an emergency medical responder, it falls outside of your scope of practice to be able to fully assess and diagnose patients with mental health issues. However, it is important that you can recognise common mental health signs, symptoms and behaviours so you know when to ask for senior help in managing these patients. Table 20.1 shows several factors that should be considered in your assessment. It is not exhaustive and similarly it is not necessary for all signs and symptoms to be present. However, it is important that you gain as much information as possible, and you should not be afraid to ask questions politely and professionally. Remember if in doubt, ask for help.

Management of Patients with Mental Disorders

Trying to assist patients with mental disorders can feel daunting. To help non-mental health professionals in assisting patients with mental disorders, a mental health first aid course was created (MHFA). The aims of MHFA are to:

- preserve life where a person may be a danger to themselves
- provide help to prevent the mental health problem becoming more serious

Table 20.1 Factors to consider during a mental health assessment

Behaviour Observe both verbal and non-verbal signs	Does the patient make eye contact? Is the patient calm and relaxed or anxious, upset, aggressive, suspicious or pre-occupied? Is the patient's body language appropriate or are they hyperactive or hypoactive?
Appearance Again assessed through observation	Is the patient dressed properly, are they unkempt or do they have poor hygiene or other evidence of poor self-care? Are there signs of self-harm, for instance cutting marks, drug and alcohol misuse or overdose?
Speech and rapport	Is the volume of speech normal or very loud or quiet? Is the rate of speech normal for the situation or is it pressured or especially slow? Is the conversation spontaneous? Does the patient talk far too much or only minimally and is it in response to questions? Is the patient friendly and co-operative or is speech forced or monotone?
Mood/affect	Does the patient present in a way that fits with their current mood; for instance, do they appear flat, restricted or blunted, or alternatively does their mood appear to vary quickly and seem inappropriate to the situation? Bearing this in mind, does the patient appear elated, anxious, angry, agitated or even disinterested and lacking any motivation? Ask the patient if they have any suicidal ideas or violent thoughts.
Cognition	Is the patient orientated to time, person and place? Is the patient able to retain and recall information and use it appropriately? Is the patient able to concentrate and pay attention as would be expected for the situation? Does the patient express a normal level of general knowledge and ability to identify familiar items, objects, people and places? Can the patient easily follow simple instructions?
Thoughts	Does the patient have any thoughts of self-harm, suicide or thoughts of harming others? Do they appear pre-occupied or to have obsessive thoughts? Do they display any unusual beliefs or delusional, unrealistic ideas about themselves, others or the world in general? Are they very anxious or very low or depressed? Do they describe feelings of hopelessness or do they appear unmotivated, even to complete small tasks like eating, drinking or appropriate levels of self-care? Does the thought process of the patient flow logically and naturally within the conversation or when taking the history, or: • Do they change subject often and quickly to unrelated topics? • Do their thoughts seem overly fast or unusually slow? • Is their speech very fast or unusually slow? • Are they very vague with answers to questions? • Are they using nonsense words or very mixed-up sentences sometimes described as a 'word salad'?

Table 20.1 *(continued)*

	The following symptoms and traits are often associated with psychosis-type illness and can feel very real and very disturbing for the patient. They are less likely to be found in children (i.e. those under 18 years of age)
	• Hallucinations:
	  • Visual disturbances and visions not apparent to others; these can be described as people, animals or objects and are individual to the patient.
	  • Auditory hallucinations, often hearing voices not belonging to the patient and outside of their head. These can be derogatory, commanding or abusive.
	• Delusions:
	  • The belief of a patient that their thoughts can be read, changed or removed from their minds.
	  • The patient may feel that they themselves are not real or that the situation they are in is not real.
	  • A patient may describe feeling detached or removed from themselves, akin to watching themselves or their situation from afar with little control.

Insight	Does the patient acknowledge that they have a current mental health problem? Do they acknowledge the need for help or further input, and are they willing to comply with this? Are they able to evaluate different treatment options and choices? Are they able to weigh up and identify any risks to themselves or others?

- promote recovery of good mental health
- provide comfort to a person suffering from a mental health problem.

To achieve this, MHFA advocates a five-point action plan (ALGEE) (Pappas, 2010):

1. **A**pproach the person, assess and assist with any crisis.
2. **L**isten non-judgementally.
3. **G**ive support and information.
4. **E**ncourage and support the person to get appropriate professional help.
5. **E**ncourage other supports, such as self-help, family and friends.

General Advice

- Don't panic: Remain calm, professional and in control. Patients are often incredibly astute at sensing any uneasiness and some may try to force your hand.
- There is no rush: Making and implementing a plan can take hours.
- Do consider their medical health: An overdose of 1 g of amitriptyline, for example, can cause serious harm and needs addressing prior to their mental health.
- Consider their mental health: If patients state that their mental health is not good, consider whether an ED attendance will really benefit anyone here, apart from relieving your own anxieties (and responsibility) about this patient group. In most cases, a risk assessment can be conducted by mental health staff and an appropriate plan put in place.
- Frontline mental health staff are not there just to 'have a chat' with patients: Several national helplines are available for that purpose, such as Rethink, Saneline and the Samaritans.
- Patients cannot be forced to go to ED unless they are detained lawfully and being taken to ED is the most appropriate course of action.
- Desperate attempts and pleas to engage can indicate you're out of your depth.
- Many known mental health patients normally have a care plan. Of course, you aren't going to know this because you can't see it, and patients may not be happy with it or may feel it doesn't address their needs 24/7. This is often the case with frequent callers who challenge the out-of-hours services when offered a different

response from that which they receive during the daytime.

- Don't tell people to pull themselves together: It can reinforce any negativity or feelings of hopelessness.
- Be objective: It can be helpful to see how patients can contradict themselves, not so you can point it out to them and make them feel stupid, but more as a reassurance that what they're saying and what they're actually doing are two different things. For example:
    - 'I feel like killing myself tonight, but I'm seeing my GP the day after tomorrow.'
    - 'I feel like killing myself, but I'm worried about the impact it would have on my children.'
    - 'I feel like killing myself, but I'm worried I'll fail and end up disabled or in pain.'
- It's okay to be human and personable. However, don't disclose too much about yourself, or try to solve their problems. Their issues may be long-term problems and highly unlikely to be solved at 03:00 with excessive personal self-disclosing.
- Don't feel you have to fill the void: Silences of a minute or two do not mean you're not being helpful. Be comfortable with silence; it's not up to you to have all the answers.
- Don't just do something, stand there! Don't confuse movement with action.
- There are no absolutes in mental health and it is never possible to state with absolute certainty that a patient isn't at risk.

Seeking Advice

As an emergency medical responder it is inevitable that you will be involved in incidents where mental health is a key feature, but it is important you recognise your own limitations in managing these patients. Mental Health is highly complex, both clinically and legally, and you should always be seeking further help and guidance. Many mental health incidents can take hours to resolve, and it is unlikely that you will need to remain at the scene for the duration of this time. Seek further help early and thoroughly document your actions, decisions and who is taking over responsibility for caring for that patient.

At worst, if mental health incidents are mishandled, patients can come to significant harm, and your actions and inactions will be scrutinised in detail afterwards; be sure that responsibility for the patient was passed on to an appropriately qualified person.

Caring for Yourself and Colleagues

Learning Objectives

At the end of this section you will be able to:

- Define mental well-being.
- List factors that may have an impact on mental well-being.
- Define resilience in terms of mental well-being.
- Describe how to improve personal mental well-being resilience.
- List sources of help for mental well-being.
- Describe how to support a colleague's mental well-being.

Introduction

As an emergency medical responder, your daily job is to help and support other people during times of crisis, but this constant exposure can have a detrimental impact on your own mental health and well-being. Research suggests that emergency service workers and volunteers are more likely to suffer mental health problems than the general workforce but are less likely to take time off work or seek help (Mind, 2015a). As many as 85% of fire and rescue staff and volunteers have experienced stress and poor mental health at work (Mind, 2015a).

Mental Well-being

Mental well-being describes your overall mental state and considers how the way you are feeling impacts on how you can cope with day-to-day life (Mind, 2016). People with good mental well-being can:

- feel confident and have positive self-esteem
- build and maintain positive relationships
- live and work productively
- cope with the stresses of daily life
- adapt to changes around them.

Impact on Mental Well-being

Mental well-being can be impacted by several factors, both inside and outside of work, including (Mind, 2015a):

- repeated exposure to traumatic incidents
- impact of physical injuries
- workload pressure
- suffering personal loss
- relationship problems
- financial worries
- loneliness.

Building Resilience

Dealing with more difficult times in life, whether they be due to personal or work related issues, can be challenging. The capacity to stay mentally well during these periods relies on your personal mental health 'resilience'. You can try to build resilience to deal with these difficult times by (Mind, 2015a):

- talking about the way you feel
- building healthy relationships
- looking after your physical health
- doing something you enjoy
- setting yourself a challenge
- relaxing
- identifying mood triggers.

Seeking Help

There will be times when you recognise either in yourself, or a colleague, that personal resilience is not enough and that further help is required. Often this decision is difficult to arrive at and can be left longer than it really should have been, as emergency service staff feel they should be the ones that stay strong as it is their role to help others. Left unsupported poor mental well-being can lead to anxiety, depression and post-traumatic stress disorder (PTSD).

Help can be sought from a range of options, outlined below.

Employer Support

Your employer is likely to have a form of internal service for supporting staff, which may include peer counselling, a multi-faith chaplain, or schemes such as Trauma Risk Management (TRiM) or external counselling support.

Medical Support

Your GP will be able to help. While a GP may be able to give a diagnosis and medications, this is not always the first step. They have a range of options, including just listening to your situation, and can refer you to other treatments, such as talking therapy or counselling if appropriate.

If you are facing a more urgent situation or crisis, you can also call 111, visit your local ED or call 999.

Specialist Fire and Rescue Organisations

The Fire Fighters Charity can provide confidential advice and support for active and retired fire fighters, and the Mind Blue Light programme is specifically designed for supporting emergency service workers with mental health illness or concerns.

Other Charities

The Samaritans provide 24-hour emotional support for anyone struggling to cope. You can call anonymously if you want, with no need to give personal details, and telephone numbers are not tracked.

Supporting a Colleague

There may be occasions where you think the mental well-being of a colleague is suffering and you may want to try and help them. The charity Mind produce information on how to do this (Mind, 2015b). In summary, you should:

- Show support by asking them how they are.
- Ask if you can help in any way.
- Treat them as you normally would.
- Don't just talk about mental health.
- Show trust and respect.

It may be helpful to remind them what support and services are available to them. If there is another colleague you know they respect that has been through a similar experience in the past it may be useful for them to talk to each other.

Your colleague may not be ready to seek help yet, so be there for them, be patient and continue to offer support and reassurance. Remember that there will be an additional emotional stress on you, so continue to look after yourself and your own resilience.

Chapter 21

Older People and Frailty

Ageing

Learning Objective

By the end of the section, you will be able to:

- Describe the anatomical and physiological changes that occur as a person ages.

Introduction

Older people are generally defined as those aged over 65; however, ageing is a highly unique process and there may be patients at a lower age that suffer from the same conditions and vulnerabilities as those aged 65 and over. So, although being aged over 65 is still the most accepted definition of older people, you should likewise consider that those aged 50–64 may also suffer from the same issues, depending on the unique progression of their own disease, vulnerabilities or risk factors (NICE, 2013b).

There are currently around 11 million people in the UK over the age of 65, a figure that is expected to increase by 50% by 2031 (Age UK, 2018). Although there are no national statistics relating to the number of older people who call the ambulance service, around 45% of the 4,374,611 people who attended an emergency department in 2012/13, and arrived by ambulance, were over the age of 65 (UKCGC 2017).

Anatomy and Physiology of Ageing

There is no single mechanism of ageing. Instead, there are a range of mechanisms that over time result in the worsening of cell function, causing cellular damage and impairing the body's ability to repair itself. This results in a range of anatomical and physiological changes (Figure 21.1).

Musculoskeletal System

Bones, joints and muscles are all affected by ageing.

Bones

Bone formation is greatest in the period from birth to adolescence, but equalises with bone absorption in a person's twenties, before bone absorption becomes more dominant. This leads to a reduction in body calcium, impairing the body's ability to create bone matrix and increasing the risk of fracture. Calcium supplements are often prescribed, as absorption of calcium from the digestive system also declines with age (Farley, 2011).

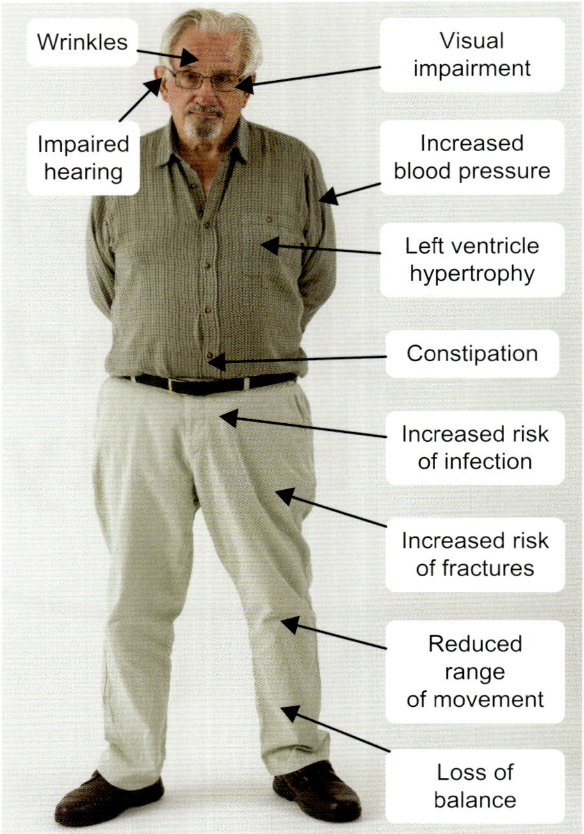

Figure 21.1 *Changes related to ageing.*

Joints

The loss of fluid in the fibrocartilage within the intervertebral discs results in kyphosis – the familiar stooped posture of older age – which also reduces the height of the person. With stooping comes a change in the person's centre of gravity and changes to their gait, which becomes slower, shorter and more cautious (Knight, 2008d).

Other joints are affected too, especially synovial joints. The reduction in synovial fluid and articular cartilage leads to bones coming into direct contact with each other (Farley, 2011).

Muscles

Muscles wasting, also known as atrophy, leads to a reduction in muscle strength and mass. The rate of decline is variable, with some muscles, such as the diaphragm, remaining unchanged, whereas the lower limbs can experience noticeable atrophy. Coupled with the decline in nervous system function, movement speed is reduced, and increased muscle rigidity results in limited movement in the neck, shoulders, hips and knees (Farley, 2011).

Respiratory System

The respiratory system is in steady decline from around the age of 25, following a functional peak at 20 years of age. There are a variety of external factors that adversely affect the respiratory system, including poor nutrition, lack of physical exercise and smoking (Farley, 2011). Changes due to ageing are fairly insignificant compared to the external factors as there is usually sufficient spare capacity in lung function to offset any decline due to older age.

Airway Changes

There are a number of changes in the airway itself as we age. Mucus becomes increasingly thick, leading to it lodging in the nasopharynx and causing recurrent coughs. The cilia that line the trachea and smaller airways flatten, reducing the clearance of secretions and other debris, thereby increasing the chance of infection (Knight, 2008a).

Ventilatory Changes

Respiratory function does deteriorate with age, in tandem with the decline of the musculoskeletal system. Costal cartilages become stiff, decreasing lung compliance and requiring the use of accessory muscles to ventilate. In addition, the strength of the respiratory system declines from around 55 years of age, with intercostal muscle wasting, increasing the work of breathing and making the respiratory system more reliant on the diaphragm (Knight, 2008a). Shortness of breath on exertion (SOBOE) is more common in older people due to (Farley, 2011):

- decreasing muscle strength
- muscles being more prone to fatigue when work of breathing increases
- muscle wasting
- decreased blood supply to the muscles of respiration.

Most measurements of lung function decline with age, but in healthy patients this is mostly offset by a large reserve capacity of the respiratory system (Farley, 2011).

Cardiovascular System

Blood Vessels

As the body ages, blood vessels (particularly the arteries) lose their elasticity and become less compliant. The tunica media of large arteries thickens, due to the increasing number and density of collagen fibres, which makes the arteries more rigid. The inner endothelial layer, normally smooth to encourage blood flow, becomes roughened by muscle fibres that have migrated from the tunica media, which increases the resistance to blood flow (Knight, 2008b).

Systolic blood pressure increases. Smaller arteries and arterioles, along with baroreceptors, become less sensitive, leading to a sluggish response to changes in posture, such as from sitting to standing, which can cause postural hypotension (Farley, 2011).

Heart

In order to overcome the increase in systemic vascular resistance, the heart needs to pump with greater force; like all muscles that are exercised, it thickens (hypertrophies), particularly the left ventricle, known as left ventricular hypertrophy (LVH).

There are also changes in the electrical conduction system, with the sino-atrial node losing around 50–75% of pacemaker cells by the age of 50. Progressive fibrosis and cell death in the bundle of His leads to cardiac conduction problems, such as a decrease in maximal heart rate and increase in arrhythmias (Knight, 2008b).

Nervous System

Brain and Senses

In healthy people the ageing brain functions normally, and learning, for example, is still able to occur. However, brain weight does decline by approximately 5–10% over a lifetime with little change up to the age of 50 years. Indeed, it is not until 60 years of age and older that there is a significant reduction in weight (Farley, 2011).

An important consequence of this is the separation of the brain from the skull, which allows increased movement and stretching of the bridging veins between the brain and the outer layer of the meninges. During trauma involving the head, this can result in tearing of the veins, with subsequent subdural haemorrhage – bleeding into the subdural space (NAEMT, 2015).

About 10% of neurons are lost by the age of 75, but this does not result in significant loss of mental function. However, the loss of sensory neurons leads to impaired hearing, vision, smelling, temperature regulation and appreciation of pain. In addition, as proprioception reduces, older people become increasingly reliant on visual, tactile and auditory cues to stay on their feet, which increases the risk of falling, particularly if any/all of these senses are impaired (Knight, 2008c).

Eyes

The muscles of the eyelids lose tone and elasticity and a reduction in orbital fat causes the eyes to become sunken, reducing the upward gaze. The cornea flattens and thickens with age, making it duller and less transparent, increasing the risk of visual blurring. At the same time, there is a reduction in the sensitivity of the cornea, decreasing the awareness of any eye injuries. Pupil diameter declines, resulting in a reduction in light entering the eye, which adversely affects vision, particularly at night. Finally, the lens thickens and stiffens, further reducing visual acuity and the ability to focus (Farley, 2011).

Ears

Hearing loss is common, although not inevitable, with around 50% of people over 75 having hearing difficulties. High-pitched sounds and consonants are particularly affected. This may be especially noticeable for the person when there are high levels of background noise, and it makes identifying the direction of sound tricky.

Immune System

From a functional peak around puberty, there is a gradual reduction in immune system capacity over a person's lifetime of between 5 and 30%, but the immune system does continue to function even in very old adults. However, older people are more likely to die of infectious diseases, such as pneumonia, influenza and gastroenteritis. In addition, older adults respond differently to infection from younger adults, including (Farley, 2011):

- Fewer microorganisms are required to cause symptomatic infection.
- Confusion prior to a raised temperature is more common.
- Symptoms can be masked and/or mistaken for other diseases.
- The immune system can be compromised by medication such as steroids and anti-inflammatories.
- There is increased risk from chronic diseases such as diabetes and chronic obstructive pulmonary disease.

Integumentary System

The skin is probably the most visible sign of older age and all layers are affected (Farley, 2011):

- **Epidermis**: Loss of skin cells leads to decreased surface contact between the dermis and epidermis, which reduces the exchange of nutrients and other products of metabolism. In addition, the epidermis atrophies, causing roughened skin that takes longer to heal and provides less of a barrier.
- **Dermis**: This layer also atrophies, becoming thinner. In addition, there is a reduction in mast cells, which play an important role in the injury and infection responses. The dramatic reduction in dermal blood vessels leads to pallor, decreased temperature and impaired thermoregulation compounded by a loss of sensory nerve endings, increasing the risk of injury.
- **Hypodermis**: A reduction in subcutaneous fat leads to increased conductive heat loss, and the redistribution of the fat leads to bony prominences, which are vulnerable to pressure ulcers and fractures following trauma. Clinically, the skin looks dry, lax and wrinkly. The wrinkles are due to a combination of gravity, decreasing subcutaneous fat and, in the face, repeated traction by facial muscles. In addition, photo-ageing caused by ultraviolet radiation from the sun increases the number of skin lesions, which are usually benign, although they can become cancerous later in life.

Digestive System

Food intake declines with age, with about a 10% reduction in calorific intake each decade after 50 years of age. Older people may experience altered taste, linked mainly to a decrease in the sense of smell and smell discrimination, as the appeal of foods is based on its smell and taste. In addition, they are more likely to have missing teeth and poorly fitting dentures, all of which contribute to weight loss and malnutrition becoming more common. Increased intake of sugar and salt can contribute to the development of diabetes and high blood pressure (Nigam, 2008).

Caring for Older Patients

Learning Objectives

By the end of this section you will be able to:

- Identify a range of common conditions associated with ageing.
- Describe the impact co-morbidities will have on your treatment plans.

Age-Related Conditions

The following is a range of conditions commonly associated with older patients; however, these conditions are not necessarily unique to older patients and can be seen in younger people as well in certain circumstances.

Parkinson's Disease

Due to the death of cells in the brain, Parkinson's patients don't have enough of the neurotransmitter dopamine. One in 500 people in the UK suffers from the disease for which there is no cure and no known cause (Parkinson's UK, 2015).

The main symptoms of Parkinson's disease are:

- tremor, rigidity and slowness of movement

but may also include:

- tiredness
- pain
- depression
- constipation.

Parkinson's disease is treated with a combination of medication, therapy and occasionally surgery to help alleviate symptoms and slow the progression of the disease.

Arthritis

Arthritis is defined as inflammation within a joint. There are many different forms of the condition, but the two main ones are inflammatory arthritis and degenerative, or mechanical, arthritis (Arthritis Research UK, 2015).

Inflammatory Arthritis

Inflammation is a normal response as part of the body's healing process, but in patients with this form of arthritis the inflammation happens for no obvious reason. This is an autoimmune condition (the body's own immune system is attacking the joints) and instead of helping to repair the body it causes damage to the joint, pain and stiffness. This type of arthritis often affects several joints at once and includes rheumatoid arthritis. As well as joint pain, other symptoms of rheumatoid arthritis include:

- tiredness
- depression
- irritability
- flu-like symptoms.

Degenerative Forms of Mechanical Arthritis

A normal joint is covered at the ends of the bone in smooth cartilage, to allow bone ends to glide across each other. In degenerative forms of arthritis, these smooth cartilage ends have been worn away (Figure 21.2). The underlying bone tries to repair this, but often overgrows, altering the shape of the joint, known as osteoarthritis.

Osteoarthritis is particularly common in joints that see heavy use, including the hips and knees, base of thumb and big toe.

Osteoporosis

Osteoporosis occurs when the mesh-like structure within bones becomes thin, causing bones to become fragile and break easily (NOS, 2015).

Bones are constantly going through a process of regenerating themselves by breaking down old matter and replacing it with new. Up to around the late twenties bone density increases slowly, and from around 35 years onwards it starts (very gradually to begin with) to decrease as part of the natural ageing process; however, in certain people this can be accelerated and lead to weaker bones, which are more likely to fracture as a result.

Women are more susceptible to osteoporosis due to increased bone loss in the years following the menopause. The main risk of osteoporosis is the increased risk of fractures from just minor forces, rather than the significant force we would normally expect to cause a fracture. Broken hips and wrists are common injuries, as is a broken neck or back in a fall from standing height.

When assessing a patient who has a history of osteoporosis, have a very low threshold for suspecting fractures and be mindful that some clinical examination tools, such as the Canadian C-Spine Rule, may not be reliable in this patient group.

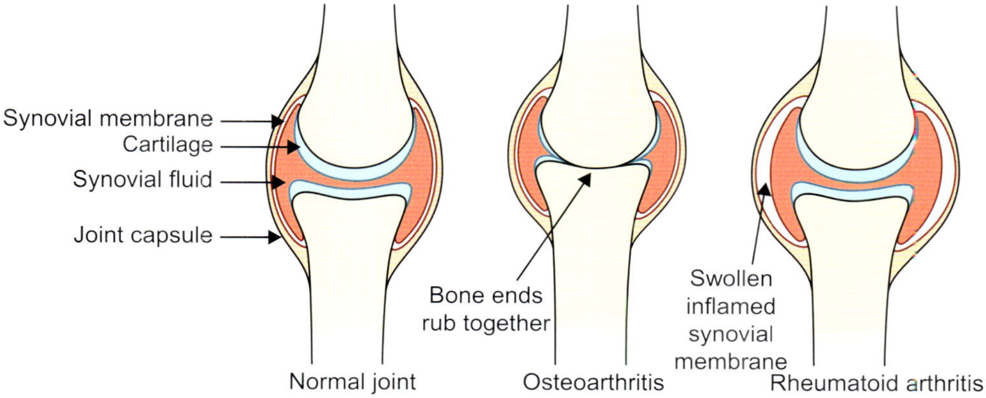

Figure 21.2 *Normal and arthritic joints.*

Mental Illness in Older People

Mental health is discussed in its own chapter, but it is worth briefly considering some specific mental health challenges facing older people.

It is thought by some that mental health problems are a normal part of ageing, but this is not necessarily the case with most older people developing no mental health problems, and many of those that do can be helped or treated, or the onset prevented with the right action (MHF, 2015).

Dementia

Dementia is one of the most common causes of mental health illness in older patients and we will look at this in some detail in the next section of this chapter.

Depression

Depression is another common mental health illness in later life that makes people feel sad and lack motivation (Age UK, 2015). We all feel like this at times, but depression occurs when these feelings are more intense and persist for weeks, months or longer. Depression is often linked to loss, which is common as people grow older. These losses can influence people's self-esteem and feelings of value and include:

- loss of job
- loss of good health
- loss of independence
- loss of spouse or friends
- loss of social network.

As with depression at any age, several treatment options, including medication and talking therapies, are available. It is also possible that certain things can be done to prevent the development of depression initially.

Many elderly people are isolated and spend prolonged periods of time on their own. Arranging for appropriate social interactions can help to alleviate these feelings of isolation and prevent the development of depression in the first place.

When treating older patients, make sure you consider the risk of depression as one of your holistic assessments. Mental and physical health are closely intertwined, and you should be aiming to always promote an individual's mental well-being as well as their physical.

Patients with Co-Morbidities

When treating older patients, it is often the case that they suffer from a number of simultaneous co-morbidities. For example, a patient suffering from cardiovascular disease and type 2 diabetes; both of them are serious long-term conditions that can be life limiting, especially if not managed correctly. They can also interact with and worsen each other. This makes caring for patients very challenging, as a number of conditions may be interacting and causing varied presentation.

Many of these patients will have specialist medical or nursing support and might be under the care of a chronic condition management team, or community matron.

When dealing with patients with a range of co-morbidities, be sure to consider all of the conditions that may be influencing the current presentation: do not become fixated on just one element of the patient's illness. These cases are complex and in elderly patients, who may already have compromised immune systems or compensatory mechanisms, can represent significant dangers. Be prepared to seek early additional help and support in such situations and recognise the limitations of your own scope of practice and knowledge where necessary.

Dementia

Learning Objectives

By the end of this section you will be able to:

- Define dementia.
- Explain the differences between dementia and delirium.
- Describe a number of strategies that can assist you when communicating with a patient with dementia.
- Identify a number of causes of challenging behaviour.
- Explain how to manage challenging behaviour.

Introduction

Dementia is a set of behaviours or 'symptoms' that suggest difficulties with cognitive function. The most common symptoms include: memory loss, confusion, mood and personality changes, and problems with planning and performing tasks in the right order. Dementia is diagnosed when the symptoms cause such problems with the tasks of daily life that the person affected can no longer carry on living independently without care.

Dementia is an 'organic' disorder, meaning there is an associated physical deterioration of the brain tissue, which can be seen via a brain scan or, after death, at autopsy, though depending on the exact type of dementia, different physical changes will be seen. Dementia is progressive – the damage and symptoms get worse over time. It is therefore not a normal result of ageing, but rather is the result of a disease (SCIE, 2013).

Dementia in Context

It is estimated that 7.1% of people over 65 have dementia, which translates to around 850,000 people in the UK in 2015 (Age UK, 2014). One in 3 people over 65 will develop some form of dementia and two-thirds of people with dementia are women (NHS Choices, 2015b). It is estimated that the cost to the UK economy stands at £26 billion a year (Alzheimer's Society, 2014).

Dementia is an increasing challenge as people are living longer, and by 2021 it is estimated that the number of people in the UK living with dementia will have reached 1 million.

Background to Dementia

Dementia tends to affect sufferers in three different ways:

- **Cognitive**: As the areas of the brain responsible for cognition are damaged and the number of cells are reduced, sufferers are less able to deal with complex thought processes or store memories so easily.
- **Behavioural**: As different areas of the brain are affected, a person's behaviour may change. This is particularly seen in frontotemporal dementia where the sufferer may lose a sense of inhibition.
- **Neurological**: Physical changes to the structure of the brain mean that the brain of dementia sufferers is not able to function appropriately. A loss of brain cells and a change to the type and quantity of chemicals in the brain leads to a vast change in neurological function. In some forms, including dementia with Lewy bodies, physical signs such as shaking may develop, showing changes to the neurological system.

Different Types of Dementia

There are over 100 types of dementia, with Alzheimer's disease being the most common single cause in the UK, making up around 66% of cases, and vascular dementia coming in second. However, multiple disease processes are even more common than single disease processes, with Alzheimer's disease and vascular dementia, and Alzheimer's disease and Lewy body dementia, being common combinations (NG, 2001).

Causes of Dementia

Different forms of dementia have different underlying causes, and here we will consider some of the most common types (Alzheimer's Society, 2018; NHS Choices, 2015b). Dementia is normally caused by gradual changes in the brain, often associated with brain cells dying more quickly than they should as part of the normal ageing process. It is thought that an abnormal protein present within the brain is responsible for a lot of this premature degeneration.

Alzheimer's Disease

In Alzheimer's disease loss of brain cells leads to the shrinking of the brain. The cerebral cortex, the area of the brain responsible for processing thought and other complex functions including memory, calculations and some communication skills, is most affected.

Clumps of protein gather in the brain and it is thought that they are responsible for the increased rate of brain cell death. Connections between brain cells are also lost and the chemicals that normally carry signals, known as neurotransmitters, are greatly reduced, all of which leads to the cognitive impairment seen.

Vascular Dementia

Vascular dementia occurs when cells are damaged as a result of a reduced blood supply and therefore oxygen reaching brain tissue. As people age their vessels tend to become narrow and harden where fatty deposits develop. This process, called atherosclerosis, means that less blood can get through the vessels, and surrounding brain tissue is starved of oxygen.

Patients who have been diagnosed with small vessel disease or have previously suffered from a stroke or a transient ischaemic attack (TIA) are at increased risk of developing vascular dementia.

Other causes include:

- infections, including encephalitis
- some brain tumours
- lack of thyroid hormone
- head injury
- long-term alcohol abuse.

Disease Progression

Every sufferer will have a unique disease progression; however, the main forms of dementia are all progressive, i.e. they will all get worse with time. The speed at which any individual's disease progresses will vary widely and is based on many factors, including their age at time of onset, genetics and other physical and mental health factors (Alzheimer's Society, 2015). Patients with a history of poorly controlled heart disease or diabetes are likely to experience a faster deterioration.

The Alzheimer's Society (2015) describe the progression of the disease in three broad stages.

Early (Mild) Stage

Dementia normally begins with mild subtle changes in a person's abilities or behaviour. The changes are often incorrectly thought to just be part of a normal ageing process, and include:

- loss of memory of recent events
- mislaying items around the house
- becoming confused easily
- losing track of the day or date.

Middle (Moderate) Stage

As the disease progresses changes become more obvious and a greater degree of help is required in day-to-day life. Changes may include:

- needing frequent reminders or help to eat, wash, dress and use the toilet
- increasing forgetfulness – especially of names
- becoming confused about where they are, and maybe trying to walk off to find somewhere else
- experiencing difficulty with perception and maybe starting to have delusions.

Changes in behaviour are more commonly seen during this stage and sufferers can become easily upset, angry or even aggressive – perhaps because they are misinterpreting events or do not understand what is happening.

Late (Severe) Stage

At this stage sufferers will need increasing levels of help with daily activities and may gradually become totally dependent on others for nursing care. Loss of memory can become severe and they may not recognise people and their surroundings, though they may have occasional moments of clarity or recognition.

Behaviour changes can become very severe with restlessness, agitation and angry outbursts, particularly during periods of close personal care, usually because the sufferer does not understand what is happening.

This stage of the disease can be very distressing for both the sufferer and their family and carers, and needs to be managed gently and tactfully.

Living with Dementia

Living with dementia is unique to every individual suffering from the disease. One of the key aims of supporting dementia patients should be to assist them in retaining independence as far as possible.

As the disease progresses, more and more help may be required but this should be matched to a person's condition, and it should not immediately be assumed that they cannot make decisions for themselves, or care for themselves, just because they have a formal diagnosis of dementia.

Dementia and Other Diseases

When assessing a dementia patient, be careful not to attribute changes in their status to the ongoing deterioration of the condition without good evidence to do so. Dementia normally progresses slowly, and any sudden changes should prompt you to search for a different cause. Many dementia patients will suffer from other co-morbidities (the presence of other diseases) and a detailed assessment will be required to identify any underlying illness.

You should ask those around you that are familiar with the patient for detailed information on their condition. For example, you may be asked to see a dementia patient with increased confusion. This is a common scenario and can be very difficult to manage. If the family or carers report a rapid change in cognitive state, it is unlikely that this is due to the dementia itself and more likely a result of another disease process. What makes your assessment increasingly difficult is the confused nature of the patient, which means it can be difficult to obtain a detailed history and examination.

Treating Patients with Dementia

Working in an emergency care environment, it is likely that you will frequently meet patients with dementia at various stages of the disease progression. Managing these patients may require some significant modifications to your usual approach, and although every encounter will be unique, you should consider the following guidance:

- **Approach all situations in a calm manner**: Your patient may be confused, scared or not understand what is happening. A calm manner on your part can help to relax your patient and make them feel safe.
- **Communicate clearly and be patient**: More details of communicating with dementia patients is included in the next section.
- Wherever possible and appropriate, **support a patient in making their own decisions** about their healthcare.
- **Use relatives, friends and carers** wherever possible to aid communication and to help the patient feel more relaxed by having a friendly familiar face present.
- **Be compassionate**: Remember that every dementia patient is different and will need different management; there is not one single way to manage 'dementia patients'.

Aggressive Behaviour

Patients with dementia may sometimes become aggressive, either verbally or physically. This can be very distressing for the person, carers, friends and family. You should understand why this happens and how to resolve it as part of your role (Alzheimer's Society, 2017).

Patients with dementia have the same needs as everyone else, including comfort, social interaction, stimulation, emotional well-being and being free from pain. However, dementia patients may not understand their own needs or be able to communicate them. This can lead to frustration and, in turn, challenging or aggressive behaviour.

Guidance for responding to such situations includes (Alzheimer's Society, 2017):

- Remain calm and avoid confrontation, as a heated response will make the situation worse.
- Reassure the person and acknowledge any feelings they are able to express.
- Listen to what they are saying.
- Try to explore what is causing the behaviour.
- Try to distract their attention if they remain angry.
- Maintain eye contact, come down to their level and try to ensure your body language and positioning is not aggressive or restrictive in any way.

Dementia and Pain Management

Pain management for dementia patients remains a difficult issue, especially for those that are not able to communicate effectively. It is well recognised that dementia patients frequently receive inadequate pain relief (Chandler, 2014), and that is especially true of emergency care patients.

One of the key challenges is that patients are unable to express their pain, so healthcare staff tend to underestimate the amount of pain a patient is suffering and therefore not provide adequate pain management techniques.

It is recommended that standardised assessment tools should be used to assess the level of pain that a patient is suffering if they are not able to communicate it themselves. One such tool designed for use with late-stage dementia patients is the Abbey pain scale (Figure 21.3) (Abbey, 2004).

The Abbey Pain Scale

For measurement of pain in people with dementia who cannot verbalise.

How to use scale: While observing the resident, score questions 1 to 6.

Name of resident:……………………………………………………

Name and designation of person completing the scale: ……………………………

Date: ………………………………… Time: ……………………………

Latest pain relief given was……………………………… at ……………… hrs.

Q1. Vocalisation
eg whimpering, groaning, crying
Absent 0 Mild 1 Moderate 2 Severe 3
Q1. ☐

Q2. Facial expression
eg looking tense, frowning, grimacing, looking frightened
Absent 0 Mild 1 Moderate 2 Severe 3
Q2. ☐

Q3. Change in body language
eg fidgeting, rocking, guarding part of body, withdrawn
Absent 0 Mild 1 Moderate 2 Severe 3
Q3. ☐

Q4. Behavioural change
eg increased confusion, refusing to eat, alteration in usual patterns
Absent 0 Mild 1 Moderate 2 Severe 3
Q4. ☐

Q5. Physiological change
eg temperature, pulse or blood pressure outside normal limits, perspiring, flushing, or pallor
Absent 0 Mild 1 Moderate 2 Severe 3
Q5. ☐

Q6. Physical changes
eg skin tears, pressure areas, arthritis, contractures, previous injuries
Absent 0 Mild 1 Moderate 2 Severe 3
Q6. ☐

Add scores for Q1 to Q6 and record here → Total pain score ☐

Now tick the box that matches the Total Pain Score →

0–2 No pain	3–7 Mild	8–13 Moderate	14+ Severe

Finally, tick the box which matches the type of pain →

Chronic	Acute	Acute on chronic

Abbey J, De Bellis A, Piller N, Esterman A, Gilles L, Parker D, Lowcay B. The Abbey Pain Scale. Funded by the JH & JD Gunn Medical Research Foundation 1998–2002. (This document may be reproduced with this reference retained.)

Figure 21.3 *The Abbey pain scale.*

Source: Abbey J, Piller N, DeBellis A et al., 2004. The Abbey pain scale: a 1-minute numerical indicator for people with end-stage dementia. *International Journal of Palliative Nursing*, 10(1), 6–13. Copyright © 2004 MA Healthcare Ltd. Reproduced by permission of MA Healthcare Ltd.

When administering pain relief to dementia patients, you should observe for a reduction in the Abbey pain scale score. This may take time and close observation will be required.

You should be aware of the different forms of pain relief available, both pharmacological and non-pharmacological, and use them appropriately, or request help from a clinician with a broader range of analgesic options as required.

When making decisions on which pain relief to use, be sure to consider side effects and any polypharmacy interactions. Many dementia patients will be on a large number of chronic medications, which may include pain relief medicines. Remember to only act within your scope of practice and to seek help and advice when you are unsure of the best option to proceed.

Dementia vs Delirium

If dementia can be thought of as chronic brain failure, then delirium is acute brain failure (Barrett, 2014). It is a common and serious condition that is characterised by disruptions in thinking, consciousness, attention, cognition and perception. Unlike dementia, its onset is over a short period of time (typically hours to days). To complicate matters, patients with dementia can also develop delirium, and this has been associated with serious complications and poor outcome, including death (Fick, 2002).

Delirium is often divided into three variants (SAS, 2014):

- **Hyperactive**: Characterised by anxiety, restlessness, irritability, anger and frustration. Patients may be easily startled and distracted, and unable to sit still. Speech can be loud, but incoherent with frequent topic hopping.
- **Hypoactive**: Patients with hypoactive delirium are typically lethargic, apathetic, slow in movement, withdrawn, drowsy and difficult to wake.
- **Mixed**: A combination of the two other variants, with patients fluctuating between hyperactive and hypoactive delirium throughout the day.

Differentiating between delirium and dementia can be difficult, so if in doubt, it is safer to assume delirium and ensure patients receive prompt medical attention (SAS, 2014).

Communication

Although the principles of communication have already been covered in Chapter 3: Communication, there are some additional points to consider when you are caring for a patient with dementia:

- **Get their attention**: Approach the patient from the front so they can see you coming. Try to make eye contact and ensure they can see your face and body movements.
- **Use their name**: Using their name can help them understand that you are not a stranger (although this may not be true), which can be reassuring.
- **Frequently remind them who you are**: This can reduce anxiety and avoid the patient becoming alarmed at being treated by a stranger.
- **Keep ambient noise and activity to a minimum**: Reducing distractions, activity and noise will help a patient with dementia (indeed most patients) to concentrate on what you are saying.
- **Don't rush**: Take your time. Slowing your rate of speech can help, but increase the time spent speaking **and** listening. It may help if you silently count to seven between short sentences, and then give the patient the same time to answer.
- **Keep calm**: Adopt a calm tone and manner to reduce distress and make the patient feel more comfortable with you. Patients with dementia maintain the ability to determine your body language even after their ability to understand speech has been lost.
- **Keep things simple**: Avoid jargon and speak in short and simple-to-understand sentences. When giving instructions, break down the task into simple stages. Give clear instructions; for example, rather than saying 'sit there' you could try saying 'sit in this blue chair, please'.
- **Use the patient's preferred method of communication**: Establish this early on from the patient and others who know them. This includes speaking to the patient in their first language or using communication aids such as pictures or talking mats.

Challenging Behaviour

Much of the time patients with dementia are placid and sweet-tempered, but over 90% will exhibit some form of challenging behaviour at some point. This behaviour includes (Barrett, 2014):

- sleeplessness
- wandering
- agitation
- pacing
- aggression (including spitting)
- disinhibition
- jealousy (especially sexual jealousy).

Challenging behaviour needs to be seen as a manifestation of unmet needs, which the patient may not be able to express, such as boredom, frustration and/or annoyance.

Managing Challenging Behaviour

It is important to appreciate that each patient will be slightly different, so the best way of managing challenging behaviour will need to be tailored to them. Advice from carers and/or relatives may help, but general principles include (YAS, 2013):

- trying to find out what is the cause of the behaviour
- reducing the stress and/or demands placed on the patient
- explaining what is happening using the patient's name and saying who you are. You are likely to have to repeat this process often
- giving patients time to respond to your requests or questions
- trying not to show criticism or irritation, and avoiding confrontation with patients
- watching for warning signs that they are becoming more anxious or agitated. Get help if the situation does not calm down quickly
- including carers and/or relatives who know the patient and who will have experience in managing the patient's challenging behaviour
- not making sudden movements or using a sharp tone. Instead, remain calm and keep your voice low.

Frailty

Learning Objectives

By the end of this section you will be able to:

- Define the term frailty.
- Describe how frailty impacts on patients.
- Describe how to recognise and support patients with frailty.

Introduction

Frailty is a distinctive health state related to the ageing process in which multiple body systems gradually lose their in-built reserves (BGS, 2014a), such that they are unable to deal with everyday or acute stresses (Xue, 2012).

Approximately 10% of patients aged over 65 are defined as suffering from frailty, rising to between a quarter and a half of those aged 85 years and older (Clegg, 2013) so as an emergency care responder you will frequently encounter older people living with frailty.

Living with Frailty

Living with frailty will be unique for each person. For some people, frailty will be the only condition they suffer, which means they are likely to only be an occasional user of health services, until such times as they become acutely unwell. For others, frailty may be one of many long-term complex conditions they live with, meaning they are a frequent user of health services (BGS, 2014b).

Frailty will mean that an individual's health reserves are diminished, so when they become unwell, they have a lesser ability to cope with acute illness/infection. As such, conditions that may normally be well tolerated and easily treated (such as a simple respiratory tract infection) can become a life-threatening illness.

Recognising Frailty

Different models of recognising frailty have been proposed and as yet no single model is preferred (BGS, 2014a). One of the simpler models, known as the phenotype model (Fried at al., 2001), describes a distinct set of characteristics:

- unintentional weight loss
- reduced muscle strength

- reduced gait speed
- self-reported exhaustion
- low energy expenditure.

Generally, individuals with three or more of these characteristics are said to be frail, though a formal diagnosis requires a far more in-depth assessment by a GP or geriatrician.

Supporting Patients with Frailty

As an emergency medical responder, it is likely you will be called to patients with frailty regularly. You should consider whether a patient already has a diagnosis of frailty and how this might impact on any other health problem they are suffering from. Equally, you may also see a patient who you believe is frail, but does not have a specific diagnosis of frailty yet.

In your management of a patient, you should consider how their frailty may impact on other medical conditions, and whether it leaves them at increased risk of other illness or injury. As mentioned above, what may be a simple infection to most people can quickly become life threatening to a frail patient without the physiological reserves to combat illness.

A common situation you may encounter would be attending an older person who has fallen at home. On arrival, they may be uninjured and not requiring medical treatment, but through your initial assessment you may identify that you believe they may be suffering from frailty. In this scenario, you should seek their consent to refer them to their GP for a fuller assessment and consideration of a care and support plan to help them and, where possible, restrict the progression of their frailty.

References

AACE and CFOA, 2016
Association of Ambulance Chief Executives and Chief Fire Officers Association, 2016. *Consensus Statement on Saving Lives and Improving Health and Wellbeing*. Available at: http://www.cfoa.org.uk/download/63854 [Accessed 30 January 2018].

AAOS, 2011
American Academy of Orthopaedic Surgeons and American College of Emergency Physicians, 2011. *Critical Care Transport*. Sudbury, MA: Jones & Bartlett Publishers.

AAP, 2013
American Academy of Pediatrics and Pediatric Education for Prehospital Professionals (Program), 2013. *Pediatric Education for Prehospital Professionals*. 3rd ed. Burlington, MA: Jones & Bartlett Learning.

Aaronson, 2004
Aaronson PI, 2004. *The Cardiovascular System at a Glance*. 2nd ed. Malden, MA: Blackwell.

Abbey, 2004
Abbey J, Piller N, DeBellis A et al., 2004. The Abbey pain scale: a 1-minute numerical indicator for people with end-stage dementia. *International Journal of Palliative Nursing*, 10(1), 6–13.

Abrassart, 2013
Abrassart S, Stern R and Peter R, 2013. Unstable pelvic ring injury with hemodynamic instability: what seems the best procedure choice and sequence in the initial management? *Orthopaedics & Traumatology: Surgery & Research*, 99(2), 175–182.

Adams, 2002
Adams JE, Davis GG, Heidepriem RW III et al., 2002. Analysis of the incidence of pelvic trauma in fatal automobile accidents. *The American Journal of Forensic Medicine and Pathology*, 23(2), 132–136.

Age UK, 2014
Age UK, 2014. *Dementia and Cognitive Decline: A review of the evidence*. Available at: http://www.ageuk.org.uk/documents/en-gb/for-professionals/research/cognitive_decline_and_dementia_evidence_review_age_uk.pdf?dtrk=true [Accessed 30 January 2018].

Age UK, 2015
Age UK, 2015. *Depression and Anxiety*. Available at: https://www.ageuk.org.uk/information-advice/health-wellbeing/conditions-illnesses/depression-anxiety/ [Accessed 30 January 2018].

Age UK, 2017
Age UK, 2017. *Safeguarding Older People from Abuse and Neglect*. Available at: https://www.ageuk.org.uk/globalassets/age-uk/documents/factsheets/fs78_safeguarding_older_people_from_abuse_fcs.pdf [Accessed 30 January 2018].

Age UK, 2018
Age UK, 2018. *Later Life in the United Kingdom*. Available at: http://www.ageuk.org.uk/documents/en-gb/factsheets/later_life_uk_factsheet.pdf?dtrk=true [Accessed 30 January 2018].

Ahmad, 2006
Ahmad F, Cheshire N and Hamady M, 2006. Acute aortic syndrome: pathology and therapeutic strategies. *Postgraduate Medical Journal*, 82(967), 305–312.

ALK-Abello, 2016
ALK-Abello, 2016. *Jext 150 and 300 Micrograms Solution for Injection in Pre-filled Pen: Patient information leaflet*. Available at: http://www.medicines.org.uk/emc/pil.23888.latest.pdf.

Allan, 2004
Allan MA and Marsh J, 2004. *History and Examination*. 2nd ed. Edinburgh: Mosby.

Allen, 2007
Allen LA and O'Connor CM, 2007. Management of acute decompensated heart failure. *Canadian Medical Association Journal*, 176(6), 797–805.

Allison, 2004
Allison K and Porter K, 2004. Consensus on the pre-hospital approach to burns patient management. *Accident and Emergency Nursing*, 12(1), 53–57.

ALSG, 2010
Advanced Life Support Group, 2010. *Pre-hospital Obstetric Emergency Training*. Chichester: Wiley-Blackwell.

Althaus, 1982
Althaus U, Aeberhard P, Schüpbach P et al., 1982. Management of profound accidental hypothermia with cardiorespiratory arrest. *Annals of Surgery*, 195(4), 492.

Alzheimer's Society, 2014
Alzheimer's Society, 2014. *Dementia UK Report*. Available at: https://www.alzheimers.org.uk/info/20025/policy_and_influencing/251/dementia_uk [Accessed 30 January 2018].

Alzheimer's Society, 2015
Alzheimer's Society, 2015. *The Progression of Alzheimer's Disease and Other Dementias*. Available at: https://www.alzheimers.org.uk/download/downloads/id/1772/factsheet_the_progression_of_alzheimers_disease_and_other_dementias.pdf [Accessed 30 January 2018].

Alzheimer's Society, 2017
Alzheimer's Society, 2017. *Aggressive Behaviour*. Available at: https://www.alzheimers.org.uk/download/downloads/id/1797/factsheet_dementia_and_aggressive_behaviour.pdf [Accessed 30 January 2018].

Alzheimer's Society, 2018
Alzheimer's Society, 2018. *Types of Dementia*. Available at: https://www.alzheimers.org.uk/info/20007/types_of_dementia [Accessed 30 January 2018].

Ambu, 2011
Ambu, 2011. *Ambu Perfit ACE: Instructions for Use*. Denmark: Ambu D/S.

Angell-James, 1975
Angell-James JE and Daly MB, 1975. Some aspects of upper respiratory tract reflexes. *Acta Oto-laryngologica*, 79(3–4), 242–252.

Arthritis Research UK, 2015
Arthritis Research UK, 2015. *What is Arthritis?* Available at: http://www.arthritisresearchuk.org/arthritis-information/conditions/arthritis/what-is-arthritis.aspx [Accessed 30 January 2018].

Asbury, 2014
Asbury S and Jacobs E, 2014. *Dynamic Risk Assessment: The Practical Guide to Making Risk-Based Decisions with the 3-Level Risk Management Model*. 1st ed. Abingdon: Routledge.

ATLS, 2008
American College of Surgeons and Committee on Trauma, 2008. *ATLS, Advanced Trauma Life Support for Doctors: Student Course Manual*. Chicago, IL: American College of Surgeons.

Austin, 2010
Austin MA, Wills KE, Blizzard L et al., 2010. Effect of high flow oxygen on mortality in chronic obstructive pulmonary disease patients in prehospital setting: randomised controlled trial. *British Medical Journal*, 341, c5462.

Baile, 2000
Baile WF, Buckman R, Lenzi R et al., 2000. SPIKES – A six step protocol for delivering bad news: application to the patient with cancer. *The Oncologist*, 5(4), 302–311.

Baker, 2009
Baker SJK, and Wass JAH, 2009. Addison's disease. *BMJ*, 339(jul02 1), b2384–b2384.

Band, 2011
Band RA, Gaieski DF, Hylton JH et al., 2011. Arriving by emergency medical services improves time to treatment endpoints for patients with severe sepsis or septic shock. *Academic Emergency Medicine*, 18(9), 934–940.

Barrett, 2014
Barrett E and Burns A, 2014. *Dementia Revealed: What primary care needs to know*. Available at: https://www.england.nhs.uk/wp-content/uploads/2014/09/dementia-revealed-toolkit.pdf [Accessed 30 January 2018].

Bartlett, 2008
Bartlett N, Yuan J, Holland AJ et al., 2008. Optimal duration of cooling for an acute scald contact burn injury in a porcine model. *Journal of Burn Care & Research: Official Publication of the American Burn Association*, 29(5), 828–834.

Benger, 2009
Benger J, Nolan J and Clancy M (eds), 2009. *Emergency Airway Management*. Cambridge and New York: Cambridge University Press.

Berry, 2001
Berry M, Evison D and Roberts AH, 2001. The influence of body mass index on burn surface area estimated from the area of the hand. *Burns*, 27(6), 591–594.

Betsy, 2012
Betsy T and Keogh JE, 2012. Microbiology Demystified. 2nd ed. New York: McGraw-Hill.

BGS, 2014a
British Geriatrics Society, 2014. *Fit for Frailty, Part 1*. Available at: http://www.bgs.org.uk/campaigns/fff/fff_full.pdf [Accessed 30 January 2018].

BGS, 2014b
British Geriatrics Society, 2014. *What is Frailty?* Available at: http://www.bgs.org.uk/frailty-explained/resources/campaigns/fit-for-frailty/frailty-what-is-it [Accessed 30 January 2018].

BHF, 2017
British Heart Foundation and Resuscitation Council (UK), 2017. *A Guide to Automated External Defibrillators (AEDs)*. Available at: http://www.resus.org.uk/pages/AED_Guide.pdf [Accessed 30 January 2018].

Biarent, 2010
Biarent D, Bingham R, Eich C et al., 2010. European Resuscitation Council Guidelines for Resuscitation 2010, Section 6. Paediatric life support. *Resuscitation*, 81(10), 1364–1388.

Bickley, 2006
Bickley LS, Szilagyi PG and Bates B, 2006. *Bates' Guide to Physical Examination and History Taking*. 9th ed. Philadelphia, PA: Lippincott Williams & Wilkins.

Blaber, 2008
Blaber A, 2008. *Foundations for Paramedic Practice: A theoretical perspective*. 1st ed. Maidenhead: Open University Press.

Bledsoe, 2014
Bledsoe BE, Porter RS and Cherry RA, 2014. *Paramedic Care: Principles and Practice*. Vol. 3. Harlow: Pearson.

BLF, 2007
British Lung Foundation, 2007. *Invisible Lives: Chronic Obstructive Pulmonary Disease (COPD) – Finding the missing millions*. Available at: http://spirohub.com/wp-content/uploads/2016/01/BLF-Invisible-Lives-report.pdf [Accessed 30 January 2018].

BMA, 2007
British Medical Association, Resuscitation Council (UK) and Royal College of Nursing, 2007. *Decisions Relating to Cardiopulmonary Resuscitation*. Available at: https://www.resus.org.uk/dnacpr/ [Accessed 30 January 2018].

BMA, 2014
British Medical Association, 2014. *Safe Handover: Safe Patients*. Available at: http://bma.org.uk/-/media/files/pdfs/practical%20advice%20at%20work/contracts/safe%20handover%20safe%20patients.pdf [Accessed 30 January 2018].

BNF, 2014
British Medical Association and Royal Pharmaceutical Society of Great Britain, 2014. *British National Formulary*. Available at: https://www.medicinescomplete.com/about/publications.htm [Accessed 30 January 2018].

BOC, 2013a
BOC Healthcare, 2013. *Medical Oxygen*. Available at: http://www.bochealthcare.co.uk/internet.lh.lh.gbr/en/images/504370-Healthcare%20Medical%20Oxygen%20Integral%20Valve%20Cylinders%20leaflet%2006409_54069.pdf [Accessed 27 February 2018].

BOC, 2013b
BOC Healthcare, 2013. *Entonox® (50% Nitrous Oxide/50% Oxygen)*. Available at: http://www.bochealthcare.co.uk/internet.lh.lh.gbr/en/images/504365-Healthcare%20Entonox%20Integral%20Valve%20Cylinder%20Instructions%20leaflet-04409_57216.pdf?v=3.0 [Accessed 27 February 2018].

Body, 2010
Body R, Carley S, Wibberley C et al., 2010. The value of symptoms and signs in the emergent diagnosis of acute coronary syndromes. *Resuscitation*, 81(3), 281–286.

Bolton, 2012
Bolton JM, Spiwak R and Sareen J, 2012. Predicting suicide attempts with the SAD PERSONS scale: a longitudinal analysis. *Journal of Clinical Psychiatry*, 73(6), e735–e741.

Bonner, 2011
Bonner TJ, Eardley WGP, Newell N et al., 2011. Accurate placement of a pelvic binder improves reduction of unstable fractures of the pelvic ring. *Journal of Bone* and *Joint Surgery*, British Volume, 93-B(11), 1524–1528.

Bont, 2014
de Bont EG, Francis NA, Dinant G-J et al., 2014. Parents' knowledge, attitudes, and practice in childhood fever: an internet-based survey. *British Journal of General Practice*, 64(618), e10–e16.

Booker, 2007
Booker R, 2007. Peak expiratory flow measurement. *Nursing Standard*, 21(39), 42–43.

Bose, 2006
Bose P, Regan F and Paterson-Brown S, 2006. Improving the accuracy of estimated blood loss at obstetric haemorrhage using clinical reconstructions. *BJOG: An International Journal of Obstetrics and Gynaecology*, 113(8), 919–924.

Bowers, 2007
Bowers B and Scase C, 2007. Tracheostomy: facilitating successful discharge from hospital to home. *British Journal of Nursing*, 16(8), 476–479.

Boyett, 2009
Boyett MR, 2009. 'And the beat goes on.' The cardiac conduction system: the wiring system of the heart. *Experimental Physiology*, 94(10), 1035–1049.

Briar, 2003
Briar C and Lasserson D, 2003. *Nervous System*. 2nd ed. London: Mosby.

Briscoe, 2006
Briscoe VJ, and Davis SN, 2006. Hypoglycemia in type 1 and type 2 diabetes: physiology, pathophysiology, and management. Clinical Diabetes, 24(3), 115 –121.

Brophy, 2012
Brophy GM, Bell R, Claassen J et al., 2012. Guidelines for the evaluation and management of status epilepticus. *Neurocritical Care*, 17(1), 3–23.

BSI, 2011
British Standards Institution, 2011. *BS EN 1089-3:2011*. London: BSI.

BTS, 2008
O'Driscoll BR, Howard LS, Davison AG et al., 2008. BTS guideline for emergency oxygen use in adult patients. *Thorax*, 63(Supplement 6), vi1–vi68.

BTS, 2017
O'Driscoll BR, Howard LS, Earis J, Mak V, British Thoracic Society Emergency Oxygen Guideline Group and BTS Emergency Oxygen Guideline Development Group, 2017. BTS guideline for oxygen use in adults in healthcare and emergency settings. *Thorax*, 72(Suppl 1), ii1–ii90.

BTS/SIGN 2016
Scottish Intercollegiate Guidelines Network and British Thoracic Society, 2016. *British Guideline on the Management of Asthma: A national clinical*

guideline. Available at: https://www.brit-thoracic.org.uk/document-library/clinical-information/asthma/btssign-asthma-guideline-2016/ [Accessed 30 January 2018].

Buss, 2010
Buss J and Thompson G (eds), 2010. *Auscultation Skills: Breath & Heart Sounds*. 4th ed. Philadelphia: Wolters Kluwer/Lippincott Williams & Wilkins Health.

Canto, 2012
Canto AJ, Kiefe CI, Goldberg RJ et al., 2012. Differences in symptom presentation and hospital mortality according to type of acute myocardial infarction. *American Heart Journal*, 163(4), 572–579.

Capps, 2010
Capps JA, Sharma V and Arkwright PD, 2010. Prevalence, outcome and pre-hospital management of anaphylaxis by first aiders and paramedical ambulance staff in Manchester, UK. *Resuscitation*, 81(6), 653–657.

CCI, 2011
Clement Clarke International, 2011. *Mini-Wright Peak Flow Meter Instructions for Use*. Edinburgh: Clement Clarke International.

Ceallaigh, 2006
Ceallaigh PÓ, Ekanaykaee K, Beirne CJ et al., 2006. Diagnosis and management of common maxillofacial injuries in the emergency department. Part 1: advanced trauma life support. *Emergency Medicine Journal*, 23(10), 796–797.

CFOA, 2017
Chief Fire Officers Association, 2017. *Safe and Well Visits*. Available at: http://www.cfoa.org.uk/21422 [Accessed 30 January 2018].

Chan, 2003
Chan MM, 2003. What is the effect of fingernail polish on pulse oximetry? *Chest*, 123(6), 2163–2164.

Chandler, 2014
Chandler R and Bruneau B, 2014. Barriers to the management of pain in dementia care. *Nursing Practice*, 110(28), 12–16.

Chapin, 2013
Chapin MM, Rochette LM, Annest JL et al., 2013. Nonfatal choking on food among children 14 years or younger in the United States, 2001–2009. *Pediatrics*, 132(2), 275–281.

Chin, 2004
Chin RFM, Neville BGR and Scott RC, 2004. A systematic review of the epidemiology of status epilepticus. *European Journal of Neurology*, 11(12), 800–810.

Clegg, 2013
Clegg A, Young J, Ili S et al., 2013. Frailty in elderly people. *The Lancet*, 381(868), 752–762.

Cook, 2006
Cook TM and Hommers C, 2006. New airways for resuscitation? *Resuscitation*, 69(3), 371–387.

Cooper, 2012
Cooper C, 2012. *Psychiatry at a Glance*. 5th Ed. Chichester: Wiley-Blackwell.

CoP, 2014
College of Paramedics, 2014. *Paramedic Curriculum Guidance*. 3rd ed. Available at: https://www.collegeofparamedics.co.uk/publications/professional-standards [Accessed 30 January 2018].

Corcoran, 2013
Corcoran N, 2013. *Communicating Health: Strategies for Health Promotion*. 2nd ed. Los Angeles: SAGE Publications Ltd.

Corwell, 2014
Corwell B, Knight B, Olivieri L et al., 2014. Current diagnosis and treatment of hyperglycemic emergencies. *Emergency Medicine Clinics of North America*, 32(2), 437–452.

Cox, 2009
Cox ED, Schreiber MA, McManus J et al., 2009. New hemostatic agents in the combat setting. *Transfusion*, 49, 248S–255S.

Crook, 2013
Crook J and Taylor RM, 2013. The agreement of fingertip and sternum capillary refill time in

children. *Archives of Disease in Childhood*, 98(4), 265–268.

CSCB, 2014
Coventry Safeguarding Children Board, 2014. *Serious Case Review: Daniel Pelka*. Available at: https://cscb-new.co.uk/downloads/Serious%20Case%20Reviews%20-%20exec.%20summaries/SCR_Archive/Coventry%20SCR%20-%20Daniel%20Pelka%20(2013).pdf [Accessed 30 January 2018].

Cure the NHS, 2018
Cure the NHS, 2018. Cure the NHS campaign. Available at: http://www.curethenhs.co.uk/ [Accessed 01 May 2018].

Cuttle, 2008
Cuttle L, Kempf M, Kravchuk O et al., 2008. The optimal temperature of first aid treatment for partial thickness burn injuries. *Wound Repair and Regeneration: Official Publication of the Wound Healing Society [and] the European Tissue Repair Society*, 16(5), 626–634.

Cuttle, 2009
Cuttle L, Pearn J, McMillan JR et al., 2009. A review of first aid treatments for burn injuries. *Burns*, 35(6), 768–775.

Cuttle, 2010
Cuttle, L, Kempf M, Liu PY et al., 2010. The optimal duration and delay of first aid treatment for deep partial thickness burn injuries. *Burns*, 36(5), 673–679.

Czura, 2011
Czura CJ, 2011. 'Merinoff Symposium 2010: Sepsis' – speaking with one voice. *Molecular Medicine*, 17(1–2), 2–3.

Daniels, 2011a
Daniels R, 2011. Surviving the first hours in sepsis: getting the basics right (an intensivist's perspective). *Journal of Antimicrobial Chemotherapy*, 66(Supplement 2), ii11–ii23.

Daniels, 2011b
Daniels R, Nutbeam T, McNamara G et al., 2011. The sepsis six and the severe sepsis resuscitation bundle: a prospective observational cohort study. *Emergency Medicine Journal*, 28(6), 507–512.

Datta, 2006
Datta A and Tipton M, 2006. Respiratory responses to cold water immersion: neural pathways, interactions, and clinical consequences awake and asleep. *Journal of Applied Physiology*, 100(6), 2057–2064.

Deakin, 2015
Deakin C, Jewkes F, Lockey D et al., 2015. *Prehospital Resuscitation*. Available at: https://www.resus.org.uk/resuscitation-guidelines/prehospital-resuscitation/ [Accessed 30 January 2018].

Deary, 1993
Deary IJ, Hepburn DA, MacLeod KM et al., 1993. Partitioning the symptoms of hypoglycaemia using multi-sample confirmatory factor analysis. *Diabetologia*, 36(8), 771–777.

DfE, 2015
Department for Education, 2015. *Working Together to Safeguard Children*. Available at: https://www.gov.uk/government/publications/working-together-to-safeguard-children [Accessed 21 May 2018].

Diabetes UK, 2016
Diabetes UK, 2016. *Diabetes Prevalence 2016*. Available at: https://www.diabetes.org.uk/professionals/position-statements-reports/statistics/diabetes-prevalence-2016/ [Accessed 30 January 2018].

Dieckmann, 2010
Dieckmann RA, Brownstein D and Gausche-Hill M, 2010. The pediatric assessment triangle: a novel approach for the rapid evaluation of children. *Pediatric Emergency Care*, 26(4), 312–315.

Dimond, 2008
Dimond BC, 2008. *Legal Aspects of Mental Capacity*. 1st ed. Oxford: Wiley-Blackwell.

Dimond, 2011
Dimond BC, 2011. *Legal Aspects of Nursing*. 6th ed. London: Pearson Education.

Dixon, 2009
Dixon M, Carmody N and O'Donnell C, 2009. The effectiveness of supraglottic airway devices in pre hospital basic life support airway management. *Emergency Medicine Journal*, 26(10), 4.

Dobson, 2009
Dobson T, Jensen J, Karim S et al., 2009. Correlation of paramedic administration of furosemide with emergency physician diagnosis of congestive heart failure. *Journal of Emergency Primary Health Care*, 7(3), 3.

DoH, 2000
Department of Health, 2000. *No Secrets: Guidance on protecting vulnerable adults in care*. Available at: https://www.gov.uk/government/publications/no-secrets-guidance-on-protecting-vulnerable-adults-in-care [Accessed 30 January 2018].

DoH, 2006a
Department of Health, 2006. *Medical Gases: Health Technical Memorandum 02-01: Medical Gas Pipeline Systems*. Available at: https://www.gov.uk/government/publications/medical-gas-pipeline-systems-part-a-design-installation-validation-and-verification [Accessed 30 January 2018].

DoH, 2006b
Department of Health, 2006. *A Review of Services for Allergy: The epidemiology, demand for and provision of treatment and effectiveness of clinical interventions*. Available at: http://webarchive.nationalarchives.gov.uk/20130107105354/http:/www.dh.gov.uk/en/publicationsandstatistics/publications/publicationspolicyandguidance/dh_4137365 [Accessed 30 January 2018].

DoH, 2007a
Department of Health, 2007. *Mass Casualties Incidents: A framework for planning*. Available at: http://webarchive.nationalarchives.gov.uk/20130107105354/http:/www.dh.gov.uk/en/publicationsandstatistics/publications/publicationspolicyandguidance/dh_073395 [Accessed 30 January 2018].

DoH, 2007b
Department of Health, 2007. *Making Experiences Count: A new approach to responding to complaints – a document for information and comment*. Available at: http://webarchive.nationalarchives.gov.uk/+/www.dh.gov.uk/en/consultations/liveconsultations/dh_075652 [Accessed 30 January 2018].

DoH, 2008
Great Britain and Department of Health 2008. Code of Practice: Mental Health Act 1983: Published Pursuant to Section 118 of the Act. London: TSO.

DoH, 2009a
Department of Health, 2009. *Reference Guide to Consent for Examination or Treatment*. Available at: https://www.gov.uk/government/uploads/system/uploads/attachment_data/file/138296/dh_103653__1_.pdf [Accessed 30 January 2018].

DoH, 2009b
Department of Health and Health Protection Agency, 2009. Pandemic (H1N1) 2009 Influenza. Available at: https://www.gov.uk/government/uploads/system/uploads/attachment_data/file/356986/pandemic_influenza_guidance_for_infection_control_in_ambulance_services.pdf [Accessed 22 December 2014].

DoH, 2010a
Department of Health, 2010. Confidentiality: NHS Code of Practice – supplementary guidance: public interest disclosures. Available at: https://www.gov.uk/government/publications/confidentiality-nhs-code-of-practicesupplementary-guidance-public-interest-disclosures [Accessed 8 December 2014].

DoH, 2010b
Department of Health, 2010. Essence of Care 2010: Benchmarks for the Fundamental Aspects of Care: Benchmarks for Personal Hygiene. London: Stationery Office.

DoH, 2010c
Australian Government, Department of Health, 2010. Personal hygiene. Available at: http://www.health.gov.au/internet/publications/publishing.nsf/content/ohpenhealth-manual-atsi-cnt-l~ohp-enhealth-manual-atsi-cnt-lch3~ohp-enhealth-manual-atsi-cnt-l-ch3.7 [Accessed 21 December 2014].

DoH, 2010d
Department of Health, 2010. Ambulance Guidelines: Reducing Infection Through Effective Practice in the Pre-Hospital Environment. Available at: http://webarchive.nationalarchives.gov.uk/20120118164404/hcai.dh.gov.uk/files/2011/03/document_ambulance_guidelines_reducing_infection_in_prehospital_final_271%e2%%80%a6.pdf[Accessed 22 December 2014].

DoH, 2011
Department of Health, 2011. *Safeguarding Adults: The role of health services*. Available at: https://www.gov.uk/government/publications/safeguarding-adults-the-role-of-health-services [Accessed 30 January 2018].

DoH, 2013a
Department of Health, 2013. *Health Technical Memorandum 07-01: Safe management of healthcare waste*. Available at: https://www.gov.uk/government/uploads/system/uploads/attachment_data/file/167976/HTM_07-01_Final.pdf [Accessed 30 January 2018].

DoH, 2013b
Department of Health, 2013. *Winterbourne View Hospital: Department of Health review and response*. Available at: https://www.gov.uk/government/publications/winterbourne-view-hospital-department-of-health-review-and-response [Accessed 30 January 2018].

DoH, 2013c
Department of Health, 2013. Berwick review into patient safety. Available at: https://www.gov.uk/government/publications/berwick-review-into-patient-safety [Accessed 31 December 2014].

DoH, 2014
Department of Health and Concordat signatories, 2014. *Mental Health Crisis Care Concordat*. Retrieved from http://www.crisiscareconcordat.org.uk/wp-content/uploads/2014/04/36353_Mental_Health_Crisis_accessible.pdf [Accessed 30 January 2018].

DoH, 2015
Department of Health, 2015. *NHS Constitution for England*. Available at: https://www.gov.uk/government/publications/the-nhs-constitution-for-england [Accessed 30 January 2018].

Dougherty, 2011
Dougherty L and Lister SE, 2011. *The Royal Marsden Hospital Manual of Clinical Nursing Procedures*. Chichester: Wiley-Blackwell.

Douglas, 2005
Douglas G, Nicol EF, Robertson C et al., 2005. *Macleod's Clinical Examination*. 11th ed. Edinburgh: Elsevier Churchill Livingstone.

Drake, 2005
Drake RL, 2005. *Gray's Anatomy for Students*. Edinburgh: Churchill Livingstone.

Dunn, 2005
Dunn L, 2005. Pneumonia: classification, diagnosis and nursing management. *Nursing Standard*, 19(42), 50–54.

Durrer, 2003
Durrer B, Brugger H, Syme D et al., 2003. The medical on-site treatment of hypothermia: ICAR-MEDCOM recommendation. *High Altitude Medicine & Biology*, 4(1), 99–103.

Durrington, 2005
Durrington HJ, Flubacher M, Ramsay CF et al., 2005. Initial oxygen management in patients with an exacerbation of chronic obstructive pulmonary disease. *QJM*, 98(7), 499–504.

DWI, 2012
Drinking Water Inspectorate, 2012. Legislation. Available at: http://dwi.defra.gov.uk/stakeholders/legislation/[Accessed 27 December 2014].

EEAST, 2013
East of England Ambulance Service NHS Trust, 2013. Major Incident Plan v1.6. Norwich: EEAST.

EEAST, 2014
East of England Ambulance Service, 2014. *Clinical Manual 2014*. Bridgwater: Class Professional Publishing.

Enoch, 2009
Enoch S, Roshan A and Shah M, 2009. Emergency and early management of burns and scalds. *BMJ*, 338, b1037.

Equality Act 2010
UK Government. *Equality Act 2010*. Available at: http://www.legislation.gov.uk/ukpga/2010/15/contents [Accessed 30 January 2018].

EROS, 2009
The European Registers of Stroke (EROS) Investigators, 2009. Incidence of stroke in Europe at the beginning of the 21st century. *Stroke*, 40(5), 1557–1563.

Evans, 2012
Evans JDW and Sutton P, 2012. *Cardiovascular System*. Edinburgh: Mosby/Elsevier.

Falk, 2003
Falk E and Thuesen L, 2003. Pathology of coronary microembolisation and no reflow. *Heart*, 89(9), 983–985.

Farley, 2011
Farley A and Hendry C, 2011. *The Physiological Effects of Ageing*. 1st ed. Chichester: Wiley-Blackwell.

Feber, 2006
Feber T, 2006. Tracheostomy care for community nurses: basic principles. *British Journal of Community Nursing*, 11(5), 186.

Ferno, 2006
Ferno-Washington, 2006. *Scoop EXL Stretcher Series User Manual*. Wilmington, OH: Ferno-Washington.

Ferreira, 2005
Ferreira J and Stanley L, 2005. *Evaluation of Manual Handling Tasks Involving the Use of Carry Chairs by UK Ambulance Personnel*. Sudbury: HSE Books.

Fick, 2002
Fick DM, Agostini JV and Inouye SK, 2002. Delirium superimposed on dementia: a systematic review. *Journal of the American Geriatrics Society*, 50(10), 1723–1732.

Fire Brigade Union, 2015
Fire Brigade Union, 2015. *Firefighters and Response to Medical Incidents*. Available at: https://www.fbu.org.uk/policy/2015/firefighters-and-response-medical-incidents [Accessed 30 January 2018].

Francis, 2013
Francis R, 2013. *Final report – Mid Staffordshire NHS Foundation Trust Public Inquiry*. Available at: http://webarchive.nationalarchives.gov.uk/20150407084003/http://www.midstaffspublicinquiry.com/report [Accessed 30 January 2018].

Frank, 2010
Frank M, Schmucker U, Stengel D et al., 2010. Proper estimation of blood loss on scene of trauma: tool or tale? *The Journal of Trauma: Injury, Infection, and Critical Care*, 69(5), 1191–1195.

Freyenhagen, 2009
Freyenhagen F, 2009. Personal autonomy and mental capacity. *Psychiatry*, 8(12), 465–467.

Fried, 2001
Fried LP, Tangen CM, Walston J et al., 2001. Cardiovascular Health Study Collaborative Research Group. Frailty in older adults: evidence for a phenotype. *J Gerontol A Biol Sci Med Sci*, 56(3), M146–156.

Frykberg, 1988
Frykberg ER and Tepas JJ, 1988. Terrorist bombings. Lessons learned from Belfast to Beirut. *Annals of Surgery*, 208(5), 569–576.

Fuchs, 2012
Fuchs S, Yamamoto L, American Academy of Pediatrics et al., 2012. *APLS: The Pediatric Emergency Medicine Resource*. Burlington, MA: Jones & Bartlett Learning.

Gabbe, 2011
Gabbe BJ, de Steiger R, Esser M et al., 2011. Predictors of mortality following severe pelvic ring fracture: results of a population-based study. *Injury*, 42(10), 985–991.

Garcia, 2004
Garcia TB and Miller GT, 2004. *Arrhythmia Recognition: The Art of Interpretation*. Sudbury, MA: Jones & Bartlett Publishers.

Garcia, 2015
Garcia TB, 2015. *12-lead ECG: The Art of Interpretation*. 2nd ed. Burlington, MA: Jones & Bartlett Learning.

Garlapati, 2012
Garlapati AK and Ashwood N, 2012. An overview of pelvic ring disruption. *Trauma*, 14(2), 169–178.

Geerts, 2012
Geerts BF, van den Bergh L, Stijnen T et al., 2012. Comprehensive review: is it better to use the Trendelenburg position or passive leg raising for the initial treatment of hypovolemia? *Journal of Clinical Anesthesia*, 24(8), 668–674.

Ginsberg, 2004
Ginsberg L, 2004. *Lecture Notes: Neurology*. 8th ed. Oxford: Wiley-Blackwell.

Gitelman, 2008
Gitelman A, Hishmeh S, Morelli BN et al., 2008. Cauda equina syndrome: a comprehensive review. *American Journal of Orthopedics*, 37(11), 556–562.

Goldberg, 2007
Goldberg A, Southern DA, Galbraith PD, et al., 2007. Coronary dominance and prognosis of patients with acute coronary syndrome. American Heart Journal, 154(6), 1116–1122.

Golden, 1997
Golden FSC, David GC and Tipton MJ et al., 1997. *Review of Rescue and Immediate Post-Immersion Problems: A medical/ergonomic viewpoint*. Sudbury: HSE Books.

Granville-Chapman, 2011
Granville-Chapman J, Jacobs N and Midwinter MJ, 2011. Prehospital haemostatic dressings: a systematic review. *Injury*, 42(5), 447–459.

Graveling, 2009
Graveling AJ and Frier BM, 2009. Hypoglycaemia: an overview. *Primary Care Diabetes*, 3(3), 131–139.

Gray, 2013
Gray A, Ward K, Lees F et al., 2013. The epidemiology of adults with severe sepsis and septic shock in Scottish emergency departments. *Emergency Medicine Journal*, 30(5), 397–401.

Greaves, 2008
Greaves I, Porter K, Ryan J et al., 2008. *Trauma Care Manual*. 2nd ed. London: Hodder Arnold.

Greaves, 2010
Greaves I, Porter K and Smith J, 2010. *Practical Prehospital Care: The Principles and Practice of Immediate Care*. 1st ed. London: Churchill Livingstone.

Gregory, 2010a
Gregory P, Ward A and Sanders MJ, 2010. *Sanders' Paramedic Textbook*. Edinburgh: Mosby.

Gregory, 2010b
Gregory P, 2010. *Manual of Clinical Paramedic Procedures*. Chichester: Wiley-Blackwell.

Harbison, 2003.
Diagnostic accuracy of stroke referrals from primary care, emergency room physicians, and ambulance staff using the face arm speech test. *Stroke*, 34(1), 71–76.

Harrison, 2007
Harrison P, 2007. *Managing Spinal Cord Injury: The First 48 Hours*. Milton Keynes: Spinal Injuries Association.

Hart, 2006
Hart CA and Thomson APJ, 2006. Meningococcal disease and its management in children. *BMJ*, 333(7570), 685–690.

Hartley, 1999
Hartley P, 1999. *Interpersonal Communication*. 2nd ed. London: Routledge.

Hasler, 2011
Hasler RM, Exadaktylos AK, Bouamra O et al., 2011. Epidemiology and predictors of spinal injury in adult major trauma patients: European cohort study. *European Spine Journal*, 20(12), 2174–2180.

HC, 2009
The Healthcare Commission, 2009. *Investigation into Mid Staffordshire NHS Foundation Trust*. Available at: http://webarchive.nationalarchives.gov.uk/20110504135228/http://www.cqc.org.uk/_db/_documents/investigation_into_mid_staffordshire_nhs_foundation_trust.pdf [Accessed 30 January 2018].

HCPC, 2016
Health and Care Professions Council, 2016. Standards of conduct, performance and ethics. Available at: https://www.hcpc-uk.org/aboutregistration/standards/standardsofconductperformanceandethics/ [Accessed 1 May 2018].

Hennes, 2006
Hennes H and Kim MK, 2006. Prehospital pain management: current status and future direction. *Clinical Pediatric Emergency Medicine*, 7(1), 25–30.

Henry, 2008
Henry C and Seymour J, 2008. *Advanced Care Planning: A guide for health and social care staff*. Available at http://www.ncpc.org.uk/sites/default/files/AdvanceCarePlanning.pdf [Accessed 30 January 2018].

Hettiaratchy, 2004
Hettiaratchy S and Papini R, 2004. Initial management of a major burn: II – assessment and resuscitation. *BMJ*, 329(7457), 101–103.

Hinkelbein, 2007
Hinkelbein J, Genzwuerker HV, Sogl R et al., 2007. Effect of nail polish on oxygen saturation determined by pulse oximetry in critically ill patients. *Resuscitation*, 72(1), 82–91.

HMG, 2015
HM Government, 2015. Disability rights. Available at: https://www.gov.uk/rights-disabled-person/overview[Accessed 6 December 2015].

Holt, 2010
Holt TA, 2010. *ABC of Diabetes*. 6th ed. ABC series. Chichester: Wiley-Blackwell/BMJ.

HO and DfE, 2016
Home Office and Department for Education, 2016. *Multi-agency Statutory Guidance on Female Genital Mutilation*. Available at: https://www.gov.uk/government/uploads/system/uploads/attachment_data/file/513205/MultiAgencyPracticeGuidelinesNov14.pdf [Accessed 30 January 2018].

Howlett, 2011
Howlett JG, 2011. Acute heart failure: sections learned so far. *Canadian Journal of Cardiology*, 27(3), 284–295.

HSCIC, 2009
Health and Social Care Information Centre 2009. *Adult Psychiatric Morbidity in England – 2007, results of a household survey*. Available from: http://www.hscic.gov.uk/pubs/psychiatricmorbidity07 [Accessed 30 January 2018].

HSCIC, 2013
Health and Social Care Information Centre, 2013. *NHS Written Complaints Data Released*. Available at: http://www.hscic.gov.uk/article/3414/nhs-written-complaintsdata-released [Accessed 30 January 2018].

HSCIC, 2015
Health and Social Care Information Centre, 2015. *Information Governance – frequently asked questions*. Available at: http://webarchive.nationalarchives.gov.uk/20160729123846/http://systems.hscic.gov.uk/infogov/igfaqs [Accessed 27 February 2018].

HSE, 2003
Health and Safety Executive, 2003. *The Principles of Good Manual Handling: Achieving a consensus*. Available at: http://www.hse.gov.uk/research/rrpdf/rr097.pdf [Accessed 30 January 2018].

HSE, 2006
Health and Safety Executive, 2006. *Essentials of Health and Safety at Work*. Sudbury: HSE Books.

HSE, 2007
Health and Safety Executive, 2007. *Managing the Causes of Work-related Stress: A Step-by-step Approach Using the Management Standards*. Suffolk: HSE.

HSE, 2008a
Health and Safety Executive, 2008. *Working Together to Reduce Stress at Work*. Available at: http://www.hse.gov.uk/pubns/indg424.pdf [Accessed 30 January 2018].

HSE, 2008b
Health and Safety Executive, (2008). Take care with oxygen. Merseyside: HSE.

HSE, 2009
Health and Safety Executive, 2009. *Health and Safety Law*. Available at: http://www.hse.gov.uk/pubns/law.pdf [Accessed 29 December 2014].

HSE, 2011
Health and Safety Executive, 2011. *Risk Factors Associated with Pushing and Pulling Loads*. Available at: http://www.hse.gov.uk/msd/pushpull/risks.htm [Accessed 30 January 2018].

HSE, 2013a
Health and Safety Executive, 2013. *Managing for Health and Safety*. Available at: http://www.hse.gov.uk/pubns/priced/hsg65.pdf [Accessed 1 May 2018].

HSE, 2013b
Health and Safety Executive, 2013. *Control of Substances Hazardous to Health: Approved Code of Practice*. Available at: http://www.hse.gov.uk/pubns/priced/l5.pdf [Accessed 1 May 2018].

HSE, 2013c
Health and Safety Executive, 2013. *Personal Protective Equipment (PPE) at Work*. Available at: http://www.hse.gov.uk/pubns/indg174.pdf [Accessed 1 May 2018].

HSE, 2014a
Health and Safety Executive, 2014. *Work Related Stress: Signs and Symptoms*. Available at: http://www.hse.gov.uk/stress/signs.htm [Accessed 1 May 2018].

HSE, 2014b
Health and Safety Executive, 2014. *Risk management*. Available at: http://www.hse.gov.uk/risk/ [Accessed 1 May 2018].

HSE, 2014c
Health and Safety Executive, 2014. *Risk Assessment – A brief guide to controlling risks in the workplace*. Available at: http://www.hse.gov.uk/pubns/indg163.htm [Accessed 1 May 2018].

HSE, 2014d
Health and Safety Executive, 2014. *Safe Use of Work Equipment*. Available at: http://www.hse.gov.uk/pubns/priced/l22.pdf [Accessed 1 May 2018].

HSE, 2015a
Health and Safety Executive, 2015. *Managing the Risks from Skin Exposure*. Available at: http://www.hse.gov.uk/skin/professional/managerisk.htm [Accessed 1 May 2018].

HSE, 2015b
Health and Safety Executive, 2015. *Methods of Decontamination*. Available at: http://www.hse.gov.uk/biosafety/blood-borne-viruses/methods-of-decontamination.htm [Accessed 2 May 2018].

HSE, 2015c
Health and Safety Executive, 2015. *Sharps Injuries*. Available at: http://www.hse.gov.uk/healthservices/needlesticks/ [Accessed 1 May 2018].

HSE, 2015d
Health and Safety Executive, 2015. *Skin Care at Work*. Available at: http://www.hse.gov.uk/healthservices/skin.htm [Accessed 1 May 2018].

HSE, 2015e
Health and Safety Executive, 2015. *Laundry Treatments at High and Low Temperatures*. Available at: http://www.hse.gov.uk/biosafety/blood-borne-viruses/laundry-treatments.htm [Accessed 2 May 2018].

HSE, 2016
Health and Safety Executive, 2016. *Manual Handling Operations Regulations 1992*. Available at: http://www.hse.gov.uk/pubns/priced/l23.pdf [Accessed 30 January 2018].

Hüpfl, 2010
Hüpfl M, Selig HF and Nagele P, 2010. Chest-compression only versus standard cardiopulmonary resuscitation: a meta-analysis. *The Lancet*, 376(9752), 1552–1557.

Hutchison, 1998
Hutchison IL, Magennis P, Shepherd JP et al., 1998. The BAOMS United Kingdom survey of facial injuries part 1: aetiology and the association with alcohol consumption. British Association of Oral and Maxillofacial Surgeons. *The British Journal of Oral & Maxillofacial Surgery*, 36(1), 3–13.

Hutchison, 2012
Hutchison C and Morrison R, 2012. Oral and maxillofacial trauma and the use of telemedicine in the Grampian region of Scotland: a retrospective study. *Journal of Oral and Maxillofacial Research*, 3(3), e2.

IASP, 2017
International Association for the Study of Pain, 2017. *IASP Taxonomy*. Available at: https://www.iasp-pain.org/Taxonomy [Accessed 30 January 2018].

Idris, 2003
Idris AH, Berg RA, Bierens J et al., 2003. Recommended guidelines for uniform reporting of data from drowning. *Circulation*, 108(20), 2565–2574.

ILAE, 1993
International League Against Epilepsy, 1993. Guidelines for epidemiologic studies on epilepsy. *Epilepsia*, 34(4), 592–596.

Ireland, 2011
Ireland S, Endacott R, Cameron P et al., 2011. The incidence and significance of accidental hypothermia in major trauma – A prospective observational study. *Resuscitation*, 82(3), 300–306.

Jalo, 2009
Jalo M, Magennis P, Ridout F et al., 2009. The second UK national facial injury survey: the demography, aetiology, nature of injury and treatment. *British Journal of Oral and Maxillofacial Surgery*, 47(7), e58.

James, 2004
James CY, Riemann BL, Munkasy BA et al., 2004. Comparison of cervical spine motion during application among 4 rigid immobilization collars. *Journal of Athletic Training*, 39(2), 138–145.

James, 2011
James B, 2011. *Lecture Notes: Ophthalmology*. 11th ed. Chichester: Wiley-Blackwell.

JCO, 2010a
Judicial Communications Office, 2010. *Coroner's Inquests into the London Bombings of 7 July 2005*. Available at: http://webarchive.nationalarchives.gov.uk/20120216072438/http:/7julyinquests.independent.gov.uk/ [Accessed 30 January 2018].

JCO, 2010b
Judicial Communications Office, 2010. *Coroner's Inquests into the London Bombings of 7 July 2005: Hearing transcripts*. Available at: http://webarchive.nationalarchives.gov.uk/20120216072438/http:/7julyinquests.independent.gov.uk/hearing_transcripts/09122010am.htm [Accessed 30 January 2018].

Jennings, 2009
Jennings PA, Cameron P and Bernard S, 2009. Measuring acute pain in the prehospital setting. *Emergency Medicine Journal*, 26(8), 552–555.

JESIP, 2013
Joint Emergency Services Interoperability Programme, 2013. *Joint Doctine: The interoperability framework*. Available at: http://www.jesip.org.uk/uploads/resources/JESIP-Joint-Doctrine.pdf [Accessed 30 January 2018].

JESIP, 2017
JESIP, 2017. *JESIP The Programme*. Available at: http://www.jesip.org.uk/jesip-the-programme [Accessed 30 January 2018].

Johnson, 2004
Johnson S and Henderson SO, 2004. Myth: the Trendelenburg position improves circulation in cases of shock. *CJEM*, 6(1), 48.

Johnson, 2012
Johnson G and Hill-Smith I, 2012. *The Minor Illness Manual*. London: Radcliffe Publishing.

JRCALC, 2016
Association of Ambulance Chief Executives, 2016. *UK Ambulance Services Clinical Practice Guidelines 2016*. Bridgwater: Class Professional Publishing.

JRCALC, 2017
Joint Royal Colleges Ambulance Liaison Committee, 2017. *Clinical Practice Supplementary Guidelines 2017*. Bridgwater: Class Professional Publishing.

Judd, 1993
Judd C and Park B, 1993. Definit on and assessment of accuracy in social stereotypes. *Psychological Review*, 100(1), 109–128.

Kaeser, 2010
Kaeser P-F and Kawasaki A, 2010. Disorders of pupillary structure and function. *Neurologic Clinics*, 28(3), 657–677.

Kalson, 2012
Kalson NS, Jenks T, Woodford M et al., 2012. Burns represent a significant proportion of the total serious trauma workload in England and Wales. *Burns: Journal of the International Society for Burn Injuries*, 38(3), 330–339.

Kapit, 2000
Kapit W, Macey RI and Meisami E, 2000. *The Physiology Coloring Book*. San Francisco, CA: Addison Wesley Longman.

Kapit, 2001
Kapit W and Elson LM, 2001. *The Anatomy Coloring Book*. 3rd ed. London: Benjamin Cummings.

Kauffman, 2014
Kauffman M, 2014. *History and Physical Examination: A Common Sense Approach*. Burlington, MA: Jones & Bartlett Learning.

Kerber, 2012
Kerber RE, 2012. Hands-on defibrillation – the end of 'I'm clear, you're clear, we're all clear'? *Journal of the American Heart Association*, 1(5), e005496.

Kilner, 2002
Kilner T, 2002. Triage decisions of prehospital emergency health care providers, using a multiple casualty scenario paper exercise. *Emergency Medicine Journal*, 19(4), 348–353.

Kimmel, 1999
Kimmel EC and Still KR, 1999. Acute lung injury, acute respiratory distress syndrome and inhalation injury: an overview. *Drug and Chemical Toxicology*, 22(1), 91–128.

King, 2014
King D, Morton R and Bevan C, 2014. How to use capillary refill time. *Archives of Disease in Childhood – Education & Practice Edition*, 99(3), 111–116.

King's Fund, 2015
The King's Fund, 2015. Life Expectancy. Available at: http://www.kingsfund.org.uk/time-to-think-differently/trends/demography/life-expectancy [Accessed 10 November 2015].

Knight, 2008a
Knight J and Nigam Y, 2008. Exploring the anatomy and physiology of ageing. Part 2 – the respiratory system. *Nursing Times*, 104(32), 24–25.

Knight, 2008b
Knight J and Nigam Y, 2008. Exploring the anatomy and physiology of ageing. Part 1 – the cardiovascular system. *Nursing Times*, 104(31), 26–27.

Knight, 2008c
Knight J and Nigam Y, 2008. Exploring the anatomy and physiology of ageing. Part 5 – the nervous system. *Nursing Times*, 104(35), 18–19.

Knight, 2008d
Knight J and Nigam Y, 2008. Exploring the anatomy and physiology of ageing. Part 10 – muscles and bone. *Nursing Times*, 104(48), 22–23.

Knops, 2011
Knops SP, 2011. Comparison of three different pelvic circumferential compression devices: a biomechanical cadaver study. *The Journal of Bone and Joint Surgery (American)*, 93(3), 230.

Kodali, 2013
Kodali BS, 2013. Capnography outside the operating rooms. *Anesthesiology*, 118(1), 192–201.

Kovacs, 2011
Kovacs G and Law JA, 2011. *Airway Management in Emergencies*. 2nd ed. Shelton: McGraw-Hill Medical.

Krell, 2006
Krell J, McCoy M, Sparto P et al., 2006. Comparison of the Ferno Scoop Stretcher with the long backboard for spinal immobilization. *Prehospital Emergency Care*, 10(1), 46–51.

Kumar, 2012
Kumar P and Clark M, 2012. *Kumar and Clark's Clinical Medicine*, 8th ed. Edinburgh: Saunders.

Layon, 2009
Layon AJ and Modell JH, 2009. Drowning: update 2009. *Anesthesiology*, 110(6), 1390–1401.

Leath, 2017
Leath C and Lowery WJ, 2017. *Assessment of Acute Abdomen*. Available at: http://bestpractice.bmj.com/topics/en-gb/503 [Accessed 30 January 2018].

Lee, 2007a
Lee C, Revell M, Porter K et al., 2007. The prehospital management of chest injuries: a consensus statement. Faculty of pre-hospital care, Royal College of Surgeons of Edinburgh. *Emergency Medicine Journal*, 24(3), 220–224.

Lee, 2007b
Lee C, Porter KM and Hodgetts TJ, 2007. Tourniquet use in the civilian prehospital setting. *Emergency Medicine Journal*, 24(8), 584–587.

Lee, 2007c
Lee C and Porter K, 2007. The prehospital management of pelvic fractures. *Emergency Medicine Journal*, 24(2), 130–133.

Lee, 2011
Lee JK and Vadas P, 2011. Anaphylaxis: mechanisms and management. *Clinical & Experimental Allergy*, 41(7), 923–938.

Leigh-Smith, 2005
Leigh-Smith S and Harris T, 2005. Tension pneumothorax – time for a re-think? *Emergency Medicine Journal*, 22(1), 8–16.

LESLP, 2015
London Emergency Services Liaison Panel, 2015. *Major Incident Procedure Manual*. Available at: https://www.met.police.uk/globalassets/foi-media/priorities_and_how_we_are_doing/corporate/specialist-crime--operations---leslp---major-incident-procedure-manual [Accessed 30 January 2018].

Levy, 2010
Levy M, Dellinger R, Townsend S et al., 2010. The Surviving Sepsis Campaign: results of an international guideline-based performance improvement program targeting severe sepsis. *Intensive Care Medicine*, 36(2), 222–231.

Lewin, 2008
Lewin J and Maconochie I, 2008. Capillary refill time in adults. *Emergency Medicine Journal*, 25(6), 325–326.

Lipman, 2013
Lipman GS, Eifling KP, Ellis MA et al., 2013. Wilderness Medical Society practice guidelines for the prevention and treatment of heat-related illness. *Wilderness & Environmental Medicine*, 24(4), 351–361.

Lissauer, 2007
Lissauer T and Clayden G, 2007. *Illustrated Textbook of Paediatrics*. 3rd ed. Edinburgh: Mosby.

Lonnecker, 2001
Lonnecker S and Schoder V, 2001. Hypothermia after burn injury – influence of pre-hospital management. *Der Chirurg*, 72(2), 164–167.

Lord, 2005
Lord SR and Davis PR, 2005. Drowning, near drowning and immersion syndrome. *Journal of the Royal Army Medical Corps*, 151(4), 250.

Luke, 2010
Leenen L, 2010. Pelvic fractures: soft tissue trauma. *European Journal of Trauma and Emergency Surgery*, 36(2), 117–123.

Lunt, 2010
Lunt H, Florkowski C, Bignall M et al., 2010. Capillary glucose meter accuracy and sources of error in the ambulatory setting. *New Zealand Medical Journal*, 123(1310), 74–85.

Lupsa, 2014
Lupsa BC and Inzucchi SE, 2014. Diabetic ketoacidosis and hyperosmolar hyperglycemic syndrome. In: Loriaux L (ed.), *Endocrine Emergencies*. Totowa, NJ: Humana Press, pp.15–31. Available from: http://link.springer.com/10.1007/978-1-62703-697-9_2 [Accessed 30 January 2018].

Mackway-Jones, 2012
Mackway-Jones K, Carley S and Advanced Life Support Group, 2012. *Major Incident Medical Management and Support: The Practical Approach at the Scene*. Chichester: Wiley-Blackwell.

Macleod, 2005
Douglas G, Nicol EF, Robertson C et al., 2005. *Macleod's Clinical Examination*. 11th ed. Edinburgh: Elsevier Churchill Livingstone.

Maconochie, 2015
Maconochie IK, Bingham R, Eich C et al., 2015. European Resuscitation Council Guidelines for Resuscitation 2015. Section 6, paediatric life support. *Resuscitation*, 95, 223–248.

Mancia, 2013
Mancia G, Fagard R, Narkiewicz K et al., 2013. 2013 ESH/ESC Guidelines for the management of arterial hypertension. The Task Force for the Management of Arterial Hypertension of the European Society of Hypertension (ESH) and of the European Society of Cardiology (ESC). *European Heart Journal*, 34(28), 2159–2219.

Mangar International, 2012
Mangar International, 2012. *ELK User Instructions and Warranty*. Available at: http://www.thelivingcentre.co.uk/fileuploader/download/download/?d=0&file=custom%2Fupload%2FFile-1425398451.pdf [Accessed 30 January 2018].

Marieb, 2013
Marieb E and Hoehn K, 2013. *Human Anatomy and Physiology*. New York: Pearson.

Martineau, 2006
Martineau L and Shek PN, 2006. Evaluation of a bi-layer wound dressing for burn care: I. Cooling and wound healing properties. *Burns*, 32(1), 70–76.

McCormack, 2010
McCormack R, Strauss EJ, Alwattar BJ et al., 2010. Diagnosis and management of pelvic fractures. *Bulletin of the NYU Hospital for Joint Diseases*, 68(4), 281.

McGrath, 2012
McGrath BA, Bates L, Atkinson D et al., 2012. Multidisciplinary guidelines for the management of tracheostomy and laryngectomy airway emergencies: Tracheostomy management guidelines. *Anaesthesia*, 67(9), 1025–1041.

McMurray, 2012
McMurray JJV, Adamopoulos S, Anker SD et al., 2012. ESC guidelines for the diagnosis and treatment of acute and chronic heart failure 2012: The Task Force for the Diagnosis and Treatment of Acute and Chronic Heart Failure 2012 of the European Society of Cardiology. Developed in collaboration with the Heart Failure Association (HFA) of the ESC. *European Heart Journal*, 33(14), 1787–1847.

Medicines Act 1968
UK Government, 1968. *Medicines Act 1968*. Available at: http://www.legislation.gov.uk/ukpga/1968/67 [Accessed 30 January 2018].

Middleton, 2012
Middleton PM, 2012. Practical use of the Glasgow Coma Scale: A comprehensive narrative review of GCS methodology. Australasian Emergency Nursing Journal, 15(3), 170–183.

MHF, 2015
Mental Health Foundation, 2015. *Mental Health in Later Life*. Available at: https://www.mentalhealth.org.uk/a-to-z/m/mental-health-later-life [Accessed 30 January 2018].

Mind, 2012
Mind, 2012. *The Mind guide to the Mental Health Act 1983*. Available at: http://www.mind.org.uk/media/7505/the-mind-guide-to-the-mental-health-act-1983-2012.pdf [Accessed 30 January 2018].

Mind, 2015a
Mind, 2015. *Fire and Rescue: How to manage your mental wellbeing*. Available at: https://www.mind.org.uk/media/2199587/managing-mental-wellbeing-firerescue.pdf [Accessed 30 January 2018].

Mind, 2015b
Mind, 2015. *Fire and Rescue: Supporting a colleague with a mental health problem*. Available at: https://www.mind.org.uk/media/3214831/12752_mind-booklets-supporting-a-colleague-fire-and-rescue-v5.pdf [Accessed 30 January 2018].

Mind, 2016
Mind, 2016. *How to Improve your Mental Wellbeing*. Available at: https://www.mind.org.uk/38566.aspx#.WbUVwLGZOu4 [Accessed 30 January 2018].

Misuse of Drugs Act 1971
UK Government, 1971. *Misuse of Drugs Act 1971*. Available at: http://www.legislation.gov.uk/ukpga/1971/38/contents [Accessed 30 January 2018].

MoD, 2008
Ministry of Defence, 2008. Health and safety risk assessment. Available at: https://www.gov.uk/government/uploads/system/uploads/system/uploads/attachment_dat a/file/28827/leaf_39.pdf [Accessed 12 December 2014].

Modell, 1999
Modell JH, Bellefleur M and David JH, 1999. Drowning without aspiration: is this an appropriate diagnosis? *Journal of Forensic Sciences*, 44, 1119–1123.

Monsieurs, 2015
Monsieurs KG, Nolan JP, Bossaert LL et al., 2015. European Resuscitation Council Guidelines for Resuscitation 2015. Section 1. Executive summary. *Resuscitation*, 95, 1–80.

Montalescot, 2013
Montalescot G, Sechtem U, Achenbach S et al., 2013. 2013 ESC guidelines on the management of stable coronary artery disease. The Task Force on the Management of Stable Coronary Artery Disease of the European Society of Cardiology. *European Heart Journal*, 34(38), 2949–3003.

Moorhouse, 2007
Moorhouse I, Thurgood A, Walker N et al., 2007. A realistic model for catastrophic external haemorrhage training. *Journal of the Royal Army Medical Corps*, 153(2), 99–101.

Moppett, 2007
Moppett IK, 2007. Traumatic brain injury: assessment, resuscitation and early management. *British Journal of Anaesthesia*, 99(1), 18–31.

Moritz, 1947
Moritz AR and Henriques FC, 1947. Studies of thermal injury. *The American Journal of Pathology*, 23(5), 695–720.

Moscati, 1999
Moscati R, Billittier AJ, Marshall B et al., 1999. Blood loss estimation by out-of-hospital emergency care providers. *Prehospital Emergency Care: official journal of the National Association of EMS Physicians and the National Association of State EMS Directors*, 3(3), 239–242.

Moye, 2007
Moye J and Marson DC, 2007. Assessment of decision making capacity in older adults: an emerging area of practice and research. *The Journals of Gerontology. Series B, Psychological Sciences and Social Sciences*, 62(1), 3–11.

Muehlberger, 2010
Muehlberger T, Ottomann C, Toman N et al., 2010. Emergency pre-hospital care of burn patients. *The Surgeon*, 8(2), 101–104.

Müller, 2006
Müller D, Agrawal R and Arntz H-R, 2006. How sudden is sudden cardiac death? *Circulation*, 114(11), 1146–1150.

Munden, 2002
Munden J and Thorn Barrows S, 2002. *Pathophysiology Made Incredibly Easy*. Philadelphia, PA: Lippincott Williams & Wilkins.

NAEMT, 2011
National Association of Emergency Medical Technicians, 2011. *Advanced Medical Life Support*. St. Louis, MO: Jones & Bartlett.

NAEMT, 2014
National Association of Emergency Medical Technicians (U.S.) and American College of Surgeons., 2014. *PHTLS: Prehospital Trauma Life Support*. 8th ed. Burlington: Jones & Bartlett Learning.

NAEMT, 2015
Snyder DR, American Geriatrics Society and National Association of Emergency Medical Technicians (US), 2015. *Geriatric Education for Emergency Medical Services: (GEMS)*. 2nd ed. Burlington, MA: Jones & Bartlett Learning.

NAO, 2005
National Audit Office, 2005. *Reducing Brain Damage: Faster Access to Better Stroke Care*. London: Stationery Office Books.

NAO, 2010
National Audit Office, 2010. *Progress in Improving Stroke Care: Department of Health*. London: Stationery Office.

NARU, 2012
National Ambulance Resilience Unit, 2012. *National Ambulance Service Command and Control Guidance*. London: Association of Ambulance Chief Executives.

NARU, 2015
National Ambulance Resilience Unit, 2015. National Ambulance Service Command and Control Guidance. Available at: https://naru.org.uk/wp-content/uploads/2016/09/NARU-CC-GUIDANCE-V.1.2.OCT-2015jm.pdf [Accessed 30 January 2018].

NASMeD, 2013
National Ambulance Service Medical Directors Group, 2013. *Triage Sieve*. Available at: http://naru.org.uk/wp-content/uploads/2014/02/NARU-TRIAGE-SIEVE-JU5A304D.pdf [Accessed 30 January 2018].

NatCen, 2013
NatCen Social Research, 2013. *British Social Attitudes research for Dying Matters*. Available at: http://www.dyingmatters.org/sites/default/files/BSA30_Full_Report.pdf [Accessed 30 January 2018].

NBCG, 2008
National Burn Care Group, 2008. UK Burn Injury Data 1986–2007. UK: UK National Burn Care Group.

NBCRC, 2001
National Burn Care Review Committee, 2001. *National Burn Care Review*. Available at: https://www.britishburnassociation.org/national-burn-care-review/ [Accessed 1 May 2018].

NEAS, 2010
North East Ambulance Service NHS Trust, 2010. Infection Prevention and Control Policy and Strategy. Available at: https://www.neas.nhs.uk/media/15946/11%20-%20infection%20prevention%20and%20control%20policy.pdf [Accessed 22 December 2014].

NEAS, 2014
North East Ambulance Service NHS Trust, 2014. *Clinical Handbook 2014*. Bridgwater: Class Professional Publishing.

Neligan, 2010
Neligan A and Shorvon SD, 2010. Frequency and prognosis of convulsive status epilepticus of different causes: a systematic review. *Archives of Neurology*, 67(8), 931–940.

Nellist, 2013
Nellist E and Lethbridge K, 2013. The need for paramedics to be able to identify cauda equina syndrome. *Journal of Paramedic Practice*, 5(7), 376–379.

NG, 2001
Neuropathology Group of the Medical Research Council Cognitive Function and Ageing Study, 2001. Pathological correlates of late-onset dementia in a multicentre, community-based population in England and Wales. Neuropathology Group of the Medical Research Council Cognitive Function and Ageing Study (MRC CFAS). *The Lancet*, 357(9251), 169–175.

Ng, 2010
Ng JM, Mellor DD, Masson EA et al., 2010. Sulphonyurea as a cause of severe hypoglycaemia in the community. *Primary Care Diabetes*, 4(1), 61–63. Available at: https://doi.org/10.1016/j.pcd.2009.12.001 [Accessed 30 January 2018].

NHS, 2017
NHS, 2017. *Low Blood Sugar (Hypoglycaemic).* Available at: http://www.nhs.uk/conditions/Hypoglycaemia/Pages/Introduction.aspx [Accessed 30 January 2018].

NHS Choices, 2011
NHS Choices, 2011. *Authorities and Trusts*. Available at: http://www.nhs.uk/servicedirectories/pages/ambulancetrustlisting.aspx [Accessed 30 January 2018].

NHS England, 2013
NHS England, 2013. A guide to the FFP3 respirator. Available at: https://www.england.nhs.uk/wp-content/uploads/2013/12/guide-ffp3-leaflet-v2.pdf [Accessed 22 December 2014].

NHS Choices, 2014a
NHS Choices, 2014. *10 Stress Busters*. Available at: https://www.nhs.uk/conditions/stress-anxiety-depression/reduce-stress/ [Accessed 1 May 2018].

NHS Choices, 2014b
NHS Choices, 2014. *Gastroenteritis in Adults*. Available at: http://www.nhs.uk/Conditions/Gastroenteritis/Pages/Causes.aspx [Accessed 2 May 2018].

NHS Choices, 2015a
NHS Choices, 2015. *Abuse and Neglect of Vulnerable Adults*. Available at: https://www.nhs.uk/conditions/social-care-and-support/vulnerable-people-abuse-safeguarding/? [Accessed 30 January 2018].

NHS Choices, 2015b
NHS Choices, 2015. About Dementia. Available at: https://www.nhs.uk/conditions/dementia/about/? [Accessed 30 January 2018].

NHS England, 2015
NHS England, 2015. *Equality, Diversity and Health Inequalities*. Available at: http://www.england.nhs.uk/about/equality/ [Accessed 30 January 2018].

NHS England, 2016
NHS England, 2016 *Confidentiality Policy*. Available at: https://www.england.nhs.uk/wp-content/uploads/2016/12/confidentiality-policy-v3-1.pdf [Accessed 30 January 2018].

NHSHWN, 2015
NHS Health at Work Network, 2015. What is Occupational Health? Available at: http://www.hse.gov.uk/skin/posters/skindermatitis.pdf [Accessed 23 November 2015].

NHS Professionals, 2010
NHS Professionals, 2010. Standard Infection Control Precautions. Available at: http://www.nhsprofessionals.nhs.uk/download/comms/cg1_nhsp_standard_infection_control_precautions_v3.pdf [Accessed 23 June 2016].

NICE, 2009
National Institute for Health and Care Excellence, 2009. *When to Suspect Child Maltreatment in Under 18s*. Available at: http://www.nice.org.uk/guidance/cg89 [Accessed 30 January 2018].

NICE, 2010a
National Institute for Health and Care Excellence, 2010. Chronic Obstructive Pulmonary Disease in over 16s: Diagnosis and management. National Clinical Guideline Centre. Available at: http://www.nice.org.uk/guidance/cg101 [Accessed 30 January 2018].

NICE, 2010b
National Institute for Health and Care Excellence, 2010. *Meningitis (bacterial) and Meningococcal septicaemia in Under 16s: Recognition, diagnosis and management*. Available at: http://www.nice.org.uk/guidance/cg102 [Accessed 30 January 2018].

NICE, 2012a
National Institute for Health and Care Excellence, 2012. *Health Inequalities and Population Health.* Available at: https://www.nice.org.uk/advice/lgb4/chapter/Introduction [Accessed 30 January 2018].

NICE, 2012b
National Institute for Health and Care Excellence, 2012. Infection: Prevention and Control of Healthcare-associated Infections in Primary and Community Care. Available at: http://www.nice.org.uk/guidance/cg139 [Accessed 21 December 2014].

NICE, 2013a
National Institute for Health and Care Excellence, 2013. *Fever in under 5s: assessment and initial management*. Available at: https://www.nice.org.uk/guidance/CG160/chapter/1-Recommendations#thermometers-and-the-detection-offever-2 [Accessed 30 January 2018].

NICE, 2013b
National Institute for Health and Care Excellence, 2013. *Falls: Assessment and prevention of falls in older people*. Available at: http://www.nice.org.uk/guidance/cg161/evidence/falls-full-guidance-190033741 [Accessed 30 January 2018].

NICE, 2014
National Institute for Health and Care Excellence, 2014. *Head Injury: Assessment and early management*. Available at: http://www.nice.org.uk/guidance/cg176/ [Accessed 30 January 2018].

NICE, 2016
National Institute for Health and Care Excellence, 2016. *Major Trauma: Assessment and initial management*. Available at: https://www.nice.org.uk/guidance/ng39/chapter/recommendations#management-of-haemorrhagein-prehospital-and-hospital-settings [Accessed 30 January 2018].

NICE, 2017
National Institute for Health and Care Excellence, 2017. *Sepsis: Recognition, diagnosis and early management*. Available at: https://www.nice.org.uk/guidance/ng51/chapter/Recommendations [Accessed 30 January 2018].

Nicerkson, 2007
Nickerson E, 2007. *Infectious Diseases*. 1st ed. Edinburgh; New York: Mosby/Elsevier.

Nienaber, 2012
Nienaber CA and Powell JT, 2012. Management of acute aortic syndromes. *European Heart Journal*, 33(1), 26–35.

Nigam, 2008
Nigam Y and Knight J, 2008. Exploring the anatomy and physiology of ageing. Part 3 – the digestive system. *Nursing Times*, 104(33), 22–23.

NIHR, 2012
National Institute for Health Research, 2012. *Diversity and Inclusion: What's it about and why is it important for public involvement in research?* Available at: http://www.invo.org.uk/posttypepublication/diversity-and-inclusion-what%E2%80%99s-it-about-and-why-is-it-important-for-public-involvement-in-research/ [Accessed 30 January 2018].

Ninis, 2010
Ninis N, Nadel S and Glennie L, 2010. *Sections from Research for Doctors in Training*. 3rd ed. Bristol: Meningitis Research Foundation.

NNBC, 2012
National Network for Burn Care, 2012. *National Burn Care Referral Guidelines*. NNBC. Available at: https://www.britishburnassociation.org/national-burn-care-referral-guidance/ [Accessed 2 May 2018].

Nolan, 2006
Nolan J, Soar J and Eikeland H, 2006. The chain of survival. *Resuscitation*, 71(3), 270–271.

Nolan, 2010
Nolan JP, Soar J, Zideman DA et al., 2010. European Resuscitation Council Guidelines for Resuscitation 2010. Section 1. Executive summary. *Resuscitation*, 81(10), 1219–1276.

Nolan, 2012
Nolan J, Soar J, Lockey A et al., 2012. *Advanced Life Support*. 6th ed. London: Resuscitation Council (UK).

Nolan, 2016
Nolan J, Soar J, Hampshire S et al., 2016. *Advanced Life Support*. 7th ed. London; Resuscitation Council (UK).

Noppen, 2010
Noppen M, 2010. Spontaneous pneumothorax: epidemiology, pathophysiology and cause. *European Respiratory Review*, 19(117), 217–219.

NOS, 2015
National Osteoporosis Society, 2015. *What is Osteoporosis?*. Available at: https://www.nos.org.uk/about-osteoporosis [Accessed 30 January 2018].

NPSA, 2007
National Patient Safety Agency, 2007. Healthcare risk assessment made easy. Available at: http://www.nrls.npsa.nhs.uk/resources/?entryid45=59825 [Accessed 9 December 2014].

NPSA, 2008
National Patient Safety Agency, 2008. Risk matrix for risk managers. Available at: http://www.npsa.nhs.uk/nrls/improvingpatientsafety/patient-safety-tools-and-guidance/risk-assessment-guides/risk-matrix-for-risk-managers/ [Accessed 9 December 2014].

NSPCC, 2018
National Society for the Prevention of Cruelty to Children, 2018. *Female Genital Mutilation (FGM): Preventing and protecting.* Available at: https://www.nspcc.org.uk/preventing-abuse/child-abuse-and-neglect/female-genital-mutilation-fgm/preventing-protecting/ [Accessed 30 January 2018].

NTSP, 2014
National Tracheostomy Safety Project (Great Britain), 2014. *Comprehensive Tracheostomy Care: The National Tracheostomy Safety Project Manual.* McGrath BA (ed.), Chichester: John Wiley & Sons.

Nutbeam, 2013
Nutbeam T and Boylan M, 2013. *ABC of Prehospital Emergency Medicine.* Chichester: John Wiley & Sons.

NZGG, 2007
New Zealand Guidelines Group, 2007. *Management of Burns and Scalds in Primary Care.* Wellington: Accident Compensation Corporation.

O'Brien, 2003
O'Brien E, Asmar R, Beilin L et al., 2003. European society of hypertension recommendations for conventional, ambulatory and home blood pressure measurement. *Journal of Hypertension*, 21(5), 821–848.

O'Donnell, 2010
O'Donnell MJ, Xavier D, Liu L et al., 2010. Risk factors for ischaemic and intracerebral haemorrhagic stroke in 22 countries (the INTERSTROKE study): a case-control study. *The Lancet*, 376(9735), 112–123.

O'Driscoll, 2008
O'Driscoll BR, Howard LS, Davison AG et al., 2008. British Thoracic Society guideline for emergency oxygen use in adult patients. *Thorax*, 63(Supplement 6), vi1–vi68.

Oluwabusi, 2012
Oluwabusi T and Sood SK, 2012. Update on the management of simple febrile seizures: emphasis on minimal intervention. *Current Opinion in Pediatrics*, 24(2), 259–265.

ONS, 2013
Office for National Statistics, 2013. *Deaths Registered in England and Wales: 2012.* Available at: https://www.ons.gov.uk/peoplepopulationandcommunity/birthsdeathsandmarriages/deaths/bulletins/deathsregistrationsummarytables/2013-07-10 [Accessed 30 January 2018].

Orlowski, 1989
Orlowski JP, Abulleil MM and Phillips JM, 1989. The hemodynamic and cardiovascular effects of near-drowning in hypotonic, isotonic, or hypertonic solutions. *Annals of Emergency Medicine*, 18(10), 1044–1049.

Osler, 2012
Osler W, 2012. Pneumonia part 1: pathology, presentation and prevention. *British Journal of Nursing*, 21(2), 103.

Pante, 2010
Pante MD and American Academy of Orthopaedic Surgeons, 2010. *Advanced Assessment and Treatment of Trauma.* Sudbury, MA: Jones & Bartlett Publishers.

Papadopoulos, 2006
Papadopoulos IN, Kanakaris N, Bonovas S, et al., 2006. Auditing 655 fatalities with pelvic fractures by autopsy as a basis to evaluate trauma care. *Journal of the American College of Surgeons*, 203(1), 30–43.

Pappas, 2010
Pappas, R and Frize, M, 2010. *Intellectual Disability: Mental Health First Aid Manual*. Available at: https://mhfa.com.au/sites/default/files/2nd-Edn-ID-MHFA-Manual-Sept-2012-small.pdf [Accessed 30 January 2018].

Parkinson's UK, 2015
Parkinson's UK, 2015. *What is Parkinson's?* Available at: http://www.parkinsons.org.uk/content/what-parkinsons [Accessed 30 January 2018].

Patel, 2008
Patel H, 2008. *Crash Course: Respiratory System*. 3rd ed. London: Elsevier Health Sciences.

Paul, 1998
Paul A, 1998. *Where Bias Begins: The truth about stereotypes*. Available at: https://www.psychologytoday.com/articles/199805/where-bias-begins-the-truth-about-stereotypes [Accessed 30 January 2018].

Peña, 2012
Peña SB and Larrard AR, 2012. Does the Trendelenburg position affect hemodynamics? A systematic review. *Emergencias*, 24, 143–150.

Perkins, 2015
Perkins GD, Handley AJ, Koster RW et al., 2015. European Resuscitation Council Guidelines for Resuscitation 2015. Section 2. Adult basic life support and automated external defibrillation. *Resuscitation*, 95, 81–99.

Perry, 2008
Perry M and Morris C, 2008. Advanced trauma life support (ATLS) and facial trauma: can one size fit all? Part 2: ATLS, maxillofacial injuries and airway management dilemmas. *International Journal of Oral and Maxillofacial Surgery*, 37(4), 309–320.

PHE, 2014
Public Health England, 2014. *Meningococcal: The green book*. Available at: https://www.gov.uk/government/publications/meningococcal-the-green-book-chapter-22 [Accessed 30 January 2018].

PHE, 2015
Public Health England, 2015. Who we are and what we do: Annual Plan 2015/16. Available at: https://www.gov.uk/government/uploads/system/uploads/attachment_data/file/452328/Annual_plan_2015-_Aug7-web.pdf [Accessed 23 November 2015].

PHE, 2017
Public Health England, 2014. *Meningococcal Disease: Guidance, data and analysis*. Available at: https://www.gov.uk/government/collections/meningococcal-disease-guidance-data-and-analysis [Accessed 30 January 2018].

Physio-Control, 2009
Physio-Control, 2009. *LifePak 15 Monitor/defibrillator Operating Instructions*. Available at: https://www.physio-control.com/uploadedFiles/Physio85/Contents/Emergency_Medical_Care/Products/Operating_Instructions/LIFEPAK15_OperatingInstructions_3306222-002.pdf [Accessed 30 January 2018].

Pickard, 2011
Pickard A, Karlen W and Ansermino JM. Capillary refill time: is it still a useful clinical sign? *Anesthesia & Analgesia*, 113(1), 120–123.

PIE, 2014
Picker Institute Europe, 2014. NHS staff surveys – 2013 results. Available at: http://www.nhsstaffsurveys.com/page/1006/latest-results/2013-results/ [Accessed 8 December 2014].

Piette, 2006
Piette MHA and De Letter EA, 2006. Drowning: still a difficult autopsy diagnosis. *Forensic Science International*, 163(1–2), 1–9.

Piirilä, 1995
Piirilä P and Sovijärvi ARA, 1995. Crackles: recording, analysis and clinical significance. *European Respiratory Journal*, 8(12), 2139–2148.

Pilbery, 2013
Pilbery R, Caroline NL, American Academy of Orthopaedic Surgeons et al., 2013. *Nancy Caroline's Emergency Care in the Streets*. United Kingdom 7th ed. Burlington: Jones & Bartlett Learning.

Pope, 2005
Pope LER and Hobbs CGL, 2005. Epistaxis: an update on current management. *Postgraduate Medical Journal*, 81(955), 309–314.

Porth, 2003
Porth CM, 2003. *Essentials of Pathophysiology: Concepts of Altered Health States*. London: Lippincott Williams & Wilkins.

Prasarn, 2014
Prasarn ML, Horodyski M, Scott NE et al., 2014. Motion generated in the unstable upper cervical spine during head tilt–chin lift and jaw thrust manoeuvres. *The Spine Journal*, 14(4), 609–614.

Prien, 1988
Prien T and Traber DL, 1988. Toxic smoke compounds and inhalation injury – a review. *Burns, Including Thermal Injury*, 14(6), 451–460.

Public Health England, 2017
Public Health England, 2017. 4. *Clinical Governance*. Available at: https://www.gov.uk/government/publications/newborn-hearing-screening-programme-nhsp-operational-guidance/4-clinical-governance. [Accessed 1 May 2018].

Pumphrey, 2000
Pumphrey R, 2000. Sections for management of anaphylaxis from a study of fatal reactions. *Clinical & Experimental Allergy*, 30(8), 1144–1150.

Purcell, 2010
Purcell D, 2010. *Minor Injuries: A Clinical Guide*. Edinburgh and New York: Elsevier Churchill Livingstone.

Ramanath, 2009
Ramanath VS, Oh JK, Sundt TM et al., 2009. Acute aortic syndromes and thoracic aortic aneurysm. *Mayo Clinic Proceedings*, 84(5), 465–481.

Ranasinghe, 2011
Ranasinghe AM, Strong D, Boland B et al., 2011. Acute aortic dissection. *BMJ*, 343, d4487.

Randle, 2009
Randle J, Coffey F and Bradbury M, 2009. *Oxford Handbook of Clinical Skills in Adult Nursing*. Oxford and New York: Oxford University Press.

RCP, 2010
Royal Society of Psychiatrists 2010. *Self-Harm, Suicide and Risk: Helping people who self-harm*. Available at: http://www.rcpsych.ac.uk/files/pdfversion/cr158.pdf [Accessed 30 January 2018].

RCP, 2015
Royal College of Physicians, 2015. *National Early Warning Score (NEWS). London: RCP*. Available from: https://www.rcplondon.ac.uk/file/38/download?token=KEp9KNl0 [Accessed 30 January 2018].

Roberts, 2003
Roberts K and Smith A, 2003. Outcome of diabetic patients treated in the prehospital arena after a hypoglycaemic episode, and an exploration of treat and release protocols: a review of the literature. *Emergency Medicine Journal*, 20(3), 274–276.

Roberts, 2014
Roberts JR, Custalow, Thomsen et al., 2014. *Roberts and Hedges' Clinical Procedures in Emergency Medicine*. 6th ed. New York: Elsevier.

Rodgers, 2004
Rodgers H, Greenaway J, Davies T et al., 2004. Risk factors for first-ever stroke in older people in the North East of England: a population-based study. *Stroke*, 35(1), 7–11.

Roguin, 2006
Roguin A, 2006. Rene Theophile Hyacinthe Laennec (1781–1826): the man behind the stethoscope. *Clinical Medicine & Research*, 4(3), 230–235.

Ross, 2014
Ross S, 2014. Rapid Infection Control Nursing. Rapid series. Chichester: Wiley-Blackwell.

Rossaint, 2010
Rossaint R, Bouillon B, Cerny V et al., 2010. Management of bleeding following major trauma: an updated European guideline. *Critical Care*, 14(2), R52.

Sampson, 2006
Sampson HA, Muñoz-Furlong A, Campbell RL et al., 2006. Second symposium on the definition and management of anaphylaxis: summary report – second National Institute of Allergy and Infectious Disease/ Food Allergy and Anaphylaxis Network Symposium. *Annals of Emergency Medicine*, 47(4), 373–380.

SAS, 2014
Scottish Ambulance Service, 2014. *Dementia Learning Resource*. Available at: http://www.nes.scot.nhs.uk/media/3064028/scottish_ambulance_service.pdf [Accessed 1 May 2018].

Savage, 2011
Savage MW, Dhatariya KK, Kilvert A et al., 2011. Joint British Diabetes Societies guideline for the management of diabetic ketoacidosis: diabetic ketoacidosis guidelines. *Diabetic Medicine*, 28(5), 508–515.

Saver, 2006
Saver JL, 2006. Time is brain – quantified. *Stroke*, 37(1), 263–266.

SCIE, 2013
Social Care Institute for Excellence, 2013. *Dementia Gateway*. Available at: https://www.scie.org.uk/dementia/ [Accessed 1 May 2018].

Scott, 2013
Scott I, Porter K, Laird C et al., 2013. The prehospital management of pelvic fractures: initial consensus statement. *Emergency Medicine Journal*, 30(12), 1070–1072.

Scott, 2015
Scott AR, the Joint British Diabetes Societies (JBDS) for Inpatient Care and the JBDS hyperosmolar hyperglycaemic guidelines group 2015. Management of hyperosmolar hyperglycaemic state in adults with diabetes. *Diabetic Medicine*, 32(6), 714–24.

Scottish Fire and Rescue, 2015
Scottish Fire and Rescue Service, 2015. *Health, Safety and Wellbeing: Annual report 2014 – 15*. Available at: http://www.firescotland.gov.uk/media/850217/20150922csgc18_15hswannualreport2014_15_appendix.pdf [Accessed 30 January 2018].

Sharma, 2008
Sharma A and Jindal P, 2008. Principles of diagnosis and management of traumatic pneumothorax. *Journal of Emergencies, Trauma and Shock*, 1(1), 34–41.

Shattock, 2012
Shattock MJ and Tipton MJ, 2012. 'Autonomic conflict': a different way to die during cold water immersion? *The Journal of Physiology*, 590(14), 3219–3230.

Sheridan, 2012
Sheridan R, 2012. *Burns: A Practical Approach to Immediate Treatment and Long-term Care*. London: Manson Publishing.

Simon, 2010
Simon C, 2010. *Oxford Handbook of General Practice*. 3rd ed. Oxford Handbooks. Oxford: Oxford University Press.

Simons, 2001
Simons FER, Gu X and Simons KJ, 2001. Epinephrine absorption in adults: intramuscular versus subcutaneous injection. *Journal of Allergy and Clinical Immunology*, 108(5), 871–873.

Simpson, 2002
Simpson T, Krieg JC, Heuer F et al., 2002. Stabilization of pelvic ring disruptions with a circumferential sheet. *The Journal of Trauma and Acute Care Surgery*, 52(1), 158–161.

Singer, 2006
Singer AJ, Freidman B, Modi P et al., 2006. The effect of a commercially available burn-cooling blanket on core body temperatures in volunteers. *Academic Emergency Medicine*, 13(6), 686–690.

Singer, 2010
Singer AJ, Taira BR, Thode Jr HC et al., 2010. The association between hypothermia, prehospital cooling, and mortality in burn victims. *Academic Emergency Medicine*, 17(4), 456–459.

SJA, SAA, BRC, 2014
St. John Ambulance, St. Andrew's Ambulance Association and British Red Cross, 2014. *First Aid Manual*. 10th ed. London: Dorling Kindersley.

Skellett, 2016
Skellett S, Hampshire S, Bingham R et al., 2016. *European Paediatric Advanced Life Support*. London: RC(UK).

Smith, 2011a
Smith I, Mackay J, Fahrid N et al., 2011. Respiratory rate measurement: a comparison of methods. *British Journal of Healthcare Assistants*, 5(1), 18–23.

Smith, 2011b
Smith J (ed.), 2011. *The Guide to the Handling of People: A systems approach*. Teddington: BackCare.

Smithson, 2012
Smithson H and Walker MC, 2012. *ABC of Epilepsy*. 1st ed. Chichester: John Wiley & Sons.

Soar, 2008
Soar J, Pumphrey R, Cant A et al., 2008. Emergency treatment of anaphylactic reactions – guidelines for healthcare providers. *Resuscitation*, 77(2), 157–169.

Soar, 2010
Soar J, Perkins GD, Abbas G, et al., 2010. European Resuscitation Council guidelines for resuscitation 2010. Section 8. Cardiac arrest in special circumstances: electrolyte abnormalities, poisoning, drowning, accidental hypothermia, hyperthermia, asthma, anaphylaxis, cardiac surgery, trauma, pregnancy, electrocution. *Resuscitation*, 81(10), 1400–1433.

Soar, 2015
Soar J, Nolan JP, Böttiger BW et al., 2015. European Resuscitation Council guidelines for resuscitation 2015. Section 3. Adult advanced life support. *Resuscitation*, 95, 100–147.

Steg, 2012
Steg G, James SK, Atar D et al., 2012. ESC guidelines for the management of acute myocardial infarction in patients presenting with ST-segment elevation. The Task Force on the Management of ST-segment elevation acute myocardial infarction of the European Society of Cardiology (ESC). *European Heart Journal*, 33(20), 2569–2619.

Stewart, 2013
Stewart M, 2013. BET 3: Pelvic circumferential compression devices for haemorrhage control: panacea or myth? *Emergency Medicine Journal*, 30(5), 425–426.

Studnek, 2012
Studnek JR, Artho MR, Garner Jr CL, et al., 2012. The impact of emergency medical services on the ED care of severe sepsis. *The American Journal of Emergency Medicine*, 30(1), 51–56.

SWAST, 2013
South Western Ambulance Service, 2013. *Infection Prevention and Control*. Available at: https://www.swast.nhs.uk/What%20We%20Do/infection-prevention-and-control.htm [Accessed 1 May 2018].

SWAST, 2014a
South Western Ambulance Service NHS Foundation Trust, 2014. *Major Incident Plan*. Available at: Exeter: SWAST.

SWAST, 2014b
South Western Ambulance Service NHS Foundation Trust, 2014. *Risk Management Strategy*. Available at: Exeter: SWAST.

SWAST, 2014c
South Western Ambulance Service NHS Foundation Trust, 2013. *Cardiac Arrest*. Available at: Exeter: SWAST.

SWAST, 2016
South Western Ambulance Service NHS Trust. (2016). *Major Haemorrhage*. SWAST. Available at: Exeter: SWAST.

Szpilman, 2012
Szpilman D, Bierens JJLM, Handley AJ et al., 2012. Drowning. *New England Journal of Medicine*, 366(22), 2102–2110.

Tall, 2003
Tall G, Wise D, Grove P et al., 2003. The accuracy of external blood loss estimation by ambulance and hospital personnel. *Emergency Medicine*, 15(4), 318–321.

Talley, 2006
Talley NJ and O'Connor S, 2006. *Clinical Examination: A systematic guide to physical diagnosis*. 5th ed. London: Elsevier.

Tapson, 2008
Tapson VF, 2008. Acute pulmonary embolism. *The New England Journal of Medicine*, 358(10), 1037–1052.

Thadepalli, 2002
Thadepalli H, 2002. Women gave birth to the stethoscope: Laennec's introduction of the art of auscultation of the lung. *Clinical Infectious Diseases*, 35(5), 587–588.

Thomassen, 2009
Thomassen O, Skaiaa SC, Brattebo G et al., 2009. Does the horizontal position increase risk of rescue death following suspension trauma? *Emergency Medicine Journal*, 26(12), 896–898.

Thompson, 2006a
Thompson MJ, Ninis N, Perera R et al., 2006. Clinical recognition of meningococcal disease in children and adolescents. *The Lancet*, 367(9508), 397–403.

Thompson, 2006b
Thompson N, 2006. *Anti-Discriminatory Practice*. 4th ed. Basingstoke: Palgrave Macmillan.

Thompson, 2008
Thompson G and Sciarra J (eds), 2008. *Wound Care Made Incredibly Visual*. Ambler: Lippincott Williams and Wilkins.

Thrumurthy, 2012
Thrumurthy SG, Karthikesalingam A, Patterson BO et al., 2012. The diagnosis and management of aortic dissection. *BMJ*, 344, d8290.

Tipton, 2011
Tipton MJ and Golden FSC, 2011. A proposed decision making guide for the search, rescue and resuscitation of submersion (head under) victims based on expert opinion. *Resuscitation*, 82(7), 819–824.

Toon, 2010
Toon MH, Maybauer MO, Greenwood JE et al., 2010. Management of acute smoke inhalation injury. *Critical Care and Resuscitation: Journal of the Australasian Academy of Critical Care Medicine*, 12(1), 53–61.

Torbicki, 2008
Torbicki A, Perrier A, Konstantinides S et al., 2008. Guidelines on the diagnosis and management of acute pulmonary embolism. *European Heart Journal*, 29(18), 2276–2315.

Tortora, 2008
Tortora GJ and Derrickson BH, 2008. *Principles of Anatomy and Physiology*. 12th ed. Hoboken: John Wiley & Sons.

Tortora, 2013
Tortora GJ, 2013. Microbiology: An Introduction. Harlow: Pearson.

Toth, 2012
Toth L, King KL, McGrath B et al., 2012. Efficacy and safety of emergency non-invasive pelvic ring stabilisation. *Injury*, 43(8), 1330–1334.

Truhlar, 2015
Truhlář A, Deakin CD, Soar J et al., 2015. European resuscitation council guidelines for resuscitation 2015. Section 4. Cardiac arrest in special circumstances. *Resuscitation*, 95, 148–201.

UK, 1983
United Kingdom, 1983. *Mental Health Act 1983*. Available at: http://www.legislation.gov.uk/ukpga/1983/20 [Accessed 1 May 2018].

UK, 2007
United Kingdom, 2007. *Mental Health Act 2007* [Text]. Available at: http://www.legislation.gov.uk/ukpga/2007/12/contents [Accessed 1 May 2018].

UKCGC, 2017
UK Caldicott Guardian Council. *A Manual for Caldicott Guardians*. Available at: https://www.gov.uk/government/uploads/system/uploads/attachment_data/file/581213/cgmanual.pdf [Accessed 27 February 2018].

UKST, 2016a
The UK Sepsis Trust, 2016. *Toolkit: Prehospital management of Sepsis in adults and young*

people over 12 years – 2016. Available at: https://sepsistrust.org/wp-content/uploads/2017/08/PH-toolkit-FINAL-2.pdf. [Accessed 1 May 2018].

UKST, 2016b
The UK Sepsis Trust, 2016. *Prehospital Sepsis Screening and Action Tool*. Available at: https://sepsistrust.org/wp-content/uploads/2017/08/PH-adult-NICE-Final-2-1.pdf [Accessed 1 May 2018].

UNICEF, 2013
UNICEF, 2013. *Female Genital Mutilation/Cutting*. Available at: http://www.childinfo.org/files/FGCM_Lo_res.pdf [Accessed 1 May 2018].

Valensi, 2011
Valensi P, Lorgis L and Cottin Y, 2011. Prevalence, incidence, predictive factors and prognosis of silent myocardial infarction: a review of the literature. *Archives of Cardiovascular Diseases*, 104(3), 178–188.

Van Ness-Otunnu, 2013
Van Ness-Otunnu R and Hack JB, 2013. Hyperglycemic crisis. *The Journal of Emergency Medicine*, 45(5), 797–805.

Vincent, 2006
Vincent J-L, Sakr Y, Sprung CL et al., 2006. Sepsis in European intensive care units: results of the SOAP study. *Critical Care Medicine*, 34(2), 344–353.

Walker, 2006
Walker A, James C, Bannister M et al., 2006. Evaluation of a diabetes referral pathway for the management of hypoglycaemia following emergency contact with the ambulance service to a diabetes specialist nurse team. *Emergency Medicine Journal*, 23(6), 449–451.

Walls, 2012
Walls RM and Murphy MF (eds), 2012. *Manual of Emergency Airway Management*. 4th ed. Philadelphia, PA: Wolters Kluwer/Lippincott Williams & Wilkins Health.

Walters, 2005
Walters TJ and Mabry RL, 2005. Issues related to the use of tourniquets on the battlefield. *Military Medicine*, 170 (9), 770–775.

Warden, 2014
Warden S, Spiwak R, Sareen J et al., 2014. The sad persons scale for suicide risk assessment: a systematic review. *Archives of Suicide Research*, 18(4), 313–326.

Waterhouse, 2009
Waterhouse C, 2009. The use of painful stimulus in relation to Glasgow Coma Scale observations. British Journal of Neuroscience Nursing, 5(5), 209–215.

Watson, 2001
Watson RS, Cummings P, Quan L et al., 2001. Cervical spine injuries among submersion victims. *The Journal of Trauma*, 51(4), 658–662.

Watson, 2009
Watson MS (ed.), 2009. *Oxford Handbook of Palliative Care*. 2nd ed. Oxford: Oxford University Press.

Wells, 2001
Wells LC, Smith JC, Weston VC et al., 2001. The child with a non-blanching rash: how likely is meningococcal disease? *Archives of Disease in Childhood*, 85(3), 218.

Weston, 2014
Weston D, 2014. Fundamentals of Infection Prevention and Control: Theory and Practice. 2nd ed. Chichester: John Wiley & Sons.

Whitaker, 2011
Whitaker DK, 2011. Time for capnography – everywhere. *Anaesthesia*, 66(7), 544–549.

WHO, 1999
World Health Organization, 1999. *Definition, Diagnosis and Classification of Diabetes Mellitus and its Complications*. Available at: http://apps.who.int/iris/handle/10665/66040 [Accessed 1 May 2018].

WHO, 2009a
World Health Organization, 2009. *WHO Guidelines on Hand Hygiene in Health Care: First global patient safety challenge: Clean care is safer care. Patient safety*. Geneva: World Health Organization.

WHO, 2009b
World Health Organization, 2009. WHO Guidelines for Safe Surgery 2009: Safe Surgery Saves Lives. Available at: http://apps.who.int/iris/bitstream/10665/44185/1/9789241598552_eng.pdf [Accessed 19 January 2015].

WHO, 2011
World Health Organization, 2011. *Pulse Oximetry Training Manual*. Available at: http://www.who.int/patientsafety/safesurgery/pulse_oximetry/who_ps_pulse_oxymetry_training_manual_en.pdf [Accessed 1 May 2018].

WHO, 2014
World Health Organization 2014. *Mental Health: A state of well being*. Available from: http://www.who.int/features/factfiles/mental_health/en/ [Accessed 1 May 2018].

WHO, 2015
World Health Organization, 2015. Infection prevention and control in health care. Available at: http://www.who.int/csr/bioriskreduction/infection_control/en/ [Accessed 23 November 2015].

Wijdicks, 2010
Wijdicks EFM, 2010. The bare essentials: coma. *Practical Neurology*, 10(1), 51–60.

Williams, 2013
Williams TA, Finn J, Celenza A et al., 2013. Paramedic identification of acute pulmonary edema in a metropolitan ambulance service. *Prehospital Emergency Care*, 17(3), 339–347.

Williams, 2014
Williams C and Roland D, 2014. Does the use of antipyretics prolong the duration of fever or illness? *Archives of Disease in Childhood – Education & Practice Edition*, 99(4), 158–159.

Wood, 2002
Wood KE, 2002. Major pulmonary embolism. *Chest*, 121(3), 877–905.

Xue, 2012
Xue QL, 2011. The frailty syndrome: definition and natural history. *Clinical Geriatric Medicine*, 27(1), 1–15.

YAS, 2013
Yorkshire Ambulance Service NHS Trust, 2013. *Dementia Learning Resource for Ambulance Staff*. Available at: http://www.yas.nhs.uk/calling999/docs/dementia%20learning%20resource%20for%20ambulance%20staff.pdf [Accessed 1 May 2018].

Young, 2018
Young GB, 2018. *Evaluation of Coma*. Available at: http://bestpractice.bmj.com/topics/en-us/417 [Accessed 30 April 2018].

Zideman, 2015
Zideman DA, De Buck EDJ, Singletary EM et al., 2015. European resuscitation council guidelines for resuscitation 2015. Section 9. First aid. *Resuscitation*, 95, 278–287.

Glossary

Medical terminology can be rather overwhelming at first. This glossary will provide an explanation of various terms.

Anterior
The front surface of the body, or situated nearer to the front of the body (particularly if comparing the position of one structure to another).

Arrhythmia
A problem with the rate or rhythm of the heartbeat.

Aspiration
Fluid or solid entering the lower respiratory tract (larynx and below).

Aspirin
Aspirin has an anti-platelet action which reduces clot formation and has analgesic (pain-relieving), antipyretic (temperature reducing) and anti-inflammatory actions.

Atelectasis
A collapse of lung tissue affecting all or part of a lung, and preventing the absorption of oxygen into the blood supply.

Auscultation
The technique of listening to sounds within the body using a stethoscope.

Autoimmune disease
Autoimmune diseases arise from an abnormal immune response of the body against itself, i.e. against substances and tissues that are normally present in the body.

Avulsion
An injury that occurs when a body structure is forcibly detached from its normal point of insertion by a traumatic force.

Body mass index
Body mass index (BMI) is defined as a person's weight divided by the square of their height in metres (kg/m2). This can be adjusted for age and gender, and supplemented with waist circumference measurements, if appropriate. A patient with a BMI of 25–29.9 kg/m2 is considered to be overweight, and if over 30 kg/m2, obese.

Bradycardia
Slow heart rate.

Brittle asthma
Brittle asthma is a rare form of severe asthma which can result in very serious and often life-threatening attacks.

BVM
Bag-valve-mask.

Care Quality Commission
An independent health and adult social care regulator for England. Its job is to make sure health and social care services provide people with safe, effective, compassionate, high-quality care. It does this by monitoring, inspecting and regulating services to make sure they meet fundamental standards of quality and safety.

Cartilage
Cartilage is a flexible connective tissue found in areas of the body, including the joints between bones, the ribcage, the ear, the nose, the bronchial tubes and the intervertebral discs. It is not as hard and rigid as bone but is stiffer and less flexible than muscle. It does not contain blood vessels, so grows and repairs slowly.

Catastrophic haemorrhage
Bleeding severe enough to cause exsanguination, i.e. blood loss causing death, typically within minutes, or less.

Cauda equina syndrome
A condition caused by a prolapse of the lumbar disc causing the roots of the lumbosacral nerve to be compressed. This causes pain, loss of feeling in the lumbar region and problems with bladder and bowel function.

Choking
A mechanical obstruction of the airway occurring anywhere between the mouth and carina.

Circadian rhythms
Circadian rhythms are physical, mental and behavioural changes that follow an approximate 24-hour cycle, responding primarily to light and darkness in a person's environment.

Cognitive function
A person's ability to process thoughts. It encompasses memories, perception, thinking and reasoning.

Connective tissue
Basic tissue type that binds, supports and separates other tissue and organs.

Crepitus
The grating, crackling or popping sounds and sensations experienced under the skin and joints, or a crackling sensation due to the presence of air under the skin. A type of crepitus, bone crepitus, can be heard and felt when two fragments of a fracture are moved against each other.

Distal
Further from the point of attachment of a limb.

Dysphagia
Difficulty swallowing.

Dysphasia
Language disorder marked by a deficiency in the generation of speech, and sometimes also in its comprehension, due to brain disease or damage.

Dyspnoea
Difficulty breathing.

$EtCO_2$
End-tidal carbon dioxide. The measurement of carbon dioxide at the end of expiration.

Fetal maceration
Degeneration and eventual disintegration of the body of a deceased unborn baby.

Focal
Affecting a specific region of the body. For example, a focal neurological deficit may result in a weakness or paralysis of a limb following an impairment of nerve, spinal cord, or brain function.

Furosemide
A commonly used diuretic (water tablet) from the group known as loop diuretics.

Glasgow Coma Scale score
The Glasgow Coma Scale (GCS) was developed in 1974 as a way of objectively testing the level of consciousness in brain-injured patients and to improve communication between healthcare professionals. It was originally a 14-point score, but the division of limb flexion into withdrawal and abnormal flexion led to the 15-point score familiar today. Although designed for in-hospital use, it is now routinely used by the ambulance service and is an important marker for the early management of traumatic brain injury (TBI).

Haematoma
A blood clot that has formed outside a blood vessel (artery or vein).

Haemoptysis
Coughing up or spitting of blood from the lungs.

Humerus
The long bone of the upper arm, reaching from shoulder to elbow.

Ileus
A partial or complete blockage of the intestine, usually the small intestine.

Intercostal
Between the ribs.

Korotkoff sounds
Turbulent blood flow that can be heard when using the manual auscultatory technique to record blood pressure. Named after a Russian surgeon, Nikolai Korotkoff, who first described them in 1905.

Kussmaul breathing
Breathing that is abnormally deep and rapid, sighing. It can be a sign of diabetic ketoacidosis,

or sometimes of kidney failure. Named after the nineteenth century Strasbourg physician Adolph Kussmaul.

Lateral
Of, at, towards, or from the side or sides.

Loop diuretics
Diuretics (water tablets) that work by inhibiting the absorption of sodium and chloride not only in the proximal and distal tubules of the kidney but also in the loop of Henle. Furosemide is an example of this class of diuretic.

Medial
Towards or at the midline of the body.

METHANE
The mnemonic METHANE is designed to provide the initial communication surrounding details of a major incident. It consists of:

- **M**ajor incident declared or standby.
- **E**xact location of the incident.
- **T**ype of incident.
- **H**azards.
- **A**ccess and egress.
- **N**umber of casualties.
- **E**mergency services.

Microorganism
A very small organism that lives outside and inside larger organisms such as the human body.

Necrosis
Death of body tissue.

Oedema
An abnormal build-up of fluid, mainly water, in the body. People with kidney failure are prone to fluid overload, leading to oedema.

Oliguria
Abnormally reduced production of urine.

Oropharyngeal airway (OPA)
A curved plastic tube, with a reinforced flange at one end and designed so that it fits between the tongue and hard palate to help keep the airway open.

Palpable
Able to be touched or felt.

Panda eyes
Bruising around both eyes that can be a sign of skull fracture.

Partial pressure
In a mixture of gases, each gas has a partial pressure which is the hypothetical pressure of that gas if it alone occupied the volume of the mixture at the same temperature. The total pressure of the gas mixture is the sum of the partial pressures of each individual gas in the mixture.

Percussion
A method of tapping on a surface to determine the underlying structure. It is used in clinical examinations to assess the condition of the thorax or abdomen.

Pleuritic chest pain
Chest pain that is usually sharp and stabbing, localised to a specific area of the chest (the patient can often point to the pain with a finger) and made worse by coughing and deep inspiration.

Polypharmacy
The administration of large numbers of prescription drugs at the same time.

Polyuria
The passing of large quantities of urine due to excess glucose in the bloodstream. It is a symptom of untreated diabetes.

Posterior
Further back in position; of or nearer the rear or hind end.

Precordium
The area over the heart and lower thorax.

Primary assessment
A swift patient assessment and management process, which can be completed within 60–90 seconds. It is designed to be a stepwise approach, meaning that any abnormalities identified in one step should be addressed before moving on to the next.

Proprioception
The sense of the relative position of neighbouring parts of the body and strength of effort being employed in movement.

Proximal
Located nearer to the centre of the body or the point of attachment.

Pulse oximetry
The technique of measuring the oxygen saturation of the haemoglobin in the blood.

Recession
In an anatomical context, the drawing away of a tissue (or part of a tissue) from its normal position.

Rigors
Shaking or exaggerated shivering which usually occurs in response to a high temperature.

Supraglottic airway devices (SADs)
Airway devices that sit just above the glottis. The most common SAD is the laryngeal mask airway.

SAMPLE
An acronym for:
- **S** Signs and symptoms of the presenting complaint
- **A** Allergies (particularly to medication but food allergies might be relevant)
- **M** Medications
- **P** Past medical history
- **L** Last oral intake
- **E** Events that led to the current illness or injury

Scope of practice
The area or areas of a person's profession where they have the knowledge, skill and experience to practise safely and effectively.

SOCRATES
An acronym for:
- **S** Site
- **O** Onset
- **C** Character. Same as Quality above
- **R** Radiation
- **A** Association. Are there any other signs and symptoms associated with the presenting complaint?
- **T** Timing
- **E** Exacerbating/relieving factors
- **S** Severity

Stridor
High-pitched (usually) inspiratory breath sound, indicating upper airway narrowing.

Superior
Located above or directed upward. In human anatomy, situated nearer to the top of the head (vertex). Opposite of inferior.

Supine
Lying face up, usually referring to a patient who is lying on their back.

Surfactant
A substance made up of lipids and proteins and produced in the lungs. It forms a coating over the surface of the alveoli to stabilise them and enable them to function effectively.

Tachycardia
Rapid heart rate.

Tachypnoea
Rapid breathing rate.

TILEE
- **T**ask. Consider if the lift:
  - Involves holding the load away from the body
  - Involves long distances
  - Requires strenuous effort or twisting
- **I**ndividual. Consider whether the lift:
  - Requires specialist training
  - Presents a hazard
  - Is within the capabilities of you and your colleagues
- **L**oad. Is the load:
  - Heavy
  - Difficult to get hold of
  - Unstable
  - Unpredictable
  - Harmful
  - Likely to grab out when alarmed at being carried down the stairs

- **E**nvironment. Determine the presence of:
  - o Constraints on posture, e.g. low ceiling, confined spaces
  - o Poor, uneven flooring
  - o Hot/cold/wet weather
  - o Poor lighting
  - o Noise
- **E**quipment. Consider what equipment:
  - o Is available
  - o Will reduce the risk to you and the patient
  - o Is safe to use
  - o You are trained and competent in the use of

Turgor
Condition of normal tension in a cell or group of cells, such as the skin.

Urticaria
(Also called nettle rash or hives.) Swelling of the superficial layers of the skin, usually as a result of an allergic reaction. The characteristic itchy lumps (called weals or hives) last for only a few hours.

Viscus
Any large organ in the interior of the abdomen.

Index